Neuroanatomy
Text and Atlas

Neuroanatomy Text and Atlas

Fourth Edition

JOHN H. MARTIN, PHD

Department of Physiology, Pharmacology, and Neuroscience
Sophie Davis School of Biomedical Education
City College of the City University of New York
New York, New York

Medical Photography by

HOWARD J. RADZYNER, RBP, AIMBI, FBCA

Illustrated by

MICHAEL E. LEONARD, MA, CMI, FAMI

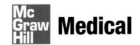 **Medical**

New York Chicago San Francisco Lisbon London Madrid Mexico City Milan
New Delhi San Juan Seoul Singapore Sydney Toronto

The McGraw·Hill Companies

Neuroanatomy Text and Atlas, Fourth Edition

2 3 4 5 6 7 8 9 0   CTP/CTP   17 16 15 14 13 12

ISBN 978-0-07-160396-6
MHID 0-07-160396-4

This book was set in Times LT Std by Cenveo Publisher Services.
The editors were Michael Weitz and Christie Naglieri.
The production supervisor was Catherine Saggese.
Project management was provided by Sandhya Gola, Cenveo Publisher Services.
The illustration manager was Armen Ovsepyan.
Illustrations created by Dragonfly Media Group.
The designer was Diana Andrews; the cover designer was Tom Lau.
Magnetic resonance tractography image on the cover courtesy of Dr. Thomas Schultz, Max Planck Institute for Intelligent Systems, Tübingen, Germany.
China Translation & Printing Services, Ltd., was printer and binder.

Library of Congress Cataloging-in-Publication Data

Martin, John H. (John Harry), 1951-
    Neuroanatomy : text and atlas / John H. Martin. -- 4th ed.
        p. ; cm.
    Includes bibliographical references and index.
    ISBN-13: 978-0-07-160396-6 (pbk. : alk. paper)
    ISBN-10: 0-07-160396-4 (pbk. : alk. paper)
        1. Neuroanatomy.   2. Neuroanatomy—Atlases.   I. Title.
[DNLM: 1. Central Nervous System—anatomy & histology—Atlases.   2.
Central Nervous System—anatomy & histology.   WL 300]
    QM451.M27 2012
    611'.8—dc23

                                                        2011025748

McGraw-Hill books are available at special quantity discounts to use as premiums and sales promotions, or for use in corporate training programs. To contact a representative please e-mail us at bulksales@mcgraw-hill.com

To Carol, Caitlin, Emma, and Rachel

Box Features

Contents

SECTION I | THE CENTRAL NERVOUS SYSTEM

SECTION II | SENSORY SYSTEMS

vii

Preface

Neuroanatomy plays a crucial role in the health science curriculum by preparing students to understand the anatomical basis of neurology and psychiatry. Imaging the human brain, in both the clinical and research setting, helps us to identify its basic structure and connections. And when the brain becomes damaged by disease or trauma, imaging localizes the extent of the injury. Functional imaging helps to identify the parts of the brain that become active during our thoughts and actions, and reveals brain regions where drugs act to produce their neurological and psychiatric effects. Complementary experimental approaches in animals—such as mapping neural connections, localizing particular neuroactive chemicals within different brain regions, and determining the effects of lesions— provide the neuroscientist and clinician with the tools to study the biological substrates of disordered thought and behavior. To interpret this wealth of information requires a high level of neuroanatomical competence.

Since the third edition of *Neuroanatomy: Text and Atlas,* clinical neuroscience has become even more dependent on localization of function for treatment of disease. Electrophysiological procedures, such as deep brain stimulation (DBS) for Parkinson disease, target small regions within the basal ganglia. DBS, as this is called, is routine in many major medical centers. Interventional neuroradiology is a chosen approach for treating many vascular abnormalities, such as repair of arterial aneurysms. Surgery to resect small portions of the temporal lobe is the treatment of choice for many patients with epilepsy. Neurosurgeons routinely use high-resolution imaging tools to characterize the functions and even the connections of regions surrounding tumors, to resect the tumor safely and minimize risk of loss of speech or motor function. Each of these innovative approaches clearly requires that the clinical team have a greater knowledge of functional neuroanatomy to design and carry out these tasks. And this demand for knowledge of brain structure, function, and connectivity will only be more critical in the future as higher-resolution and more effective approaches are developed to repair the damaged brain.

Neuroanatomy helps to provide key insights into disease by providing a bridge between molecular and clinical neural science. We are learning the genetic and molecular bases for many neurological and psychiatric diseases, such as amyotrophic lateral sclerosis and schizophrenia. Localizing defective genes to particular brain regions and neural circuits helps to further our understanding of how pathological changes in brain structure alter brain function. And this knowledge, in turn, will hopefully lead to breakthroughs in treatments and even cures.

An important goal of *Neuroanatomy: Text and Atlas* is to prepare the reader for interpreting the new wealth of human brain images—structural, functional, and connectivity—by developing an understanding of the anatomical localization of brain function. To provide a workable focus, this book is largely restricted to the central nervous system. It takes a traditional approach to gaining neuroanatomical competence: Because the basic imaging picture is a two-dimensional slice through the brain, the locations of structures are examined on two-dimensional myelin-stained sections through the human central nervous system.

What is new for the fourth edition of *Neuroanatomy: Text and Atlas?* All chapters have been revised to reflect advances in neural science since the last edition. In addition to full color illustrations, there are many new features:

- Chapters begin with a clinical case to illustrate the connections and function of the key material. Some of these cases are specialized and not apt to be seen in routine practice. They were chosen to show how human behavior can change in remarkable ways following damage to a localized brain region; sometimes a very small region.
- Chapters end with a series of multiple choice review questions.
- Material on central nervous system development is now included in the relevant individual chapters rather than a single development chapter.
- There are separate chapters on touch and pain.

Designed as a self-study guide and resource for information on the structure and function of the human central nervous system, this book can serve as both text and atlas for an introductory laboratory course in human neuroanatomy.

For over 23 years, both at Columbia University's College of Physicians and Surgeons and now at the City University of New York's Medical School, we use this book in conjunction with a series of neuroanatomy laboratory exercises during the neuroscience teaching block in the curriculum. Rather than presenting the material in a traditional lecture format, we have successfully taught neuroanatomy in a dynamic small group learning environment. Supplemented with use of brain models and specimens, neuroanatomy small group sessions complement neural science lecture material and round-out medical, graduate, and allied health science students' learning experience.

The organization of *Neuroanatomy: Text and Atlas* continues to parallel that of *Principles of Neural Science,* edited by Eric R. Kandel, James H. Schwartz, Thomas Jessell, Steven A. Siegelbaum, and A. James Hudspeth (McGraw-Hill). Like *Principles of Neural Science, Neuroanatomy: Text and Atlas* is aimed at medical students, and graduate students in neuroscience, biology, and psychology programs. The content of many of the chapters is geared to dental students, such as a chapter focus on the trigeminal system, as well as physical therapy and occupational therapy students by considering the motor systems in detail.

John H. Martin

Acknowledgments

I take this opportunity to recognize the help I received in the preparation of the fourth edition of *Neuroanatomy: Text and Atlas.* I am grateful to the following friends and colleagues who have read portions of the manuscript or have provided radiological or histological materials for this or previous editions: Dimitris Agamanolis, David Amaral, Richard Axel, Bertil Blok, Eric Bushong, Bud Craig, Mike Crutcher, Maurice Curtis, Adrian Danek, Aniruddha Das, Sam David, Mony deLeon, John Dowling, Mark Ellisman, Susan Folstein, Blair Ford, Peter Fox, Stephen Frey, Eitan Friedman, Guido Gainotti, Lice Ghilardi, Mickey Goldberg, James Goldman, Pat Goldman-Rakic, Suzanne Haber, Shaheen Hamdy, Andrei Holodny, Jonathan Horton, David Hubel, Matilde Inglese, Sharon Juliano, Joe LeDoux, Kevin Leung, Marge Livingstone, Camillo Marra, Randy Marshall, Etienne Olivier, Elizabeth Pimentel, Jesús Pujol, Josef Rauschecker, David Ruggiero, Neal Rutledge, Thomas Schultz, Brian Somerville, Bob Vassar, Bob Waters, Torsten Wiesel, Rachel Wong, and Semir Zeki. I also would like to thank Alice Ko for help with the three-dimensional reconstructions that provided the basis for various illustrations. I am grateful to Dr. Frank Galliard, who created the Radiopaedia.com website, for selection of many fine MRIs illustrating neurological damage. I would especially like the to highlight and thank Dr. Joy Hirsch—and her associates at the College of Physicians and Surgeons of Columbia University, Steve Dashnaw and Glenn Castilo—for many of the high-resolution MRIs used in the fourth edition.

I would like to extend a special note of thanks to members of the neuroanatomy teaching faculty at the College of Physicians and Surgeons and the Sophie Davis School of Biomedical Education at the City University of New York for many helpful discussions. For the illustrations, I thank the Dragonfly Media Group, and especially Rob Fedirko for bringing to fruition the many facets of the complex art program, notably adding color to the illustrations and all of the new artwork. For artwork carried over from previous editions, I also thank Michael Leonard, the original illustrator and Dragonfly Media Group. I especially thank Howard Radzyner for the superb photographs of myelin-stained brain sections that have helped to define *Neuroanatomy: Text and Atlas* from its first edition. At McGraw-Hill, I am indebted to Armen Ovespyan for his careful management of the art program. I greatly appreciate the hard work and patience of Christie Naglieri, Senior Project Development Editor, and Catherine Saggese, Senior Production Supervisor. I thank Sandhya Gola at Cenveo Publisher Services and Sheryl Krato for permissions. Finally, I would like to thank my editor Michael Weitz for his support, patience, and guidance—not to mention timely pressure—in the preparation of the fourth edition. Last, and most important, I thank Carol S. Martin for her untiring support during the preparation of this edition and all previous editions of the book.

Guide to Using This Book

Neuroanatomy: Text and Atlas takes a combined regional and functional approach to teaching neuroanatomy: Knowledge of the spatial interrelations and connections between brain regions is developed in relation to the functions of the brain's various components. The book first introduces the major concepts of central nervous system organization. Subsequent chapters consider neural systems subserving particular sensory, motor, and integrative functions. At the end of the book is an atlas of surface anatomy of the brain and myelin-stained histological sections, and a glossary of key terms and structures.

Overview of Chapters

The general structural organization of the mature central nervous system is surveyed in Chapter 1. This chapter also introduces neuroanatomical nomenclature and fundamental histological and imaging techniques for studying brain structure and function. The three-dimensional shapes of key deep structures are also considered in this chapter. The functional organization of the central nervous system is introduced in Chapter 2. This chapter considers how different neural circuits, spanning the entire central nervous system, serve particular functions. The circuits for touch perception and voluntary movement control are used as examples. The major neurotransmitter systems are also discussed.

Central nervous system vasculature and cerebrospinal fluid are the topics of Chapter 3. By considering vasculature early in the book, the reader can better understand why particular functions can become profoundly disturbed when brain regions are deprived of nourishment. These three chapters are intended to provide a synthesis of the basic concepts of the structure of the central nervous system and its functional architecture. A fundamental neuroanatomical vocabulary is also established in these chapters.

The remaining 13 chapters examine the major functional neural systems: sensory, motor, and integrative. These chapters reexamine the views of the surface and internal structures of the central nervous system presented in the introductory chapters, but now from the perspective of the different functional neural systems. As these latter chapters on functional brain architecture unfold, the reader gradually builds a neuroanatomical knowledge of the regional and functional organization of the spinal cord and brain, one system at a time.

These chapters on neural systems have a different organization from that of the introductory chapters: Each is divided into two parts, functional and regional neuroanatomy. The initial part, on functional neuroanatomy, considers how the brain regions that comprise the particular neural system work together to produce their intended functions. This part of the chapter presents an overall view of function in relation to structure before considering the detailed anatomical organization of the neural system. Together with descriptions of the functions of the various components, diagrams illustrate each system's anatomical organization, including key connections that help to show how the particular system accomplishes its tasks. Neural circuits that run through various divisions of the brain are depicted in a standardized format: Representations of myelin-stained sections through selected levels of the spinal cord and brain stem are presented with the neural circuit superimposed.

Regional neuroanatomy is emphasized in the latter part of the chapter. Here, structures are depicted on myelin-stained histological sections through the brain, as well as magnetic resonance images (MRIs). These sections reveal the locations of major pathways and neuronal integrative regions. Typically, this part examines a sequence of myelin-stained sections ordered according to the flow of information processing in the system. For example, coverage of regional anatomy of the auditory system begins with the ear, where sounds are received and initially processed, and ends with the cerebral cortex, where our perceptions are formulated. In keeping with the overall theme of the book, the relation between the structure and the function of discrete brain regions is emphasized.

Emphasis is placed on the close relationship between neuroanatomy and neuroradiology especially through use of MRI scans. These scans are intended to facilitate the transition from learning the actual structure of the brain, as revealed by histological sections, to that which is depicted on radiological images. This is important in learning to "read" the scans, an important clinical skill. However, there is no substitute for actual stained brain sections for developing an understanding of three-dimensional brain structure.

Atlas of the Central Nervous System

This book's atlas, in two parts, offers a complete reference of anatomical structure. The first part presents key views of the surface anatomy of the central nervous system. This collection of drawings is based on actual specimens but emphasizes common features. Thus, no single brain has precisely the form illustrated in the atlas. The second part of the atlas presents a complete set of photographs of myelin-stained sections through the central nervous system in three anatomical planes.

With few exceptions, the same surface views and histological sections used in the chapters are also present in the atlas. In this way, the reader does not have to cope with anatomical variability and is thus better able to develop a thorough understanding of a limited, and sufficiently complete, set of materials. Moreover, brain views and histological sections shown in the chapters have identified only the key structures and those important for the topics discussed. In the atlas, all illustrations are comprehensively labeled as a reference. The atlas also serves as a useful guide during a neuroanatomy laboratory.

Didactic Boxes

Selected topics that complement material covered in the chapters are presented in boxes. In many of the boxes, a new perspective on neuroanatomy is presented, one that has emerged only recently from research. The neuroscience community is enthusiastic that many of these new perspectives may help explain changes in brain function that occur following brain trauma or may be used to repair the damaged nervous system.

Clinical Cases

Each chapter begins with a clinical case, chosen to highlight a fascinating clinical feature of the neural system discussed in the chapter. Whereas some of these cases are rare and not apt to be seen in routine medical practice, they show how perception, motor behavior, or personality and emotions can change after a stroke or tumor damages the brain, or how brain structure and function change after a selective gene mutation. The case description is followed by an explanation of what structures and neural systems are damaged that produce the neurological signs. Questions are posed that can be answered on the basis of reading the case explanations and the chapter text. Detailed answers are provided at the end of the book.

Study Questions

Each chapter ends with a set of study questions. Answers are provided at the end of the book. A brief explanation of the more integrative and difficult questions also is provided.

Glossary

The glossary contains a listing of key terms and structures. Typically, these terms are printed in boldface within the chapters. Key terms are defined briefly in the context of their usage in the chapters. Key structures are identified by location and function.

Additional Study Aids

This book offers three features that can be used as aids in learning neuroanatomy initially, as well as in reviewing for examinations, including professional competency exams:

- Summaries at the end of each chapter, which present concise descriptions of key structures in relation to their functions.
- A glossary of key terms.
- The atlas of key brain views and myelin-stained histological sections, which juxtapose unlabeled and labeled views. The unlabeled image can also be used for self-testing, such as for structure identification.

These study aids are designed to help the reader assimilate efficiently and quickly the extraordinary amount of detail required to develop a thorough knowledge of human neuroanatomy.

THE CENTRAL NERVOUS SYSTEM

I

Organization of the Central Nervous System

CLINICAL CASE | Alzheimer Disease

A 79-year-old man has become forgetful, often misplacing items at home, and sometimes is confused when paying for his groceries. His family reports that his forgetfulness seems to be getting worse. On neurological examination, he reports the correct date and knows where he is and why he is there; he has normal speech. However, he is unable to recall the names of three unrelated words 5 minutes after correctly repeating them. When asked to perform simple addition and subtraction, he is slow and has difficulty. His mental status was further evaluated, which revealed additional cognitive impairment. He was diagnosed with Alzheimer disease, based on his neuro-psychiatric examinations and brain imaging studies.

Figure 1–1 shows, side by side, a photograph of a brain from a person that had Alzheimer disease (A1) and a normal brain (B1). Magnetic resonance images (MRIs) are presented below (A2–5; B2–5). The appearance of brain slices will be explored further, beginning with Chapter 2, as we learn about the brain's internal structure. But we can take this opportunity to consider changes to the cortex and ventricular system as revealed on slices of the living brain. Parts 2–4 present a series of MRIs close to the transverse plane (see inset; also, Figures 1–16 and 1–17). On these images, white and gray matter appear as different shades of gray and cerebrospinal fluid, black. Cranial fatty substances (for example, skin and in the bony orbits) are white. Note how the ventricles are thin in the healthy brain (right column), but dilated in the diseased brain (left column).

The hippocampal formation (Figure 1-10A; see Chapter 16) also becomes atrophic in Alzheimer disease. This is seen in the coronal MRIs in Figure 1–1. The generalized cortical atrophy and ventricular enlargement are also apparent on the transverse MRI.

You should try to answer the following questions based on your reading of the chapter and inspection of the images. Note that the description of key neurological signs that follow the questions also will provide the answers.

1. **Why is the ventricular system affected, even though it is a non-neuronal structure?**

2. **Are some brain areas more severely affected than others?**

—Continued next page

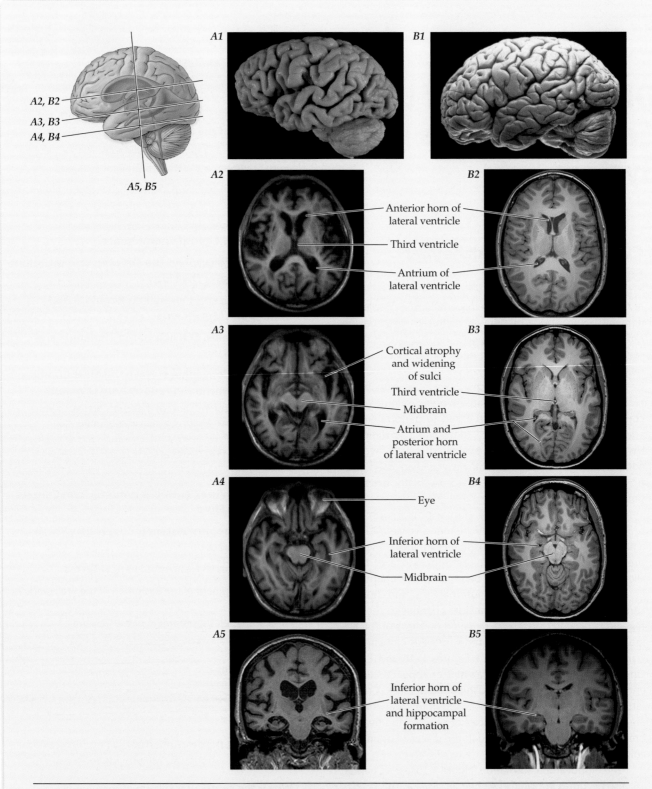

FIGURE 1–1 Brain (top) and MRIs (transverse plane, 2-4; coronal plane, 5) from a person with Alzheimer disease (**A**) and a healthy person (**B**). The brain views show generalized atrophy in Alzheimer disease. The MRIs (2-5) show cortical atrophy and ventricular enlargement. The MRIs are T1 images; brain tissues are shades of gray and cerebrospinal fluid, black. (**A1,** Image courtesy of Dr. Mony J de Leon [NYU School of Medicine], Dr. Jerzy Wegiel [Institute for Basic Research], and Dr. Thomas Wisniewski [NYU School of Medicine]; NIH Alzheimer's Disease Center P30 AG08051. **A2, A3, A4,** Images reproduced with permission from Dr. Frank Galliard, Radiopaedia. com. **A5,** Image courtesy of The Dementia Research Center, UCL Institute of Neurology.)

Key neurological signs and corresponding damaged brain structures

Brain of person with Alzheimer disease and healthy brain

No description is necessary; the amount and extent of cortical atrophy is obvious in the brain of the person that had Alzheimer disease (A1). Cortical atrophy is accompanied by atrophy in subcortical structures as well. Because the volume of the skull is fixed, as brain tissues decrease in volume, there is a corresponding increase in ventricular volume. Thus, ventricular enlargement is a consequence of loss of neural tissue.

Magnetic resonance images

Both the generalized cortical atrophy and ventricular enlargement can be seen on magnetic resonance images (MRIs) of the brain. A superior-to-inferior sequence of three images in the transverse plan (see insets) is shown. The MRI in part 2 slices through the anterior horn and atrium of the lateral ventricles, where enlargement is enormous. Because of the extensive cortical atrophy, the cortical sulci are wider

and filled with more cerebral spinal fluid. Note the region around lateral sulcus and insular cortex (Figure 1–1A2), where the mixture of a greater amount of cerebrospinal fluid and thinned cortex produces a large dark region. The inset in Figure 1–11A illustrates the insular cortex. The hippocampal formation is key to consolidation of short-term to long-term memory (see Chapter 16). Its reduction in Alzheimer disease, together with degeneration of temporal lobe cortex, leaves a gaping hole in the temporal lobe. Hippocampal degeneration can explain why the patient has poor word recall. These images also reveal that the brain stem is not grossly affected. Although not visible on these images, a small nucleus on the inferior brain surface, the basal nucleus, is severely affected early in Alzheimer disease. This nucleus contains neurons that use acetylcholine. Since these neurons project widely throughout the cortex, with their loss many cortical neurons are deprived of a strong excitatory input. This, together with the gross degeneration, helps to explain the cognitive impairments in the patient. The sizes of the midbrain (parts 3 and 4) and pons (part 5) appear normal.

Reference

Brust, JCM. *The Practice of Neural Science*. New York, NY: McGraw-Hill; 2000.

The human nervous system carries out an enormous number of functions by means of many subdivisions. Indeed, the brain's complexity has traditionally made the study of neuroanatomy a demanding task. This task can be greatly simplified by approaching the study of the nervous system from the dual perspectives of its regional and functional anatomy. **Regional neuroanatomy** examines the spatial relations between brain structures within a portion of the nervous system. Regional neuroanatomy defines the major brain divisions as well as local, neighborhood relationships within the divisions. In contrast, **functional neuroanatomy** examines those parts of the nervous system that work together to accomplish a particular task, for example, visual perception. Functional systems are formed by specific neural connections within and between regions of the nervous system; connections that form complex neural circuits. A goal of functional neuroanatomy is to develop an understanding of the neural circuitry underlying behavior. By knowing regional anatomy together with the functions of particular brain structures, the clinician can determine the location of nervous system damage in a patient who has a particular neurological or psychiatric impairment. Combined knowledge of what structures do and where they are located is essential for a complete understanding of nervous system organization. The term *neuroanatomy* is therefore misleading because it implies that knowledge of structure

is sufficient to master this discipline. Indeed, in the study of neuroanatomy, structure and function are tightly interwoven, so much so that they should not be separated. The interrelationships between structure and function underlie **functional localization,** a key principle of nervous system organization.

This chapter examines the organization of the nervous system and the means to study it by developing the vocabulary to describe its regional anatomy. First, the cellular constituents of the nervous system are described briefly. Then the chapter focuses on the major regions of the nervous system and the functions of these regions. This background gives the reader insight into functional localization.

Neurons and Glia Are the Two Principal Cellular Constituents of the Nervous System

The nerve cell, or **neuron,** is the functional cellular unit of the nervous system. Neuroscientists strive to understand the myriad functions of the nervous system partly in terms of the interconnections between neurons. The other major cellular constituent of the nervous system is the neuroglial cell, or **glia.** Glia provide structural and metabolic support for neurons during development and in maturity.

All Neurons Have a Common Morphological Plan

It is estimated that there are about 100 billion neurons in the adult human brain. Although neurons come in different shapes and sizes, each has four morphologically specialized regions with particular functions: dendrites, cell body, axon, and axon terminals (Figure 1–2A). **Dendrites** receive information from other neurons. The **cell body** contains the nucleus and cellular organelles critical for the neuron's survival and function. The cell body also receives information from other neurons and serves important integrative functions. The **axon** conducts information, which is encoded in the form of action potentials, to the **axon terminal.** Connections between two neurons in a neural circuit are made by the axon terminals of one and the dendrites and cell body of the other, at the synapse (discussed below).

Despite a wide range of morphology, we can distinguish three classes of neuron based on the configuration of their dendrites and axons: unipolar, bipolar, and multipolar (Figure 1–2B). These neurons were drawn by the distinguished Spanish neuroanatomist Santiago Ramón y Cajal at

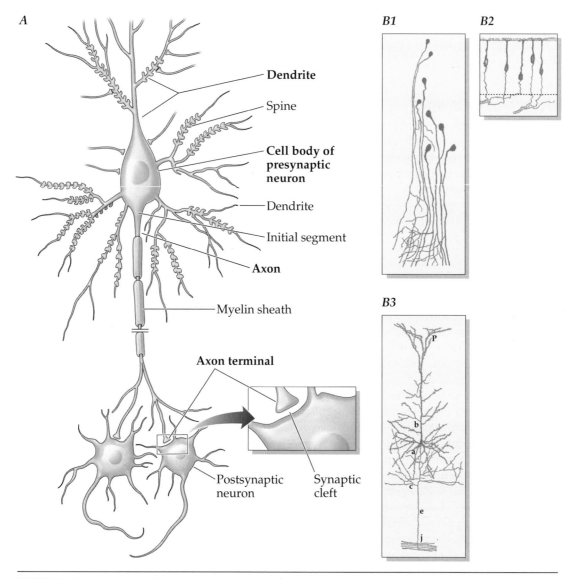

FIGURE 1–2 Neurons are the functional cellular unit of the nervous system. **A.** A schematic nerve cell is shown, illustrating the dendrites, cell body, and axon. Dendritic spines are located on the dendrites. These are sites of excitatory synapses. Inhibitory synapses are located on the shaft of the dendrites, the cell body, and the initial segment. The axon can be seen to emerge from the cell body. The presynaptic terminals of the neuron are shown synapsing on the cell bodies of the postsynaptic neurons. The inset shows the spatial relations of three components of the synapse: the presynaptic axon terminal, the synaptic cleft, and the postsynaptic neuron. **B.** Selected examples of three neuron classes: (**B1**) unipolar, (**B2**) bipolar, and (**B3**) multipolar. (**A,** Adapted from Kandel ER, Schwartz JH, and Jessell TM, eds. *Principles of Neural Science*, 4th ed. New York, NY: McGraw-Hill, 2000. **B,** Reproduced with permission from from Cajal SR. *Histologie du système nerveux de l'homme et des vertébres.* 2 vols. Maloine, 1909-1911.)

the beginning of the twentieth century. **Unipolar neurons** are the simplest in shape (Figure 1–2B1). They have no dendrites; the cell body of unipolar neurons receives and integrates incoming information. A single axon, which originates from the cell body, gives rise to multiple processes at the terminal. In the human nervous system, unipolar neurons are the least common. They control exocrine gland secretions and smooth muscle contractility.

Bipolar neurons have two processes that arise from opposite poles of the cell body (Figure 1–2B2). The flow of information in bipolar neurons is from one of the processes, which function like a dendrite, across the cell body to the other process, which functions like an axon. A bipolar neuron subtype is a pseudounipolar neuron (see Figure 6–2 top). During development the two processes of the embryonic bipolar neuron fuse into a single process in the pseudounipolar neuron, which bifurcates a short distance from the cell body. Many sensory neurons, such as those that transmit information about odors or touch to the brain, are bipolar and pseudounipolar neurons.

Multipolar neurons feature a complex array of dendrites on the cell body and a single axon that branches extensively (Figure 1–2B3). Most of the neurons in the brain and spinal cord are multipolar. Multipolar neurons that have long axons, with axon terminals located in distant sites, are termed **projection neurons.** Projection neurons mediate communication between regions of the nervous system and between the nervous system and peripheral targets, such as striated muscle cells. The neuron in Figure 1–2B3 is a particularly complex projection neuron. The terminals of this neuron are not shown because they are located far from the cell body. For this type of neuron in the human, the axon may be up to 1-m long, about 50,000 times the width of the cell body! Other multipolar neurons, commonly called **interneurons,** have short axons that remain in the same region of the nervous system in which the cell body is located. Interneurons help to process neuronal information within a local brain region.

Neurons Communicate With Each Other at Synapses

Information flow along a neuron is polarized. The dendrites and cell body receive and integrate incoming information, which is transmitted along the axon to the terminals. Communication of information from one neuron to another also is polarized and occurs at specialized sites of contact called **synapses.** The neuron that sends information is the **presynaptic neuron** and the one that receives the information is the **postsynaptic neuron.** The information carried by the presynaptic neuron is most typically transduced at the synapse into a chemical signal that is received by specialized membrane receptors on the dendrites and cell body of the postsynaptic neuron.

The synapse consists of three distinct elements: (1) the **presynaptic terminal,** the axon terminal of the presynaptic neuron, (2) the **synaptic cleft,** the narrow intercellular space between the neurons, and (3) the **receptive membrane** of the postsynaptic neuron. Synapses are present on dendrites, the cell body, the **initial segment** of the axon, or the portion of the axon closest to the cell body, and the presynaptic axon terminal. Synapses located on different sites can serve different functions.

To send a message to its postsynaptic neurons, a presynaptic neuron releases **neurotransmitter,** packaged into vesicles, into the synaptic cleft. Neurotransmitters are small molecular weight compounds; among these are amino acids (eg, glutamate; glycine; and γ-aminobutyric acid, or GABA), acetylcholine, and monoaminergic compounds such as norepinephrine and serotonin. Larger molecules, such as peptides (eg, enkephalin and substance P), also can function as neurotransmitters. After release into the synaptic cleft, the neurotransmitter molecules diffuse across the cleft and bind to receptors on the postsynaptic membrane. Neurotransmitters change the permeability of particular ions across the neuronal membrane. A neurotransmitter can either excite the postsynaptic neuron by depolarizing it, or inhibit the neuron by hyperpolarizing it. For example, excitation can be produced by a neurotransmitter that increases the flow of sodium ions into a neuron (ie, depolarization), and inhibition can be produced by a neurotransmitter that increases the flow of chloride ions into a neuron (ie, hyperpolarization). Glutamate and acetylcholine typically excite neurons, whereas GABA and glycine typically inhibit neurons. Many neurotransmitters, like dopamine and serotonin, have more varied actions, exciting some neurons and inhibiting others. Their action depends on a myriad of factors, such as the particular receptor subtype that the neurotransmitter engages and whether the binding of the neurotransmitter leads directly to the change in ion permeability or if the change is mediated by the actions on second messengers and other intracellular signaling pathways (eg, G protein coupled receptors). For example, the dopamine receptor subtype 1 is depolarizing, whereas the type 2 receptor is hyperpolarizing; both act through G protein coupled mechanisms. A neurotransmitter can even have opposing actions on the same neuron depending on the composition of receptor subtypes on the neuron's membrane. Action through second messengers and other intracellular signaling pathways can have short-term effects, such as changing membrane ion permeability, or long-term effects, such as gene expression. Many small molecules that produce strong effects on neurons are not packaged into vesicles; they are thought to act through diffusion. These compounds, for example, nitric oxide, are produced in the postsynaptic neuron and are thought to act as retrograde messengers that serve important regulatory functions on pre- and postsynaptic neurons, including maintaining and modulating the strength of synaptic connections. These actions are important for learning and memory.

Although chemical synaptic transmission is the most common way of sending messages from one neuron to another, purely electrical communication can occur between neurons. At such **electrical synapses,** there is direct cytoplasmic continuity between the presynaptic and postsynaptic neurons.

Glial Cells Provide Structural and Metabolic Support for Neurons

Glial cells comprise the other major cellular constituent of the nervous system; they outnumber neurons by about 10 to 1. Given this high ratio, the structural and metabolic support that glial cells provide for neurons must be a formidable task! There are two major classes of glia: microglia and macroglia. **Microglia** subserve a phagocytic or scavenger role, responding to nervous system infection or damage. They are rapidly mobilized—they become activated—in response to different pathophysiological conditions and trauma. Activated microglia can destroy invading microorganisms, remove debris, and promote tissue repair. Interestingly, they also mediate changes in neuronal properties after nervous system damage; sometimes maladaptive changes, so they may also hinder recovery after injury. For example, neurons often become hyperexcitable after nervous system damage, and microglia can be involved in this process. **Macroglia,** of which there are four separate types—oligodendrocytes, Schwann cells, astrocytes, and ependymal cells—have a variety of support and nutritive functions. **Schwann cells** and **oligodendrocytes** form the **myelin sheath** around peripheral and central axons, respectively (Figures 1–2A and 1–3). The myelin sheath increases

A

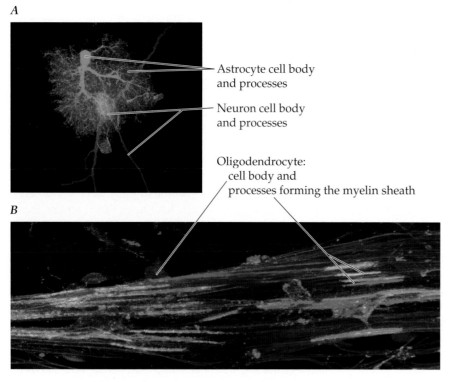

Astrocyte cell body and processes

Neuron cell body and processes

Oligodendrocyte: cell body and processes forming the myelin sheath

B

C

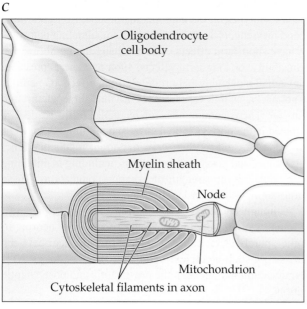

Oligodendrocyte cell body

Myelin sheath

Node

Mitochondrion

Cytoskeletal filaments in axon

FIGURE 1–3 Astrocytes and oligodendrocytes are the most ubiquitous types of glial cells in the central nervous system. Parts *A* and *B* are histological sections showing examples of these cell types. *A.* An astrocyte (green) is shown enveloping a neuronal cell body (red). *B.* Oligodendrocytes are shown forming the myelin sheaths surrounding axons. A blue stain (DAPI) marks nuclei in the cell bodies. The processes (green) are stained for an important component of the myelin sheath, myelin basic protein (MBP). (Part *A,* Image courtesy of Ellisman M and Bushong E, Univ. California, San Diego. Allen NJ, Barres BA. Neuroscience Glia: More than just brain glue. *Nature.* 2009;457 [7230]:675-677. Part *B,* Reproduced with permission from Lee PR, Fields RD. Regulation of myelin genes implicated in psychiatric disorders by functional activity in axons. *Front Neuroanat.* 2009;3:4. Part *C,* Adapted from Kandel ER, Schwartz JS, and Jessell TM, eds. *Principles of Neural Science,* 4th ed. New York, NY: McGraw-Hill, 2000.).

the velocity of action potential conduction. It is whitish in appearance because it is rich in a fatty substance called **myelin,** which is composed of many different kinds of myelin proteins. Schwann cells also play important roles in organizing the formation of the connective tissue sheaths surrounding peripheral nerves during development and in axon regeneration following damage in maturity. **Astrocytes** have important structural and metabolic functions. For example, in the developing nervous system, astrocytes act as scaffolds for growing axons and guides for migrating immature neurons. Many synapses are associated with astrocyte processes that may monitor synaptic actions and provide chemical feedback. Astrocytes also contribute to the blood-brain barrier, which protects the vulnerable environment of the brain from invasion of chemical from the periphery, which can influence neuronal firing. The last class of macroglia,

ependymal cells, line fluid-filled cavities in the central nervous system (see below). They play an important role in regulating the flow of chemicals from these cavities into the brain.

The Nervous System Consists of Separate Peripheral and Central Components

Neurons and glial cells of the nervous system are organized into two anatomically separate but functionally interdependent parts: the **peripheral** and the **central nervous systems** (Figure 1–4A). The peripheral nervous system is subdivided into **somatic** and **autonomic** divisions. The somatic division contains the sensory neurons that innervate the skin, muscles,

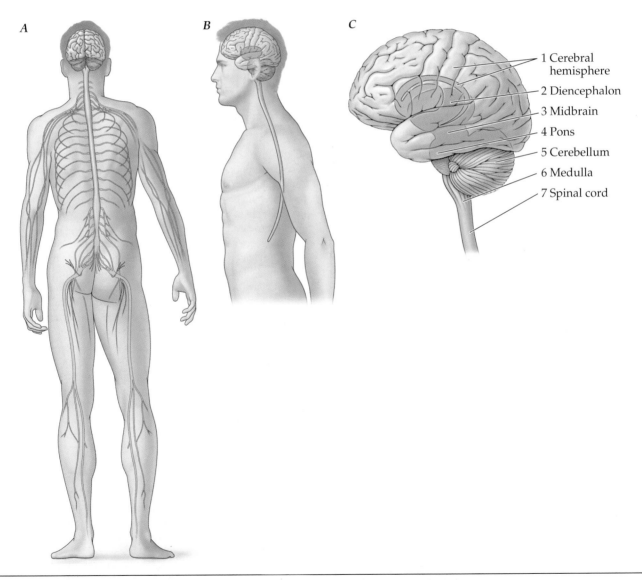

1 Cerebral hemisphere
2 Diencephalon
3 Midbrain
4 Pons
5 Cerebellum
6 Medulla
7 Spinal cord

FIGURE 1–4 A. Location of the central and peripheral nervous system in the body. Major peripheral nerves are shown in yellow. **B.** The brain and spinal cord, viewed laterally. **C.** There are seven major divisions of the central nervous system: (1) cerebral hemispheres, (2) diencephalon, (3) midbrain, (4) pons, (5) cerebellum, (6) medulla, and (7) spinal cord. The midbrain, pons, and medulla comprise the brain stem.

and joints. These neurons detect and, in turn, inform the central nervous system of stimuli. This division also contains the axons of motor neurons that innervate skeletal muscle, although the cell bodies of motor neurons lie within the central nervous system. These axons transmit control signals to muscle to regulate the force of muscle contraction. The autonomic division contains the neurons that innervate glands and the smooth muscle of the viscera and blood vessels (see Chapter 15). This division, with its separate **sympathetic, parasympathetic,** and **enteric** subdivisions, regulates body functions based, in part, on information about the body's internal state.

The central nervous system consists of the **spinal cord** and **brain** (Figure 1–4B), and the brain is further subdivided into the medulla, pons, cerebellum, midbrain, diencephalon, and cerebral hemispheres (Figure 1–4C). Within each of the seven central nervous system divisions resides a component of the **ventricular system,** a labyrinth of fluid-filled cavities that serve various supportive functions (see Figure 1–13). Box 1–1 shows how all of the divisions of the central nervous system and the components of the ventricular system are present from very early in development, from about the first month after conception.

Neuronal cell bodies and axons are not distributed uniformly within the nervous system. In the peripheral nervous system, cell bodies collect in peripheral **ganglia** and axons are contained in **peripheral nerves.** In the central nervous system, neuronal cell bodies and dendrites are located in **cortical** areas, which are flattened sheets of cells (or laminae) located primarily on the surface of the cerebral hemispheres, and in **nuclei,** which are clusters of neurons located beneath the surface of all of the central nervous system divisions. Nuclei come in various sizes and shapes; they are commonly oval and columnar but sometimes occur in complex three-dimensional configurations (see Figure 1–10). Regions of the central nervous system that contain axons have an unwieldy number of names, the most common of which is **tract.** In fresh tissue, nuclei and cortical areas appear grayish and tracts appear whitish, hence the familiar terms **gray matter** and **white matter.** The whitish appearance of tracts is caused by the presence of the myelin sheath surrounding the axons (Figure 1–3). The gray and white matter can be distinguished in fixed tissue using anatomical methods and in the living brain using radiological methods (see Chapter 2, Boxes 2–1, 2–2).

Box 1–1

Development of the Basic Plan of the Brain and Spinal Cord

The central nervous system develops from a specialized portion of the embryonic ectoderm, the neural plate. Originally a flattened sheet of cells, the neural plate forms a tube-like structure—termed the neural tube—as the neurons and glial cells proliferate. The walls of the neural tube form the neuronal structure of the central nervous system. The cavity in the neural tube forms the ventricular system.

Very early in development the rostral portion of the neural tube forms the three hollow swellings, or vesicles, corresponding to where there is an enormous proliferation of developing neurons (Figure 1–5): (1) the **prosencephalon,** or **forebrain,** (2) the **mesencephalon,** or **midbrain,** and (3) the **rhombencephalon,** or **hindbrain.** The caudal portion of the neural tube remains relatively undifferentiated and forms the **spinal cord.** Two secondary vesicles emerge from the prosencephalon later in development, the **telencephalon** (or cerebral hemisphere) and the **diencephalon** (or thalamus and hypothalamus). Whereas the mesencephalon remains undivided throughout further brain development, the rhombencephalon gives rise to the **metencephalon** (or pons and cerebellum) and the **myelencephalon** (or medulla). The five brain vesicles and primitive spinal cord, already identifiable by the fifth week of fetal life, give rise to the seven major divisions of the central nervous system (see Figure 1–4).

The complex configuration of the mature brain is determined in part by how the developing brain bends, or **flexes.** Flexures occur because proliferation of cells in the brain stem and cerebral hemispheres is enormous, and the space that the developing brain occupies in the cranium is constrained. At the three-vesicle stage, there are two prominent flexures: the **cervical flexure,** at the junction of the spinal cord and the caudal hindbrain (or future medulla), and the **cephalic flexure,** at the level of the midbrain

(Figure 1–5, bottom). At the five-vesicle stage, a third flexure becomes prominent, the **pontine flexure.** By birth the cervical and pontine flexures have straightened out. The cephalic flexure, however, remains prominent and causes the longitudinal axis of the forebrain to deviate from that of the midbrain, hindbrain, and spinal cord (see Figure 1–16B).

The large cavities within the cerebral vesicles develop into the ventricular system of the brain, and the caudal cavity becomes the central canal of the spinal cord (Figure 1–5). The ventricular system contains **cerebrospinal fluid,** which is produced mainly by the **choroid plexus** (see Chapter 3). As the brain vesicles develop, the cavity within the cerebral hemispheres divides into the two **lateral ventricles** (formerly termed the first and second ventricles) and the **third ventricle** (Figure 1–5B). The lateral ventricles, which develop as outpouchings from the rostral portion of the third ventricle, are each interconnected with the third ventricle by an **interventricular foramen** (of Monro) (Figure 1–5, inset). The **fourth ventricle,** the most caudal ventricle, develops from the cavity within the hindbrain. It is connected to the third ventricle by the **cerebral aqueduct** (of Sylvius) and merges caudally with the **central canal** (of the caudal medulla and spinal cord).

Cerebrospinal fluid normally exits from the ventricular system into the space overlying the central nervous system's surface through foramina in the fourth ventricle (discussed in Chapter 3). (The central canal does not have such an aperture for the outflow of cerebrospinal fluid.) Pathological processes can prevent flow of cerebrospinal fluid from the ventricular system. For example, later in development the cerebral aqueduct becomes narrowed because of cell proliferation in the midbrain. Its narrow diameter makes it vulnerable to the constricting effects of congenital abnormalities, tumors, or swelling from trauma. Occlusion can occur; however, cerebrospinal fluid continues to be produced despite occlusion. If occlusion occurs before the bones of the skull are fused (ie, in embryonic life or in infancy), ventricular volume will increase, the brain will enlarge rostral to the occlusion, and head size will increase. This condition is called **hydrocephalus.** If occlusion occurs after the bones of the skull are fused, ventricular size cannot increase without increasing intracranial pressure. This is a life-threatening condition.

The Spinal Cord Displays the Simplest Organization of All Seven Major Divisions

The spinal cord participates in processing sensory information from the limbs, trunk, and many internal organs; in controlling body movements directly; and in regulating many visceral functions (Figure 1–6). It also provides a conduit for the transmission of both sensory information in the tracts that ascend to the brain and motor information in the descending tracts. The spinal cord is the only part of the human central nervous system that has an external **segmental** organization (Figure 1–6B,C).

The spinal cord has a modular organization, in which every segment has a similar basic structure (Figure 1–6C).

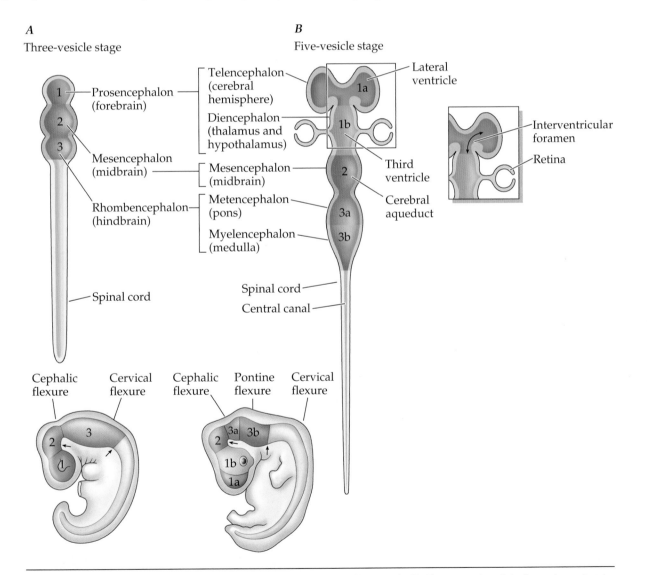

FIGURE 1–5. Schematic illustration of the three- and five-vesicle stages of the neural tube. The top portion of the figure shows dorsal views of the neural tube drawn without flexures. The bottom portion of the figure presents lateral views. ***A.*** Three-vesicle stage. ***B.*** Five-vesicle stage. Note that the lineage of each vesicle at the five-vesicle stage is indicated by the shading. The two secondary vesicles from the forebrain have different green shades, and the two vesicles that derived from the hindbrain have different blue shades. The inset shows the location of the intraventricular foramen on one side in the five-vesicle stage. (Adapted from Kandel ER, Schwartz JH, and Jessell TM, eds. *Principles of Neural Science*, 3rd ed. McGraw-Hill, 1991.)

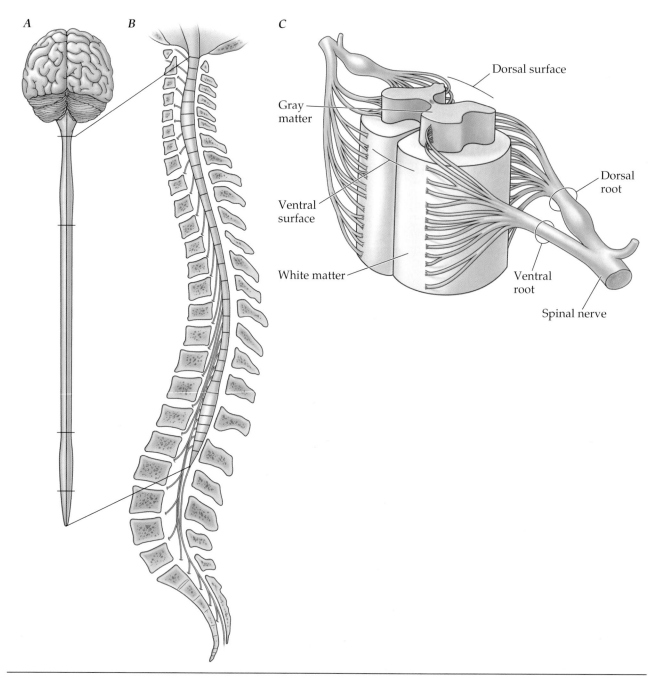

FIGURE 1–6 Spinal cord organization. **A.** A dorsal view of the central nervous system. The horizontal lines over the spinal cord mark the locations of the different spinal cord divisions. These will be considered in more detail in later chapters. **B.** A lateral view of the spinal cord and the vertebral column. **C.** Surface topography and internal structure of the spinal cord.

Each spinal cord segment contains a pair of nerve roots (and associated rootlets) called the **dorsal** and **ventral roots.** (The terms *dorsal* and *ventral* describe the spatial relations of structures; these and other anatomical terms are explained later in this chapter.) Dorsal roots contain only sensory axons, which transmit sensory information into the spinal cord. By contrast, ventral roots contain motor axons, which transmit motor commands to muscle and other body organs. Dorsal and ventral roots exemplify the separation of function in the nervous system, a principle that is examined further in subsequent chapters. These sensory and motor axons, which are part of the peripheral nervous system, become intermingled in the **spinal nerves** en route to their peripheral targets (Figure 1–6C).

The Brain Stem and Cerebellum Regulate Body Functions and Movements

The next three divisions—medulla, pons, and midbrain—comprise the **brain stem** (Figure 1–7). The brain stem has three general functions. First, it receives sensory information from cranial structures and controls the muscles of the head. These functions are similar to those of the spinal cord. **Cranial nerves,** the sensory and motor nerve roots that enter and exit the brain stem, are parts of the peripheral nervous system and are analogous to the spinal nerves (Figure 1–7). Second, similar to the spinal cord, the brain stem is a conduit for information flow because ascending sensory and descending motor tracts travel through it. Finally, nuclei in the brain stem integrate information from a variety of sources for arousal and other higher brain functions.

In addition to these three general functions, the various divisions of the brain stem each subserve specific sensory and motor functions. For example, portions of the **medulla** participate in essential blood pressure and respiratory regulatory mechanisms. Indeed, damage to these parts of the brain is almost always life threatening. Parts of the **pons** and **midbrain** play a key role in the control of eye movement.

The principal functions of the **cerebellum** are to regulate eye and limb movements and to maintain posture and balance (Figure 1–8). Limb movements become poorly coordinated when the cerebellum is damaged. In addition, parts of the cerebellum play a role in higher brain functions, including language, cognition, and emotion (Chapter 13).

The Diencephalon Consists of the Thalamus and Hypothalamus

The two principal parts of the **diencephalon** participate in diverse sensory, motor, and integrative functions. One component, the **thalamus** (Figure 1–9), is a key structure for transmitting information to the cerebral hemispheres. The thalamus is composed of numerous nuclei. Neurons in separate thalamic nuclei transmit information to different cortical areas. In the brains of most people, a small portion of the thalamus in each half adheres at the midline, the **thalamic adhesion.** The other component of the diencephalon, the **hypothalamus** (Figure 1–9A; see also Figure 1–12A), controls endocrine hormone release from the pituitary gland and the overall functions of the autonomic nervous system.

The Cerebral Hemispheres Have the Most Complex Shape of All Central Nervous System Divisions

The **cerebral hemispheres** are the most highly developed portions of the human central nervous system. Each hemisphere is a distinct half, and each has four major components:

cerebral cortex, hippocampal formation, amygdala, and basal ganglia. Together, these structures mediate the most sophisticated of human behaviors, and they do so through complex anatomical connections.

The Subcortical Components of the Cerebral Hemispheres Mediate Diverse Motor, Cognitive, and Emotional Functions

The **hippocampal formation** is important in learning and memory, whereas the **amygdala** not only participates in emotions but also helps to coordinate the body's response to stressful and threatening situations, such as preparing to fight (Figure 1–10A). These two structures are part of the **limbic system** (see Chapter 16), which includes other parts of the cerebral hemispheres, diencephalon, and midbrain. Because parts of the limbic system play a key role in mood, it is not surprising that psychiatric disorders are often associated with limbic system dysfunction.

The **basal ganglia** are another deeply located collection of neurons. The portion of the basal ganglia that has the most complex shape is called the **striatum** (Figure 1–10B). The importance of the basal ganglia in the control of movement is clearly revealed when they become damaged, as in Parkinson disease. Tremor and a slowing of movement are some of the overt signs of this disease. The basal ganglia also participate in cognition and emotions in concert with the cerebral cortex and are key brain structures involved in addiction.

The Four Lobes of the Cerebral Cortex Each Have Distinct Functions

The **cerebral cortex,** which is located on the surface of the brain, is highly convoluted (Figures 1–11 and 1–12). The human cerebral cortex is approximately 2,500 cm². Convolutions are an evolutionary adaptation to fit a greater surface area within the confined space of the cranial cavity. In fact, only one quarter to one third of the cerebral cortex is exposed on the surface. The elevated convolutions on the cortical surface, called **gyri,** are separated by grooves called **sulci** or **fissures** (which are particularly deep sulci). The cerebral hemispheres are separated from each other by the **sagittal** (or interhemispheric) **fissure** (Figure 1–12B).

The four **lobes** of the cerebral cortex are named after the cranial bones that overlie them: frontal, parietal, occipital, and temporal (Figure 1–11, inset). The functions of the different lobes are remarkably distinct, as are the functions of individual gyri within each lobe.

The **frontal lobe** serves diverse behavioral functions, from thoughts to action, cognition, and emotions. The **precentral gyrus** contains the **primary motor cortex,** which participates in controlling the mechanical actions of movement, such as the direction and speed of reaching. Many projection neurons in the

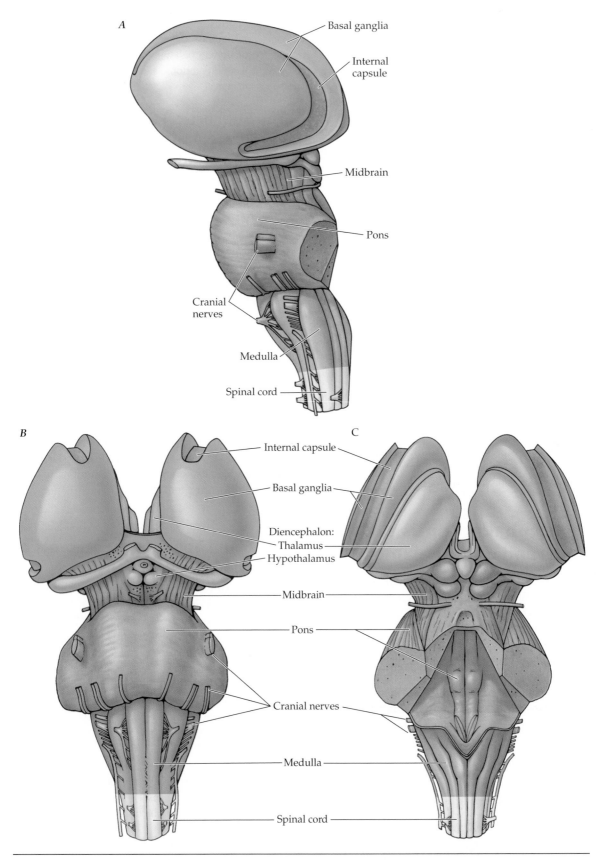

FIGURE 1–7. Lateral (**A**), ventral (**B**), and dorsal (**C**) surfaces of the brain stem. The thalamus and basal ganglia are also shown. The different divisions of the brain are shaded in different colors.

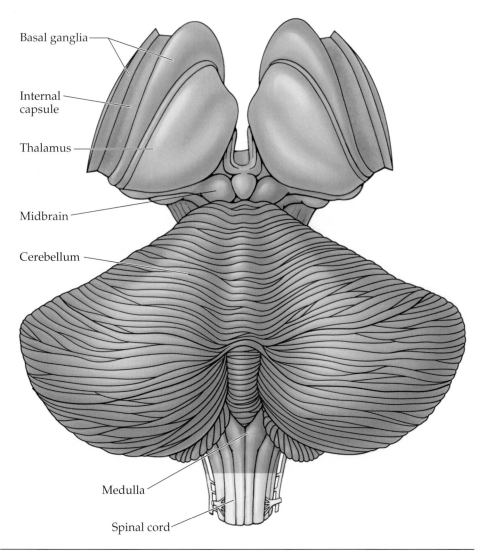

Basal ganglia

Internal capsule

Thalamus

Midbrain

Cerebellum

Medulla

Spinal cord

FIGURE 1-8 Dorsal view of the brain stem, thalamus, and basal ganglia, together with the cerebellum.

primary motor cortex have an axon that terminates in the spinal cord. The superior, middle, and inferior frontal gyri form most of the remaining portion of the frontal lobe. The premotor areas, which are important in motor decision making and planning movements, are adjacent to the primary motor cortex in these gyri. The inferior frontal gyrus in the left hemisphere in most people contains Broca's area, which is essential for the articulation of speech. Much of the frontal lobe is **association cortex.** Association cortical areas are involved in the complex processing of sensory and other information for higher brain functions, including emotions, organizing behavior, thoughts, and memories. Areas closer to the frontal pole comprise the **frontal association cortex.** The **prefrontal association cortex** is important in thought, cognition, and emotions. The **cingulate gyrus** (Figure 1–11B), medial frontal lobe, and most of the **orbital gyri** (Figure 1–12A) are important in emotions. Psychiatric disorders of thought, as in schizophrenia, and mood disor-

ders, such as depression, are linked with abnormal functions of frontal association cortex. The **basal forebrain,** which is on the ventral surface of the frontal lobe (Figure 1–12A), contains a special population of neurons that uses acetylcholine to regulate cortical excitability. These neurons are examined further in Chapter 2. Although the olfactory sensory organ, the **olfactory bulb,** is located on the ventral surface of the frontal lobe, its connections are predominantly with the temporal lobe (Figure 1–12A).

The **parietal lobe,** which is separated from the frontal lobe by the **central sulcus,** mediates our perceptions of touch, pain, and limb position. These functions are carried out by the **primary somatic sensory cortex,** which is located in the **postcentral gyrus.** Primary sensory areas are the initial cortical processing stages for sensory information. The remaining portion of the parietal lobe on the lateral brain surface consists of the superior and inferior parietal lobules, which are separated

A

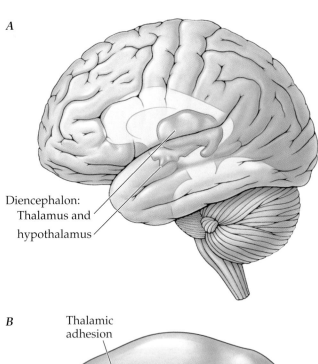

Diencephalon:
Thalamus and
hypothalamus

B   Thalamic
adhesion

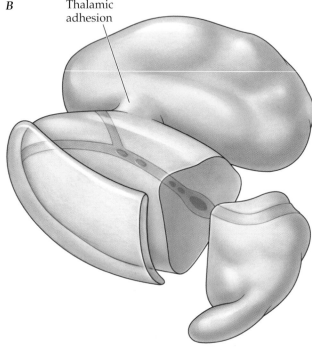

FIGURE 1–9 *A.* Lateral surface of the cerebral hemispheres and brain stem, illustrating the location of the thalamus and hypothalamus. *B.* Three-dimensional structure of the thalamus. The separate structure lateral to the main portion of the thalamus is the thalamic reticular nucleus, which forms a lamina over the lateral sides of the thalamus.

by the intraparietal sulcus. The **superior parietal lobule** contains higher-order somatic sensory areas, for further processing of somatic sensory information, and other sensory areas. Together these areas are essential for a complete self-image of the body, and they mediate behavioral interactions with the world around us. A lesion in this portion of the parietal lobe

in the right hemisphere, the side of the human brain that is specialized for spatial awareness, can produce bizarre neurological signs that include neglecting a portion of the body on the side opposite the lesion. For example, a patient may not dress one side of her body or comb half of her hair. The **inferior parietal lobule** is involved in integrating diverse sensory information for perception and language, mathematical reasoning, and visuospatial cognition.

The **occipital lobe** is separated from the parietal lobe on the medial brain surface by the **parietooccipital sulcus** (Figure 1–11B). On the lateral and inferior surfaces, there are no distinct boundaries, only an imaginary line connecting the **preoccipital notch** (Figure 1–11A) with the parietooccipital sulcus. The occipital lobe is the most singular in function, subserving vision. The **primary visual cortex** is located in the walls and depths of the **calcarine fissure** on the medial brain surface (Figure 1–11B). Whereas the primary visual cortex is important in the initial stages of visual processing, the surrounding higher-order visual areas play a role in elaborating the sensory message that enables us to see the form and color of objects. For example, on the ventral brain surface is a portion of the occipitotemporal gyrus in the occipital lobe (also termed the fusiform gyrus) that is important for recognizing faces (Figure 1–12A). Patients with a lesion of this area can confuse faces with inanimate objects, a condition termed *prosopagnosia.*

The **temporal lobe,** separated from the frontal and parietal lobes by the **lateral sulcus** (or **Sylvian fissure)** (Figure 1–11A), mediates a variety of sensory functions and participates in memory and emotions. The **primary auditory cortex,** located on the **superior temporal gyrus,** works with surrounding areas on the superior temporal gyrus and within the lateral sulcus and the superior temporal sulcus for perception and localization of sounds (Figure 1–11A). The superior temporal gyrus on the left side is specialized for speech. Lesion of the posterior portion of this gyrus, which is the location of Wernicke's area, impairs the understanding of speech. The **middle temporal gyrus,** especially the portion close to the occipital lobe, is essential for perception of visual motion. The **inferior temporal gyrus** mediates the perception of visual form and color (Figures 1–11A and 1–12A). The cortex located at the **temporal pole** (Figure 1–12A), together with adjacent portions of the medial temporal lobe and inferior and medial frontal lobes, is important for emotions.

Deep within the lateral sulcus are portions of the frontal, parietal, and temporal lobes. This territory is termed the **insular cortex** (Figure 1–11, inset). It becomes buried late during prenatal development (see Figure 1-14). Portions of the insular cortex are important in taste, internal body senses, pain, and balance.

The **corpus callosum** contains axons that interconnect the cortex on the two sides of the brain (Figure 1–11B). Tracts containing axons that interconnect the two sides of the brain are called **commissures,** and the corpus callosum is the largest of the brain's commissures. To integrate the functions of the two halves of the cerebral cortex, axons

A

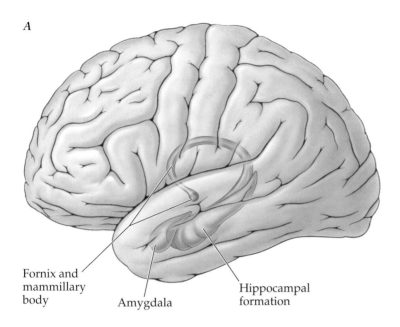

Fornix and mammillary body

Amygdala

Hippocampal formation

B

Striatum

Ventricular system

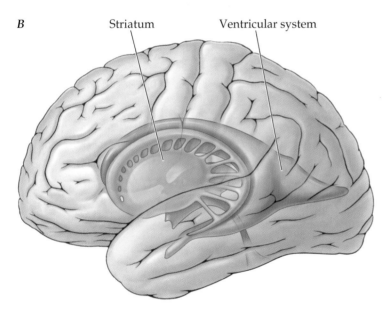

FIGURE 1–10 Three-dimensional views of deep structures of the cerebral hemisphere. **A.** The hippocampal formation (red) and amygdala (orange). The fornix (blue) and mammillary body (purple) are structures that are anatomically and functionally related to the hippocampal formation. **B.** Striatum is a component of the basal ganglia with a complex three-dimensional shape. The ventricular system is also illustrated. Note the similarity in overall shapes of the striatum and the lateral ventricle.

of the corpus callosum course through each of its four principal parts: rostrum, genu, body, and splenium (Figure 1–11B). Information between the occipital lobes travels through the splenium of the corpus callosum, whereas information from the other lobes travels through the rostrum, genu, and body.

Cavities Within the Central Nervous System Contain Cerebrospinal Fluid

The central nervous system has a tubular organization. Within it are cavities, collectively termed the **ventricular system,** that contain **cerebrospinal fluid** (Figure 1–13). Cerebrospinal fluid is a watery fluid that cushions the central nervous system from physical shocks and is a medium for chemical communication. An intraventricular structure, the **choroid plexus,** secretes most of the cerebrospinal fluid. Cerebrospinal fluid production is considered in Chapter 3.

The ventricular system consists of ventricles, where cerebrospinal fluid accumulates, and narrow communication channels. There are two **lateral ventricles,** each within one cerebral hemisphere, the **third ventricle,** between the two halves of the diencephalon, and the **fourth ventricle,** which is located between the brain stem and cerebellum. Development of the lateral ventricles, along with the sulci

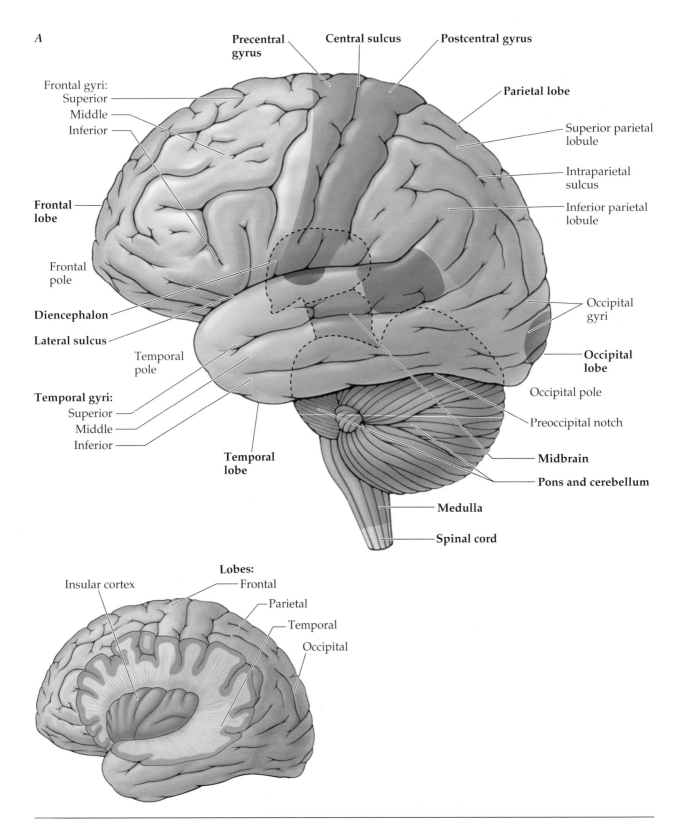

A

Precentral gyrus

Central sulcus

Postcentral gyrus

Frontal gyri:
Superior
Middle
Inferior

Parietal lobe

Superior parietal lobule

Intraparietal sulcus

Frontal lobe

Inferior parietal lobule

Frontal pole

Diencephalon

Lateral sulcus

Temporal pole

Occipital gyri

Occipital lobe

Occipital pole

Temporal gyri:
Superior
Middle
Inferior

Preoccipital notch

Temporal lobe

Midbrain

Pons and cerebellum

Medulla

Spinal cord

Lobes:

Insular cortex

Frontal

Parietal

Temporal

Occipital

FIGURE 1–11. *A.* Lateral surface of cerebral hemisphere and brain stem and a portion of the spinal cord. The different colored regions correspond to distinct functional cortical areas. The primary motor and somatic sensory areas are located in the pre- and postcentral gyri, respectively. The primary auditory cortex lies in the superior temporal gyrus adjacent to the sensory and motor areas. Broca's area comprises most of the inferior frontal gyrus, and Wernicke's area is in the posterior part of the superior temporal gyrus. Boldface labeling indicates key structures. The inset shows the four lobes of the cerebral cortex and the insular cortex in relation to the four lobes.

B

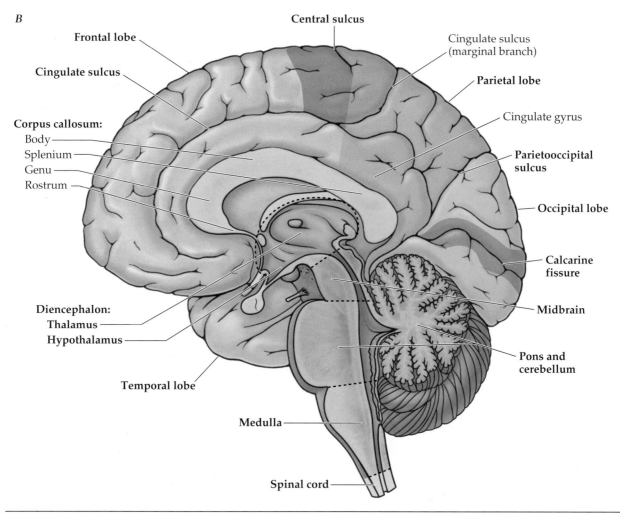

Central sulcus

Frontal lobe

Cingulate sulcus
(marginal branch)

Cingulate sulcus

Parietal lobe

Corpus callosum:
Body
Splenium
Genu
Rostrum

Cingulate gyrus

Parietooccipital
sulcus

Occipital lobe

Calcarine
fissure

Diencephalon:
Thalamus
Hypothalamus

Midbrain

Pons and
cerebellum

Temporal lobe

Medulla

Spinal cord

Continued—**FIGURE 1–11** *B.* Medial surface. The primary visual cortex is located in the banks of the calcarine fissure. A small portion extends onto the lateral surface. The divisions of the brain stem and the cerebellum are also shown in A and B.

and gyri of the cerebral cortex, is discussed in Box 1-2. The ventricles are interconnected by narrow channels: The **interventricular foramina** (of Monro) connect each of the lateral ventricles with the third ventricle, and the **cerebral aqueduct (of Sylvius),** in the midbrain, connects the third and fourth ventricles. The ventricular system extends into the spinal cord as the **central canal.** Cerebrospinal fluid exits the ventricular system through several apertures in the fourth ventricle and bathes the surface of the entire central nervous system.

The Central Nervous System Is Covered by Three Meningeal Layers

The **meninges** consist of the dura mater, the arachnoid mater, and the pia mater (Figure 1–15). (The meninges are more commonly called the dura, arachnoid, and pia, without using the term *mater.*) The **dura mater** is the thickest and outermost of these membranes and serves a protective function. (*Dura mater* means "hard mother" in Latin.) Ancient surgeons knew that patients could survive even severe skull fractures if bone fragments had not penetrated the dura. Two important partitions arise from the dura and separate different components of the cerebral hemispheres and brain stem (Figure 1–15B): (1) The **falx cerebri** separates the two cerebral hemispheres, and (2) the **tentorium cerebelli** separates the cerebellum from the cerebral hemispheres.

The **arachnoid mater** adjoins but is not tightly bound to the dura mater, thereby allowing a potential space, the **subdural space,** to exist between them. This space is important clinically. Because the dura mater contains blood vessels, breakage of one of its vessels due to head trauma can lead to subdural bleeding and to the formation of a blood clot (a **subdural hematoma).** In this condition the blood clot pushes the arachnoid mater away from the dura mater, fills the subdural space, and compresses underlying neural tissue.

Box 1-2

C-shaped Development of the Cerebral Hemisphere

The structure of the cerebral hemispheres is transformed markedly during development, in contrast to the spinal cord, brain stem, and diencephalon, which largely retain their longitudinal organization. This transformation is primarily the result of the enormous proliferation of cells of the **cerebral cortex,** the principal component of the cerebral hemispheres, and their subsequent migration along predetermined axes. This leads to the distinctive shape of the cerebral cortex and many underlying structures.

The surface area of the cerebral cortex increases enormously during development. As the cortex develops, it encircles the diencephalon and takes on a **C-shape.** First, the surface area of the parietal lobe increases, followed by an increase in the frontal lobe. Next, the cortex expands posteriorly and inferiorly, forming the occipital and temporal lobes (Figure 1–14; 50–100 days). Because the cranial cavity does not increase in size in proportion to the increase in cortical surface area, this expansion is accompanied by tremendous infolding. Apart from the lateral sulcus, the cerebral cortex remains smooth, or lisencephalic, until the sixth or seventh month, when it develops gyri and sulci. About one third of the cerebral cortex is exposed, and the remainder is located within sulci. Interestingly, the hippocampal formation (Figure 1–10A) is located on the medial brain surface very early in development. As it develops, it becomes infolded beneath the cortex of the temporal lobe.

Even before most of the gyri and sulci are present on the cortical surface, a lateral region becomes buried by the developing frontal, parietal, and temporal lobes. This region, the **insular cortex** (Figure 1–14; 7–9 months; see Figure 1–11), is located deep within the lateral sulcus, one of the earliest grooves to form on the lateral surface. In the mature brain, the insular cortex is revealed only when the banks of the lateral sulcus are partially separated or when the brain is sectioned (see Figure 8–7). The portions of the frontal, parietal, and temporal cortices that cover the insular cortex are termed the **opercula.** The frontal operculum of the dominant hemisphere (typically the left hemisphere in right-handed individuals) contains Broca's area, which is important in speech articulation (see Chapter 8). The parietal and temporal opercular regions and the insular cortex have important sensory functions.

As the cerebral cortex grows, it also forces many of the underlying subcortical structures to assume a C-shape, including the lateral ventricle (Figure 1–10B), the striatum (Figure 1–10B), and hippocampal formation and fornix (Figure 1–10A). The lateral ventricle is roughly spherical in shape at 2 months and is transformed into a C-shape as the cortex develops (Figure 1–14; 100 days). By about 5 and 6 months, the lateral ventricle expands anteriorly to form the **anterior** (or frontal) **horn,** caudally to form the body and **posterior** (or occipital) **horn,** and inferiorly to form the **inferior** (or temporal) **horn** (Figure 1–14; noted on 9-month brain).

The **hippocampal formation** together with the **fornix,** its output path, as well as the **striatum** also develop C-shapes (Figure 1–10), like that of the lateral ventricle. The hippocampal formation (Figure 1–10A) is critical for consolidating our short-term into long-term memories, and the striatum (Figure 1–10B) plays a key role in such diverse higher brain functions as cognition, limb and eye movement control, and emotions.

The innermost meningeal layer, the **pia mater,** is very delicate and adheres to the surface of the brain and spinal cord. (*Pia mater* means "tender mother" in Latin.) The space between the arachnoid mater and pia mater is the **subarachnoid space.** Filaments of arachnoid mater pass through the subarachnoid space and connect to the pia mater, giving this space the appearance of a spider's web. (Hence the name *arachnoid,* which derives from the Greek word *arachne,* meaning "spider.")

An Introduction to Neuroanatomical Terms

The terminology of neuroanatomy is specialized for describing the brain's complex three-dimensional organization. The central nervous system is organized along the **rostrocaudal** and **dorsoventral** axes of the body (Figure 1–16). These axes are most easily understood in animals with a central nervous system that is simpler than that of humans. In the rat, for example, the rostrocaudal axis runs approximately in a straight line from the nose to the tail (Figure 1–16A). This axis is the **longitudinal axis** of the nervous system and is often termed the **neuraxis** because the central nervous system has a predominant longitudinal organization. The dorsoventral axis, which is perpendicular to the rostrocaudal axis, runs from the back to the abdomen. The terms **posterior** and **anterior** are synonymous with dorsal and ventral, respectively.

The longitudinal axis of the human nervous system is not straight as it is in the rat (Figure 1–16B). During development the brain—and therefore its longitudinal axis—undergoes a prominent bend, or **flexure,** at the midbrain. Instead of describing structures located rostral to this flexure as dorsal or ventral, we typically use the terms **superior** and **inferior.** As described in Box 1–1, this axis bend reflects the persistence of the cephalic flexure (see Figure 1–5).

We define three principal planes relative to the longitudinal axis of the nervous system in which anatomical sections are made (Figure 1–17). **Horizontal** sections are cut parallel to the longitudinal axis, from one side to the other. **Transverse** sections are cut perpendicular to the longitudinal axis, between the dorsal and ventral surfaces. Transverse sections through the cerebral hemisphere are roughly parallel to the coronal suture of the skull and, as a consequence,

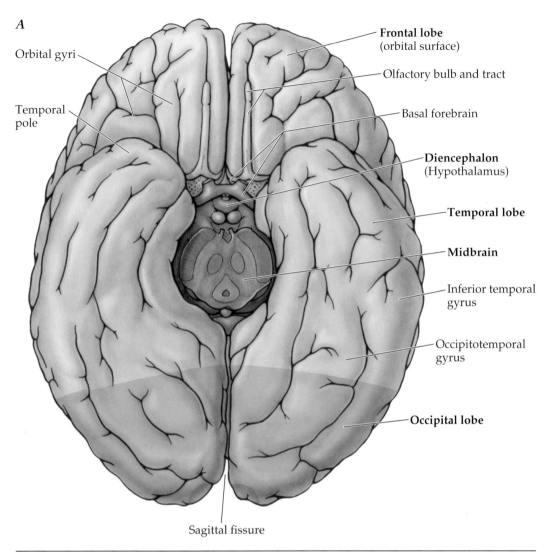

A

Orbital gyri

Temporal
pole

Frontal lobe
(orbital surface)

Olfactory bulb and tract

Basal forebrain

Diencephalon
(Hypothalamus)

Temporal lobe

Midbrain

Inferior temporal
gyrus

Occipitotemporal
gyrus

Occipital lobe

Sagittal fissure

FIGURE 1–12. *A.* Ventral surface of the cerebral hemisphere and diencephalon; the midbrain is cut in cross section. The primary visual cortex is shown at the occipital pole.

are also termed **coronal** sections. **Sagittal** sections are cut parallel both to the longitudinal axis of the central nervous system and to the midline, between the dorsal and ventral surfaces. A **midsagittal** section divides the central nervous system into two symmetrical halves, whereas a **parasagittal** section is cut off the midline. Radiological images are also obtained in these planes. This will be described in Chapter 2.

Summary

Cellular Organization of the Nervous System

The cellular constituents of the nervous system are *neurons* (Figure 1–2) and *glia* (Figure 1–3). Neurons have four specialized regions: (1) the *dendrites,* which receive information, (2) the *cell body,* which receives and integrates information,

and (3) the *axon,* which transmits information from the cell body to (4) the *axon terminals.* There are three neuron classes: *unipolar, bipolar,* and *multipolar* (Figure 1–2B). Intercellular communication occurs at *synapses,* where a *neurotransmitter* is released. The glia include four types of *macroglia. Oligodendrocytes* and *Schwann cells* form the myelin sheath in the central and peripheral nervous systems, respectively. *Astro-*

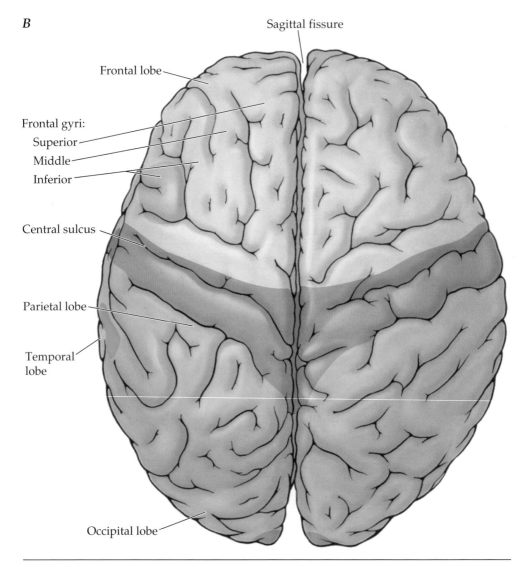

Continued—**FIGURE 1-12** **B.** Dorsal surface of the cerebral hemisphere. The primary motor and somatic sensory cortical areas are located anterior and posterior to the central sulcus. Broca's area is in the inferior frontal gyrus, and Wernicke's area is located in the posterior temporal lobe. The primary visual cortex is shown at the occipital pole.

cytes serve as structural and metabolic support for neurons. *Ependymal cells* line the ventricular system. The glia also consist of the *microglia*, which are phagocytic.

Regional Anatomy of the Nervous System

The nervous system contains two separate divisions, the *peripheral nervous system* and the *central nervous system* (Figure 1–4). Each system may be further subdivided. The *autonomic* division of the peripheral nervous system controls the glands and smooth muscle of the viscera and blood vessels, whereas the *somatic* division provides the sensory innervation of body tissues and the motor innervation of skeletal muscle. There are seven separate components of the central nervous system (Figures 1–4 and 1–6 through

1–12): (1) *spinal cord*, (2) *medulla*, (3) *pons*, (4) *cerebellum*, (5) *midbrain*, (6) *diencephalon*, which contains the *hypothalamus* and *thalamus*, and (7) *cerebral hemispheres*, which contain the *basal ganglia, amygdala, hippocampal formation*, and *cerebral cortex*. The external surface of the cerebral cortex is characterized by *gyri* (convolutions), *sulci* (grooves), and *fissures* (particularly deep grooves) (Figure 1–14). The cerebral cortex consists of four lobes: *frontal, parietal, temporal*, and *occipital*. The *insular cortex* is buried beneath the frontal, parietal, and temporal lobes. The *corpus callosum*, a *commissure*, interconnects each of the lobes. Three sets of structures lie beneath the cortical surface: the *hippocampal formation*, the *amygdala*, and the *basal ganglia*. The *limbic system* comprises a diverse set of cortical and subcortical structures. The *olfactory bulbs* lie on the orbital surface of the frontal lobes.

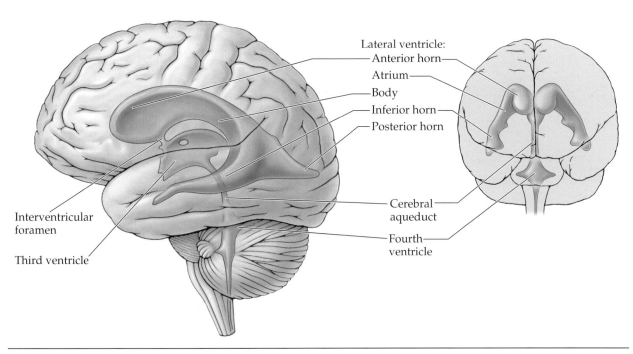

FIGURE 1–13 Ventricular system. The lateral ventricles, third ventricle, cerebral aqueduct, and fourth ventricle are seen from the lateral brain surface (left) and the front (right). The lateral ventricle is divided into four main components: anterior (or frontal) horn, body, inferior (or temporal) horn, and posterior (or occipital) horn. The atrium of the lateral ventricle is the region of confluence of the body, inferior horn, and posterior horn. The interventricular foramen (of Monro) connects each lateral ventricle with the third ventricle. The cerebral aqueduct connects the third and fourth ventricles.

Ventricular System

Cavities comprising the *ventricular system* are filled with *cerebrospinal fluid* and are located within the central nervous system (Figure 1–13). One of the two *lateral ventricles* is located in each of the cerebral hemispheres, the *third ventricle* is located in the diencephalon, and the *fourth ventricle* is between the brain stem (pons and medulla) and the cerebellum. The *central canal* is the component of the ventricular system in the spinal cord. The *interventricular foramina* connect the two lateral ventricles with the third ventricle. The *cerebral aqueduct* is in the midbrain and connects the third and fourth ventricles.

Meninges

The central nervous system is covered by three meningeal layers, from outermost to innermost: *dura mater, arachnoid mater,* and *pia mater* (Figure 1–15). Arachnoid mater and pia mater are separated by the *subarachnoid space,* which also contains cerebrospinal fluid. Two prominent flaps in the dura separate brain structures: *falx cerebri* and the *tentorium cerebelli* (Figure 1–15). Also located within the dura are the *dural sinuses,* low-pressure blood vessels (Figure 1–15).

Axes and Planes of Section

The central nervous system is oriented along two major axes (Figure 1–16): the *rostrocaudal axis,* which is also termed the *longitudinal axis,* and the *dorsoventral axis,* which is perpendicular to the longitudinal axis. Sections through the central nervous system are cut in relation to the rostrocaudal axis (Figure 1–17). *Horizontal* sections are cut parallel to the rostrocaudal axis, from one side to the other. *Transverse,* or *coronal,* sections are cut perpendicular to the rostrocaudal axis, between the dorsal and ventral surfaces. *Sagittal* sections are cut parallel to the longitudinal axis and the midline, also between the dorsal and ventral surfaces.

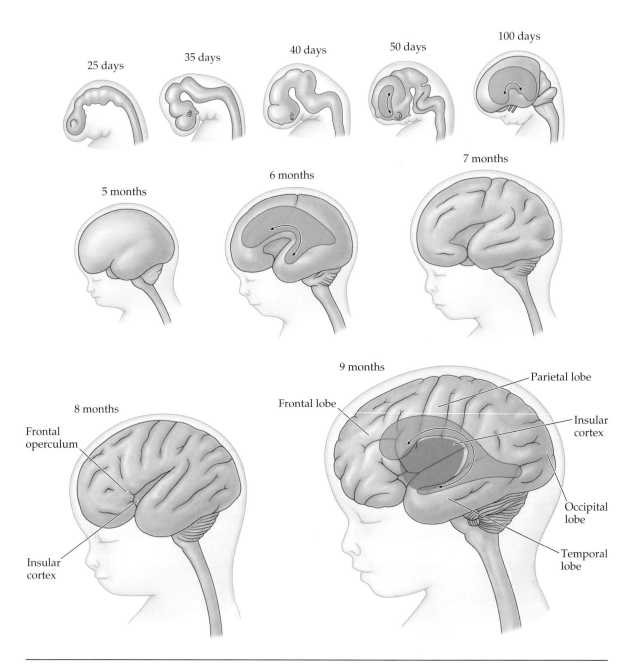

FIGURE 1–14 The development of the human brain is shown from the lateral surface in relation to the face and the general shape of the cranium. The lateral ventricle is colored green. The arrows drawn over the lateral ventricle show its emerging C-shape. (Courtesy Tom Prentiss, illustrator.)

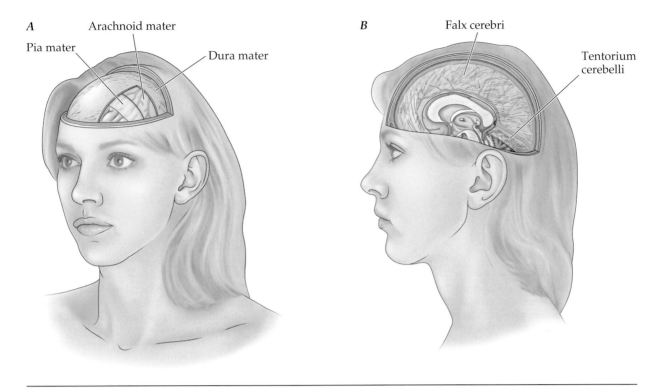

FIGURE 1–15 *A.* The meninges consist of the dura mater, arachnoid mater, and pia mater. *B.* The two major dural flaps are the falx cerebri, which incompletely separates the two cerebral hemispheres, and the tentorium cerebelli, which separates the cerebellum from the cerebral hemisphere. (**A,** Adapted with permission from Snell RS. *Clinical Neuroanatomy*. 7th ed. Lippincott Williams & WIlkins, 2010)

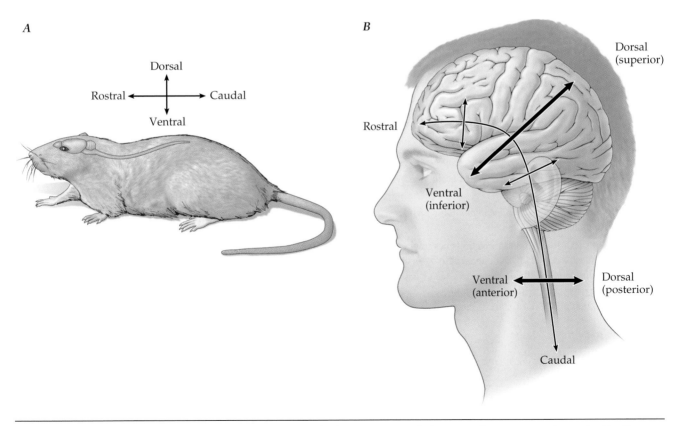

FIGURE 1–16 The axes of the central nervous system are illustrated for the rat (*A*), an animal whose central nervous system is organized in a linear fashion, and the human (*B*), whose central nervous system has a prominent flexure at the midbrain. (Reproduced with permission from Martin JH. *Neuroanatomy: Text & Atlas*, 2nd ed. Stamford, CT: Appleton & Lange, 1996.)

A Horizontal plane

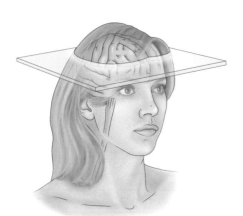

B Coronal plane

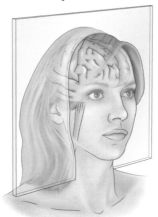

C Sagittal plane

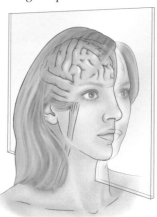

FIGURE 1–17 The three main anatomical planes: (*A*) horizontal, (*B*) coronal, and (*C*) sagittal. Note that the horizontal plane is shown through the cerebral hemispheres and diencephalon. A section in the same plane but through the brain stem or spinal cord is called a transverse section because it cuts the neuraxis at a right angle (see Figure 1–16B). The coronal plane is sometimes termed transverse because it is also at a right angle to the neuraxis (see Figure 1–16B). Unfortunately the terminology becomes even more confusing. A coronal section through the cerebral hemispheres and diencephalon will slice the brain stem and spinal cord parallel to their long axis. Strictly speaking this would be a horizontal section. However, this term is not useful for the human brain because such a "horizontal" section is oriented vertically.

Selected Readings

Amaral DG, Strick PL. The organization of the central nervous system. In: Kandel ER, Schwartz JH, Jessell TM, Siegelbaum SA, and Hudspeth AJ, eds. *Principles of Neural Science*. 5th ed. New York, NY: McGraw-Hill, in press.

Kandel ER, Hudspeth AJ. The brain and behavior. In: Kandel ER, Schwartz JH, Jessell TM, Siegelbaum SA, and Hudspeth AJ, eds.

Principles of Neural Science. 5th ed. New York, NY: McGraw-Hill, in press.

Suk I, Tamargo RJ. Concealed neuroanatomy in Michelangelo's separation of light from darkness in the Sistine Chapel. *Neurosurgery*. 2010;66(5):851-861.

References

Allen NJ, Barres BA. Glia: More than just brain glue. *Nature*. 2009;457:675-677.

Duvernoy HM. *The Human Hippocampus*. Munich, Germany: J. F. Bergmann Verlag; 1988.

Lee PR, Fields RD. Regulation of myelin genes implicated in psychiatric disorders by functional activity in axons. *Front Neuroanat*. 2009;3:4.

Paxinos G, Mai JK, eds. *The Human Nervous System*. London: Elsevier; 2004.

Raichle ME. A brief history of human brain mapping. *TINS*. 2009;32(2):118-126.

Sherman DL, Brophy PJ. Mechanisms of axon ensheathment and myelin growth. *Nat Rev Neurosci*. 2005;6(9): 683-690.

Volterra A, Meldolesi J. Astrocytes, from brain glue to communication elements: The revolution continues. *Nat Rev Neurosci*. 2005;6(8):626-640.

1. Which of the following analogies best describes the functional relationship between two different parts of a neuron?
    A. A dendrite is to an axon terminal, as presynaptic input signaling is to postsynaptic output
    B. A cell body is to a dendrite, as synaptic output is to synaptic integration
    C. A cell body is to synaptic output, as an axon is to action potential conduction
    D. A dendrite is to neurotransmitter release, as an axon terminal is to postsynaptic membrane neurotransmitter receptors

2. Which of the following neuron components is located within a white matter tract?
    A. Dendrite
    B. Cell body
    C. Axon
    D. Axon termination

3. Which of the following best lists the parts of neurons that are located in a nucleus?
    A. Cell bodies only
    B. Cell bodies and dendrites
    C. Cell bodies, axons, and dendrites
    D. Cell bodies, dendrites, axons, and axon terminals

4. Which of the following analogies best describes the function of Schwann cells and oligodendrocytes?
    A. The myelin sheath of central nervous system axons is to the myelin sheath of peripheral nervous system axons
    B. The myelin sheath of peripheral nervous system axons is to the myelin sheath of central nervous system axons
    C. Central nervous system action potential conduction is to peripheral nervous system action potential conduction
    D. Peripheral nervous system axon structure is to central nervous system axon structure

5. A person suffers from a traumatic brain injury. There is bleeding and inflammation at the injury site. Which of the following cell types plays a phagocytic role in eliminating blood and tissue debris?
    A. Astrocytes
    B. Microglia
    C. Schwann cells
    D. Neurons

6. Ependymal cells are located in which of the following nervous system structures?
    A. Cerebral arteries
    B. Ventricles
    C. Cerebral cortex
    D. Sensory ganglia

7. Which of the following is NOT part of the peripheral nervous system?
    A. Motor neuron cell body
    B. Sympathetic ganglia
    C. Dorsal root
    D. Ventral root

8. Which of the following is NOT a feature of the autonomic nervous system?
    A. Innervation of glands
    B. Innervation of smooth muscle of the gut
    C. Innervation of somatic motor neurons that innervate limb muscles
    D. Innervation of smooth muscle in blood vessel walls.

9. Which of the following best describes sulci and gyri?
    A. Functional regions of the brain are located on gyri.
    B. Sulci separate the lobes of the brain.
    C. Gyri are the bumps and sulci are the grooves that separate the gyri.
    D. Sulci are the bumps and gyri are the grooves that separate the sulci.

10. Which of the following best describes the location of major brain regions?
    A. The thalamus is located rostral to the midbrain..
    B. The basal ganglia are located ventral to the cerebellum.
    C. The midbrain is located caudal to the medulla.
    D. The cerebellum is located ventral to the pons.

11. A patient has a tumor in the region of the insular cortex. Which of the following choices best describes the location of the tumor?
    A. It is buried beneath the brain surface, under the frontal lobe.
    B. It is buried beneath the frontal and parietal lobes.
    C. It is buried beneath the frontal, parietal, and temporal lobes.
    D. It is buried beneath the frontal, parietal, temporal, and occipital lobes.

12. A pitcher was hit in the head with a baseball. The impact of the ball hitting his head caused a skull fracture over his left orbit. Which of the following brain structures is located closest to the site of fracture?
    A. Inferior frontal lobe
    B. Postcentral gyrus
    C. Calcarine fissure
    D. Anterior horn of lateral ventricle

13. Complete the following using the most appropriate choice:
    The falx cerebri separates
    A. the occipital lobes and the cerebellum
    B. the cerebellum and the medulla
    C. the two cerebral hemispheres
    D. the two halves of the diencephalon

14. The atrium of the lateral ventricle is located within which major central nervous system division?
    A. Pons
    B. Cerebellum
    C. Cerebral cortex
    D. Diencephalon

15. A brain MRI in the coronal plane would not image, on a single slice, which pair of listed brain regions?
    A. Frontal lobe and temporal lobe
    B. Frontal lobe and occipital lobe
    C. Parietal lobe and cerebellum
    D. Temporal lobe and lateral ventricle

Chapter 2

Structural and Functional Organization of the Central Nervous System

CLINICAL CASE | Horizontal Gaze Palsy With Progressive Scoliosis

Horizontal gaze palsy with progressive scoliosis (HGPPS) is an extremely rare genetic syndrome. It is the result of mutation in the ROBO3 gene, essential for normal axon guidance in many developing neurons, including those of the corticospinal tract and the medial lemniscus. Mutations in this gene are associated with a failure of axonal crossing in certain regions of the brain. Because it is so rare, this syndrome is not likely to be encountered in routine medical practice. Nevertheless, by examining brain images from patients with HGPPS, we have the opportunity to see how brain structure changes when decussation does not occur. Further, by assessing their neurological signs and the results of electrophysiological testing, we have the opportunity to see how mutation can affect the way sensory and motor information is processed by the brain.

A 12-year-old boy with a genetically determined mutation of the ROBO3 gene was examined for somatic sensory, limb motor, and ocular motor functions. Sensory testing did not reveal impairment. He has mild gait instability and a tremor during reaching (**intention tremor**). He is able to follow a visual stimulus moving vertically with his eyes. He is unable to follow a horizontal moving stimulus. His eyes remain fixated in the forward direction, bilaterally.

Figure 2–1A1 is a midsagittal magnetic resonance imaging (MRI) from a person with HGPPS. Brain tissue is shades of gray (gray matter darker than white matter) and cerebrospinal fluid, black. The bracket is located dorsal to the pons and medulla. Cerebrospinal fluid penetrates into this region on the midline because there is a shallow groove (sulcus). Note that this is not present in the control MRI (Figure 2–1B1). The transverse MRI through the upper medulla (A2) reveals an abnormally flattened appearance in the patient with HGPPS

—Continued next page

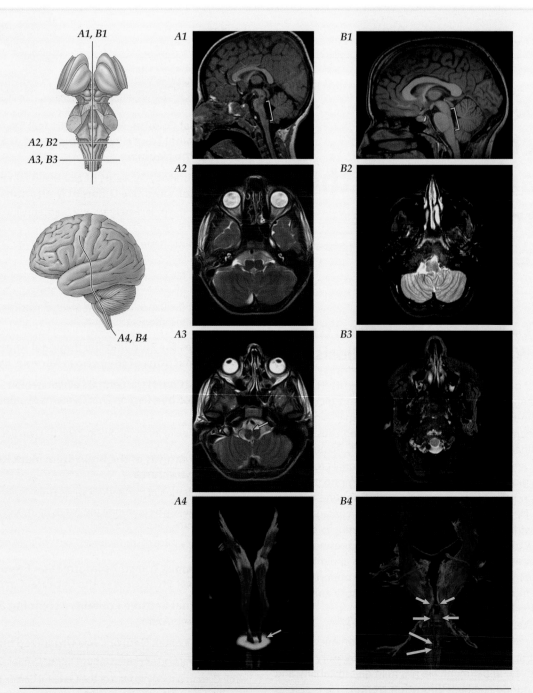

FIGURE 2–1 Brain images from patients with horizontal gaze palsy with progressive scoliosis (HGPPS) are shown on the left and images from a healthy person's brain, on the right. 1. Midsagittal MRI. The bracket marks the region of a midline groove in an HGPPS patient. 2. Transverse MRI sections through the medulla. There is abnormal flattening of the rostral medulla (*A2*) and a ventral groove in the caudal medulla (*A3*). 4. Diffusion tensor image (DTI) of the corticospinal tracts. The tracts are shown from about the level of the internal capsule (top) to the caudal medulla (bottom). The patient's corticospinal tracts (A4) show no crossing fibers, whereas the tract from the healthy person (B4) shows many sites of crossing fibers. The corticospinal tract decussation (red) is at the level of the two large arrows. Other decussations are identified by the smaller arrows. The insets in the bottom right show the imaging planes for parts 1-4. (**A1,** Reproduced with permission from Bosley TM, Salih MA, Jen JC, et al. Neurologic features of horizontal gaze palsy and progressive scoliosis with mutations in ROBO3. *Neurology.* 2005;64(7):1196-1203. **A2, A3, A4,** Reproduced with permission from Haller S, Wetzel SG, and Lutschg J. Functional MRI, DTI, and neurophysiology in horizontal gaze palsy with progressive scoliosis. *Neuroradiology.* 2008;50(5):453-459. **B1, B2, B3,** Courtesy of Dr. Joy Hirsch, Columbia University. **B4,** Reproduced with permission from Poretti A, Boltshauser E, Loenneker T, et al. Diffusion tensor imaging in Joubert syndrome. *AJNR. Am J Neuroradiol.* 2007;28(10):1929-1933.)

compared with the control brain (B2). A section through the caudal medulla reveals an aberrant deep midline groove (A3, arrow; B3).

Neurophysiological testing was conducted to assess the integrity of the touch and corticospinal motor pathways (see Figure 2–2). To determine the function of the sensory pathway, the skin is electrically stimulated and the overall change in on-going neuronal activity of parietal lobe (ie, EEG) is recorded. Recording the EEG in the region of the somatic sensory cortex in response to electrical stimulation of skin revealed ipsilateral activation, not the customary contralateral activation. To determine the function of the corticospinal tract, transcranial magnetic stimulation (TMS) is used to activate the motor cortex, and the evoked change in muscle activity is recorded. TMS of the motor cortex activated muscles on the ipsilateral side, not the typical contralateral side.

Finally, **diffusion tensor imaging** (DTI; this is discussed in Box 2–2) was performed on the patient's MRIs in order to follow the corticospinal tract. This method permits imaging of neural pathways in the brain. Figure 2–1A4 shows the DTI image from a HGPPS patient. There are two parallel pathways. The arrow points to the caudal medulla, where the decussation normally occurs. Furthermore, there are no other decussations along the pathway. B4 is a DTI from a healthy control. The large arrows point to the pyramidal decussation (red) and the smaller arrows, to other brain stem decussations of the pathway. We will learn about these pathways in later chapters.

After reading the explanations below, you should be able to answer the following questions.

1. **At what dorsoventral level do the axons of the sensory and motor pathways cross the midline?**

2. **Is the crossing of all central nervous system axons prevented in this genetic syndrome?**

Key neurological signs and corresponding damaged brain structures

Dorsal and ventral midline grooves

Pathways decussate at the midline. In addition to the presence of many structural proteins, decussating axons also provide some physical attachment of the two sides of the brain stem. It is reasoned that without the decussation, or with a reduced number of decussating axons, the two

sides of the brain at that spot do not adhere. A space is revealed indirectly because cerebrospinal fluid is present. This is much like seeing cerebrospinal fluid in sulci of the cerebral cortex. Because this syndrome is so rare, there are no histological pathological specimens. Importantly, Figure 2–1A1 shows that the corpus callosum is present in the patient. This indicates that not all decussation is prevented in this genetic syndrome. Callosal neurons use a different mechanism for guiding their axons across the midline than corticospinal tract and medial lemniscal neurons. It is not yet understood how this genetic defect produces scoliosis, which is curving of the vertebral column.

Absence of horizontal eye movements

As we will learn in Chapter 12, horizontal eye movements are coordinated by neurons that have an axon that decussates in the dorsal pons. Normally, there is an important decussation where the dorsal midline groove is present (Figure 2–1A1). Without this decussation and other circuit change, the eyes are prevented from moving horizontally.

Ipsilateral corticospinal tract and dorsal column–medial lemniscal signaling

Both the corticospinal tract and dorsal column–medial lemniscal system have a decussation in the caudal medulla; the motor decussation is caudal to the somatic sensory decussation. Again, the structurally-abnormal cleft in the ventral medulla points to the absence or fewer decussating axons of the two systems. This is consistent with the results of electrophysiological testing and the DTI for the corticospinal tract. The tremor is probably due to an abnormal circuit between the cortex and the cerebellum. Brain stem neurons transmit signals from the cortex on one side to the cerebellum on the other. This decussation is also prevented in HGPPS.

References

Bosley TM, Salih MA, Jen JC, et al. Neurologic features of horizontal gaze palsy and progressive scoliosis with mutations in ROBO3. *Neurology.* 2005;64(7):1196-1203.

Haller S, Wetzel SG, Lutschg J. Functional MRI, DTI and neurophysiology in horizontal gaze palsy with progressive scoliosis. *Neuroradiology.* 2008;50(5):453-459.

Jen JC, Chan WM, Bosley TM, et al. Mutations in a human ROBO gene disrupt hindbrain axon pathway crossing and morphogenesis. *Science.* 2004;304(5676):1509-1513.

Martin J, Friel K, Salimi I, Chakrabarty S. Corticospinal development. In: Squire L, ed. *Encyclopedia of Neuroscience.* Vol 3. Oxford: Academic Press; 2009:302-214.

From a consideration of the regional and functional anatomy of the central nervous system, the principle of **functional localization** emerges. Each major division of the central nervous system, each lobe of the cortex, and even the gyri within the lobes perform a limited and often unique set of functions. In contrast to most organs of the body—like the heart, stomach, or limb muscles, where their structure helps to predict their function—the gross structure of the brain provides little insight into its overall function, much less the nuances of its role in perception, movement, thought, or emotions. For example, the inferior frontal lobe and the superior parietal lobe look much the same; both have a complex rolling topography of gyri and sulci. Microscopically, they too are remarkably similar, each with neurons organized into six layers. Yet the inferior frontal lobe functions to produce speech and the superior parietal lobe is important in attention. These functional differences come about largely as a result of their connections with other brain regions. The inferior frontal lobe receives information about speech sounds, and connects with brain motor centers, principally those controlling the muscles of the face and mouth. By contrast, the superior parietal lobe receives diverse sensory information, especially visual information, and connects with brain areas important for planning behavior, in particular looking to what interests us. Whereas the logic of functional localization can be understood on the basis of how neural circuits develop specific connections, we have little insight into the logic of why functions are localized where they are.

In addition to the specific connections between structures, there are neural circuits with widespread connections that modulate the actions of neural systems with particular functions. Consider how the quiescent state of a mother's brain can be mobilized by the sound of her infant's cry during the night. In an instant, perception is keen, movements are coordinated, and judgments are sound. The neural systems mediating arousal and other generalized functions involve the integrated actions of different parts of the brain stem. Importantly, these regulatory systems use particular neurotransmitters, such as serotonin or dopamine, to exert their actions. These neurotransmitter-specific regulatory systems are also particularly important in human behavioral dysfunction because many of their actions are abnormal in psychiatric disease.

By considering the patterns of neural connections between specific structures, this chapter begins to explain how the various components of the spinal cord and brain acquire their particular sensory, motor, or integrative functions. First, it examines the overall organization of the neural systems for touch and limb position sense and for voluntary movement control. Limb position sense is our ability to detect the location and orientation of our limbs without looking at them. Because these systems travel through all of the major brain divisions to execute their functions, they are excellent for introducing general structure-function relations. Second, the chapter examines the different modulatory systems. Finally,

key anatomical and radiological sections through the spinal cord and brain are examined. An understanding of the different neural systems is reinforced by identifying the locations of these systems in the central nervous system. Knowledge of the location of nuclei and tracts in these anatomical sections is important not only for understanding neuroanatomy but also for learning to identify brain structure on radiological images.

The Dorsal Column–Medial Lemniscal System and Corticospinal Tract Have a Component at Each Level of the Neuraxis

The principal pathway for touch and limb position sense, the **dorsal column–medial lemniscal system**, and the key pathway for voluntary movement, the **corticospinal tract,** each have a longitudinal organization, spanning virtually the entire neuraxis. These two pathways are good examples of how particular patterns of connections between structures at different levels of the neuraxis produce a circuit with a limited number of functions. This does not mean that there are no other neural systems for these body senses and control functions. Indeed, many systems work together for even the simplest perceptions and movements. Analyzing the basic functions of circuits in isolation, as we are here, provides a starting point for understanding functional neuroanatomy.

The dorsal column–medial lemniscal system is termed an **ascending pathway** because it brings information from sensory receptors in the periphery to lower levels of the central nervous system, such as the brain stem, and then to higher levels, such as the thalamus and cerebral cortex. In contrast, the corticospinal tract, a **descending pathway,** carries information from the cerebral cortex to a lower level of the central nervous system, the spinal cord.

The dorsal column–medial lemniscal system (Figure 2–2A) consists of a three-neuron circuit that links the periphery with the cerebral cortex. Even though there are minimally three neurons in this circuit, many thousands of neurons at each level are typically engaged during normal tactile experiences. Each of the neurons in the figure stands for many hundred or thousands. The first neurons in the circuit are the dorsal root ganglion neurons, which translate stimulus energy into neural signals and transmit this information directly to the spinal cord and brain stem. This component of the system is a fast transmission line that is visible on the dorsal surface of the spinal cord as the **dorsal column** (see Figure 2–5B).

The first synapse is made in the **dorsal column nucleus,** a relay nucleus in the medulla. A **relay nucleus** processes incoming signals and transmits this information to the next component of the circuit. The cell bodies of the second

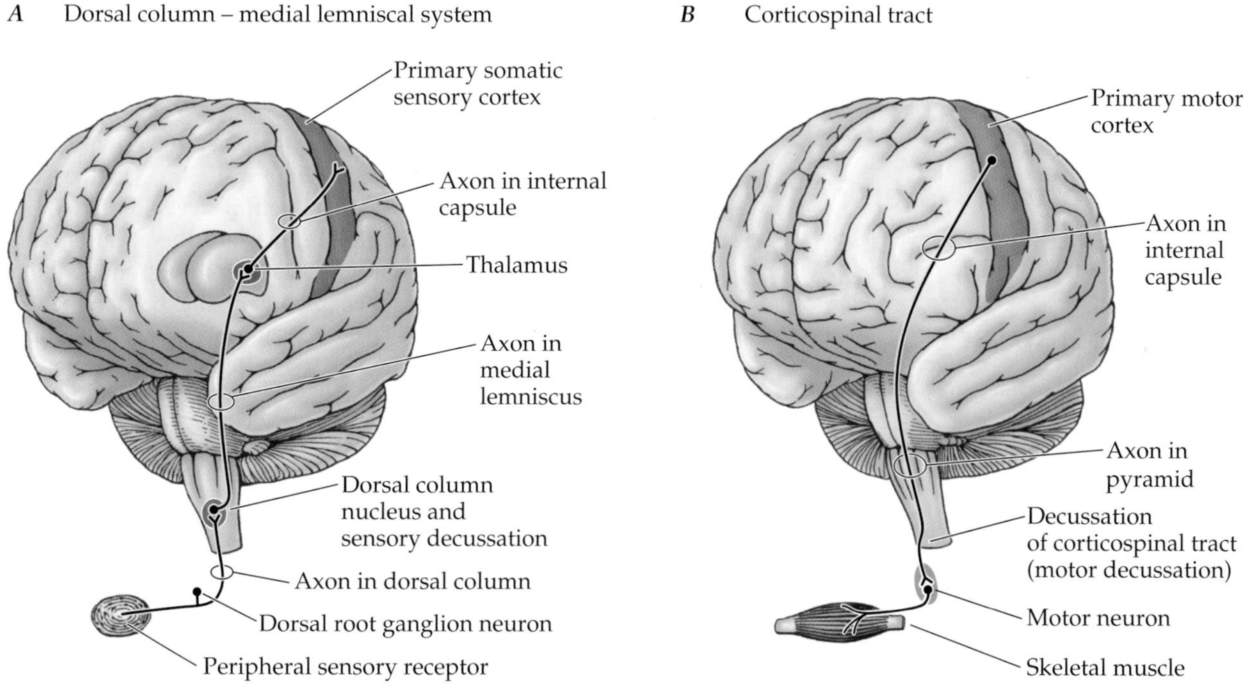

A   Dorsal column – medial lemniscal system

B   Corticospinal tract

Primary somatic
sensory cortex

Axon in internal
capsule

Thalamus

Axon in
medial
lemniscus

Dorsal column
nucleus and
sensory decussation

Axon in dorsal column

Dorsal root ganglion neuron

Peripheral sensory receptor

Primary motor
cortex

Axon in
internal
capsule

Axon in
pyramid

Decussation
of corticospinal tract
(motor decussation)

Motor neuron

Skeletal muscle

FIGURE 2–2 The dorsal column–medial lemniscal system (**A**) and corticospinal tract (**B**) are longitudinally organized.

neurons in the pathway are located in the dorsal column nucleus. The axons of these second-order neurons cross the midline, or **decussate.** Because of this decussation, sensory information from one side of the body is processed by the opposite side of the brain. Most sensory (and motor) pathways decussate at some point along their course. While we understand the molecular mechanisms of how some axons cross the midline and others do not, surprisingly, we do not know the reason why particular neural systems decussate. The case presented in this chapter describes the loss of decussation of the dorsal column-medial lemniscal system due to a genetic defect.

After crossing the midline, the axons ascend in the brain stem tract, the **medial lemniscus,** to synapse in a particular relay nucleus in the **thalamus.** From here, the third-order neurons send their axons through the white matter underlying the cortex, in the **internal capsule.** These axons synapse on neurons in the **primary somatic sensory cortex,** which is located in the postcentral gyrus of the parietal lobe (Figure 2–2A). Each sensory system has a primary cortical area and several higher-order areas. The primary area processes basic sensory information, and the higher-order areas participate in the elaboration of sensory processing leading to perception. Damage to this system, more commonly at the spinal level, makes fine tactile discriminations difficult and impairs our limb position sense.

Axons of the corticospinal tract descend from the cerebral cortex to terminate on motor neurons in the spinal cord (Figure 2–2B). In contrast to the dorsal column–medial

lemniscal system, in which fast transmission lines are interrupted by series of synapses in relay nuclei, the corticospinal tract consists of single neurons that link the cortex directly with the spinal cord. The cell bodies of many corticospinal tract neurons are located in the primary motor cortex on the **precentral gyrus** of the frontal lobe, just rostral to the primary somatic sensory cortex. The axons of these neurons leave the motor cortex and travel down in the internal capsule, near the thalamic axons transmitting information to the somatic sensory cortex.

The corticospinal tract emerges from beneath the cerebral hemisphere to course ventrally within the brain stem. In the medulla, the corticospinal axons form the **pyramid,** a prominent landmark on the ventral surface. In the caudal medulla, most corticospinal axons decussate (pyramidal, or motor, decussation). In the case study, a genetic impairment resulted in the loss of the pyramidal decussation (Figure 2-1A4). The corticospinal tract axons descend into the spinal cord, where they travel within the white matter before terminating on motor neurons in the gray matter. These motor neurons innervate skeletal muscle; they are sometimes termed lower motor neurons. Motor cortex neurons that give rise to the corticospinal tract are often termed upper motor neurons. Patients with corticospinal tract damage, commonly caused by interruption of the blood supply to the internal capsule or a spinal cord injury, demonstrate a range of impairment, depending on the amount of damage, ranging from impaired fine motor skills and muscle weakness to paralysis. Following these pathways shows how many different brain regions are recruited into action for simple sensory and motor functions.

The Modulatory Systems of the Brain Have Diffuse Connections and Use Different Neurotransmitters

Specificity of neural connections characterizes the somatic sensory and motor pathways. The dorsal column–medial lemniscal system can mediate our sense of touch because it specifically connects touch receptors in the skin with a particular region of the cerebral cortex. Similarly, the corticospinal tract's role in controlling movement is conferred by its particular connections with motor circuits in the spinal cord. Several major exceptions exist in which systems of neurons have more widespread projections; and in each case these systems are thought to serve more generalized functions, including motivation, arousal, and facilitation of learning and memory. The cell bodies of **diffuse-projecting neurons** are located throughout the brain stem, diencephalon, and basal forebrain; some are clustered into distinct nuclei and others are scattered. They terminate throughout all divisions of the central nervous system.

Four systems of diffuse-projecting neurons are highlighted here because of their importance in the sensory, motor, and integrative systems examined in subsequent chapters. Each system uses a different neurotransmitter: acetylcholine, dopamine, noradrenalin (norepinephrine), or serotonin. Many of the neurons that use one of these neurotransmitters also contain other neuroactive compounds, such as peptides, that are released at the synapse at the same time. Dysfunction of these systems occurs in many psychiatric and neurological diseases.

Neurons in the Basal Forebrain and Diencephalon Contain Acetylcholine

The axons of **acetylcholine**-containing neurons in the basal forebrain (ie, at the base of the cerebral hemispheres) and several other sites, including the lateral hypothalamus, project throughout the cerebral cortex and hippocampal formation (Figure 2–3A). Acetylcholine augments the excitability of cortical neurons, especially in association areas. In **Alzheimer disease,** a neurological disease in which individuals lose memories and cognitive functions, these cholinergic neurons degenerate. There are also cholinergic neurons in the pedunculopontine nucleus, which is located in the pons. These cholinergic neurons are implicated in disordered movement control in Parkinson disease.

The Substantia Nigra and Ventral Tegmental Area Contain Dopaminergic Neurons

The cells of origin of the dopaminergic system are located mostly in the midbrain (Figure 2–3B1), in the **substantia nigra** and **ventral tegmental area**; the major targets of these dopaminergic neurons are the striatum and portions of the frontal lobe. Dopamine strongly influences brain systems engaged in organizing behavior and planning movements. There are at least five major dopamine receptor types, which have different distributions within the central nervous system and different cellular actions. More is known of the clinical consequences of damage to brain dopamine systems than of the other neurotransmitter-specific systems. In **Parkinson disease,** for example, there is a loss of the dopamine-containing neurons in the substantia nigra. Movements become slowed in patients with Parkinson disease, and they develop tremor (see Chapter 14). These motor signs improve with dopamine replacement therapy. Dopamine is also implicated in schizophrenia, through the actions of the ventral tegmental area. The hypothalamus also contains dopaminergic neurons that are important in neuroendocrine control and, through descending projections, regulation of the autonomic nervous system and skeletal muscle control.

Neurons in the Locus Ceruleus Give Rise to a Noradrenergic Projection

Although there are numerous brain stem nuclei with noradrenergic neurons (Figure 2–3B2), the **locus ceruleus** has the most widespread projections. Based on the connections and the physiological properties of locus ceruleus neurons, this noradrenergic projection is thought to play an important role in the response of the brain to stressful stimuli, particularly those that evoke fear. The locus ceruleus, through its widespread noradrenergic projections to the cerebral cortex, has been implicated in depression and in panic attacks, an anxiety disorder. Additional noradrenergic cell groups are located in the caudal pons and medulla; these neurons are critically involved in maintaining the function of the sympathetic nervous system, especially in blood pressure regulation.

Neurons of the Raphe Nuclei Use Serotonin as Their Neurotransmitter

The **raphe nuclei** (Figure 2–3B3) consist of numerous distinct groups of brain stem neurons located close to the midline. Neurons in the raphe nuclei use serotonin as a neurotransmitter. The actions of the serotonin systems are diverse because, as with dopamine, there are many different serotonin receptor types. The raphe nuclei from the rostral pons and midbrain give rise to ascending projections.

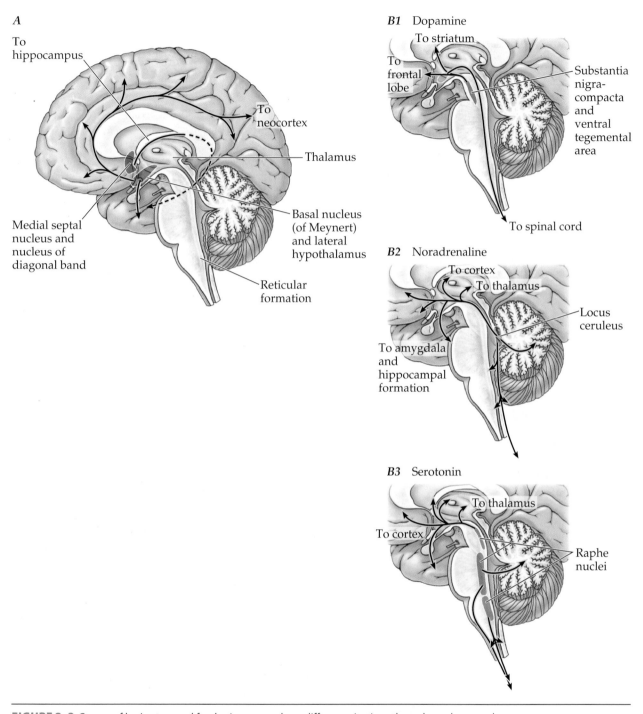

FIGURE 2–3 Groups of brain stem and forebrain neurons have diffuse projections throughout the central nervous system. **A.** Schematic illustration of the diffuse projection pattern of acetylcholine-containing neurons in the basal nucleus (of Meynert), septal nuclei, and nucleus of the diagonal band (of Broca). Many of the axons projecting to the hippocampal formation course in the fornix (dashed line). **B1.** Dopamine-containing neurons in the substantia nigra and ventral tegmental area. Yellow marks the location of dopamine neurons in the hypothalamus. **B2.** Noradrenaline-containing neurons in the locus ceruleus. **B3.** Serotonin-containing neurons in the raphe nuclei.

Dysfunction of the ascending serotonergic projection to the diencephalon and telencephalon has been implicated in disorders of thought and mood. Projections from the raphe nuclei in the medulla target other brain stem regions and the spinal cord. One function of the serotonergic projection to the spinal cord is to control the flow of information about pain from our limbs and trunk to the central nervous system.

Box 2–1

Anatomical Techniques for Studying the Regional and Microscopic Anatomy of the Human Central Nervous System

There are two principal anatomical methods for studying normal regional human neuroanatomy using postmortem tissue. **Myelin stains** use dyes that bind to the myelin sheath surrounding axons. Unfortunately, in myelin-stained material, the white matter of the central nervous system stains black and the gray matter stains light. (The terms white matter and gray matter derive from their appearance in fresh tissue.) **Cell stains** use dyes that bind to components within a neuron's cell body. Tissues prepared with either a cell stain or a myelin stain have a characteristically different appearance (Figure 2–4A, B). The various staining methods are used to reveal different features of the nervous system's organization. For example, cell stains are used to characterize the cellular architecture of nuclei and cortical areas, and myelin stains are used to reveal the general topography of brain regions. Myelin staining is also used to reveal the location of damaged axons because, after such damage, the myelin sheath degenerates. This results in unstained tissue that otherwise ought to stain darkly (see Figure 2–5D).

Other staining methods reveal the detailed morphology of neurons—their dendrites, cell body, and axon (Figure 2–4C)—or the presence of specific neuronal chemicals such as neurotransmitters, receptor molecules, or enzymes (see Figure 14–12A). Certain lipophilic dyes that diffuse preferentially along neuronal membranes can be applied directly to a human postmortem brain specimen. This technique allows delineation of some neural connections in the human brain because the axons of neurons at the site of application of the tracer are labeled.

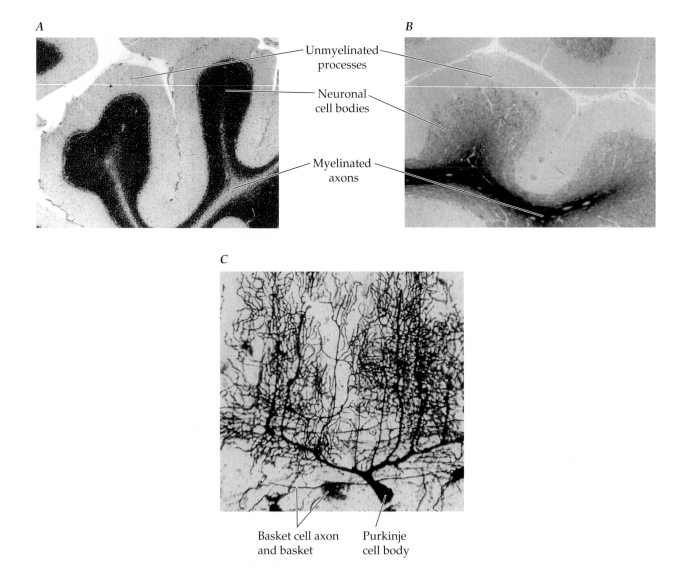

FIGURE 2–4 Anatomical staining of central nervous system. **A.** Nissl-stained section through the cerebellar cortex; **B.** Myelin-stained section through the cerebellar cortex; **C.** Golgi stain of a cerebellar Purkinje cell.

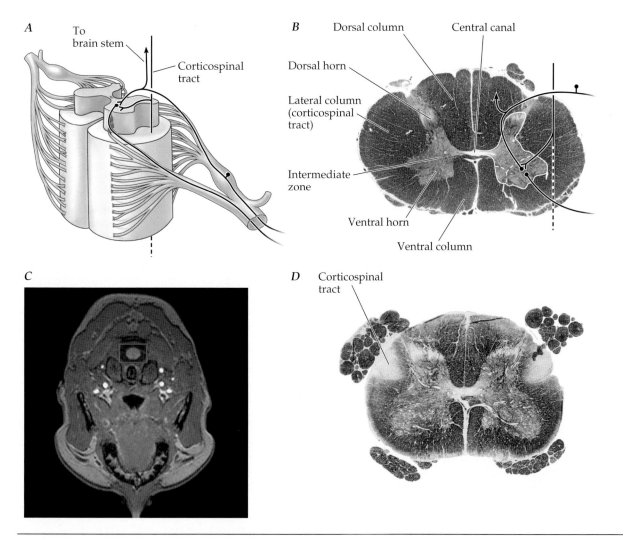

FIGURE 2–5 Spinal cord. **A.** Three-dimensional schematic view of a spinal cord segment showing key spinal cord structures, the circuit for the knee-jerk reflex, and a connection from the corticospinal tract to a motor neuron. **B.** Myelin-stained transverse section through the cervical spinal cord. The three parts of the spinal gray matter—the dorsal horn, intermediate zone, and ventral horn—are distinguished. The circuits for the reflex and corticospinal tract are also shown. **C.** MRI through the cervical spinal cord. The red box pinpoints the spinal cord. **D.** Myelin-stained section through the spinal cord showing unmyelinated regions in the dorsolateral portion of the lateral columns, where the corticospinal tracts are located.

Guidelines for Studying the Regional Anatomy and Interconnections of the Central Nervous System

The rest of this chapter focuses on central nervous system organization from the perspective of its internal structure. In this and subsequent chapters, myelin-stained sections and magnetic resonance images (MRIs) are used to help illustrate the structural and functional organization of the central nervous system. For myelin-stained sections, while many structures are distinguished clearly from their neighbors because of morphological changes at boundaries, locating other structures can be difficult because neighboring structures stain alike. The only way to distinguish like structures on myelin-stained sections is

by examining tissue from a person who had sustained nervous system damage during life. Damaged and intact structures, as discussed in the next section, appear different. Similarly, neighboring structures on MRIs from healthy people may or may not look different, depending on whether they have the same hydrogen ion content (see Box 2–2), the key tissue property in magnetic resonance imaging. Here too, images from the healthy and damaged nervous systems must be compared to reveal systems. In addition, MRIs often do not provide sufficient detail for learning neuroanatomy. To obviate these limitations, we use a combination of radiological and histological images throughout this book, including functional images. In this chapter, radiological and histological images of the spinal cord, brain stem (five levels), and diencephalon and telencephalon (two levels) are used to illustrate the functions and locations of nuclei and tracts.

Box 2-2

Magnetic Resonance Imaging Visualizes the Structure and Function of the Living Human Brain

Several radiological techniques are routinely used to image the living human brain. **Computerized tomography** (CT) produces scans that are images of a single plane, or "slice," of tissue. The image produced is a computerized reconstruction of the degree to which different tissues absorb transmitted x-rays. Although CT scans are commonly used clinically to reveal intracranial tumors and other pathological changes, the overall level of anatomical resolution is poor. **Magnetic resonance imaging** (MRI) probes the regional and functional anatomy of the brain in remarkably precise detail. Routine MRI of the nervous system reveals the proton constituents of neural tissues and fluids; most of the protons are contained in water. Protons in different tissue and fluid compartments, when placed in a strong magnetic field, have slightly different properties. MRI takes advantage of such differences to construct an image of brain structure or even function.

MRI relies on the simple property that protons can be made to emit signals that reflect the local tissue environment. Hence, protons in different tissues emit different signals. This is achieved by exciting protons with low levels of energy, which is delivered to the tissue by electromagnetic waves emitted from a coil placed over the tissue while the person is in the MRI scanner. Once excited, protons emit a signal with three components, or parameters, that depend on tissue characteristics. The first parameter is related to proton density (ie, primarily a measure of water content) in the tissue. The second and third parameters are related to proton relaxation times; that is, the times it takes protons to return to the energy state they were in before excitation by electromagnetic waves. The two relaxation times are termed T1 and T2. T1 relaxation time (or spin-lattice relaxation time) is related to the overall tissue environment, and T2 relaxation time (or spin-spin relaxation time), to interactions between protons. When an MRI scan is generated, it can be made to be dominated by one of these parameters. This differential dependence is accomplished by fine-tuning the electromagnetic waves used to excite the tissue. The choice of whether to have an image reflect proton density, T1 relaxation time, or T2 relaxation time depends on the purpose of the image. For example, in T2-weighted images, which are dominated by T2 relaxation time, watery constituents of the brain produce a stronger signal than fatty constituents (eg, white matter); hence, cerebrospinal fluid (CSF) is bright and white matter, dark. These images can be used to distinguish an edematous region of the white matter after stroke, for example, from a normal region.

Four constituents of the central nervous system are distinguished using MRI: (1) cerebrospinal fluid, (2) blood, (3) white matter, and (4) gray matter. The exact appearance of these central nervous system constituents depends on whether the image reflects proton density, T1 relaxation time (Figure 2–6A), or T2 relaxation time (Figure 2–6B). For T1 images, the signals produced by protons in cerebrospinal fluid are weak, and, on this image, cerebrospinal fluid is shaded black. Cerebrospinal fluid in the ventricles and overlying the brain surface, in the subarachnoid space, has the same dark appearance. On T2 images, cerebrospinal fluid appears white, because the signal it generates is strong. In T1 images, protons in blood in arteries and veins produce a strong signal, and these tissue constituents appear white. In T2 images, blood produces a weak signal. This weak signal derives from two factors: tissue motion (ie, normally blood flows and the signals from flowing blood are dispersed and weak) and the presence of hemoglobin, an iron-containing protein that attenuates the MRI signal because of its paramagnetic properties. The gray and white matter are also distinct because their protons emit signals of slightly different strengths. For example, on the T1-weighted image (Figure 2–6A), the white matter appears white and the gray matter appears dark.

Several major deep structures can be seen on the MRI scans in Figure 2–6A, B: the thalamus, the striatum, another component of the basal ganglia termed the lenticular nucleus, and the internal capsule. Figure 2–6D shows a T1-weighted MRI in the sagittal plane, close to the midline. The gyri and cerebrospinal fluid in the sulci look like the drawn image of the medial surface of the brain (Figure 2–6C). The image of the brain stem and cerebellum is a "virtual slice."

There have been two major advances in the basic MRI technique. **Diffusion-weighted MRI (DTI)** takes advantage of a component of the MRI signal that depends on the direction of diffusion of water protons within the tissue, which is highly restricted within white matter tracts. This approach can be used to examine fiber pathways in the brain, or **tractography.** The DTI in Figure 2–7A demonstrates the extensive networks of connections between different regions of the cerebral cortex. The other approach is **functional MRI** (or **fMRI;** Figure 2–7B). This technique provides an image of the changes in blood flow–related neural activity in different brain regions. This MRI was obtained while the subject was experiencing the hurt of social exclusion. The image shows that the anterior cingulate gyrus is activated, suggesting it is important in this kind of emotion.

The Spinal Cord Has a Central Cellular Region Surrounded by a Region That Contains Myelinated Axons

A spinal segment is shown in Figure 2–5A. The gray matter of the spinal cord contains two functionally distinct regions, the **dorsal** and **ventral horns** (Figure 2–5B). The dorsal horn is the receptive, or sensory, portion of the spinal gray matter, and the ventral horn, the motor portion. The white matter of the spinal cord, which surrounds the gray matter, contains three rostrocaudally oriented columns in which axons ascend or descend: the dorsal, lateral, and ventral columns. Between the gray matter on the two sides of the spinal cord is the **central canal,** a component of the ventricular system. Portions of the central canal become closed in the adult.

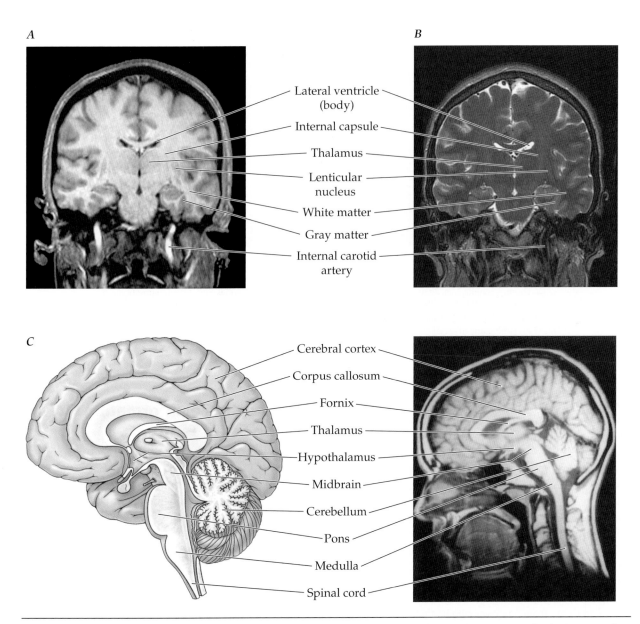

A

B

Lateral ventricle (body)

Internal capsule

Thalamus

Lenticular nucleus

White matter

Gray matter

Internal carotid artery

C

Cerebral cortex

Corpus callosum

Fornix

Thalamus

Hypothalamus

Midbrain

Cerebellum

Pons

Medulla

Spinal cord

FIGURE 2–6 MRI. T1 (*A*) and T2 (*B*) MRI scans produce opposite images. Cerebrospinal fluid appears white on T1-weighted MRI scans and dark on T2-weighted images. T1-weighted images look like a brain slice because gray matter appears dark and white matter appears white. The imaging planes for the two MRI scans are the same, and similar to Figure 2–17. **C.** Schematic and corresponding T1 midsagittal MRI. (Courtesy of Dr. Neal Rutledge, University of Texas at Austin.)

Somatic sensory receptor neurons, **dorsal root ganglion neurons,** innervate peripheral tissue and transmit this sensory information to neurons in the central nervous system (Figure Figure 2–5A, B). The axons of the dorsal root ganglion neurons enter the spinal cord through a dorsal rootlet, branch, and project their axons directly into the spinal gray and white matter. The dorsal root ganglion neurons that sense touch and limb position have an axon branch that enters the dorsal column to ascend to the brain stem for perception (Figure 2–5A, B). These sensory receptor neurons also terminate in the spinal cord, for mediating reflexes.

Neurons of the ventral horn subserve limb and trunk movements. A special class of neurons, motor neurons,

are located here; they have axons that exit the spinal cord through the **ventral root** to innervate muscle. Monosynaptic connections occur between a certain type of dorsal root ganglion neuron that innervates stretch receptors in muscles and motor neurons (Figure 2–5A, B). In certain segments of the spinal cord, this circuit mediates the **knee-jerk reflex.** A tap to the patella tendon of the knee stretches the quadriceps muscle, thereby stretching the receptors in the muscle. Within the spinal gray matter, the branches of dorsal root ganglion cells that innervate these receptors synapse on quadriceps motor neurons. Because this synapse is excitatory, it uses glutamate as its transmitter, the quadriceps motor neurons are discharged, and the muscle

A

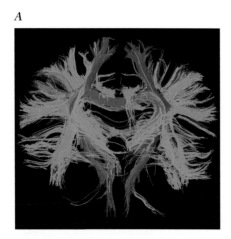

B

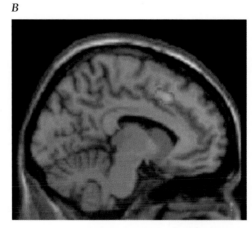

FIGURE 2–7 *A*. Diffusion tensor image (DTI) of connections between different areas of cortex. (Courtesy of Dr. Thomas Schultz, Max Planck Institute for Intelligent Systems, Tübingen.) *B*. Functional magnetic resonance image (fMRI) showing the region in the anterior cingulate gyrus that became active in a subject experiencing the hurt of social exclusion. (From Eisenberger NI, Lieberman MD, Williams KD. Does rejection hurt? An FMRI study of social exclusion. *Science.* 2003;302[5643]:290-292.)

contracts. Many other leg muscles and arm muscles have similar stretch reflexes. The axon branch that enters the dorsal column transmits information to the brain about limb position. This is an example of a dorsal root ganglion neuron that has both local spinal and ascending connections and, as a consequence, can serve both reflexes and perception.

Motor neurons also receive direct connections from the corticospinal tract, whose axons descend in the **lateral column** of the white matter (Figure 2–5A). A myelin-stained section from a healthy person is shown in Figure 2–5B. Whereas the location of the corticospinal tract can only be inferred on a myelin-in the healthy adult nervous system (Figure 2–5B), its location in tissue from a person who had a lesion involving the tract is clearly revealed as a lightly stained region (Figure 2–5D). This is because after an axon has been damaged, such as by a physical injury or stroke, consistent structural changes occur. The portion of the axon distal to the cut, now isolated from the neuronal cell body, degenerates because it is deprived of nourishment. This process is termed **Wallerian (or anterograde) degeneration.** In the central nervous system, when a myelinated axon degenerates, the myelin sheath around the axon also degenerates. The tissue can be stained for the presence of myelin, in which case the territory with the degenerated axons will remain unstained, creating a negative image of their locations (Figure 2–5D). The ventral column contains the axons of both ascending sensory and descending motor pathways and is considered in later chapters. An MRI through the spinal cord in the neck reveals little of its anatomical and functional organization (Figure 2–5C). However, we see the small size of the spinal cord in relation to the size of the neck.

The Direction of Information Flow Has Its Own Set of Terms

For spinal circuits, the terms *afferent* and *efferent* are often used in place of *sensory* and *motor* to describe the direction of information flow. The term **afferent** means that axons transmit information toward a particular structure. For the dorsal root ganglion neurons, information flow is from the periphery to the central nervous system. Dorsal root ganglion neurons are often called primary afferent fibers. The term **efferent** indicates that the axons carry information away from a particular structure. For motor neurons, information flow is from the central nervous system to muscle fibers. The terms *afferent* and *efferent* are also commonly used to describe direction of information flow within the central nervous system in relation to a particular target. For example, with respect to the motor neuron, both dorsal root ganglion axons and axons in the corticospinal tract carry afferent information. There is a distinction, however, because only the former transmits sensory information.

Surface Features of the Brain Stem Mark Key Internal Structures

The rostral spinal cord merges with the brain stem (Figure 2–8). On the dorsal brain stem surface are four major landmarks: dorsal columns, dorsal column tubercles, the fourth ventricle, and the colliculi. The dorsal columns and **tubercles** are part of the dorsal column–medial lemniscal system and are discussed further in the next section of this chapter. With the cerebellum removed, the floor of the **fourth**

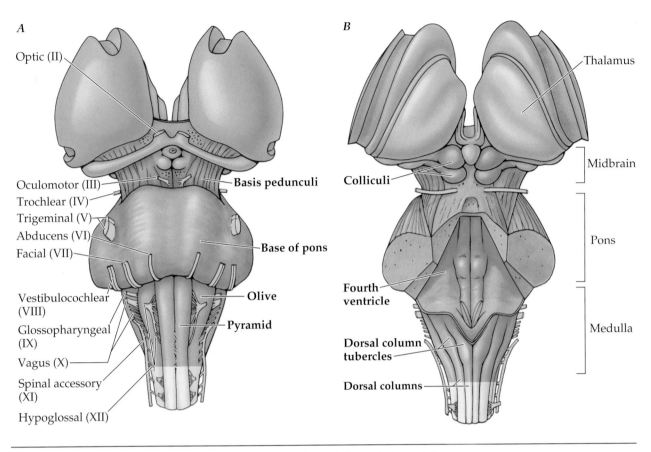

FIGURE 2–8 Ventral (**A**) and dorsal (**B**) surfaces of the brain stem, diencephalon, and telencephalon.

ventricle can be identified by its rhomboid shape. The **colliculi** are four bumps located on the dorsal surface of the midbrain. The rostral pair of bumps, termed the *superior colliculi*, are important in controlling eye movements. The caudal pair, called the *inferior colliculi*, are involved in the processing of sounds.

Four major landmarks also can be identified on the ventral surface (Figure 2–8A): pyramids, olives, base of the pons, and basis pedunculi; all four are key components of the motor system. In the medulla, the axons of the corticospinal tract are located in the **pyramids** and, just lateral to them, the **olives.** Neurons in the olives together with those in the **base of the pons,** the large basal surface of the pons, are major sources of afferent information to the cerebellum. Using this information, the cerebellum controls the accuracy of movement. Finally, many of the axons immediately beneath the ventral midbrain surface in the **basis pedunculi** are corticospinal tract axons, the same as those in the pyramid. These axons descend through the base of the pons and emerge on the medullary surface in the pyramid. Another characteristic of the brain stem is the presence of the **cranial nerves** (Figure 2–8). Knowledge of their locations helps develop a general understanding of brain stem anatomy. There are 12 pairs of cranial nerves, which, like the spinal nerves, mediate sensory and motor function, but of cranial structures.

The **reticular formation,** which comprises the central core of most of the brain stem, contains neurons that regulate arousal by influencing the excitability of neurons throughout the central nervous system. Some neurons of the modulatory systems described above are located in the reticular formation. Receiving input from all of the sensory modalities, neurons of the reticular formation can affect neuronal excitability through diffuse projections throughout the nervous system.

Many of the nuclei of the brain stem are analogous in connections and functions to regions of spinal cord gray matter. For example, nuclei in the brain stem receive sensory input directly from the receptor neurons innervating cranial structures. These are the cranial nerve sensory nuclei, which have general functions similar to neurons of the dorsal horn. Similarly, cranial nerve motor nuclei in the brain stem innervate cranial muscles and are similar to motor nuclei of the ventral horn.

The next several sections address brain stem regional and functional anatomy by examining transverse sections through five key levels: (1) the spinal cord–medullary junction, (2) the caudal medulla, (3) the middle medulla, (4) the caudal pons,

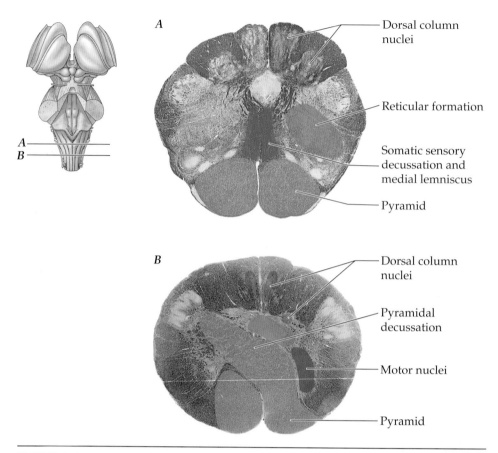

FIGURE 2–9 Myelin-stained sections through two levels of the medulla, through the dorsal column nuclei (**A**) and pyramidal decussation (**B**). Planes of the sections are indicated in the inset. Key medullary structures are highlighted.

and (5) the rostral midbrain. Knowledge of the surface features of the brain stem helps in recognizing the level of a particular section.

The Organization of the Medulla Varies From Caudal to Rostral

There are three characteristic levels through the medulla. The caudal-most level is at the junction with the spinal cord. The key feature of this level is the **pyramidal** (or motor) **decussation** (Figure 2–9B), which is where the corticospinal tract decussates. Because of this decussation, one side of the brain controls muscles of the opposite side of the body (see Figure 2–2B).

The next level is in the midmedulla, through the dorsal column nuclei (Figure 2–9A), which relay information about touch to the thalamus. At this level, the dorsal column nuclei bulge to form the dorsal surface landmarks, the dorsal column tubercles (Figure 2–9A). The second-order neurons of the dorsal column–medial lemniscal system originate in these nuclei. Their axons decussate and ascend to the thalamus in the medial lemniscus (Figure 2–9A). Because of this decussation, sensory information from one side of the body is

processed by the other side of the brain (see Figure 2–2A). This is similar to the motor decussation.

The third key medullary level is through the olive, a bulge located on the ventral medullary surface lateral to the medullary pyramid, which marks the position of the **inferior olivary nucleus** (Figure 2–10A). This nucleus contains neurons whose axons project to the cerebellum, where they form one of the strongest excitatory synapses in the entire central nervous system (see Chapter 13). Throughout the medulla, the corticospinal tract is located ventral to the medial lemniscus, in the medullary pyramid (Figure 2–9A and Figure 2–10). The medullary section in Figure 2–10B is from a person who sustained a corticospinal system injury by a stroke where it is located in the cerebral hemisphere (discussed further in the section on the internal capsule). Axons in the pyramid on one side, which is the same side as the lesion, have degenerated. Because of the absence of staining of that pyramid, the ventral border of the medial lemniscus is apparent.

An MRI through the rostral medulla and cerebellum is shown in Figure 2–10C. This level provides a clear view of the ventricular system. The central canal, which is a microscopic structure in the spinal cord, expands to form the fourth ventricle in the rostral medulla. Whereas the ventricular floor is formed by the medulla, the roof is formed by the cerebellum.

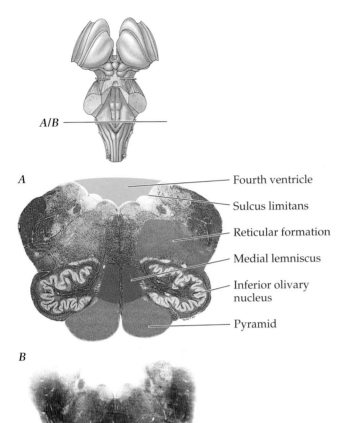

A/B

A
- Fourth ventricle
- Sulcus limitans
- Reticular formation
- Medial lemniscus
- Inferior olivary nucleus
- Pyramid

B
Pyramid:
- Degenerated
- Normal

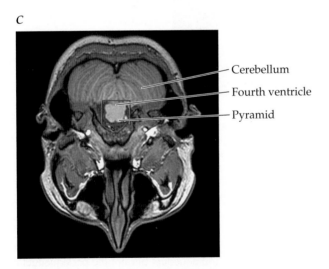

C
- Cerebellum
- Fourth ventricle
- Pyramid

FIGURE 2–10 Images of the medulla. *A.* Myelin-stained section through medulla. *B.* Myelin-stained transverse section through the medulla from someone who had a large lesion of the internal capsule that destroyed the corticospinal tract on one side. Compare this section to the one in A. The border between the medial lemniscus and the pyramid is estimated in A but is revealed clearly in B. *C.* MRI through the level show in A. Key regions are highlighted in A. Imaging plane is shown in the inset.

> **INFO Box: Radiological image convention**
>
> Whereas the dorsal brain surface in anatomical slices is, as a matter of convention, shown as the top of the image, MRIs, as well as other radiological images in humans, display dorsal down. For brain stem sections, this can result in confusion as one is initially learning neuroanatomy. For sections through the cerebral hemispheres and diencephalon, anatomical and radiological conventions are the same (dorsal up). Another radiological convention is that the right side of an image is the left side of the person. This switch derives from the traditional setting that the physician views a patient from the foot of the bed; hence, looking at an image is like standing at the foot of the patient's bed.

The Pontine Nuclei Surround the Axons of the Corticospinal Tract in the Base of the Pons

The dorsal surface of the pons forms part of the floor of the fourth ventricle; the cerebellum forms the roof, which can be seen both on the myelin-stained section and on the normal MRI of the same level (Figure 2–11A, B). The medial lemniscus, which is less distinct than in the medulla because neighboring myelinated fibers obscure its borders, is displaced dorsally by the **pontine nuclei.** Neurons in the pontine nuclei, which transmit information from the cerebral cortex to the cerebellum, participate in skilled movement control. The pontine nuclei surround the corticospinal axons; both nuclei and axons are located within the base of the pons (Figure 2–8A). The other MRI scan (Figure 2–11C) is from a patient who sustained injury to the corticospinal system at a more rostral level. The region containing degenerating fibers is revealed by a bright signal.

The Dorsal Surface of the Midbrain Contains the Colliculi

The midbrain can be divided into three regions, moving from the dorsal surface to the ventral surface (Figure 2–12A): (1) the **tectum** (Latin for "roof"), (2) the **tegmentum** (Latin for "cover"), and (3) the **basis pedunculi** (Latin for "base stalk or support"). The tegmentum and basis pedunculi comprise the **cerebral peduncle.** The colliculi are located in the tectum (Figure 2–8B). The superior colliculi (Figure 2–12) play an important role in controlling saccadic eye movements, rapid eye movements that dart from one region of interest to the next, and the inferior colliculi (located more caudally;

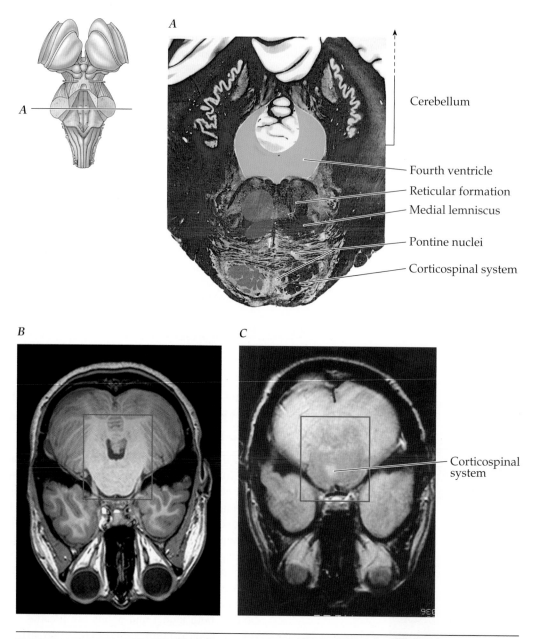

FIGURE 2–11 Images of the pons. Myelin-stained section through the mid-pons (**A**); MRI through the pons at approximately the same level as in A (**B**); MRI of patient with corticospinal tract injury (**C**). The imaging plane is shown in the inset. Note, in these images, dorsal is the upper part of the figure, for both the myelin-stained sections and the MRIs. (C, Courtesy of Dr. Jesús Pujol; from Pujol J, Martí-Vilalta JL, Junque C, Vendrell P, Fernández J, Capdevila A. Wallerian degeneration of the pyramidal tract in capsular infarction studied by magnetic resonance imaging. *Stroke.* 1990;21:404-409.)

see Atlas II-13) are important in hearing. All of these major regions of the midbrain can be seen on the MRI.

The **cerebral aqueduct (of Sylvius),** which connects the third and fourth ventricles, is located at the border of the tectum and tegmentum. This ventricular conduit is surrounded by a nuclear region, termed the **periaqueductal gray,** which contains neurons that are part of the circuit for endogenous pain suppression. For example, pain may be perceived as less severe during intense emotional experiences such as childbirth or military combat, and this neural system participates in this

pain diminution. The medial lemniscus is located within the tegmentum. The cerebral aqueduct but not the periaqueductal gray can be seen on the MRI (Figure 2–12B).

The corticospinal tract is located in the basis pedunculi. This pathway is therefore seen on the ventral surface of the midbrain; it descends on the ventral surface of the medulla as the pyramid. The corticospinal tract fibers are damaged in the MRI in Figure 2–12C. The approximate ventral border of the basis pedunculi is drawn in the image. The substantia nigra, which contains dopaminergic neurons important in movement

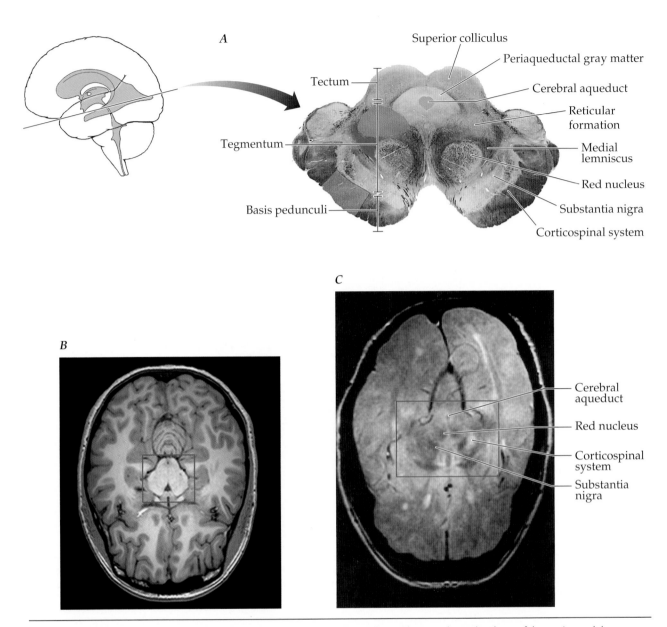

FIGURE 2–12 Myelin-stained section (**A**) and MRI scans (**B, C**) through the midbrain. The inset shows the planes of the section and the approximate plane for the MRI scans in relation to the ventricular system (aqua). The cerebral aqueduct, reticular formation, medial lemniscus, and corticospinal system are highlighted in **A**. Note that the descending cortical axons in **C** have degenerated. (**C,** Courtesy of Dr. Jesús Pujol; from Pujol J, Martí-Vilalta JL, Junqué C, Vendrell P, Ternández J, Capdevila A. Wallerian degeneration of the pyramidal tract in capsular infarction studied by magnetic resonance imaging. *Stroke.* 1990;21:404-409.)

control (see Figure 2–3B1), separates the corticospinal fibers and the medial lemniscus. The **red nucleus** is another midbrain nucleus that helps control movement.

The Thalamus Transmits Information From Subcortical Structures to the Cerebral Cortex

Most sensory information reaches the cortex indirectly by relay neurons in the thalamus (Figure 2–13). This is also the case for neural signals for controlling movements, cognitive processes, learning and memory, and emotions. Neurons in each half of the thalamus project to the cerebral cortex on the same (ipsilateral) side. Thalamic neurons are clustered into discrete nuclei. The organization of thalamic nuclei can be approached from anatomical and functional perspectives. Based on their locations, six nuclear groups are distinguished in the thalamus (Figure 2–13). The four major groups are named according to their locations with respect to bands of myelinated axons, called the **internal medullary laminae:**

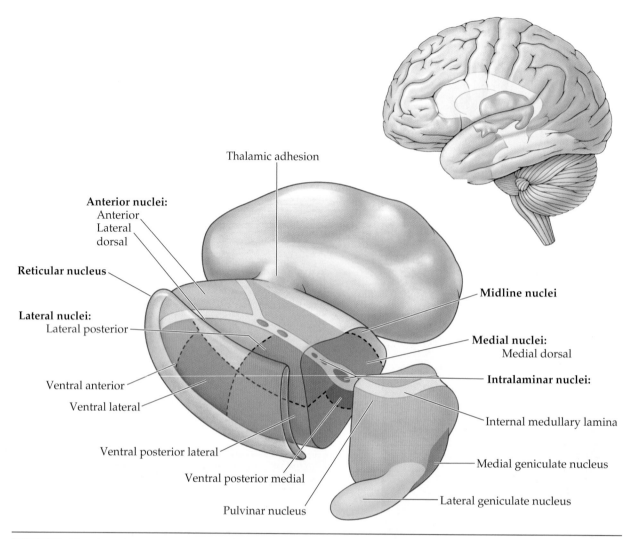

FIGURE 2–13 A three-dimensional view of the thalamus as well as its approximate location in the cerebral hemispheres. The major nuclei are labeled. Nuclei of the lateral group of nuclei are numbered. The inset shows the diencephalon, with the hypothalamus located ventral, and extending rostral, to the thalamus.

(1) anterior nuclei, (2) medial nuclei, (3) lateral nuclei, and (4) intralaminar nuclei, which lie within the laminae. The two other nuclear groups are (5) the midline nuclei and (6) the reticular nuclei (Table 2–1).

On the basis of the functions and the extent of their cortical connections, we divide the various thalamic nuclei into two major functional classes: (1) relay nuclei and (2) diffuse-projecting nuclei (Table 2–1). **Relay nuclei** transmit information from particular subcortical inputs to a restricted portion of the cerebral cortex. Because of this specificity of connections, each relay nucleus serves a distinct role in perception, volition, emotion, or cognition. By contrast, the **diffuse-projecting nuclei** are thought to function in arousal and in regulating the excitability of wide regions of the cerebral cortex. The patterns of termination of neurons in diffuse-projecting nuclei are described as regional because they may cross functional boundaries in the cortex. By contrast, the terminations of an individual relay nucleus are confined to a single functional cortical area.

The cortical projections of some of the major thalamic relay nuclei are shown in Figure 2–14. Relay nuclei that mediate sensation and movement are located in the lateral portion of the thalamus and project their axons to the sensory and motor cortical areas. For each sensory modality, there is a different relay nucleus. The only exception is olfaction, in which information from the periphery is transmitted directly to the cortex on the medial temporal lobe (see Chapter 9). Each sensory modality has a primary area that receives input directly from the thalamic relay nucleus for that modality. For example, the ventral posterior lateral nucleus is the relay nucleus for the dorsal column–medial lemniscal system. It transmits somatic sensory information from the medial lemniscus to the primary somatic sensory cortex for touch and other mechanical sensations (Figure 2–14,

Table **2-1** Thalamic nuclei: major connections and functions

Nucleus	Functional class	Major inputs	Major outputs	Functions
Anterior Group				
Anterior	Relay	Hypothalamus (mammillary body), hippocampal formation	Cingulate gyrus (limbic association cortex)	Learning, memory, and emotions
Lateral dorsal	Relay	Hippocampal formation; pretectum	Cingulate gyrus	
Medial Group				
Medial dorsal	Relay	Basal ganglia, amygdala, olfactory system, hypothalamus	Prefontal association cortex	Emotions, cognition, learning, and memory
Lateral Group				
Ventral anterior	Relay	Basal ganglia	Supplementary motor cortex	Movement planning
Ventral lateral	Relay	Cerebellum	Premotor and primary motor cortex	Movement planning and control
Ventral posterior	Relay	Spinal cord, brain stem, medial lemniscus, trigeminal lemniscus	Primary somatic sensory cortex	Touch, limb position sense, pain, and temperature sense
Lateral geniculate	Relay	Retina	Primary visual cortex	Vision
Medial geniculate	Relay	Inferior colliculus	Primary auditory cortex	Hearing
Pulvinar	Relay	Superior colliculus; parietal, temporal, occipital lobes	Parietal, temporal, occipital association cortex	Sensory integration, perception, language
Lateral posterior	Relay	Superior colliculus, pretectum, occipital lobe	Posterior parietal association cortex	Sensory integration
Intralaminar Nuclei				
Centromedian	Diffuse-projecting	Brain stem, basal ganglia, spinal cord	Cerebral cortex, basal ganglia	Regulation of cortical activity
Central lateral	Diffuse-projecting	Spinal cord, brain stem	Cerebral cortex, basal ganglia	Regulation of cortical activity
Parafascicular	Diffuse-projecting	Spinal cord, brain stem	Cerebral cortex, basal ganglia	Regulation of cortical activity
Midline Nuclei	Diffuse-projecing	Reticular formation, hypothalamus	Cerebral cortex, basal forebrain allocortex	Regulation of forebrain neuronal excitability
Reticular Nucleus		Thalamus, cortex	Thalamus	Regulation of thalamic neuronal activity

dark gray). The different motor areas of the frontal lobe also receive input directly from motor relay nuclei. An important nucleus for controlling voluntary movement, the ventral lateral nucleus, transmits signals from the cerebellum to the motor cortex (Figure 2–14), which gives rise to the corticospinal tract.

Relay nuclei located in the anterior, medial, and other parts of the lateral thalamus project to the **association cor-** **tex,** the cortical regions that lie outside the sensory and motor areas. There are three major regions of association cortex, which subserve distinct sets of functions: (1) the parietal-temporal-occipital cortex, (2) the prefrontal cortex, and (3) the limbic cortex. The **parietal-temporal-occipital associa-** **tion cortex,** located at the juncture of these lobes (Figure 2–14, blue), receives information primarily from the pulvinar nucleus as well as from different sensory cortical areas.

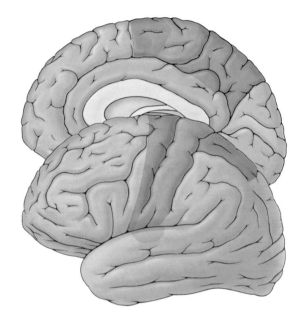

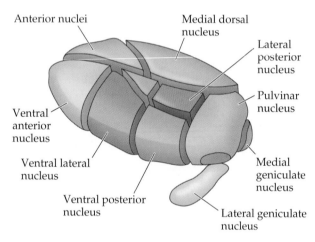

Anterior nuclei

Medial dorsal nucleus

Lateral posterior nucleus

Pulvinar nucleus

Ventral anterior nucleus

Ventral lateral nucleus

Ventral posterior nucleus

Medial geniculate nucleus

Lateral geniculate nucleus

FIGURE 2–14 The relationship between the major thalamic nuclei and the cortical regions to which they project.

This area is crucial for perception and for the sensory guidance of movement, such as reaching for a glass of water or looking at an object of interest. The **prefrontal association cortex** is important for cognitive functions and for organizing behavior, including the memories and motor plans necessary for interacting with the environment (Figure 2–14, light stipple). For example, patients with damage to the prefrontal cortex blindly repeat motor acts irrespective of their efficacy. The prefrontal association cortex receives a major projection from the medial dorsal nucleus, with a smaller input from the pulvinar nucleus. The **limbic association cortex** is essential for emotions as well as for learning and memory. It is located primarily on the medial brain surface, in the cingulate gyrus and medial frontal lobe, and on the orbital surface of the frontal lobe (Figure 2–14). Patients with structural or functional abnormalities of the limbic cortex, such

as temporal lobe epilepsy, often also have mood disorders such as depression, and personality changes (see clinical case, Chapter 16). The limbic association cortex receives input from the anterior nucleus, medial dorsal nucleus, and pulvinar nucleus.

The Internal Capsule Contains Ascending and Descending Axons

The internal capsule (Figure 2–14) is a tract, but unlike the medial lemniscus and corticospinal tract, it is a two-way path for transmission of information from the thalamus to the cerebral cortex and from the cerebral cortex to subcortical structures. The axons of the thalamic neurons that receive input from the medial lemniscus pass through the internal capsule en route to the primary somatic sensory cortex. The corticospinal axons descend through the internal capsule. The descending fibers of the internal capsule that project into the brain stem, or farther into the spinal cord, form the basis pedunculi in the midbrain. Although it appears as though the axons of the internal capsule condense as they course toward the brain stem, their numbers actually decrease: The contingent of ascending axons is not present in the basis pedunculi, accounting for a large reduction, and descending axons terminate in the thalamus, brain stem, and spinal cord, resulting in further decreases in numbers.

When the cerebral hemispheres are sliced horizontally (see line of section in Figure 2–16A), the internal capsule resembles an arrowhead with the tip pointing medially. This configuration gives the internal capsule three divisions: (1) anterior limb, (2) genu (Latin for "knee"), and (3) posterior limb. The thalamus is located medial to the posterior limb. The internal capsule also separates various components of the basal ganglia. The different parts of the internal capsule contain axons with somewhat different functions. For example, damage to the posterior limb can produce profound limb weakness or paralysis, because this is where the corticospinal tract descends. The corresponding MRI scan from a healthy person (Figure 2–16B) shows many of the structures present on the myelin-stained section. The path of the descending fibers of the internal capsule, from the cerebral hemispheres to the pons, can be followed on a myelin-stained coronal section (Figure 2–17A) and on the corresponding MRI scan from the patient with the corticospinal tract lesion (Figure 2–17B).

Cerebral Cortex Neurons Are Organized Into Layers

The dorsal column–medial lemniscal system projects to the cerebral cortex, which is also the origin of the corticospinal tract. Its neurons are organized into discrete

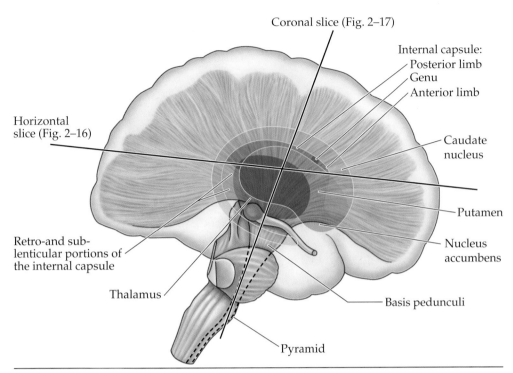

FIGURE 2-15 Schematic three-dimensional view of the internal capsule and other ascending and descending cortical axons. The three limbs of the internal capsule are distinguished, as are the retro- and sublenticular portions. The descending cortical axons collect into a discrete tract in the brain stem. Lines indicate planes of horizontal (eg, Figure 2–16) and coronal (eg, Figure 2–17) sections. Part of the basal ganglia is also shown. (Adapted with permission from Parent A. *Carpenter's Human Neuroanatomy*, 9th ed. Williams & Wilkins, 1996.).

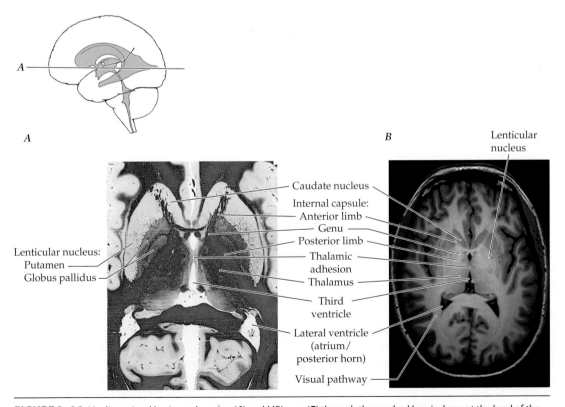

FIGURE 2-16 Myelin-stained horizontal section (**A**) and MRI scan (**B**) through the cerebral hemisphere, at the level of the thalamus. The inset shows the planes of the section and the MRI scan.

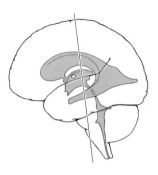

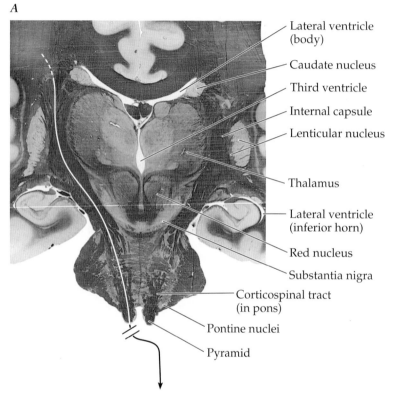

A

Lateral ventricle (body)

Caudate nucleus

Third ventricle

Internal capsule

Lenticular nucleus

Thalamus

Lateral ventricle (inferior horn)

Red nucleus

Substantia nigra

Corticospinal tract (in pons)

Pontine nuclei

Pyramid

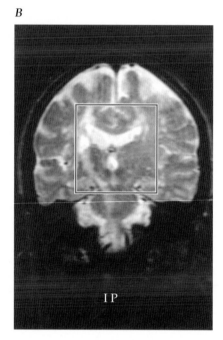

B

IP

FIGURE 2–17 Myelin-stained section (*A*) and MRI scan (*B*) through the cerebral hemisphere, at the level of the thalamus. The path of the descending cortical axons is drawn on *A*. The inset shows the planes of the section and the MRI scan. The light region in *B* contains degenerated descending cortical axons in the posterior limb of the internal capsule, basis pedunculi, and pyramid. (Courtesy of Dr. Jesús Pujol; from Pujol J, Martí-Vilalta JL, Junqué C, Vendrell P, Fernández J, Capdevila A. Wallerian degeneration of the pyramidal tract in capsular infarction studied by magnetic resonance imaging. *Stroke.* 1990;21:404-409.)

layers. Lamination is a feature of all cortical regions. Approximately 95% of the cerebral cortex contains at least six cell layers; this cortex is commonly called **neocortex** because it dominates the cerebral cortex of phylogenetically higher vertebrates such as mammals. The somatic sensory and motor cortical areas are part of the neocortex. The remaining 5% of cortex, which is termed **allocortex,** is morphologically distinct (see Figure 16–16). Allocortex, which is located mostly on the ventral brain surface, is involved in olfaction and aspects of learning and memory.

The Cerebral Cortex Has an Input-Output Organization

The thickness of each of the six cell layers of neocortex varies, as does the density of neurons in each layer. Each region of neocortex that subserves a different function has its own microscopic anatomy, which is an important determinant of function. Thalamic neurons that project to the cortex send their axons primarily to layer IV (Figure 2–18B). This is the input layer of cortex, which is thickest in sensory areas. There they synapse on dendrites of layer IV neurons, as well

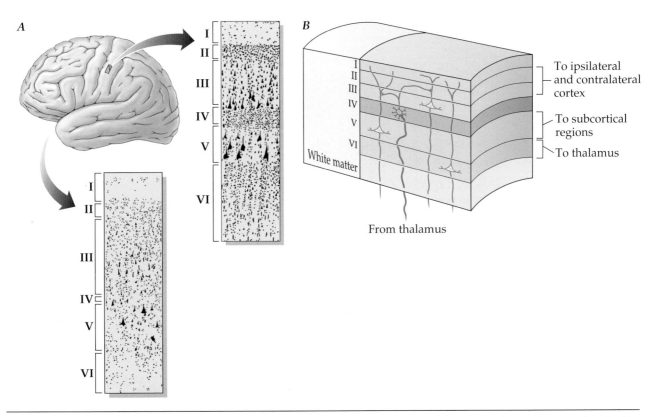

FIGURE 2–18 Three-dimensional schematic of a portion of the cerebral cortex. The pieces are from the postcentral and and precentral gyri. Within the cortex are six layers in which cells and their processes are located. **A.** Lamination pattern of neurons from the somatic sensory cortex (postcentral gyrus) is shown to the right, and from the motor cortex (precentral gyrus) is shown below. **B.** Neurons whose cell bodies are located in layers II and III project to other cortical areas, those in layer V project their axons to subcortical regions, and those in layer VI project back to the thalamus.

as neurons whose cell bodies are located in other layers, but they have dendrites in layer IV. Neurons in layer IV distribute this incoming information to neurons in other layers. Layers II, III, V, and VI are the output layers of cortex. Layer I does not contain many neurons in the mature brain, mostly dendrites of neurons located in deeper layers and elsewhere.

Pyramidal neurons in layers II, III, V, and VI project to other cortical areas as well as to subcortical structures. There are three separate classes of pyramidal neurons, each with their own projection pattern: (1) corticocortical association, (2) callosal, and (3) descending projection. The efferent projection neurons with different targets are located in different cortical layers:

- **Corticocortical association neurons,** located predominantly in layers II and III, project to cortical areas on the same side.

- **Callosal neurons** are also located in layers II and III. They project their axons to the contralateral cortex via the **corpus callosum** (see Figure 1–11B).

- **Descending projection neurons** are separate classes of projection neurons whose axons descend to (1) parts of the basal ganglia (striatum), (2) the thalamus, (3) the brain stem, or (4) the spinal cord. Descending

projection neurons that terminate in the striatum, brain stem, and spinal cord are found in layer V, whereas those projecting to the thalamus are located in layer VI.

The Cytoarchitectonic Map of the Cerebral Cortex Is the Basis for a Map of Cortical Function

The German anatomist Korbinian Brodmann identified over 50 morphologically distinct divisions of cortex (now termed **Brodmann's areas;** Figure 2–16, bottom). These divisions are based only on differences in the neuronal architecture, or **cytoarchitecture,** of the cortex, such as the sizes and shapes of neurons in the different laminae and their packing densities (Figure 2–19, top). It is remarkable that research on the functions of the cerebral cortex has shown that different functional areas of the cortex have a different cytoarchitecture. In humans, by noting the particular behavioral changes that follow discrete cortical lesions and using functional imaging approaches, such as functional MRI (Box 2–2; Figure 2–7B), we have gained some insight into the functions of most of the cytoarchitectonic divisions identified by Brodmann (Table 2–2).

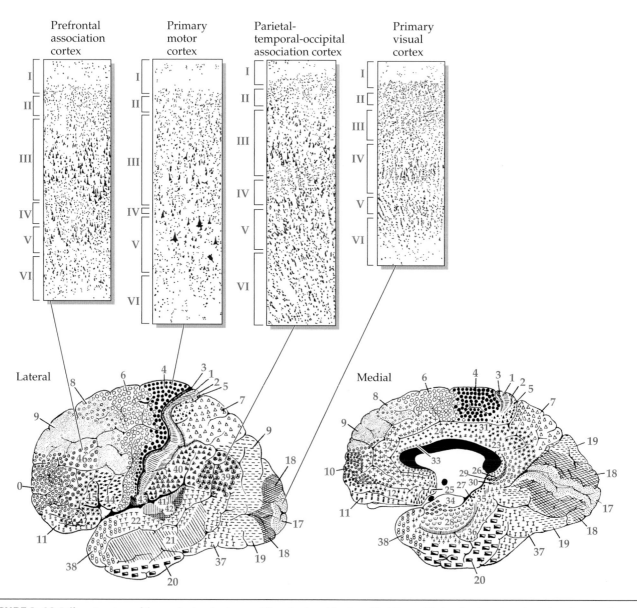

FIGURE 2–19 Different regions of the cerebral cortex have a different cytoarchitecture. (***Top***) Drawn Nissl-stained sections through various portions of the cerebral cortex. (***Bottom***) Brodmann's cytoarchitectonic areas of the cerebral cortex. (**Top,** Adapted from Campbell AW. *Histological Studies on the Localisation of Cerebral Function*. Cambridge University Press, 1905. **Bottom,** Adapted from Campbell 1905 and Brodmann K. *Vergleichende Lokalisationslehre der Grosshirnrinde in ihren Prinzipien dargestellt auf Grund des Zellen-baues*. Barth, 1909.)

Table **2-2** Brodmann's areas

Brodmann's area	Functional area	Location	Function
1, 2, 3	Primary somatic sensory cortex	Postcentral gyrus	Touch proprioception
4	Primary motor cortex	Precentral gyrus	Voluntary movement control
5	Higher-order somatic sensory cortex; posterior parietal association area	Superior parietal lobule	Sterognosia
6	Supplementary motor cortex; supplementary eye field; premotor cortex; frontal eye fields	Precentral gyrus and rostral adjacent cortex	Limb and eye movement planning
7	Posterior parietal association area	Superior parietal lobule	Visuomotor, spatial awareness, perception
8	Frontal eye fields	Superior, middle frontal gyri, medial frontal lobe	Saccadic eye movements
9, 10, 11, 12	Prefrontal association cortex; frontal eye fields	Superior, middle frontal gyri, medial frontal lobe	Thought, cognition, movement planning
17[1]	Primary visual cortex	Banks of calcarine fissure	Vision
18	Secondary visual cortex	Medial and lateral occipital gyri	Vision, depth
19	Higher-order visual cortex, middle temporal visual area	Medial and lateral occipital gyri	Vision, color, motion, depth
20	Visual inferotemporal area	Inferior temporal gyrus	Form vision
21	Visual inferotemporal area	Middle temporal gyrus	From vision
22	Higher-order auditory cortex	Superior temporal gyrus	Hearing, speech
23, 24, 25, 26, 27	Limbic association cortex	Cingulate gyrus, subcallosal area, retrosplenial area, and parahippocampal gyrus	Emotions, learning and memory
28	Primary olfactory cortex; limbic association cortex	Parahippocampal gyrus	Smell, emotions, learning and memory
29, 30, 31, 32, 33	Limbic association cortex	Cingulate gyrus and retrosplenial area	Emotions
34, 35, 36	Primary olfactory cortex; limbic association cortex	Parahippocampal gyrus	Smell, emotions
37	Parietal-temporal-occipital association cortex; middle temporal visual area	Middle and inferior temporal gyri at junction temporal and occipital lobes	Perception, vision, reading, speech
38	Primary olfactory cortex; limbic association cortex	Temporal pole	Smell, emotions, personality
39	Parietal-temporal-occipital association cortex	Inferior parietal lobule (angular gyrus)	Perception, vision, reading, speech
40	Parietal-temporal-occipital association cortex	Inferior parietal lobule (supramarginal gyrus)	Perception, vision, reading, speech
41	Primary auditory cortex	Heschl's gyri and superior temporal gyrus	Hearing
42	Secondary auditory cortex	Heschl's gyri and superior temporal gyrus	Hearing
43[2]	Gustatory cortex	Insular cortex, frontoparietal operculum	Taste
44	Broca's area; lateral premotor cortex	Inferior frontal gyrus (frontal operculum)	Speech, movement planning
45	Prefrontal association cortex	Inferior frontal gyrus (frontal operculum)	Thought, cognition, planning behavior
46	Prefrontal association cortex (dorsolateral prefrontal cortex)	Middle frontal gyrus	Thought, cognition, planning behavior, aspects of eye movement control
47	Prefrontal association cortex	Inferior frontal gyrus (frontal operculum)	Thought, cognition, planning behavior

[1]Areas 13, 14, 15, and 16 are part of the insular cortex. The relationship between cytoarchitecture and function is not established for the insular cortex.

[2]Area 43 may serve gustatory (taste) function, which is represented deeper in the insular cortex (see Chapter 9).

Brain Modulatory Systems

Four major neurotransmitter-specific systems have cell bodies located throughout the brain stem, diencephalon, and basal forebrain and terminate throughout the central nervous system (Figure 2–3). *Acetylcholine*-containing neurons in the pons, basal forebrain, and the lateral hypothalamus project throughout the cerebral cortex and hippocampal formation. Loss of many of these neurons occurs in Alzheimer disease. *Dopamine*-containing neurons in the substantia nigra and ventral tegmental area target the striatum and frontal lobe. These cells degenerate in Parkinson disease. *Noradrenergic* neurons in the locus ceruleus have widespread cortical projections, and those in the pons and medulla project to the spinal cord. *Serotonergic* neurons in the raphe nuclei of the brain stem have diffuse projections that are important for pain suppression and aspects of mood and arousal.

Spinal Cord Organization

The spinal cord, the most caudal of the major central nervous system divisions, has a central region that contains predominantly cell bodies of neurons (gray matter), surrounded by a region that contains mostly myelinated axons (white matter) (Figure 2–5). Both of these regions can be further subdivided. The *dorsal horn* of the gray matter subserves somatic sensation, and the *ventral horn,* skeletal motor function. The *dorsal column* of the white matter carries somatic sensory information to the brain; the *lateral* and *ventral columns* carry both somatic sensory and motor information (Figure 2–5).

Brain Stem Organization

The caudal medulla (Figure 2–8 and Figure 2–9B) is similar in its organization to the spinal cord. At a more rostral level (Figure 2–8 and Figure 2–9A), the medulla contains nuclei on its dorsal surface—the *dorsal column nuclei*—that subserve tactile sensation, and a pathway on its ventral surface—the corticospinal tract, located in the *pyramid*—that subserves voluntary movement. The *medial lemniscus* is located dorsal to the pyramid. The somatic sensory pathway decussates rostral to the motor pathway. At the level of the *inferior olivary nucleus* (Figure 2–10), the fourth

ventricle forms the dorsal surface of the medulla. The pons (Figure 2–11) contains nuclei in its ventral portion—the *pontine nuclei*—that transfer information from the cerebral cortex to the cerebellum. The midbrain (Figure 2–12) contains the *colliculi* on its dorsal surface (Figure 2–8B) and the *basis pedunculi* on its ventral surface (Figure 2–8A).

Organization of the Diencephalon and Cerebral Hemispheres

The *diencephalon* and the *cerebral hemispheres* have a more complex organization than that of the brain stem or spinal cord. The *thalamus,* which relays information from subcortical structures to the cerebral cortex, contains two different functional classes of nuclei: (1) *relay* and (2) *diffuse-projecting* (Table 2–1). Three of the four main anatomical divisions of the thalamus serve relay functions (Figure 2–13): (1) *anterior nuclei,* (2) *medial nuclei,* and (3) *lateral nuclei.* The fourth main anatomical division of the thalamus, the *intralaminar nuclei,* contains diffuse-projecting nuclei. The anatomical divisions are based on the spatial location of nuclei with respect to the *internal medullary lamina,* bands of myelinated fibers in the thalamus. A topographical relationship exists between the projections of the different thalamic nuclei and the cerebral cortex (Figure 2–14). Thalamocortical projections (as well as descending cortical projections) course through the *internal capsule* (Figure 2–15, Figure 2–16, and Figure 2–17).

The principal type of cortex is *neocortex* (or isocortex). It has six layers and the different layers have different thicknesses depending on the function of the particular cortical area (Figure 2–18). Layer IV is the principal input layer (Figure 2–18B). Layers II and III contain corticocortical association and callosal neurons and project to other cortical areas. Layer V contains descending projection neurons that terminate in the striatum, brain stem, and spinal cord. Layer VI contains descending projection neurons that terminate in the thalamus. Based on cortical layering patterns as well as the sizes and shapes of cortical neurons, or *cytoarchitecture,* about 50 different areas of the cerebral cortex have been identified (Figure 2–19; Table 2–2). These are termed *Brodmann's areas.*

Selected Readings

Amaral D. The functional organization of perception and movement. In: Kandel ER, Schwartz JH, Jessell TM, Siegelbaum SA, and Hudspeth AJ, eds. *Principles of Neural Science*. 5th ed. New York, NY: McGraw-Hill, in press.

Raichle ME. A brief history of human brain mapping. *TINS*. 2009;32(2):118-126.

References

Berman JI, Berger MS, Mukherjee P, Henry RG. Diffusion-tensor imaging-guided tracking of fibers of the pyramidal tract combined with intraoperative cortical stimulation mapping in patients with gliomas. *J Neurosurg*. 2004;101:66.

Brodmann K. *Vergleichende Lokalisationslehre der Grosshirnrinde in ihren Prinzipien dargestellt auf Grund des Zellenbaues*. Leipzig: Barth, 1909.

Campbell AW. *Histological Studies on the Localisation of Cerebral Function*. New York, NY: Cambridge University Press; 1905.

Dillon WP. Neuroimaging in neurologic disorders. In: Fauci AS, Braunwald E, Kasper D, et al., eds. *Harrison's Principles of Internal Medicine*. 17th ed. New York, NY: McGraw-Hill; 2008.

Gorman DG, Unützer J. Brodmann's missing numbers. *Neurology*. 1993;43:226-227.

Haber SN, Johnson GM. The basal ganglia. In: Paxinos G, Mai JK, eds. *The Human Nervous System*. London: Elsevier; 2004.

Halliday G. Substantia nigra and locus coeruleus. In: Paxinos G, Mai JK, eds. *The Human Nervous System*. London: Elsevier; 2004:451-464.

Hassler R. Architectonic organization of the thalamic nuclei. In: Shaltenbrand G, Warhen WW, eds. *Stereotaxy of the Human Brain*. Stuttgart, New York: G. Thieme Verlag; 1982:140-180.

Hornung J-P. Raphe nuclei. In: Paxinos G, Mai JK, eds. *The Human Nervous System*. London: Elsevier; 2004:424-450.

Koutcherov Y, Juang X-F, Halliday G, Paxinos G. Organization of human brain stem. In: Paxinos G, Mai JK, eds. *The Human Nervous System*. London: Elsevier; 2004.

Percheron G. Thalamus. In: Paxinos G, Mai JK, eds. *The Human Nervous System*. London: Elsevier; 2004:592-676.

Pujol J, Martí-Vilalta JL, Junqué C, Vendrell P, Fernández J, Capdevila A. Wallerian degeneration of the pyramidal tract in capsular infarction studied by magnetic resonance imaging. *Stroke*. 1990;21:404-409.

Rexed B. The cytoarchitectonic organization of the spinal cord in the cat. *J Comp Neurol*. 1952;96:415-495.

Saper CB. Hypothalamus. In: Paxinos G, Mai JK, eds. *The Human Nervous System*. London: Elsevier; 2004.

Zilles K. Architecture of the human cerebral cortex. In: Paxinos G, Mai JK, eds. *The Human Nervous System*. London: Elsevier; 2004:997-1055.

Study Questions

1. A 72-year-old man is brought to the emergency room with left-sided weakness and impaired touch sensation on the left side of the body. Which of the following statements best describes the location of the brain damage producing these neurological signs?
   A. Stroke in the left cerebral cortex
   B. Stoke in the right cerebral cortex
   C. Stoke affecting the right side of the spinal cord
   D. Damage to peripheral nerves on the left side of the body

2. A person was in a car accident and injured the lateral white matter of the spinal cord and became partly paralyzed. Which of the following choices best explains why the person became paralyzed as a consequence of the injury?

   A. The injury produced extensive damage to neuronal cell bodies within the white matter.
   B. The injury produced extensive damage to astrocytes in the white matter.
   C. The injury destroyed the component of the ventricular system that is located in the spinal cord.
   D. The injury extensively damaged axons within the white matter.

3. A patient has Alzheimer disease, which, among other impairments, is associated with a loss of acetylcholine in the forebrain. Which of the following is a major forebrain source of acetylcholine?
   A. Basal nucleus
   B. Ventral tegmental area

C. Locus ceruleus

D. Raphe nuclei

4. Which of the following is a major source of noradrenaline?

    A. Medial septal nucleus

    B. Substantia nigra compacta

    C. Locus ceruleus

    D. Raphe nuclei

5. Many of the neurological signs of Parkinson disease are produced by a loss of brain dopamine. Which of the following is a major source of dopamine?

    A. Basal nucleus

    B. Ventral tegmental area and substantia nigra compacta

    C. Locus ceruleus and reticular formation

    D. Raphe nuclei

6. Which of the following is a major source of serotonin (5-HT)?

    A. Basal nucleus

    B. Dorsal column nuclei

    C. Locus ceruleus

    D. Raphe nuclei

7. Damage to the dorsal columns and dorsal horn cord, such as what might occur after a traumatic spinal cord injury, would result in disrupting which of the following circuits?

    A. Somatic sensory

    B. Somatic motor

    C. Visceral motor function

    D. All of the above choices

8. Which of the following choices lists correctly the rostro-caudal order of the brain stem divisions?

    A. Medulla, midbrain, pons

    B. Midbrain, pons, medulla

    C. Midbrain, medulla, pons

    D. Pons, midbrain, medulla

9. A patient has a cerebellar stroke. The major motor sign that the person presents with is termed ataxia, a characteristic incoordination after cerebellar damage. Which of the following statements accurately describes the location of the stroke in the brain?

    A. Caudal to the tentorium and dorsal to the pons

    B. Rostral to the tentorium and dorsal to the pons

    C. Caudal to the tentorium and ventral to the pons

    D. Rostral to the tentorium and ventral to the pons

10. A person is shot in the head. The bullet entered the skull above the right ear. In sequence, which of the following choices best describes the brain structures the bullet would encounter, from lateral to medial?

    A. Parietal cortex, insular cortex, putamen, globus pallidus, anterior limb of the internal capsule, thalamus

    B. Parietal cortex, insular cortex, putamen, globus pallidus, posterior limb of the internal capsule, thalamus

    C. Insular cortex, putamen, posterior limb of the internal capsule, globus pallidus, thalamus

    D. Insular cortex, putamen, globus pallidus, anterior limb of the internal capsule, thalamus

Chapter 3

Vasculature of the Central Nervous System and the Cerebrospinal Fluid

CLINICAL CASE | Middle Cerebral Artery Occlusion, Right Side Paralysis, and Global Aphasia

A 57-year-old male was brought to the emergency room after being discovered by his wife to be unable to move his right arm or leg. On testing, his right upper limb strength was 0/5 and the lower limb, 1/5. The left limbs had normal strength and spontaneous movements. In addition, there was drooping of the right side of the lower face. Pinch of the nail beds—a mildly noxious stimulus that elicits a withdrawal—revealed withdrawal of the left arm but no response for the right arm. The patient was able to look to the left but not the right; there were no saccadic (rapid, conjugate) eye movements to the right. The patient was unable to speak and only followed simple commands.

Figure 3–1A shows a horizontal MRI. The large white territory corresponds to the infarcted region on the left side of the cerebral hemisphere. Figure 3–18B is a magnetic resonance angiogram (MRA), showing the distribution of arteries with flowing blood. Note the asymmetry in the MRA, with an absence of middle cerebral artery perfusion on the left side.

Answer the following questions based on your readings of the case report and this chapter.

1. **The patient's lesion is large. Occlusion of which cerebral artery produced the lesion, and what was the contribution of its deep and superficial branches?**

2. **Damage to what single key structure could produce the major limb and facial motor signs?**

—Continued next page

A

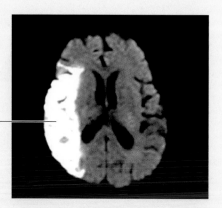

Middle cerebral ——— artery infarct

B

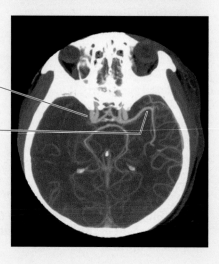

Middle cerebral
artery absent on
infracted side

but present on the ———
unaffected side

FIGURE 3–1 Neuroradiological imaging after stroke. **A.** Diffusion-weighted image (DWI) showing a large left middle cerebral artery infarction. The white region corresponds to the infarcted territory of the middle cerebral artery. **B.** Magnetic resonance angiogram (MRA) showing a complete lack of perfusion of the left middle cerebral artery. This demonstrates occlusion at its proximal portion. (Reproduced with permission from Ropper AH et al. *Adams & Victor's Principles of Neurology*, 9th ed. AccessMedicine; 2009, Fig. 34–3.)

Key neurological signs and corresponding damaged brain structures

Paralyzed right arm and leg

The corticospinal tract, which is key to controlling the contralateral arm and leg, descends subcortically and then travels in the posterior limb of the internal capsule (see Figure 2–17). This subcortical white matter and the more dorsal parts of the posterior limb of the internal capsule are supplied by deep branches of the middle cerebral artery. The infarction also would have destroyed part of the lateral precentral gyrus, where the corticospinal tract to the arm segments of the spinal cord originates. This is supplied by superficial branches of the middle cerebral artery. By contrast, the infarction spares the leg area of motor cortex (see Figure 10–8). Whereas the descending axons are destroyed when they are in the internal capsule, as we shall see in later chapters sparing of the cortex may help during neurorehabilitation.

Right lower facial droop

The corticobulbar tract controls facial muscles. This is the component of the descending cortical motor pathway that controls cranial motor nuclei in the brain stem. (Bulb is an archaic term to describe the lower brain stem.) The tract travels subcortically from lateral part of the precentral gyrus (face area of motor cortex) to the genu and posterior limb of the internal capsule, rostral to the corticospinal tract axons. The subcortical white matter and dorsal parts of the internal capsule are largely supplied by the deep branches of the middle cerebral artery. The face-controlling area of motor cortex is supplied by superficial branches of the middle cerebral artery. Interestingly, control of the lower face—like that of the arms and legs—is strictly contralateral, but upper facial muscle control is bilateral. Damage to the corticobulbar tract on one side thus eliminates control of lower face on the opposite side, resulting in paralysis or major weakness. Upper facial muscles, because they receive control by both sides of the brain, are functional after a unilateral corticobulbar tract lesion.

Absence of limb withdrawal to noxious stimulation

Damage to the internal capsule can destroy the ascending thalamocortical projection, carrying somatic sensory information to the postcentral gyrus. This results in the loss of somatic sensation. However, in the case of our patient, there were no spontaneous right arm movements and there was no upper limb strength. Therefore, it is unlikely that he would have been able to move the limb had noxious stimulation been felt.

Absence of eye movement to the right

The infarction damaged the cortical regions, and their descending control pathways, for saccadic eye movements. These are the rapid, darting, eye movements we use to shift our gaze from one object of interest to another.

Inability to speak and understand language

The cortical centers controlling speech are in the left hemisphere in most right-handed individuals. These areas are Wernicke's area in the superior temporal gyrus, for sensory processing in speech, and Broca's area in the inferior frontal lobule, for producing speech. Both areas are supplied by superficial branches of the middle cerebral artery. Their axonal interconnections are also supplied, in large part, by the middle cerebral artery. In the absence of these structures, there is loss of language, both spoken and understanding.

Brain vasculature disorders constitute a major class of nervous system disease. The principal source of nourishment for the central nervous system is glucose, and because neither glucose nor oxygen is stored in appreciable amounts, when the blood supply of the central nervous system is interrupted, even briefly, brain functions become severely disrupted.

Much of what is known about the arterial supply to the central nervous system derives from three approaches. First, classical studies in normal postmortem tissue used colored dye injected into a blood vessel to identify the areas it supplies. Second, in postmortem tissue or on radiological examination, the portion of the central nervous system supplied by a particular artery can be inferred by observing the extent of damage that occurred after the artery became occluded. Third, radiological techniques, such as cerebral angiography and magnetic resonance angiography, make it possible to view the arterial and venous circulation in the living brain (see Box 3–1). These important clinical tools also permit localization of a vascular obstruction or other pathology.

As discussed in previous chapters, brain vasculature is closely related to the ventricular system and the watery fluid contained within it, the cerebrospinal fluid. This is because most cerebrospinal fluid is produced by active secretion of ions from blood plasma by the choroid plexus. Moreover, to maintain a constant brain volume, cerebrospinal fluid is returned to the blood through valves between the subarachnoid space and the dural sinuses.

This chapter initially focuses on arterial supply because of the importance of distributing oxygenated blood to the brain and spinal cord for normal function, followed by venous drainage. The blood-brain barrier, which isolates the intravascular compartment from the extracellular compartment of the central nervous system, is considered next. Finally, cerebrospinal fluid production and circulation within the different components of the ventricular system is examined.

Neural Tissue Depends on Continuous Arterial Blood Supply

Local regions of the central nervous system receive blood from small sets of penetrating arteries that receive their blood from the major arteries (Table 3–1). Cessation or reduction of the arterial supply to an area results in decreased delivery of oxygenated blood to the tissue, a condition termed **ischemia.** Decreased blood supply typically occurs when an artery becomes occluded or when systemic blood pressure drops substantially, such as during a heart attack. Occlusion commonly occurs because of an acute blockade, such as from an embolus, or the gradual narrowing of the arterial lumen (stenosis), as in atherosclerosis.

A brief reduction in blood flow produces transient neurological signs, attributable to lost functions of the oxygen-deprived area. This event is termed a **transient ischemic attack (TIA).** If ischemia is persistent and is uncorrected for several minutes, it can cause death of the tissue it normally supplies, termed an **infarction.** This can result in more enduring or even permanent impairments. These events describe an **ischemic stroke.** Under special circumstances, the local reduction in arterial blood flow may not produce an ischemic stroke and infarction because the tissue receives a redundant supply from another artery. This is termed **collateral circulation,** which is covered further in the section on the anterior and posterior circulations.

Hemorrhagic stroke can occur when an artery ruptures, thereby releasing blood into the surrounding tissue. A hemorrhagic stroke not only produces a loss of downstream flow but also can damage brain tissue at the rupture site because of the volume now occupied by the blood outside of the vessel. A common cause of a hemorrhagic stroke is when an **aneurysm,** or ballooning of an artery due to weakening of the muscular wall, ruptures.

Table **3–1** **Blood supply of the central nervous system**

Structure	Level	System	Major artery[1]	Structure	Level	System	Major artery[1]
Spinal Cord		P	Anterior spinal artery	Subthalamus		A	Anterior choroidal
		P	Posterior spinal artery			A	Posterior communicating
		S	Radicular arteries			P	Posterior choroidal
Medulla	Caudal	P	Anterior spinal artery			P	Posterior cerebral
		P	Posterior spinal artery	**Basal Ganglia**			
	Rostral	P	Vertebral	Globus pallidus	Superior	A	Middle cerebral: lenticulostriate
		P	Vertebral: PICA		Middle, inferior	A	Anterior choroidal
Pons	Caudal and middle	P	Basilar	Striatum	Superior	A	Middle cerebral: lenticulostriate
		P	Basilar: AICA		Inferior	A	Anterior cerebral: lenticulostriate
	Rostral	P	Basilar: SCA	**Septal Nuclei**		A	Anterior cerebral
Cerebellum	Caudal	P	Vertebral: PICA			A	Anterior communicating
	Middle	P	Basilar: AICA			A	Anterior choroidal
	Rostral	P	Basilar: SCA	**Amygdala**		A	Anterior choroidal
Midbrain	Caudal (inferior colliculi)	P	Basilar	**Hippocampal Formation**		A	Posterior cerebral
		P	Basilar: SCA	**Internal Capsule**			
	Rostral (superior colliculi)	P	Posterior cerebral	Anterior limb	Superior	A	Middle cerebral
					Middle	A	Anterior cerebral
					Inferior	A	Internal capsule
Diencephalon					Inferior	A	Anterior choroidal
Thalamus		A	Posterior communicating	Genu	Superior	A	Middle cerebral
		P	Posterior cerebral: posterior choroidal		Middle	A	Anterior cerebral
		P	Posterior cerebral: thalamogeniculate		Inferior	A	Anterior choroidal; anterior cerebral
		P	Posterior cerebral: thalamoperforating	Posterior limb	Superior	A	Middle cerebral
Hypothalamus		A	Anterior cerebral		Inferior	A	Anterior choroidal
		A	Anterior communicating	Retrolenticular		A	Anterior choroidal
		A	Posterior communicating	**Cerebral Cortex**			
		P	Posterior cerebral	Frontal lobe		A	Anterior cerebral
						A	Middle cerebral
				Parietal lobe		A	Anterior cerebral
						A	Middle cerebral
				Occipital lobe		P	Posterior cerebral
				Temporal lobe		P	Posterior cerebral

[1]Artery distributions based on radiological and dye-fill data; artery supplying more than approximately 80% of structure.

Abbreviation key: A, anterior circulation; AICA, anterior inferior cerebellar artery; P, posterior circulation; PICA, posterior inferior cerebellar artery; S, systemic circulation; SCA, superior cerebellar artery.

The Vertebral and Carotid Arteries Supply Blood to the Central Nervous System

The principal blood supply for the brain comes from two arterial systems that receive blood from different systemic arteries: the **anterior circulation,** fed by the **internal carotid arteries,** and the **posterior circulation,** which receives blood from the **vertebral arteries** (Figure 3–2, inset; Table 3–1). The vertebral arteries join at the junction of the medulla and pons (or pontomedullary junction) to form the **basilar artery,** which lies unpaired along the midline (Figure 3–2). The anterior circulation is also called the **carotid circulation,** and the posterior circulation, the **vertebral-basilar circulation.** The anterior and posterior circulations are not independent but are connected by

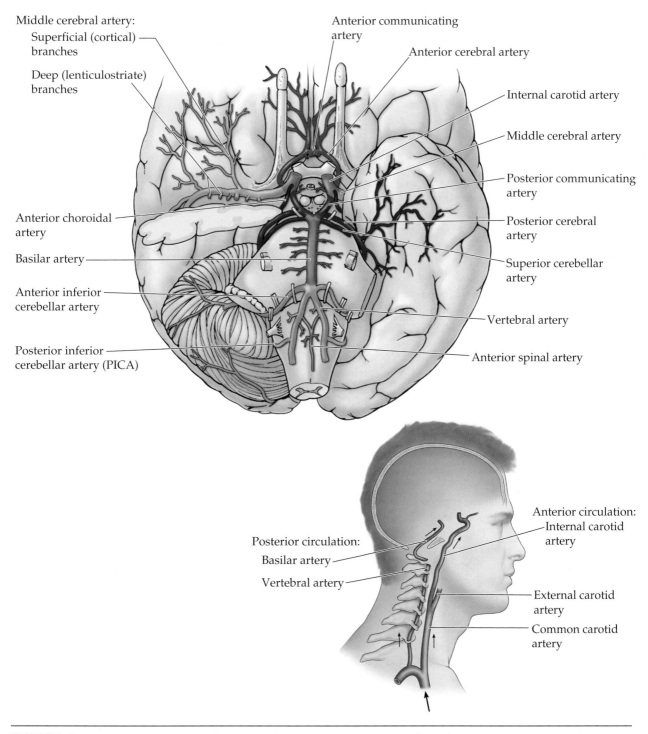

Middle cerebral artery:
Superficial (cortical) branches
Deep (lenticulostriate) branches

Anterior choroidal artery

Basilar artery

Anterior inferior cerebellar artery

Posterior inferior cerebellar artery (PICA)

Anterior communicating artery

Anterior cerebral artery

Internal carotid artery

Middle cerebral artery

Posterior communicating artery

Posterior cerebral artery

Superior cerebellar artery

Vertebral artery

Anterior spinal artery

Posterior circulation:
Basilar artery
Vertebral artery

Anterior circulation:
Internal carotid artery

External carotid artery

Common carotid artery

FIGURE 3–2 Diagram of the ventral surface of the brain stem and cerebral hemispheres, illustrating the key components of the anterior (carotid) circulation and the posterior (vertebral-basilar) circulation. The anterior portion of the temporal lobe of the right hemisphere is removed to illustrate the course of the middle cerebral artery through the lateral (Sylvian) fissure and the penetrating branches (lenticulostriate arteries). The circle of Willis is formed by the anterior communicating artery, the two posterior communicating arteries, and the three cerebral arteries. The inset (**bottom**) shows the extracranial and cranial courses of the vertebral, basilar, and carotid arteries. Arrows indicate normal direction of blood flow.

networks of arteries on the ventral surface of the diencephalon and midbrain and on the cortical surface (see below).

Whereas the cerebral hemispheres receive blood from both the anterior and posterior circulations, the brain stem receives blood only from the posterior circulation. The arterial supply for the spinal cord is provided by the systemic circulation—which also supplies muscle, skin, and bones—and, to a lesser degree, by the vertebral arteries. Cerebral and spinal arteries drain into veins. Although spinal veins are part of the general systemic circulation and return blood directly to the heart, most cerebral veins drain first into the **dural sinuses,** a set of large venous collection channels in the dura mater.

The Spinal and Radicular Arteries Supply Blood to the Spinal Cord

The spinal cord receives blood from two sources. First are the **anterior** and **posterior spinal arteries** (Figure 3–2), branches of the vertebral arteries. Second are the **radicular arteries**, which are branches of segmental vessels, such as the cervical, intercostal, and lumbar arteries. Neither anterior nor posterior spinal arteries typically form a single continuous vessel along the entire length of the ventral or dorsal spinal cord. Rather, each forms a network of communicating channels oriented along the rostrocaudal axis of the spinal cord. The radicular arteries feed into this network along the entire length of the spinal cord.

Although the spinal and radicular arteries supply blood to all spinal cord levels, different spinal cord segments are preferentially supplied by one or the other set of arteries. The cervical spinal cord is supplied by both the vertebral and radicular arteries (in particular, the ascending cervical artery). In contrast, the thoracic, lumbar, and sacral segments are nourished primarily by the radicular arteries (the intercostal and lumbar arteries). When spinal cord segments are supplied by a single artery, they are particularly susceptible to injury after arterial occlusion. In contrast, segments that receive a redundant (or collateral) blood supply tend to fare better following single vessel occlusion. For example, individual rostral thoracic segments are supplied by fewer radicular arteries than are more caudal segments. When a radicular artery that serves the rostral thoracic segments becomes occluded, serious damage is more likely to occur because there is no backup system for perfusion of oxygenated blood. Interruption of the blood supply to critical areas of the spinal cord can produce sensory and motor control impairments similar to those produced by traumatic mechanical injury, such as that resulting from an automobile accident.

The Vertebral and Basilar Arteries Supply Blood to the Brain Stem

Each of the three divisions of the brain stem and the cerebellum receives its arterial supply from the posterior circulation (Figure 3–3A). In contrast to the spinal arteries, which are located both ventrally and dorsally, arteries supplying most of the brain stem arise from the ventral surface only. Branches emerge from these ventral arteries and either penetrate directly or run around the circumference of the brain stem to supply dorsal brain stem structures and

the cerebellum. Three groups of branches arise from the vertebral and basilar arteries: (1) paramedian, (2) short circumferential, and (3) long circumferential (Figure 2–3B). The **paramedian branches** supply regions close to the midline. The **short circumferential branches** supply lateral, often wedge-shaped regions, and the **long circumferential branches** supply the dorsolateral portions of the brain stem and cerebellum.

Even though the spinal arteries primarily supply the spinal cord, they also supply a small portion of the caudal medulla. The spinal arteries lie close to the dorsal and ventral midline and nourish the most medial areas (Figure 3–3B4). The more lateral area is served by direct branches of the vertebral arteries, which are equivalent to the more rostral short circumferential branches.

The rest of the medulla is supplied by the vertebral arteries. Small (unnamed) branches that exit from the main arteries supply the medial medulla (ie, paramedian and short circumferential branches). Because these arteries supply axons of the corticospinal tract and the medial lemniscus (see Figure 2–2), when the arteries become occluded, patients develop impairments in voluntary limb movement and mechanosensation. The major laterally emerging (long circumferential) branch from the vertebral artery, the **posterior inferior cerebellar artery (PICA),** nourishes the most dorsolateral region (Figure 3–3B3). This region of the medulla does not receive blood from any other artery. The absence of a collateral arterial supply makes the posterior inferior cerebellar artery particularly important because occlusion almost always results in significant tissue damage. When this occurs, patients commonly develop characteristic sensory and motor impairments due to destruction of nuclei and tracts in the dorsolateral medulla. Common neurological signs include loss of facial pain sensation and uncoordinated limb movements, both on the side of the occlusion, and loss of limb and trunk pain on the opposite side. An understanding of this complex pattern of sensory and motor loss will be achieved when pain and motor control circuits are described in later chapters.

The two vertebral arteries join to form the basilar artery at the pontomedullary junction (Figure 3–3A), from which paramedian and short circumferential arteries supply the base of the pons, where corticospinal fibers are located. The dorsolateral portion of the caudal pons is supplied by a long circumferential branch of the basilar artery, termed the **anterior inferior cerebellar artery (AICA).** The region in the pons rostral to that supplied by the anterior inferior cerebellar artery is nourished by the **superior cerebellar artery,** another long circumferential branch of the basilar artery (Figure 3–3A).

Long circumferential branches of the vertebral and basilar arteries supply the cerebellum. The posterior inferior cerebellar artery supplies the caudal portion of the cerebellum. More rostral portions are supplied by the anterior inferior cerebellar artery and the superior cerebellar artery (Figure 3–2 and Figure 3–3A).

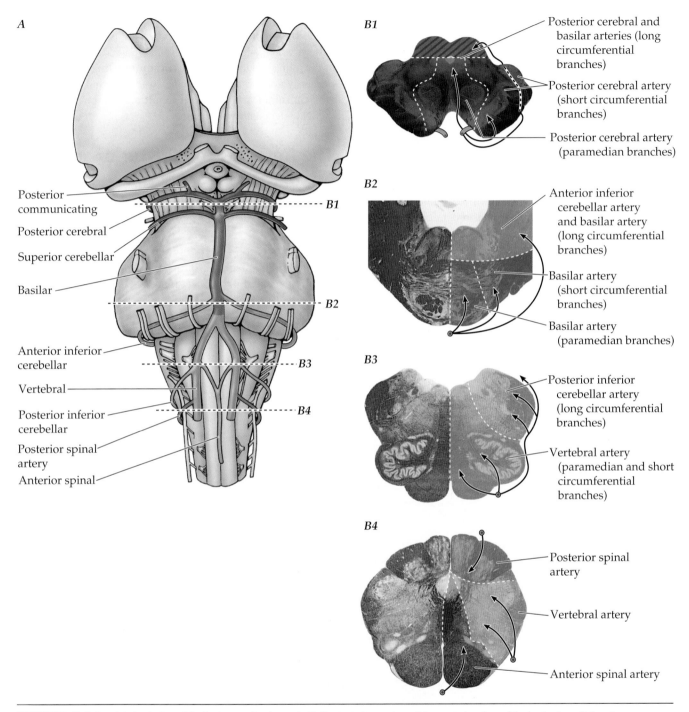

FIGURE 3–3 A. Arterial circulation of the brain stem is schematically illustrated on a view of the ventral surface of the brain stem. **B.** Four transverse sections through the brain stem are shown, illustrating the distribution of arterial supply. In the upper medulla (**B3**), pons (**B2**), and midbrain (**B1**), portions of tissue from medial to dorsolateral are supplied by paramedian, short circumferential, and long circumferential branches. The caudal medulla receives its arterial supply from the vertebral and spinal arteries (**B4**). The dashed lines in **A** indicate the planes of section in **B**.

The basilar artery splits at the pons-midbrain border into the two posterior cerebral arteries. While the **posterior cerebral artery** is part of the vertebral-basilar system, it develops from the anterior system, thereby receiving blood from the carotid arteries. However, later in development much more blood comes from the basilar artery, making the posterior cerebral artery functionally part of the posterior circulation in maturity. The posterior cerebral artery nourishes most of the midbrain (Figure 3–3B1). Paramedian and short circumferential branches supply the base and tegmentum, whereas long circumferential branches supply the tectum. The colliculi, the principal portion of the tectum, also receive a small supply by the superior cerebellar artery.

The Internal Carotid Artery Has Four Principal Portions

The **internal carotid artery** consists of four segments (Figure 3–4A): (1) The **cervical segment** extends from the bifurcation of the common carotid (into the external and internal carotid arteries; see Figure 3–2) to where it enters the carotid canal; (2) the **intrapetrosal segment** courses through the petrous portion of the temporal bone; (3) the **intracavernous segment** courses through the cavernous sinus, a venous structure overlying the sphenoid bone (see Figure 3–15); and (4) the **cerebral segment** extends to where the internal carotid artery bifurcates into the anterior and middle cerebral arteries. The intracavernous and cerebral portions form the **carotid siphon,** an important radiological landmark.

Branches emerging directly from the cerebral segment of the internal carotid artery supply deep cerebral and other cranial structures. The major branches of this artery (Figure 3–4B), in caudal to rostral order, are (1) the **ophthalmic artery,** which supplies the optic nerve and the inner portion of the retina, (2) the **posterior communicating artery,** which primarily nourishes diencephalic structures, and (3) the **anterior choroidal artery,** which supplies diencephalic and subcortical telencephalic structures.

The Anterior and Posterior Circulations Supply the Diencephalon and Cerebral Hemispheres

The internal carotid artery divides near the basal surface of the cerebral hemisphere to form the **anterior cerebral** and **middle cerebral arteries** (Figure 3–2). Thus, the anterior

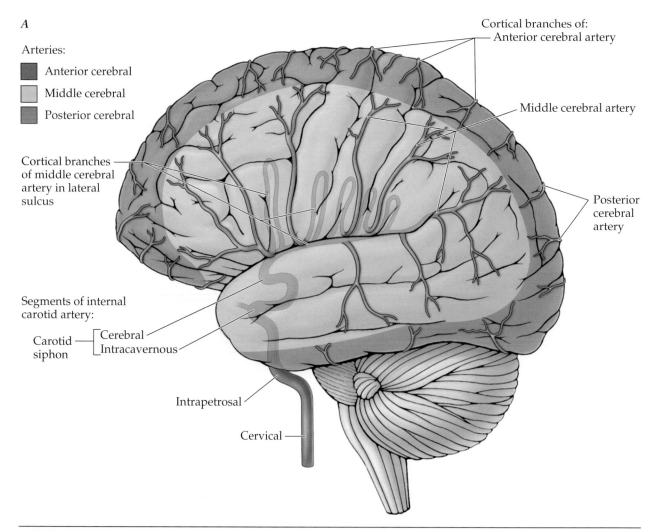

FIGURE 3–4 The courses of the three cerebral arteries are illustrated in views of the lateral (**A**) and midsagittal (**B**) surfaces of the cerebral hemisphere. The territories supplied by each cerebral artery are shown in different colors. Note that the anterior cerebral artery (**B**) courses around the genu of the corpus callosum.

B

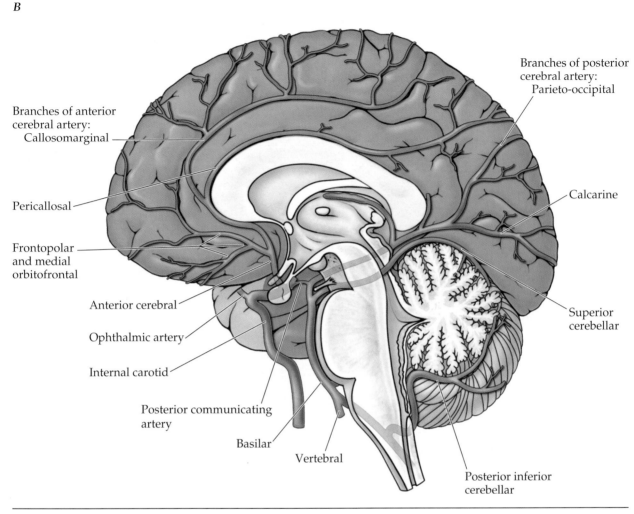

Branches of anterior
cerebral artery:
   Callosomarginal

Pericallosal

Frontopolar
and medial
orbitofrontal

Anterior cerebral

Ophthalmic artery

Internal carotid

Posterior communicating
artery

Basilar

Vertebral

Branches of posterior
cerebral artery:
   Parieto-occipital

Calcarine

Superior
cerebellar

Posterior inferior
cerebellar

Continued—**FIGURE 3–4**

and middle cerebral arteries receive their blood from the anterior circulation and, as described, the posterior cerebral artery receives blood from the posterior circulation. The three cerebral arteries each comprise deep and cortical branches. The deep branches come off the arteries proximally. The deep branches of the three cerebral arteries, together with the arteries that branch from the cerebral segment of the internal carotid artery, supply deep brain gray matter and white matter regions. The cortical branches are the distal, or terminal, endings of the cerebral arteries; they supply the various neuronal laminae of the cerebral cortex.

Collateral Circulation Can Rescue Brain Regions Deprived of Blood

There are two sites where the anterior and posterior circulations communicate, on the ventral and dorsal brain surfaces. Communication between the circulations is clinically

important because decreased flow in one system can be compensated by increased flow in the other. At the ventral site, the proximal portions of the cerebral arteries and the communicating arteries form the **circle of Willis.** This is an example of a network of interconnected arteries, or an **anastomosis.** The two **posterior communicating arteries** allow blood to flow between the middle and posterior cerebral arteries on each side, and the **anterior communicating artery** allows blood to flow between the anterior cerebral arteries (Figure 3–2). When either the posterior or the anterior arterial circulation becomes occluded, collateral circulation may occur through the circle of Willis to rescue the region deprived of blood. Many individuals, however, lack one of the components of the circle of Willis. In these individuals, a functional "circle" may not be achieved, resulting in incomplete cerebral perfusion by the surviving system.

The second site for communication is where the terminal ends of the cerebral arteries anastomose on the dorsal convexity of the cerebral hemisphere (Figure 3–5). These

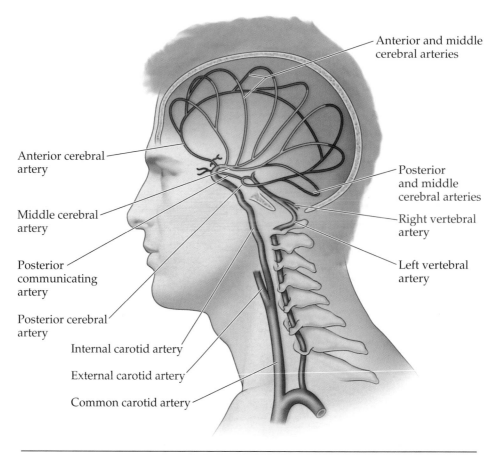

FIGURE 3–5 Paths for collateral blood supply and the course of the major cerebral arteries over the lateral and medial cortical surfaces. Anastomotic channels between the middle and anterior cerebral arteries, and the middle and posterior cerebral arteries are depicted. The left side of the circle of Willis is shown: anterior communicating artery (purple; unlabeled), posterior communicating artery, and posterior cerebral artery (see also Figure 3–1).

interconnections occur between branches only when they are located on the cortical surface, not when the artery has penetrated the brain. When a major artery becomes compromised, these anastomoses limit the extent of damage. For example, if a branch of the posterior cerebral artery becomes occluded, tissue with compromised blood supply in the occipital lobe may be rescued by collateral circulation from the middle cerebral artery that connects anastomotically with the blocked vessel. This collateral circulation can rescue the gray matter of the cerebral cortex. In contrast, little collateral circulation exists in the white matter.

Although collateral circulation provides the cerebral cortex with a safety margin during arterial occlusion, the dorsal anastomotic network that provides such insurance also creates a vulnerability. When systemic blood pressure is reduced, the region served by this network is particularly susceptible to ischemia because such anastomoses occur at the terminal ends of the arteries, regions where perfusion is lowest. The peripheral borders of the territory supplied by major vessels are termed **border zones,** and an infarction occurring in these regions is termed a **border zone infarct.**

Deep Branches of the Anterior and Posterior Circulations Supply Subcortical Structures

The arterial supply of the diencephalon, basal ganglia, and internal capsule derives from both the anterior and posterior circulations (Figures 3–6 and 3–7; Table 3–1). This supply is complex, and there are many individual variations. As discussed, the branches supplying these structures emerge from the proximal portions of the cerebral arteries or directly from the internal carotid artery. The superior half of the **internal capsule** is supplied primarily by branches of the middle cerebral artery (Figure 3–7). The inferior half of the anterior limb and genu of the internal capsule is supplied primarily by the anterior cerebral artery and the posterior limb, by the anterior choroidal artery (see Figures 4–5 and 4–6). The **basal ganglia** receive their arterial blood supply from the anterior and middle cerebral arteries and the anterior choroidal artery (Figure 3–6). Many of the proximal branches of the anterior and middle cerebral arteries are also termed the **lenticulostriate arteries.** The **thalamus** is nourished by branches of the posterior cerebral and posterior communicating arteries. The

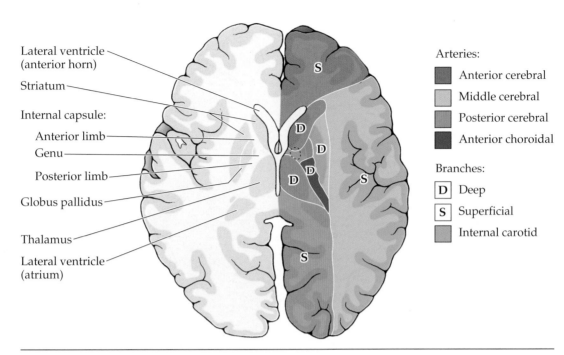

FIGURE 3–6 The arterial circulation of deep cerebral structures is illustrated in schematic horizontal section. Distributions of deep and superficial branches of the cerebral arteries are shown.

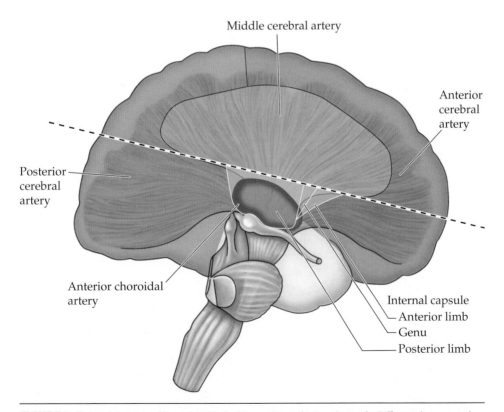

FIGURE 3–7 Arterial supply of the subcortical white matter and internal capsule. Different dorsoventral levels of the internal capsule and limbs receive their arterial supply from different cerebral arteries. The dashed line indicates the plane of the horizontal section in Figure 3–6. The territories supplied by each cerebral artery are shown.

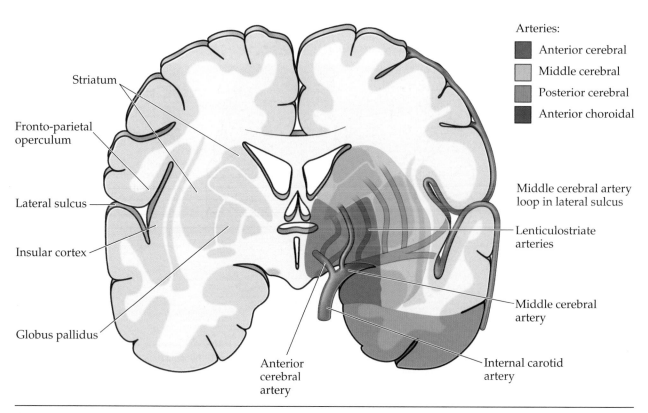

Arteries:

- ■ Anterior cerebral
- ■ Middle cerebral
- ■ Posterior cerebral
- ■ Anterior choroidal

FIGURE 3–8 The course of the middle cerebral artery through the lateral sulcus and along the insular and opercular surfaces of the cerebral cortex is shown in a schematic coronal section. (Adapted from DeArmond SJ, Fusco MM, Dewey MM. *Structure of the Human Brain,* 3rd ed. Oxford University Press; 1989).

hypothalamus is fed by branches of the anterior and posterior cerebral arteries and the two communicating arteries.

Different Functional Areas of the Cerebral Cortex Are Supplied by Different Cerebral Arteries

The cerebral cortex is supplied by the distal, or cortical, branches of the anterior, middle, and posterior cerebral arteries (Figure 3–8 and Figure 3–4). The **anterior cerebral artery** is C-shaped, like many parts of the cerebral hemispheres (see Box 1–2). It originates where the internal carotid artery

bifurcates and courses within the sagittal fissure and around the rostral end (termed the *genu*; see Figure 1–11B) of the corpus callosum (Figure 3–4B). Knowledge of the approximate boundaries of the cortical regions supplied by the different cerebral arteries helps explain the functional disturbances that follow vascular obstruction, or other pathology, of the cerebral vessels. As its gross distribution would suggest, the anterior cerebral artery supplies the dorsal and medial portions of the frontal and parietal lobes (Figure 3–4B).

The **middle cerebral artery** supplies blood to the lateral convexity of the cortex (Figure 3–4A). The middle cerebral artery begins at the bifurcation of the internal carotid artery

Box 3–1

Radiological Imaging of Cerebral Vasculature

Cerebral vessels can be observed in vivo using **cerebral angiography.** First, radiopaque material is injected into either the anterior or the posterior arterial system. Then a series of skull x-ray images are taken in rapid repetition as the material circulates. Images obtained while the radiopaque material is within cerebral arteries are called **angiograms** or **arteriograms.** Images can also be obtained later, after the radiopaque substance has reached the cerebral veins or the dural sinuses **(venograms).** The entire course of the internal carotid artery is shown in cerebral angiograms in Figure 3–9. Images can be obtained from different angles

with respect to the cranium. Two views are common—from the front (frontal projection, Figure 3–9A) and from the side (lateral projection, Figure 3–9B). The lateral view shows the C-shape of the anterior cerebral artery (and its branches). The medial-to-lateral course of the middle cerebral artery is revealed in the frontal view.

The rostrocaudal course of the middle cerebral artery, from the point at which it enters the lateral sulcus to the point at which it emerges and distributes over the lateral surface of the cerebral cortex, is revealed in the lateral view (Figure 3–9B). The middle cerebral artery forms loops at the dorsal junction of the insular cortex and the opercular surface of the frontal and parietal lobes (see Figure 3–8). These loops serve as radiological landmarks that aid in estimating the position of the brain in relation to the skull. Figure 3–10 shows the posterior circulation viewed from a lateral perspective. Figure 3–11 shows the two vertebral arteries joining to form the basilar artery and the subsequent bifurcation of the basilar artery into the two posterior cerebral arteries.

Cerebral angiography involves intravascular injection of radiopaque material. The process of injecting this material, and the material itself, can produce neurological complications; therefore, its use is not without risk. Magnetic resonance imaging has also been applied to the study of brain vasculature because it can detect motion of water molecules. This application, termed **magnetic resonance angiography** (MRA), selectively images blood in motion. The MRA scan in Figure 3–12 is a dorsoventral reconstruction (ie, as if looking up from the bottom). The posterior communicating artery is present only on the left side. This patient does not have a complete circle of Willis. The entire cerebral circulation can be reconstructed from the locations of cerebral arteries or veins at multiple levels.

and takes an indirect course through the lateral sulcus (Figure 3–8), along the surface of the **insular cortex,** and over the inner opercular surfaces of the frontal, temporal, and parietal lobes. It finally emerges on the lateral convexity. This complex configuration of the middle cerebral artery can be seen on radiological images of brain vasculature (Box 3–1).

The **posterior cerebral artery,** originating where the basilar artery bifurcates (Figure 3–2 and Figure 3–3A), courses around the lateral margin of the midbrain (Figure 3–4B). This artery supplies the occipital lobe and portions of the medial and inferior temporal lobes (Figure 3–4B).

Cerebral Veins Drain Into the Dural Sinuses

Venous drainage of the cerebral hemispheres is provided by superficial and deep cerebral veins (Figure 3–13). Superficial veins, arising from the cerebral cortex and underlying white matter, are variable in distribution. Among the more prominent and consistent are the superior anastomotic vein, lying across the parietal lobe, and the inferior anastomotic vein, on the surface of the temporal lobe. The **deep cerebral veins,** such as the internal cerebral vein (Figure 3–13, inset), drain the more interior portions of the white matter, including the basal ganglia and parts of the diencephalon. Many deep cerebral veins drain into the **great cerebral vein (of Galen)** (Figure 3–13, inset, and Figure 3–15).

Drainage of blood from the central nervous system into the major vessels emptying into the heart—the systemic circulation—is achieved through either a direct or an indirect path. Spinal cord and caudal medullary veins drain directly, through a network of veins and plexuses, into the systemic circulation. By contrast, the rest of the central nervous system drains by an indirect path: The veins first empty into the **dural sinuses** before returning

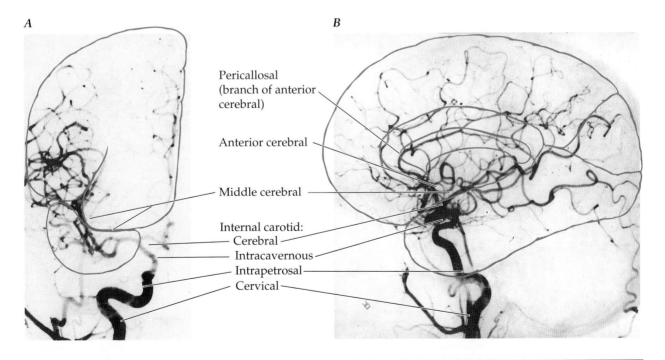

A

B

Pericallosal (branch of anterior cerebral)

Anterior cerebral

Middle cerebral

Internal carotid:
Cerebral
Intracavernous
Intrapetrosal
Cervical

FIGURE 3–9 Cerebral angiograms of the anterior circulation are shown in frontal (**A**) and lateral (**B**) projections. Overlaying each angiogram is a schematic drawing of the cerebral hemispheres, showing the approximate location of surface landmarks in relation to the arteries. (Angiograms courtesy of Dr. Neal Rutledge, University of Texas at Austin.)

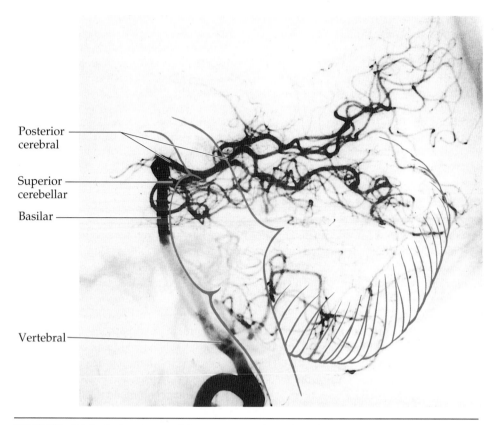

FIGURE 3–10 Cerebral angiogram of the posterior circulation (lateral projection). The overlay drawing is a schematic illustration of the brain stem and cerebellum in relation to the distribution of the posterior circulation. (Angiogram courtesy of Dr. Neal Rutledge, University of Texas at Austin.)

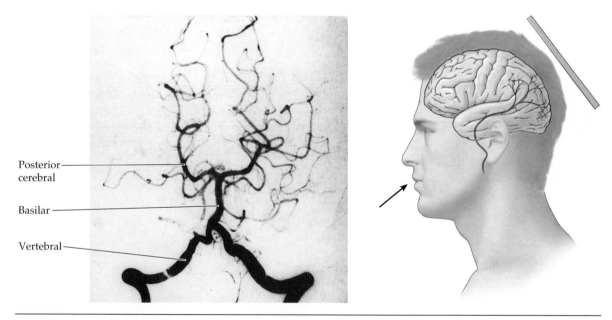

FIGURE 3–11 Cerebral angiogram of the posterior circulation (viewed anteriorly and inferiorly). The inset shows the head and selected cerebral vasculature on the left side (vertebral, basilar, and posterior cerebral arteries) in relation to the direction of transmitted x-rays and the imaging plane. (Angiogram courtesy of Dr. Neal Rutledge, University of Texas at Austin.)

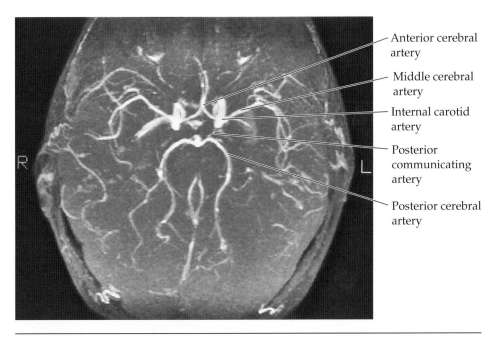

Anterior cerebral artery

Middle cerebral artery

Internal carotid artery

Posterior communicating artery

Posterior cerebral artery

FIGURE 3–12 Magnetic resonance angiogram. This image is a reconstruction of arteries of the anterior and posterior circulations as if viewed from below. As with conventional angiograms, magnetic resonance angiograms are two-dimensional representations of the three-dimensional arterial system.

blood to the systemic circulation. The dural sinuses function as low-pressure channels for venous blood flow back to the systemic circulation. They are located within layers of the dura. The portion of the dura mater overlying the cerebral hemispheres and brain stem contains two separate layers: (1) an outer periosteal layer, which is attached to the bone, and (2) an inner meningeal layer, which apposes the arachnoid (Figure 3–14A, B). The dural sinuses are located between the periosteal and meningeal layers of the dura (Figure 3–14A, B).

The superficial cerebral veins drain into the superior and inferior sagittal sinuses (Figure 3–15A). The **superior sagittal sinus** runs along the midline at the superior margin of the falx cerebri. The **inferior sagittal sinus** courses along the inferior margin of the falx cerebri just above the corpus callosum. The inferior sagittal sinus, together with the great cerebral vein (of Galen), returns venous blood to the **straight** (sometimes called *rectus*) **sinus** (Figure 3–15). At the occipital pole, the superior sagittal sinus and the straight sinus join to form the two **transverse sinuses.** Finally, these sinuses drain into the **sigmoid sinuses** (Figure 3–15B), which return blood to the internal jugular veins. The cavernous sinus, into which drain the ophthalmic and facial veins, is also illustrated in Figure 3–15B.

Veins of the midbrain drain into the great cerebral vein (Figure 3–13, Figure 3–15A), which empties into the straight sinus, whereas the pons and rostral medulla drain into the **superior petrosal sinus** (Figure 3–15B). Cerebellar veins drain into the great cerebral vein and the superior petrosal sinus.

The Blood-Brain Barrier Isolates the Chemical Environment of the Central Nervous System From That of the Rest of the Body

The intravascular compartment is isolated from the extracellular compartment of the central nervous system (Figure 3–16A). This feature, the **blood-brain barrier,** was discovered when intravenous dye injection stained most tissues and organs of the body but not the brain. This permeability barrier protects the brain from neuroactive compounds in the blood as well as rapid changes in the ionic constituents of the blood that can affect neuronal excitability.

The blood-brain barrier results from two unique characteristics of endothelial cells in the capillaries of the brain and spinal cord (Figure 3–16A). First, in peripheral capillaries, endothelial cells have fenestrations (pores) that allow large molecules to flow into the extracellular space. Moreover, the intercellular spaces between adjacent endothelial cells are leaky. In contrast, in central nervous system capillaries, adjacent endothelial cells are tightly joined, preventing movement of compounds into the extracellular compartment of the central nervous system (Figure 3–16A). Second, there is little transcellular movement of compounds from intravascular to extracellular compartments in the central nervous system because the endothelial cells lack the required transport mechanisms. Moreover, relatively nonselective transport may occur by pinocytosis in peripheral but not central nervous system capillaries.

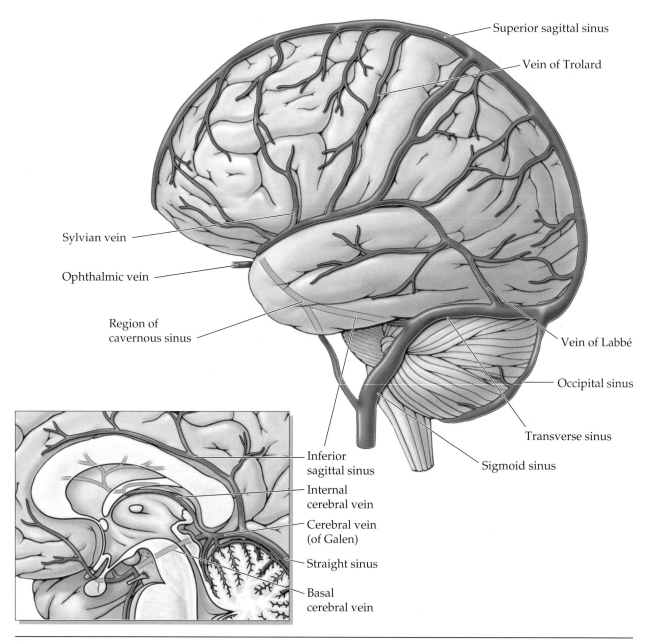

FIGURE 3–13 Lateral view of the brain, showing major superficial veins and the dural sinuses. Inset shows veins on midline.

Although most of the central nervous system is protected by the blood-brain barrier, eight brain structures lack a blood-brain barrier. These structures are close to the midline, and because they are closely associated with the ventricular system, they are collectively termed **circumventricular organs** (Figure 3–16B). At each of these structures, either neurosecretory products are secreted into the blood or local neurons detect blood-borne compounds as part of a mechanism for regulating the body's internal environment. One circumventricular organ, the area postrema (Figure 3–16B), is important for trigger vomiting in response to circulating blood-borne chemicals. A band of

specialized glial cells with tight junctions is present that forms a blood-brain barrier between the area postrema and the rest of the medulla.

Cerebrospinal Fluid Serves Many Diverse Functions

Cerebrospinal fluid fills the ventricles. It also fills the subarachnoid space and thus bathes the external brain surface. Together, the ventricles and subarachnoid space contain approximately 140 mL of cerebrospinal fluid, of which 25 mL are in the

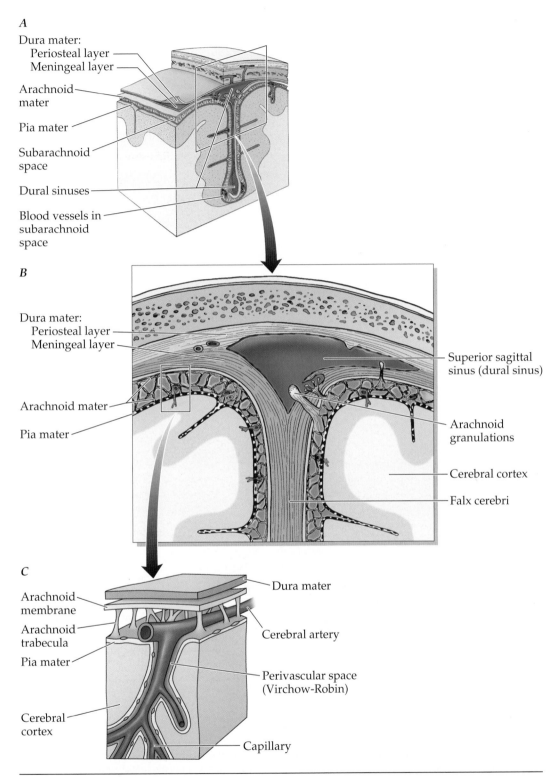

A

Dura mater:
  Periosteal layer
  Meningeal layer
Arachnoid mater
Pia mater
Subarachnoid space
Dural sinuses
Blood vessels in subarachnoid space

B

Dura mater:
  Periosteal layer
  Meningeal layer

Arachnoid mater
Pia mater

Superior sagittal sinus (dural sinus)

Arachnoid granulations

Cerebral cortex

Falx cerebri

C

Arachnoid membrane
Arachnoid trabecula
Pia mater

Cerebral cortex

Dura mater

Cerebral artery

Perivascular space (Virchow-Robin)

Capillary

FIGURE 3–14 Meningeal layers. **A.** Low magnification view of the three meningeal layers: pia mater, arachnoid mater, and dura mater. **B.** Higher magnification view of the boxed region in **A** showing a schematic cut through the superior sagittal sinus, illustrating the arachnoid granulations and collections of arachnoid villi containing the unidirectional valves through which cerebrospinal fluid passes to the venous circulation. **C.** Arterial invagination of brain in relation to the meninges and associated spaces. (**B,** Adapted with permission from Parent A. *Carpenter's Human Neuroanatomy,* 9th ed. Williams & Wilkins; 1996. **C,** Adapted with permission from Parent A. *Carpenter's Human Neuroanatomy,* 9th ed. Williams & Wilkins; 1996.)

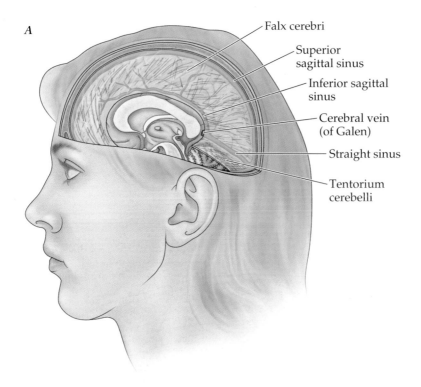

A

Falx cerebri

Superior sagittal sinus

Inferior sagittal sinus

Cerebral vein (of Galen)

Straight sinus

Tentorium cerebelli

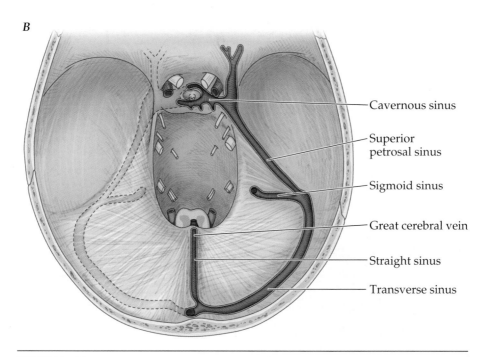

B

Cavernous sinus

Superior petrosal sinus

Sigmoid sinus

Great cerebral vein

Straight sinus

Transverse sinus

FIGURE 3–15 Falx cerebri and superior sagittal sinus from a lateral perspective (**A**). **B.** View of cranial cavity with the brain removed showing the return of blood from the sinuses to the venous system.

ventricles and the remaining in the subarachnoid space. Intra-ventricular pressure is normally around 10–15 mm Hg.

Cerebrospinal fluid serves at least three essential functions. First, it provides physical support for the brain, which floats within the fluid. Cerebrospinal fluid cushions the brain from physical shocks. Second, it serves an excretory function and regulates the chemical environment of the central nervous system. Because the brain has no lymphatic system, water-soluble metabolites, which have limited ability to cross the blood-brain barrier, diffuse from the brain into the cerebrospinal fluid. Third, it acts as a channel for chemical communication within the central nervous system. Neurochemicals released by neurons can

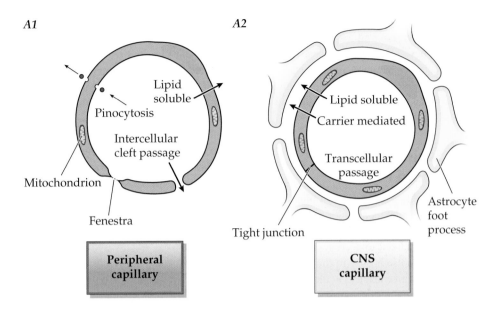

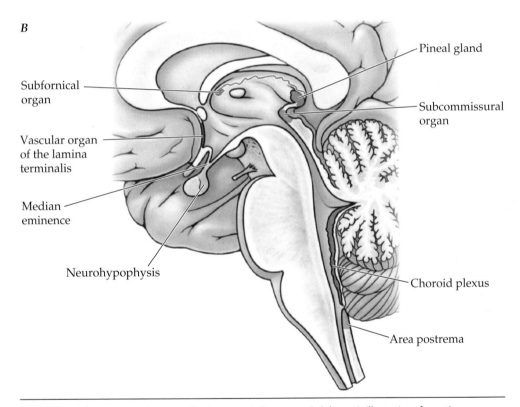

FIGURE 3–16 Blood-brain barrier and circumventricular organs. **A.** Schematic illustration of a section through a peripheral (**A1**) and central nervous system (**A2**) capillary. There is less restricted transport across the endothelium of the peripheral than central capillary. **B.** Circumventricular organs are brain regions that do not have a blood-brain barrier. The locations of the eight circumventricular organs are shown on a view of the midsagittal brain: neurohypophysis (also termed posterior lobe of pituitary gland), median eminence, vascular organ of the lamina terminalis, subfornical organ, pineal gland, subcommissural organ, choroid plexus, and area postrema. Note that all circumventricular organs are located centrally, in close association with the components of the ventricular system.

enter the cerebrospinal fluid and be taken up by cells on the ventricular floor and walls. Moreover, once in the cerebrospinal fluid, these compounds also have relatively free access to neural tissue adjacent to the ventricles because, in contrast to the blood-brain barrier, most of the ventricular lining presents no barrier between the cerebrospinal fluid compartment and the extracellular compartment of the brain.

Most of the Cerebrospinal Fluid Is Produced by the Choroid Plexus

Cerebrospinal fluid is secreted mainly by the **choroid plexus.** The cellular constituents of choroid plexus are blood vessels and pia, which form the core of the choroid plexus, and the **choroid epithelium,** which is specialized to secrete cerebrospinal fluid. The choroid plexus is present only in the ventricles; in the roof of the third and fourth ventricles. In the lateral ventricles, the choroid plexus is located in the ventricular roof and floor. A barrier imposed by the choroidal epithelium prevents the transport of materials from blood into the cerebrospinal fluid. This is the **blood–cerebrospinal fluid barrier,** analogous to the blood-brain barrier. The choroidal epithelium is innervated by autonomic fibers, which serve a regulatory function. For example, denervation of the sympathetic fibers produces hydrocephalus in animals. A second blood–cerebrospinal fluid barrier exists between the arachnoid and the dural blood vessels.

The rest of the cerebrospinal fluid is secreted by brain capillaries. This extrachoroidal source of cerebrospinal fluid enters the ventricular system through ependymal cells, the ciliated cuboidal epithelial cells that line the ventricles. Total cerebrospinal fluid production by both sources is approximately 500 mL per day. Although the principal function of the choroid plexus is cerebrospinal fluid secretion, the plexus also has a reabsorptive function. The choroid plexus can eliminate from the cerebrospinal fluid a variety of compounds introduced into the ventricles.

Cerebrospinal Fluid Circulates Throughout the Ventricles and Subarachnoid Space

Cerebrospinal fluid produced by the choroid plexus in the lateral ventricles (Figure 3–17) flows through the interventricular foramina and mixes with cerebrospinal fluid produced in the third ventricle. The lateral ventricle is a C-shaped structure, as are many deep neuronal regions of the cerebral hemispheres (see Box 1–2). From the lateral ventricles, CSF flows through the cerebral aqueduct and into the fourth ventricle, another major site for cerebrospinal fluid production because the choroid plexus is also located there. Three apertures in the roof of the fourth ventricle drain cerebrospinal fluid from the ventricular system into the subarachnoid space: the **foramen of Magendie,** located on the midline, and the two **foramina of Luschka,** located at the lateral margins of the fourth ventricle (Figure 3–17, inset).

The subarachnoid space is dilated in certain locations, termed **cisterns;** cerebrospinal fluid pools here. Five prominent cisterns are located on the midline: (1) the **interpeduncular cistern,** between the basis pedunculi on the ventral midbrain surface, (2) the **quadrigeminal cistern,** dorsal to the superior and inferior colliculi (which are also called the quadrigeminal bodies), (3) the **pontine cistern,** at the ventral portion of the pontomedullary junction, (4) the **cisterna magna,** dorsal to the medulla, and (5) the **lumbar cistern,** in the caudal vertebral canal. The subarachnoid space also contains the blood vessels of the central nervous system (Figure 3–18B). Blood vessels penetrate the brain together with the pia, creating a perivascular space between the vessels and pia for a short distance, and a path for CSF flow from the subarachnoid space to interstitial spaces within the brain and spinal cord. These spaces, termed the *Virchow-Robin spaces,* contain cerebrospinal fluid (Figure 3–17B).

Cerebrospinal Fluid Is Drawn From the Lumbar Cistern

Cerebrospinal fluid can be safely withdrawn from the lumbar cistern, without risking spinal cord damage. This can be understood by considering how the caudal vertebral column and spinal cord develop. Throughout the first 3 months of development, the spinal cord grows at about the same rate as the vertebral column (Figure 3–18A). During this period, the spinal cord occupies the entire **vertebral canal,** the space within the vertebral column. The dorsal and ventral roots associated with each segment pass directly through the intervertebral foramina to reach their target structures. Later, the growth of the vertebral column exceeds that of the spinal cord. In the adult, the most caudal spinal cord segment is located at the level of the **first lumbar vertebra.** This differential growth produces the **lumbar cistern,** an enlargement of the subarachnoid space in the caudal portion of the spinal canal (Figure 3–18B). The dorsal and ventral roots from the lumbar and sacral segments, which subserve sensation and movement of the legs, travel within the lumbar cistern before exiting the vertebral canal (Figure 3–18B). These roots resemble a horse's tail in gross dissection, hence the name **cauda equina.** Cerebrospinal fluid can be withdrawn from the lumbar cistern without risk of damaging the spinal cord by inserting a needle through the intervertebral space between the third and fourth (or fourth and fifth) vertebrae (Figure 3–18B). The roots are displaced by the needle rather than being pierced. This procedure is known as a **spinal** or **lumbar tap.**

The Dural Sinuses Provide the Return Path for Cerebrospinal Fluid

Cerebrospinal fluid passes from the subarachnoid space to the venous blood through specialized structures termed **arachnoid villi.** Arachnoid villi are microscopic evaginations of the arachnoid mater that protrude into the **dural sinuses** as well

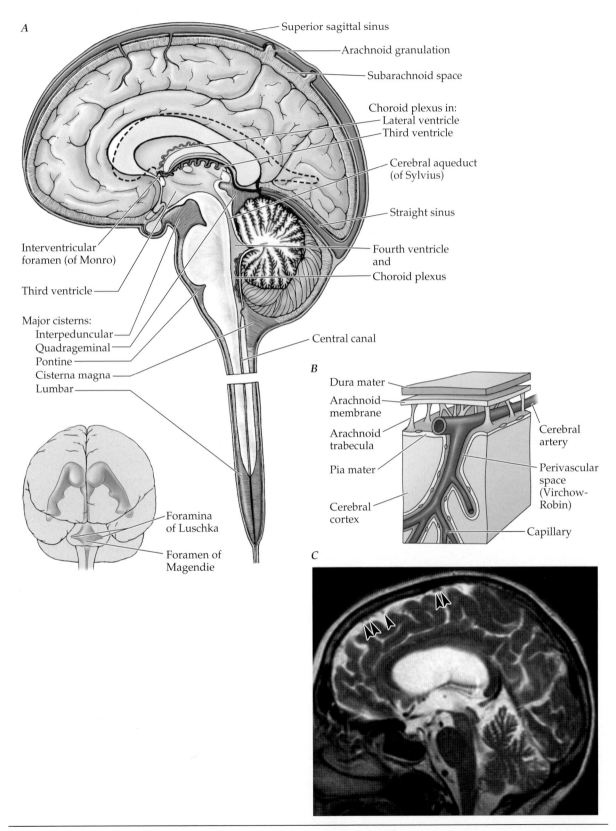

FIGURE 3–17 **A.** The subarachnoid space and ventricular system are shown on a view of the midsagittal surface of the central nervous system. (Adapted from Nicholls JG et al. *From Neuron to Brain*. Sinauer Associates Inc., 3rd ed. Publishers; 1992.) The inset (below, left) shows the locations of the foramina through which cerebrospinal fluid exits the ventricular system. **B.** The relationship between the meningeal layers and the compartment in which CSF flows, which is between the pia and arachnoid membrane. **C.** T2-weighted MRI showing the locations of arachnoid granulations (arrowheads). (**B,** Adapted with permission from Parent A. *Carpenter's Human Neuroanatomy,* 9th ed. Williams & Wilkins; 1996. C, Adapted from Brodbelt A, Stoodley M. CSF pathways: A review. *Br J Neurosurg.* 2007;21[5]:510-520.)

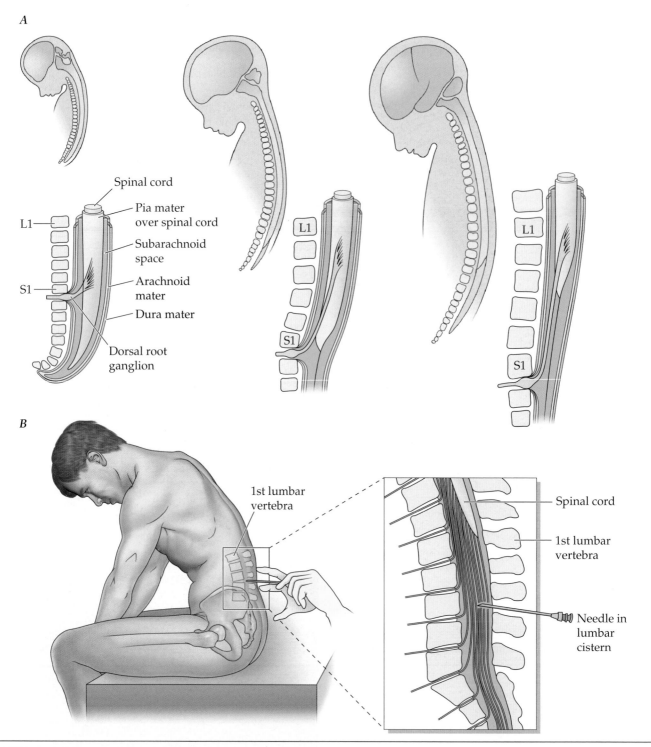

FIGURE 3-18 The lumbar cistern forms because the vertebral column grows in length more than the spinal cord. **A.** Side view of the lumbosacral spinal cord and vertebral column at three developmental stages: 3 months, 5 months, and in the newborn. The insets show the fetus at these stages. **B.** Schematic showing principle of withdrawal of cerebrospinal fluid from the lumbar cistern (lumbar puncture). The needle is inserted into the subarachnoid space of the lumbar cistern. The view on the right shows the relationship between the needle and the roots in the cistern. Note that the lumbar puncture is performed with the patient lying on his or her side. In this figure, the patient is sitting upright to simplify visualization of the procedure and comparison with the anatomy of the vertebrae. (**A,** Adapted from House EL, Pansky B, and Siegel A. *A Systematic Approach to Neuroscience,* 3rd ed. New York, NY: McGraw-Hill; 1979. **B,** Adapted from House EL, Pansky B, Siegel A. *A Systematic Approach to Neuroscience.* 3rd ed. New York, NY: McGraw-Hill; 1979.)

as directly into certain veins. The cerebrospinal fluid flows through a system of large vacuoles in the arachnoid cells of the villi and through an extracellular path between cells of the villi; they are not actually valves. Numerous clusters of arachnoid villi are present over the dorsal (superior) convexity of the cerebral hemispheres in the superior sagittal sinus, where they form a macroscopic structure called the **arachnoid granulations** (Figures 4–13B and 4–16). The arachnoid granulations can be imaged on MRI (Figure 3–17C). The arachnoid villi are also present where the spinal nerves exit the spinal dural sac. These villi direct the flow of cerebrospinal fluid into the radicular veins.

Summary

Arterial Supply of the Spinal Cord and Brain Stem

The arterial supply of the spinal cord is provided by the *vertebral* (Figure 3–3A) *and radicular arteries.* The brain is supplied by the *internal carotid arteries* (the *anterior circulation)* and the *vertebral arteries,* which join at the ponto-medullary junction to form the *basilar artery* (collectively termed the *posterior circulation)* (Figure 3–2). The brain stem and cerebellum receive blood only from the posterior system (Figure 3–3 and Figure 3–4B; Table 3–1). The medulla receives blood directly from small branches of the *vertebral arteries* and from the *spinal arteries* and the *posterior inferior cerebellar artery (PICA)* (Figure 3–3B3,4). The pons is supplied by *paramedian* and *short circumferential branches* of the *basilar artery.* Two major long circumferential branches are the *anterior inferior cerebellar artery (AICA)* and the *superior cerebellar artery* (Figure 3–3B2). The midbrain receives its arterial supply primarily from the *posterior cerebral artery* as well as from the basilar artery (Figure 3–3B1). The PICA supplies the caudal cerebellum, and the AICA and superior cerebellar artery supply the rostral cerebellum (Figure 3–4B).

Stroke and Collateral Circulation

Neural tissue depends on a continuous supply of arterial blood. Cessation or reduction of the arterial supply to an area can produce *ischemia* and an *infarction.* A brief interruption in blood flow produces a *transient ischemic attack (TIA),* or temporary loss of function of the affected region. Persistent loss of blood flow by arterial occlusion produces an *ischemic stroke.* When an artery ruptures, a *hemorrhagic stroke* occurs. An *aneurysm,* which is a ballooning of an artery, can rupture to produce a hemorrhagic stroke. The anterior and posterior systems are interconnected by two networks of arteries that can provide redundant arterial supply, or *collateral circulation:* (1) the *circle of Willis*—which is formed by the anterior, middle, and posterior *cerebral arteries;* the *posterior communicating arteries;* and the *anterior communicating artery* (Figure 3–2); and (2) terminal branches of the cerebral arteries, which anastomose on the superior convexity of the cerebral cortex (Figure 3–5).

Arterial Supply of the Diencephalon and Cerebral Hemispheres

The diencephalon and cerebral hemispheres are supplied by the *anterior* and *posterior circulations* (Figure 3–2 and Figures 3–4 to 3–8). The cerebral cortex receives its blood supply from the three cerebral arteries: the *anterior and middle cerebral arteries,* which are part of the anterior circulation, and the *posterior cerebral artery,* which is part of the posterior circulation (Figure 3–2). The diencephalon, basal ganglia, and internal capsule receive blood from branches of the *internal carotid artery,* the three *cerebral arteries,* and the *posterior communicating artery* (Figure 3–2; Table 4–1).

Venous Drainage

The venous drainage of the spinal cord and caudal medulla is direct to the systemic circulation. By contrast, veins draining the cerebral hemispheres, diencephalon, midbrain, pons, cerebellum, and rostral medulla (Figure 3–13) drain into the *dural sinuses* (Figures 3–14 and 3–15). The major dural sinuses are as follows: *superior sagittal, inferior sagittal, straight, transverse, sigmoid, superior,* and *inferior petrosal.*

Blood-Brain Barrier

The internal environment of most of the central nervous system is protected from circulating neuroactive agents in blood by the *blood-brain barrier* (Figure 3–16A). This barrier is formed by a number of specializations in the *capillary endothelium* of the central nervous system. Brain regions without a blood-brain barrier, termed the *circumventricular organs* (Figure 3–16B), include the (1) *area postrema* in the medulla, (2) *subcommissural organ,* (3) *subfornical organ,* (4) *vascular organ of the lamina terminalis,* (5) *median eminence,* (6) *neurohypophysis,* (7) *choroid plexus,* and (8) *pineal gland.*

Production and Circulation of Cerebrospinal Fluid

Most of the cerebrospinal fluid is produced by the *choroid plexus,* which is located in the *ventricles* (Figure 3–17). It exits from the ventricular system, through foramina in the fourth ventricle—the two *foramina of Luschka* (located laterally) and the *foramen of Magendie (located on the midline)*—directly into the *subarachnoid space.* Cerebrospinal fluid pools in cisterns of the subarachnoid space over the brain and caudal to the spinal cord (Figure 3–18). Cerebrospinal fluid passes into the *dural sinuses* (Figure 3–14) through unidirectional valves termed *arachnoid villi* clustered in the *arachnoid granulations* (Figure 3–17).

Selected Readings

Laterra J, Goldstein GW. The blood-brain barrier, choroid plexus, and cerebrospinal fluid. In: Kandel ER, Schwartz JH, Jessell TM, Siegelbaum SA, and Hudspeth AJ, eds. *Principles of Neural Science.* 5th ed. New York, NY: McGraw-Hill, in press.

References

Abbott NJ, Ronnback L, Hansson E. Astrocyte-endothelial interactions at the blood-brain barrier. *Nat Rev Neurosci.* 2006;7(1):41-53.

Bourque CW. Central mechanisms of osmosensation and systemic osmoregulation. *Nat Rev Neurosci.* 2008;9(7): 519-531.

Brodbelt A, Stoodley M. CSF pathways: A review. *Br J Neurosurg.* 2007;21(5):510-520.

Choi JH, Mohr JP. Brain arteriovenous malformations in adults. *Lancet Neurol.* 2005;4:299.

Davson H, Keasley W, Segal MB. *Physiology and Pathophysiology of the Cerebrospinal Fluid.* New York, NY: Churchill Livingstone; 1987.

Duvernoy HM. *The Superficial Veins of the Human Brain.* Heidelberg, Germany: Springer-Verlag; 1975.

Duvernoy HM. *The Human Brain Stem and Cerebellum: Surface, Structure, Vascularization, and Three-dimensional Sectional Anatomy with MRI.* Vienna, Austria: Springer-Verlag; 1995.

Duvernoy HM. *Human Brain Stem Vessels: Including the Pineal Gland and Information on Brain Stem Infarction.* Springer; 1999.

Fisher CM. Modern concepts of cerebrovascular disease. In: Meyer JS, ed. *The Anatomy and Pathology of the Cerebral Vasculature.* Spectrum Publications; 1975:1-41.

Fishman RT. *Cerebrospinal Fluid in Diseases of the Nervous System.* 2nd ed. Saunders; 1992.

Gross PM. Morphology and physiology of capillary systems in subregions of the subfornical organ and area postrema. *Can J Physiol Pharmacol.* 1991;69(7):1010-1025.

Karibe H, Shimizu H, Tominaga T, Koshu K, Yoshimoto T. Diffusion-weighted magnetic resonance imaging in the early evaluation of corticospinal tract injury to predict functional motor outcome in patients with deep intra-cerebral hemorrhage. *J Neurosurg.* 2000;92:58-63.

McKinley MJ, Clarke IJ, Oldfield BJ. Circumventricular organs. In: Paxinos G, ed. *The Human Nervous System.* London: Elsevier; 2004:563-591.

McKinley MJ, McAllen RM, Davern P, et al. The sensory circumventricular organs of the mammalian brain. *Adv Anat Embryol Cell Biol.* 2003;172:III-XII, 1-122.

Noda M. The subfornical organ, a specialized sodium channel, and the sensing of sodium levels in the brain. *Neuroscientist.* 2006;12(1):80-91.

Price CJ, Hoyda TD, Ferguson AV. The area postrema: A brain monitor and integrator of systemic autonomic state. *Neuroscientist.* 2008;14(2):182-194.

Ropper AH, Samuels MA. Cerebrovascular diseases. In: *Adams & Victor's Principles of Neurology.* 9th ed. McGraw-Hill; 2009.

Savitz SI, Caplan LR. Vertebrobasilar disease. *N Engl J Med.* 2005;352:2618.

Scremin OU. Cerebral vascular system. In: Paxinos G, Mai JK, eds. *The Human Nervous System.* London: Elsevier; 2004:1326-1348.

Segal MB. The choroid plexuses and the barriers between the blood and the cerebrospinal fluid. *Cell Mol Neurobiol.* 2000;20:183-196.

Smith WS, English JD, Johnston SC. Cerebrovascular diseases. In: Fauci AS, Braunwald E, Kasper D, et al., eds. *Harrison's Principles of Internal Medicine.* New York, NY: McGraw-Hill; 2008.

Study Questions

1. Which of the following best completes the following analogy: Anterior circulation is to posterior circulation, as
   A. anterior cerebral hemispheres, basal ganglia, thalamus, ventral brain stem, and ventral spinal cord are to the posterior cerebral hemispheres, cerebellum, dorsal brain stem, and dorsal spinal cord
   B. internal carotid artery is to the vertebral and basilar arteries
   C. vertebral and basilar arteries are to the internal carotid artery
   D. anterior inferior cerebellar artery is to the posterior inferior cerebral artery

2. Which of the following statements best describes the normal path blood takes from one vertebral artery to the left occipital lobe?
   A. Basilar artery, left posterior cerebral artery
   B. Basilar artery, left posterior communicating artery, left middle cerebral artery
   C. Basilar artery, left superior cerebellar artery, left posterior cerebral artery
   D. Left posterior inferior cerebellar artery, left posterior cerebral artery

3. Which of the following arteries is NOT a branch of the internal carotid artery?
   A. Posterior inferior cerebellar artery
   B. Ophthalmic artery
   C. Anterior choroidal artery
   D. Posterior communicating artery

4. Which of the following best completes the analogy about cerebral arterial distributions:
   The middle cerebral artery is to the anterior cerebral artery, as
   A. the basal ganglia is to the thalamus
   B. the inferior frontal lobule is to the occipital pole
   C. the cingulate gyrus is to the superior temporal gyrus
   D. the lateral postcentral gyrus is to the medial postcentral gyrus

5. Which description of the brain stem arterial distributions is most accurate?
   A. Arterial branches supply pie-shaped wedges of tissue, beginning at dorsal midline and extending circumferentially.
   B. Short circumferential branches supply the dorsal brain stem; long circumferential branches supply the ventral brain stem.
   C. Arteries course on the ventral surface and send branches dorsally.
   D. The basilar artery supplies the midline; the vertebral arteries, the next lateral territory; and the cerebellar arteries supplying most laterally.

6. Which arterial interfaces are not locations of collateral circulation?
   A. Anterior cerebral artery and middle cerebral artery
   B. Middle cerebral artery and posterior cerebral artery
   C. Anterior cerebral artery and posterior cerebral artery
   D. Posterior inferior cerebellar artery and vertebral arteries

7. Which of the following arteries supplies part of the posterior limb of the internal capsule?
   A. Anterior choroidal artery
   B. Posterior cerebral artery
   C. Posterior choroidal artery
   D. Ophthalmic artery

8. Lenticulostriate arteries do not supply the
   A. internal capsule
   B. postcentral gyrus
   C. globus pallidus
   D. putamen

9. The course of the anterior cerebral artery is best shown with an arteriogram that provides a
   A. frontal view of the brain
   B. medial or lateral view of the brain
   C. frontal-inferior view of the brain
   D. posterior view of the brain

10. A patient has a subdural hematoma. Which of the following best describes the space within which blood accumulates?
    A. The space between the dura and the arachnoid
    B. The space between the dura and the pia
    C. The space between the dura and the cortex surface
    D. Any space within a part of the central nervous system covered by the dura

11. Which of the following best describes the principal source of cerebrospinal fluid (CSF)?
    A. Choroid plexus in the lateral ventricles
    B. Choroid plexus in the lateral and third ventricles
    C. Choroid plexus in the lateral, third, and fourth ventricles
    D. Choroid plexus in the ventricles and central canal of the spinal cord

12. CSF exits the ventricles through the _____ and then from the subarachnoid space to the venous sinuses through the _____.
    A. foramen of Luschka; foramen of Magendie
    B. foramen of Magendie; foramen of Luschka
    C. foramina of Luschka and Magendie; arachnoid granulations
    D. arachnoid granulations; foramina of Luschka and Magendie

13. A baby was born with hydrocephalus. This likely was caused by constriction of the cerebral aqueduct during early development. In which part of the central nervous system would this constriction have occurred?
    A. Olfactory bulb
    B. Diencephalon
    C. Midbrain
    D. Medulla

14. Which of the following best describes the most likely cause of congenital hydrocephalus?
    A. Most CSF is produced by the choroid plexus. With cerebral aqueduct constriction, CSF continues to be produced. This leads to enlargement of the lateral and third ventricles.
    B. More CSF is produced by the choroid plexus than can be released by the arachnoid granulations.
    C. Production of CSF that comes from nonchoroid plexus sources is increased.
    D. There is enlargement of the subarachnoid space, after CSF exits from the arachnoid granulations.

15. A 38-year-old male suspected of having Guillain-Barré syndrome will have a lumbar tap to sample protein content in CSF. Which of the following best explains why CSF sampling is by lumbar tap?
    A. CSF pools within the subarachnoid space located at the most inferior portion of the central nervous system.
    B. CSF exits from the ventricular system at the caudal terminus of the vertebral column.
    C. The lumbar cistern is the only part of the subarachnoid space in which there is sufficient CSF for sampling.
    D. CSF collects in multiple subarachnoid cisterns. The lumbar cistern is safe to sample because it contains only nerve roots since the caudal termination of the spinal cord is rostral to the lumbar cistern.

SENSORY SYSTEMS

Somatic Sensation: Spinal Mechanosensory Systems

CLINICAL CASE | Neurosyphilis and Loss of Vibration Sense and Limb Proprioception

A 36-year-old man was admitted to the hospital for unsteadiness of gait and several other sensory and motor signs, including pain and limb strength impairments. Sensation to touch, pinprick, and temperature was normal. Perception of vibration and limb position sense were absent. When he was asked to stand upright with his eyes closed, he swayed and lost balance. This is a positive "Romberg sign." His gait was broad based, clumsy, and staggering. MRI of his brain was normal but MRI of his spinal cord showed an intense signal in the dorsal columns, bilaterally (Figure 4–1A), that appeared to be the same as CSF.

The man had an untreated syphilitic infection for 10 or more years. He was diagnosed with neurosyphilis, also called tabes dorsalis, on the basis of several laboratory and neurological tests, including the MRI and sensory loss indicated above. This is the advanced stage of syphilis, when it infects the nervous system.

Try to answer the following questions based on your reading of the chapter, inspection of the images, and consideration of the neurological signs.

1. **What functional system becomes impaired when there is neuronal degeneration in the dorsal columns?**

2. **Why does the patient demonstrate Romberg's sign?**

Key neurological signs and corresponding damaged brain structures

Neurosyphilis

Syphilis is normally treated with penicillin. Left untreated, the infectious agent—the spirochete, *Treponema pallidum*—

infects the nervous system. In time, this can result in dysfunction or degeneration of its neuronal targets. Common target neurons are the dorsal root ganglion sensory neurons, which are important for mechanosensation. Especially vulnerable is limb position sense (or limb proprioception), which is signaled by muscle and joint sensory receptors, and vibration sense, which is signaled by Pacinian corpuscles. At autopsy, tabetic patients can show degeneration of the dorsal columns. This can be revealed by staining histological sections of the spinal cord for myelin. Oligodendrocytes also degenerate in regions where axons have degenerated, therefore showing demyelination (Figure 4–1B). The region of intense signal on the MRI demonstrates damaged dorsal column fibers.

—Continued next page

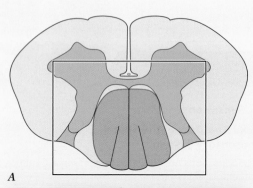

A

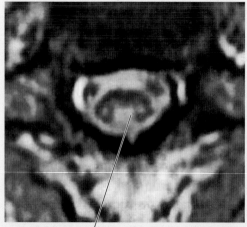

Region of degeneration
in the dorsal columns

B

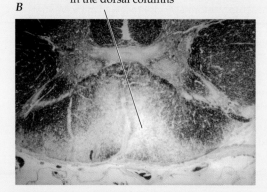

FIGURE 4–1. Degenerative changes in the dorsal columns with neurosyphilis. **A.** MRI (T2-weighted) at the level of the second thoracic vertebra. **B.** A section through the spinal cord of a person that had neurosyphilis while alive. This is a myelin-stained section. The white regions in the dorsal column correspond to demyelination because of axonal degeneration. A schematic drawing of the spinal cord is shown on top and highlights the degenerated region in the dorsal column (red) and the area of the histological image (box) in B. Note, the dorsal spinal cord surface is down in these illustrations. (**A,** Reproduced with permission from Stepper F, Schroth G, Sturzenegger M. Neurosyphilis mimicking Miller-Fisher syndrome: a case report and MRI findings. *Neurology*. 1998;51[1]: 269-271.)

Loss of limb proprioception and vibration sense

Both of these senses are mediated by dorsal root ganglion neurons that have a large-diameter axon, which project rostrally within the dorsal columns. In the absence of limb proprioceptive afferents, patients rely on vision to compensate for the loss of sensory awareness of their limbs. This explains the loss of balance when the patient closed his eyes. Touch is preserved in this patient; there may be diminished sensitivity, but this was not tested. Dorsal root ganglion mechanosensory neurons with a small-diameter axon may play more of a role in touch after degeneration of dorsal root ganglion neurons with large-diameter axons. This residual sensation is termed crude touch.

Reference

Stepper F, Schroth G, Sturzenegger M. Neurosyphilis mimicking Miller-Fisher syndrome: A case report and MRI findings. *Neurology*. Jul 1998;51(1):269-271.

The somatic sensory systems mediate our bodily sensations, including mechanical sensations, protective senses, as well as a wide range of visceral sensory experiences. Apart from our basic sensory capabilities—like discriminating textures and shapes of grasped objects or ensuring that we do not become hurt when we hold something too hot—somatic sensations are also critical for many integrative functions. Consider the capacity of touch to quiet the cry of a newborn baby or awaken us from a deep sleep. Somatic sensory information is critical for controlling movements, from the simplest reflexes—such as the stretch or withdrawal reflexes—to fine voluntary movements. Recall how awkward speech and facial muscle control become when sensation of our jaw and lips is blocked by local anesthetic injection in preparation for dental work. Somatic sensations are clinically important: pain typically brings a person to the doctor; touch, vibratory sense, a mechanosensory component, and pin prick are routinely used to probe sensory function in humans suspected of having peripheral nerve or central nervous system damage.

Spinal somatic sensory systems receive information from the limbs, neck, and trunk, while the trigeminal systems receive information from the head. The spinal and trigeminal systems remain distinct as they travel to the cerebral cortex, contacting separate populations of neurons at each processing stage. However, even though the ascending spinal and trigeminal pathways are anatomically distinct, their general organization is remarkably similar.

This and the next two chapters focus on the somatic sensory systems. The first two chapters consider the spinal systems mediating mechanosensation and the protective senses, because they have distinctive anatomical organizations. The third chapter examines the trigeminal and viscerosensory systems. We consider these two somatic sensory functions together because they are both mediated in large part by particular cranial nerves and their key central nervous system processing centers are closely aligned.

In this chapter, somatic sensations and the overall functional organization of the spinal sensory systems are discussed first. Then the regional anatomy of the mechanosensory system is examined at different levels through the nervous system, beginning with the morphology of the somatic sensory receptor neurons and continuing to the cerebral cortex.

Somatic Sensations

The somatic senses consist of many distinct components that can be further subdivided, termed modalities and submodalities. This diversity adds to the richness of somatic sensations (Table 4–1). A somatic sensory submodality is thought to be mediated by a single type of sensory receptor.

Table **4–1** Modalities and submodalities of somatic sensation and afferent fiber groups

Modality and submodality	Receptor type	Fiber diameter (µm)	Group	Myelination
Touch				
Texture/superficial	Meissner's and Merkel's receptors	6-12	A-β (2)	Myelinated
Deep pressure	Mechanoreceptors			
Vibration	Pacinian			
Sensual touch	Mechanoreceptors	0.2-1.5	C	Unmyelinated
Limb proprioception				
Static/dynamic (kinesthesia)	Muscle stretch and tendon force (primary and secondary; Golgi tendon organs)	13-20; 6-12	A-α (1), A-β (2)	Myelinated
Thermal Sense				
Cold	Cold receptors	1-5	A-δ (3), C (4)	Myelinated; unmyelinated
Warmth	Warmth receptors	0.2-1.5		
Pain				
Sharp (pricking; fast)	Nociceptors	1-5	A-δ (3), C (4)	Myelinated; unmyelinated
Dull (burning; slow)		0.2-1.5		Myelinated; unmyelinated
Itch	Pruritic receptor	0.2-1.5	C (4)	Unmyelinated
Visceral sensation				
Blood pressure, chemosensory; ion sensing, etc.	Mechano, thermo, chemoreceptors	Various; not well understood	Various; not well understood	Myelinated; unmyelinated

- **Touch** comprises distinct superficial and deep submodalities that allow us to sense smooth and rough textures, the shapes of objects, and the pressure exerted by objects pressed onto the skin over muscle (deep pressure). Vibration sensitivity is used routinely for sensory testing. People with impairments in these modalities experience clumsiness and incoordination. Sensual touch is a soothing, but poorly localized, form of touch. It is important more in affecting our emotions than discrimination. These various submodalities are mediated by different types of mechanoreceptors.

- **Proprioception** is our sense of limb position and limb movement (kinesthesia). Whereas vision supplements proprioception, healthy individuals are also keenly aware of where their limbs are relative to the body axis, gravity, and to each other. Together with touch, proprioception is critical for movement control.

- Thermal senses, separate warmth and cold, provide critical information about the safety and comfort of our environment, as well as enable us to maintain our body temperature within narrow limits.

- **Pain** alerts the individual of tissue damage, present or impending. Pain is mediated by specific nociceptors. It comprises sharp pricking pain and a dull burning pain.

- **Itch** is triggered selectively by chemical irritation of the skin, especially in response to particular tissue inflammatory agents. Itch provokes the urge to scratch, thereby tending to remove the offending substance.

- Visceral sensation provides not only awareness of the internal state of our body but also the information for regulating many bodily functions, such as blood pressure and breathing. Many aspects of visceral sensation are never conscious, such as arterial pressure, and others are only so under special circumstances, such as nausea and fullness.

Many of these modalities and submodalities are engaged during routine activity. For example, in picking up a cup of coffee, you use proprioception in identifying the location of your hand as you reach to grasp the handle; contact with the cup is detected by touch. If the cup is warm, your temperature sense is recruited, and if it is hot, you experience pain. After consuming caffeine in the coffee, your heart may beat faster, which is sensed by both visceral sensory receptors and mechanoreceptors in the chest.

Functional Anatomy of the Spinal Mechanosensory System

Mechanical Sensations Are Mediated by the Dorsal Column–Medial Lemniscal System

Touch and limb position sense are mediated by the **dorsal column–medial lemniscal system** (Figure 4–2), named after its two principal components. After a lesion of the dorsal column–medial lemniscal system, the person's tactile thresholds become elevated and discriminative capabilities are markedly reduced. An individual with such a lesion, for example, may not be able to distinguish gradations of rough and smooth (eg, grades of sandpaper). Moreover, this individual also would have difficulty maintaining balance with his or her eyes closed because of the absence of leg position sense. This set of impairments occurs in **tabes dorsalis,** an advanced stage of neurosyphilis, because dorsal root ganglion neurons with large-diameter axons degenerate. Fortunately, tabes dorsalis is rare today because of antibiotics. A crude sense of touch remains after a dorsal column lesion, indicating that other spinal pathways receive input from mechanoreceptor neurons but that this information is not organized for fine discriminations. This is discussed briefly in Chapter 5 with pain and temperature senses.

A three neuron circuit transmits sensory information from the periphery to the cerebral cortex. Figure 4–2A overlays the circuit on the views of the spinal cord, dorsal brain stem, and thalamus; Figure 4–2B presents the circuit in relation to a sequence of slices through the spinal cord and the brain. **Mechanoreceptors,** a specialized kind of dorsal root ganglion neuron, provide the major sensory input to the dorsal column–medial lemniscal system. The central branches of mechanoreceptors synapse both in the spinal cord, which is primarily important for bringing information to spinal motor circuits for reflex function, and in the medulla. The synapse in the medulla is located in the first major relay in the dorsal column–medial lemniscal system, in the **dorsal column nuclei.** Here, the first-order neurons in the pathway, the primary mechanosensory neurons, synapse on the second-order neurons in the central nervous system (Figure 4–2). The axons of the second-order neurons decussate in the medulla. These axons travel in the **medial lemniscus,** which transmits information primarily to the **ventral posterior lateral nucleus** of the thalamus. Thalamic neurons in this nucleus project their axons to the **primary somatic sensory cortex** in the postcentral gyrus (Figure 4–2). This cortical area is important in localization of mechanical stimuli and in identifying the quality of such stimuli.

From the primary somatic sensory cortex, information is transmitted to higher-order cortical areas located ventrally and dorsally that play a role in more complex aspects of touch and position sense. Cortical areas that are located ventrally, including the secondary somatic sensory cortex (see Figure 4–2, inset), are important for recognizing objects by touch and grasp alone, or "what" something is. Dorsal areas, including area 5 (see Figure 4–12), are important in spatial localization, or "where" something is located. The dorsal areas are also important in using mechanosensory information for guiding hand and arm movements. We will learn that the visual and auditory cortical areas also have dorsal, or "where," and ventral, "what," areas.

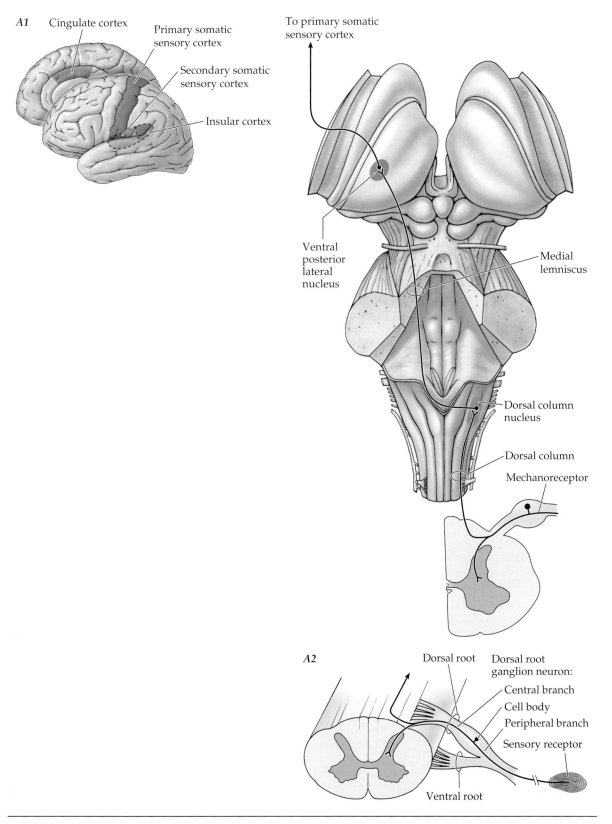

A1
Cingulate cortex
Primary somatic sensory cortex
Secondary somatic sensory cortex
Insular cortex

To primary somatic sensory cortex

Ventral posterior lateral nucleus

Medial lemniscus

Dorsal column nucleus

Dorsal column

Mechanoreceptor

A2
Dorsal root
Dorsal root ganglion neuron:
Central branch
Cell body
Peripheral branch
Sensory receptor
Ventral root

FIGURE 4–2 Organization of the dorsal column–medial lemniscal system. **A.** Dorsal view of the brain stem without the cerebellum, illustrating the course of the dorsal column–medial lemniscal system. A2 shows the dorsal root ganglion neuron and the organization of the primary afferent fiber. The sensory receptor illustrated in A2 is a mechanoreceptor, a Pacinian corpuscle. The inset shows views of lateral and medial surfaces of the cerebral cortex.

B
Cerebral cortex
and thalamus

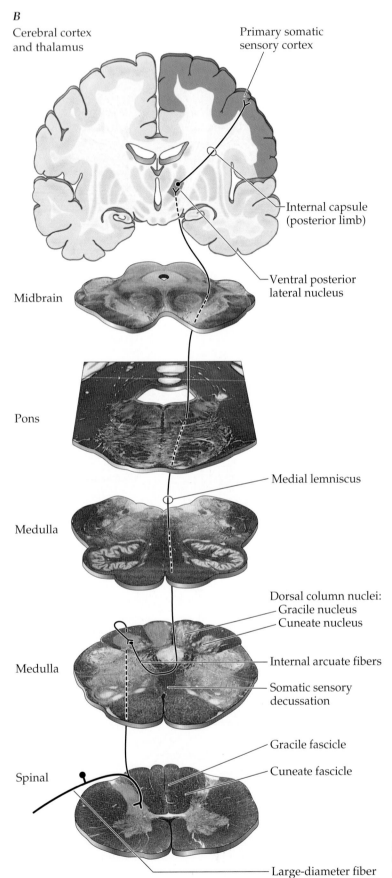

Primary somatic
sensory cortex

Internal capsule
(posterior limb)

Midbrain

Ventral posterior
lateral nucleus

Pons

Medial lemniscus

Medulla

Dorsal column nuclei:
Gracile nucleus
Cuneate nucleus

Medulla

Internal arcuate fibers

Somatic sensory
decussation

Gracile fascicle

Cuneate fascicle

Spinal

Large-diameter fiber

FIGURE 4–2 *B.* The dorsal column-medial lemniscal pathway,
as viewed by a series of transverse slices through the brain stem
and a coronal slice through the thalamus and cerebral cortex.

Regional Anatomy of the Spinal Mechanosensory System

The rest of this chapter takes a regional approach to the spinal mechanosensory system. Progressing in sequence from the periphery to the cerebral cortex, the chapter examines the key components of the dorsal column–medial lemniscal system. Knowledge of the regional anatomy is important for understanding how injury to a discrete portion of the central nervous system affects different functional systems.

The Peripheral Axon Terminals of Dorsal Root Ganglion Neurons Contain the Somatic Sensory Receptors

The **dorsal root ganglion neurons,** named for the **dorsal root ganglia** in which their cell bodies are located, are **pseudounipolar neurons** (Figure 4–2A2). A single axon emerges from the cell body and bifurcates; one axonal branch is directed toward the periphery, where it innervates the skin or other tissues, and the other, directed centrally, synapses on central nervous system neurons. The peripheral and central axon branches of dorsal root ganglion neurons are often called **primary sensory (or afferent) fibers.**

The peripheral axon terminal is the receptive portion of the neuron. Here, stimulus energy is transduced into neural signals by membrane receptor-channel complexes that respond to a particular stimulus energy (eg, mecanical or thermal). **Mechanoreceptors** are activated when mechanical energy is conducted from the body surface, where stimulation occurs, to the membrane of the receptors, where stretch-activated channels are located. Mechanoreceptors for limb position sense are sensitive to muscle or tendon stretch as well as mechanical changes in the tissues around muscles and joints.

Mechanoreceptors have **encapsulated axon terminals.** Five major types of encapsulated sensory receptor neurons are located in the skin and underlying deep tissue that mediate mechanosensations: Ruffini's corpuscles, Merkel's receptors, Meissner's corpuscles, Pacinian corpuscles, and hair receptors (Figure 4–3A). Merkel's receptors and Meissner's corpuscles are located at the epidermis-dermis border. These receptors are sensitive to stimulation within a very small region of overlying skin; hence they have very small receptive fields. These receptors are important for fine tactile discrimination, such as reading Braille. Ruffini's and Pacinian corpuscles are located in the dermis. Ruffini's corpuscles are sensitive to skin stretch and are important in discriminating the shape of grasped objects. Pacinian corpuscles are the most sensitive mechanoreceptor, responding to skin displacement of as little as 500 nM. Merkel's receptors and Pacinian corpuscles are **rapidly adapting,** responding to changes in the stimulus, such as when it comes on or shuts off. Meissner's corpuscles and Ruffini's receptors are **slowly adapting,** firing action potentials for the duration of the stimulus. Hair receptors may be either slowly or rapidly adapting. Each primary sensory fiber has multiple terminal branches and, therefore, multiple receptive endings.

The principal receptor for proprioception is the **muscle spindle receptor,** which is located within the muscle belly. It measures muscle stretch (Figure 4–3B). This structure is innervated by multiple sensory fibers with different properties. The muscle spindle is more complicated than the other encapsulated mechanoreceptors because it also contains tiny muscle fibers, controlled by the central nervous system, that regulate the receptor neuron's sensitivity. There is another deep mechanoreceptor, the **Golgi tendon receptor,** which is entwined within the collagen fibers of tendon and is sensitive to the force generated by contracting muscle. It may have a role in an individual's sense of how much effort it takes to produce a particular motor act. The muscle spindle and Golgi tendon receptors also play key roles in the reflex control of muscle. The joints are innervated by mechanoreceptors, but they play more of a role in sensing joint pressure and the extremes of joint motion than proprioception.

The capsule covering Pacinian, Ruffini's, and Meissner's corpuscles and non-neural structures associated with muscle spindle and Golgi tendon receptors do not participate directly in stimulus transduction. Rather, they modify the mechanoreceptor's response to a stimulus. For example, Pacinian corpuscles are normally rapidly adapting but become slowly adapting when the capsule is dissected away. Merkel's receptors are different in their organization. The peripheral terminals of the sensory fiber contacts Merkel's cells, located in the skin. Merkel's cells appear to form a synapse-like apposition with the fiber terminal, suggesting that mechanosensory transduction is accomplished by the Merkel's cell, which synaptically activates the sensory fiber.

The protective senses have their own specialized receptors. **Nociceptors** respond to noxious stimuli and mediate pain, whereas **itch**-sensitive neurons, or **pruritic receptor,** respond to histamine. Receptor neurons sensitive to cold or warmth are termed **thermoreceptors.** The morphology of these three classes of receptor neurons is simple; they are **bare nerve endings** (Figure 4–3A). The viscera are also innervated. These receptors will be discussed in Chapter 6.

The modality sensitivity of a receptor neuron also determines the diameter of its axon and the patterns of connections it makes in the central nervous system. Most mechanoreceptors have a **large-diameter axon** covered by a thick myelin sheath. The larger the diameter of the axon, the faster it conducts action potentials. The mechanoreceptors are the fastest conducting sensory receptor neurons in the somatic sensory system. The dorsal column–medial lemniscal system receives sensory input principally from these fast conducting mechanoreceptors with large-diameter axons. By contrast, dorsal root ganglion neurons that are sensitive to noxious stimuli, temperature, and itch have **small-diameter axons** that are either thinly myelinated or unmyelinated. Table 4–1 lists the functional categories of primary sensory fibers, including the two fiber nomenclatures based on axonal diameter: A-α (group 1), A-β (group 2), A-δ (group 3), and C (group 4).

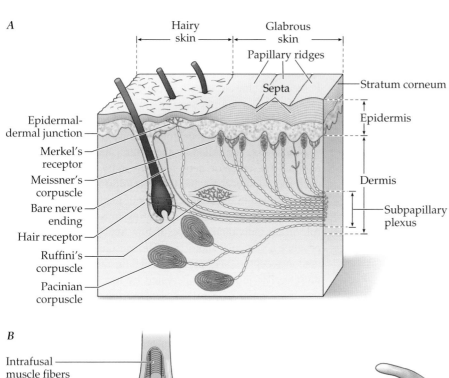

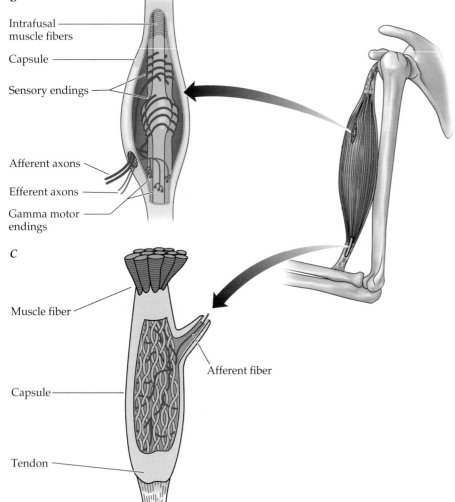

FIGURE 4–3   A. The morphology of peripheral somatic sensory receptors on hairy skin *(left)* and hairless, or glabrous, skin *(right)*. **B.** The muscle spindle organ *(top inset)* is a stretch receptor located within the muscle. It receives an efferent innervation from the spinal cord that maintains receptor sensitivity during muscle contraction. Specialized motor neurons, termed gamma motor neurons, innervate muscle fibers (intrafusal fibers) within the receptor's capsule. The synapse between the gamma motor neuron and the intrafusal fiber is termed the gamma motor ending. **C.** The Golgi tendon organ, located within tendons, is most sensitive to active force generated by contracting muscle. (**A,** Adapted from Light AR, Perl ER. Peripheral sensory systems. In: Dyck P, Thomas PK, Lambert EH, Bruge R, eds. *Peripheral Neuropathy*, 3rd ed. Vol 1. Philadelphia, PA: W. B. Saunders; 1993. **B,** Adapted from Schmidt RF. *Fundamentals of Neurophysiology*, 3rd ed. Berlin, Heidelberg, New York: Springer; 1985.)

Dermatomes Have a Segmental Organization

The central branches of dorsal root ganglion neurons collect into the dorsal roots (Figure 4–2A2). The spinal cord has a rostrocaudal segmental organization, which forms early during development. Mesodermal tissue breaks up into 38 to 40 pairs of repeating units, called **somites** (Figure 4–4A). These somites—from which the muscles, bones, and other structures of the neck, limbs, and trunk develop—have a rostrocaudal organization. There are 8 cervical, 12 thoracic, 5 lumbar, 5 sacral, and 8 to 10 coccygeal somites. Importantly, for each

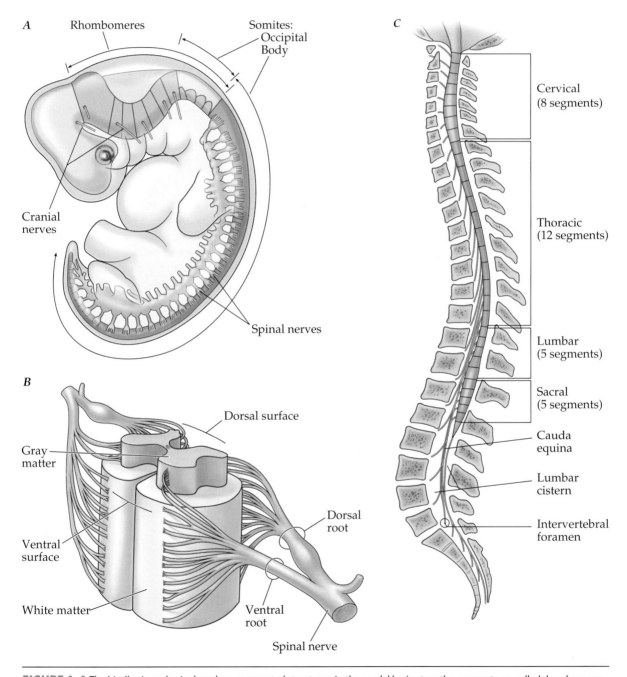

FIGURE 4–4 The hindbrain and spinal cord are segmented structures. In the caudal brain stem the segments are called rhombomeres; in the spinal cord they are called body somites. Four occipital somites form structures of the head. These are shown in the caudal medulla (A). **A.** The position of the developing nervous system in the embryo is illustrated as well as the segmental organization of rhombomeres and somites. The cranial nerves that contain the axons of brain stem motor neurons are also shown. From rostral to caudal the following cranial nerves are illustrated: IV, V VI, VII, IX, X, and XII. The two mesencephalic segments and the segment between the metacephalon and mesencephalon are not shown. **B.** Drawing of a single spinal cord segment from the mature nervous system. **C.** Lateral view of the mature spinal cord in the vertebral canal. Note that the spinal nerves exit from the vertebral canal through intervertebral foramina. (**A,** Adapted from Lumsden A. The cellular basis of segmentation in the developing hindbrain. *Trends Neurosci.* 1990;13[8]:329–335.)

of these somites, there is a corresponding vertebra and spinal cord segment, with associated dorsal and ventral roots. Each spinal cord segment (Figure 4–4B) provides the sensory and motor innervation of the skin and muscle of the body part derived from its associated somite. Thus, each segment contains repeated elements of somatic sensory and motor circuits that are present in adjacent rostral and caudal segments. In the mature spinal cord, segmentation is apparent as the series of dorsal and ventral roots emerging from its surface. The cervical segments (Figure 4–4C) innervate the skin and muscles of the back of the head, neck, and arms. The thoracic segments innervate the trunk, and the lumbar and sacral segments innervate the legs and perineal region. (Most of the coccygeal segments disappear later in development.) The segments providing the sensory and motor innervation of the upper and lower extremities are enlarged to accommodate more dorsal horn neurons, needed for the greater sensitivity of the extremities, and more motor neurons, for finer control; the cervical (C5-T1) and lumbosacral (L1-S2) enlargements (Figures 4–4C and 4–5).

The area of skin innervated by the axons in a single dorsal root is termed a **dermatome.** Since the roots have a segmental organization, so too do the dermatomes. Dermatomes of adjacent dorsal roots overlap extensively with those of their neighbors (Figure 4–5, inset). This is because the primary sensory fibers have extensive rostro-caudal branches in the spinal cord. This explains the common clinical observation that, when a physician probes sensory capacity after injury to a single dorsal root, typically no anesthetic area is observed, although patients with such damage sometimes experience tingling or even a diminished sensory capacity. Single dorsal root injury commonly produces **radicular pain,** which is localized to the dermatome of the injured root. By comparing the location of radicular pain or other sensory disturbances with a dermatomal map, such as in Figure 4–5, the clinician can localize the site and extent of damage.

The Spinal Cord Gray Matter Has a Dorsoventral Sensory-Motor Organization

Very early during development, the dorsal and ventral halves of the spinal cord gray matter become committed to mediating somatic sensory and motor functions. The dorsal half becomes the **dorsal horn,** which mediates sensory functions; many dorsal horn neurons project to the brain stem or diencephalon; others are interneurons. The ventral half becomes the **ventral horn,** which mediates motor functions. Motor neurons are located in the ventral horn; they project their axons to the periphery via the ventral roots (Figure 4–6). Because the spinal cord has a longitudinal organization, the dorsal and ventral horns form columns of neurons that run rostrocaudally. Between the dorsal and ventral horns is an overlapping region (intermediate zone; Figure 4–6B) that will be considered further in Chapters 5 and 10. The spinal gray matter has a laminar organization (I-X; Figure 4–6A);

this is important for pain and motor function and also will be considered in Chapters 5 and 10.

Dorsal root ganglion neurons that are sensitive to mechanical stimuli, on the one hand, and pain, temperature, and itch, on the other, synapse in different parts of the dorsal horn. We will see in later chapters that somatic motor neurons controlling striated muscle are located in different parts of the ventral horn than are neurons controlling visceral structures.

Mechanoreceptor Axons Terminate in Deeper Portions of the Spinal Gray Matter and in the Medulla

The central branch of a dorsal root ganglion neuron enters the spinal cord at its dorsolateral margin (Figure 4–6A). Once inside the spinal cord, dorsal root ganglion axons branch extensively. Mechanosensory fibers, which have a large diameter, enter the spinal cord medial to Lissauer's tract (Figure 4-6B), a region containing mostly unmyelinated and thinly myelinated fibers for pain and temperature senses (see Chapter 5). The axons skirt over the cap of the gray matter to enter the dorsal column (Figure 4–6A), where they give off an ascending branch into the dorsal column and numerous segmental branches into the gray matter. The segmental branches terminate in the deeper layers of the dorsal horn and in the ventral horn (Figure 4–6A) and play complex roles in limb and trunk reflexes. Whereas all mechanoreceptor classes have branches that terminate within the dorsal horn, the muscle spindle receptors are the only mechanoreceptors to terminate within the motor nuclei (Figure 4–6A). The muscle spindle receptor mediates the monosynaptic stretch (eg, knee jerk) reflex (see Figure 2–5A).

The ascending branch of a dorsal root ganglion neuron is the principal one for perception, and it relays information to the dorsal column nuclei. Whereas the majority of axons in the dorsal column are the central branches of mechanoreceptors, a small number of dorsal horn neurons project their axons into the dorsal columns, comprising approximately 10%-15% of the axons in the path. Surprisingly, these are important for visceral pain (Chapter 5). The branching patterns of the pain, temperature, and itch fibers, which have a small-diameter axon, are different from that of the mechanosensory fibers, terminating within the more dorsal portion of the dorsal horn (see Figure 5–3).

The Ascending Branches of Mechanoreceptive Sensory Fibers Travel in Dorsal Columns

Each dorsal column transmits somatic sensory information from the ipsilateral side of the body to the ipsilateral medulla. Axons from each dermatome lie within thin sheets that are parallel to the midline. Axons innervating the most caudal dermatomes are located close to the midline. Axons from progressively more rostral dermatomes are added on laterally. Axons transmitting information from the lower limb ascend

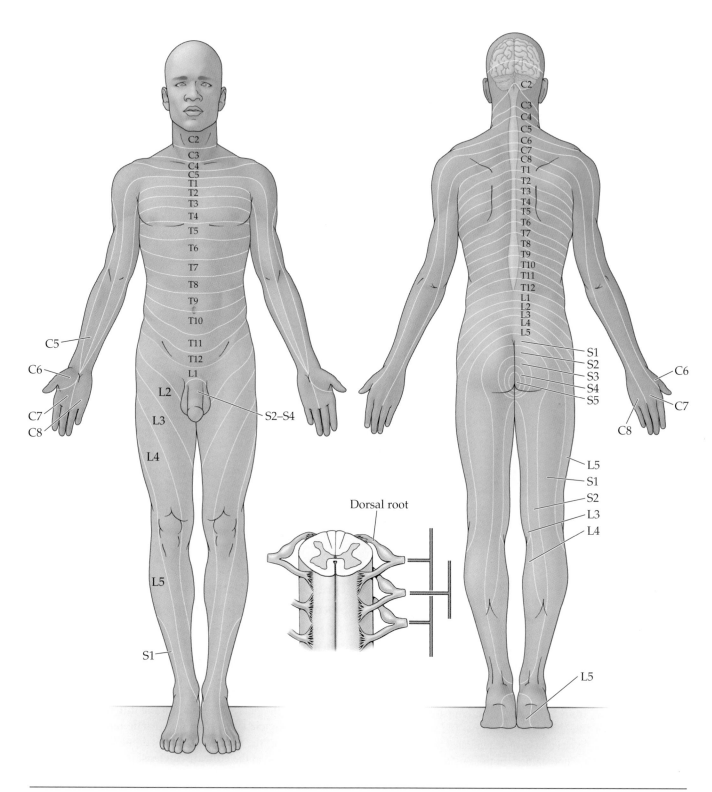

FIGURE 4–5 The dermatomes of the body have a segmental organization. The inset illustrates dermatomal overlap. The brain and spinal cord are visible on the dorsal view (right). Note that the spinal cord ends at L1 segment. This is where cerebrospinal fluid can be withdrawn by lumbar tap (Figure 3-18B).

in the most medial portion of the dorsal column, termed the **gracile fascicle** (Figure 4–7A). Axons from the lower trunk ascend lateral to those from the lower limb, but still within the gracile fascicle. Within the **cuneate fascicle,** axons from the upper trunk, upper limb, neck, and occiput ascend. The

cuneate fascicle begins approximately at the level of the sixth thoracic segment. The gracile and cuneate fascicles are separated by the **dorsal intermediate septum,** and the dorsal columns of the two halves of the spinal cord are separated by the **dorsal median septum** (Figure 4–7A). Spinal cord injury

A

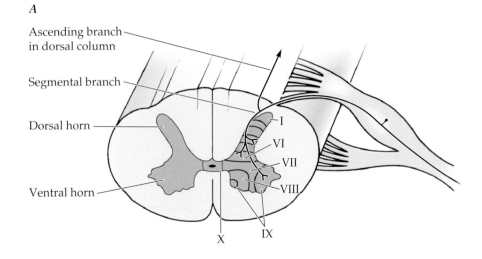

B

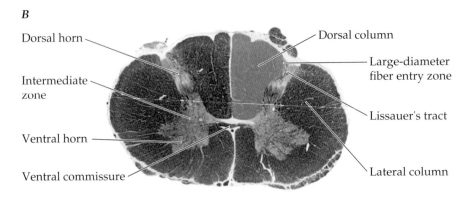

FIGURE 4–6 Organization of spinal cord segment. ***A.*** Terminations and spinal projections of a large-diameter fiber. Note that small-diameter fibers also terminate in other laminae. ***B.*** Myelin-stained section through the cervical spinal cord.

can interrupt the dorsal column axons, resulting in a mechanosensory loss below the level of the injury. This is discussed in Chapter 5, where we will learn that a spinal cord injury typically produces a complex pattern of ipsilateral mechanosensory and contralateral pain impairment (see Box 5–1).

The dermatomal organization of the dorsal columns can be examined in postmortem tissue from individuals who sustained spinal cord trauma. The sections shown in Figure 4–7B1 were taken from a person whose lumbar spinal cord was crushed in a traumatic spinal injury. The sections are stained for myelin. Axons that have degenerated have lost their myelin sheath and are not stained. In the caudal thoracic spinal cord (Figure 4–7B1, bottom section), close to the crushed region, nearly all of the axons in both gracile fascicles have degenerated. At more rostral levels, the degenerated region becomes confined medially as new contingents of healthy axons continue to enter the spinal cord lateral to the degenerated axons from the lumbar cord. The pattern by which axons enter and ascend in the dorsal columns is shown schematically in Figure 4–7B2. This injury also affects pain and temperature pathways (Figure 4–7; anterolateral system), which is considered in Chapter 5.

The Dorsal Column Nuclei Are Somatotopically Organized

Dorsal column axons synapse on neurons in the **dorsal column nuclei** (Figure 4–8D), the first major relay in the ascending pathway for touch and limb position senses. These and other somatic sensory relay nuclei have local circuits that enhance sensitivity so that when adjacent portions of the skin are touched, the person can discern the difference. Axons of the gracile fascicle synapse in the **gracile nucleus,** which is located close to the midline, whereas those from the cuneate fascicle synapse in the **cuneate nucleus.**

Throughout the somatic sensory systems a systematic relationship exists between the position of axons in tracts and neurons in nuclei and cortex. This organization is termed **somatotopy.** Beginning with the sequential ordering of the dorsal roots (Figure 4–5) and the dermatomal organization of the dorsal columns, the organizational plan adheres to a simple rule: Adjacent body parts are represented in adjacent sites in the central nervous system. This is the somatotopic organization, an arrangement that ensures that local neighborhood relations in the periphery are preserved in the central nervous

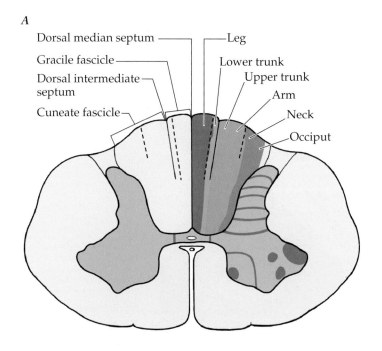

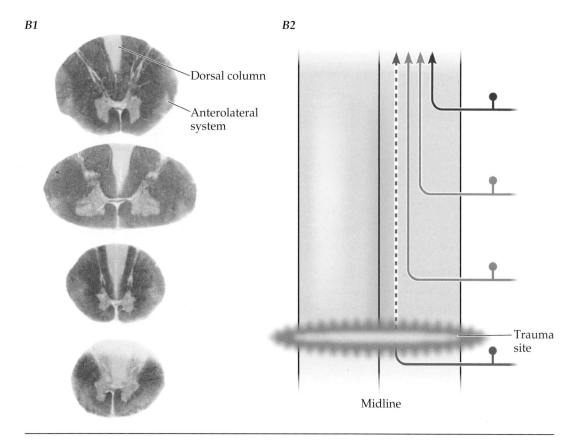

FIGURE 4–7 Somatotopic organization of the dorsal columns. **A.** Somatotopic arrangement of incoming axons. Dorsal spinal landmarks are shown on the left. **B.** The somatotopic organization of the dorsal columns can be demonstrated by examining spinal cord sections from a patient who sustained damage to the lumbar spinal cord. **B1.** Four levels through the spinal cord are shown, rostrocaudally from top to bottom: a section rostral to the cervical enlargement, a section through the cervical enlargement, and two thoracic sections. **B2.** The course taken by the central branches of the dorsal root fibers as they enter the spinal cord and ascend in the dorsal columns. The dashed line depicts the course of a degenerated axon transected by the crush. The anterolateral system is for pain and temperature sense; this will be considered in Chapter 5.

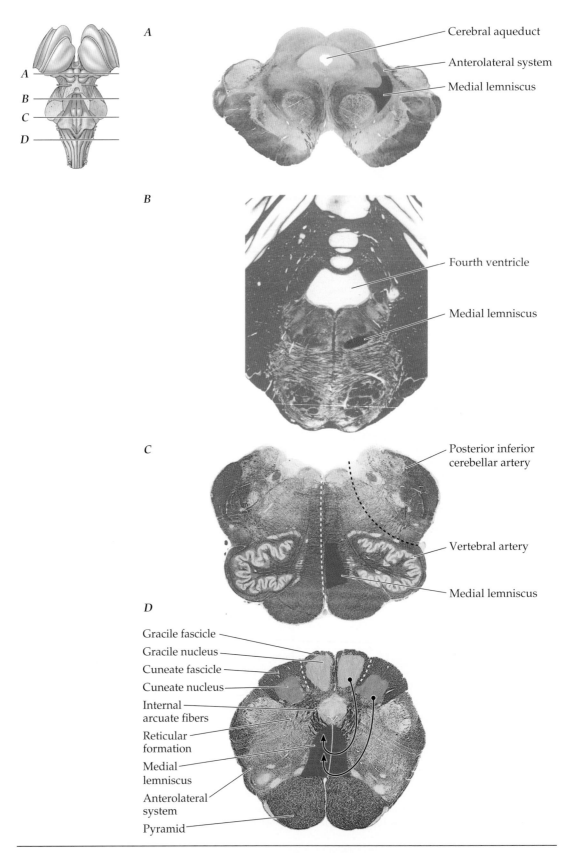

FIGURE 4–8 Course of medial lemniscus through brain stem. **A.** Myelin-stained transverse section through the midbrain. **B.** Pons. **C.** Mid-medulla. The pattern of arterial perfusion of the rostral medulla is shown at this level. **D.** Caudal medulla. Myelin-stained transverse section through the dorsal column nuclei. Trajectories of internal arcuate fibers from the gracile and cuneate nuclei are shown. The inset shows the approximate plane of section.

system. In the dorsal column nuclei, there is a coherent map of the body surface. Similar principles apply to the topographic organization of the peripheral receptive sheet in the visual system (retinotopy) and in the auditory system (tonotopy).

The Decussation of the Dorsal Column–Medial Lemniscal System Is in the Caudal Medulla

From the dorsal column nuclei, the axons of the second-order neurons sweep ventrally through the medulla, where they are called the **internal arcuate fibers,** and decussate (Figure 4–8D). Immediately after crossing the midline, the fibers ascend to the thalamus in the **medial lemniscus.** Axons from the gracile nucleus decussate ventral to axons from the cuneate nucleus and ascend in the ventral part of the medial lemniscus, compared with axons from the cuneate nucleus. Because of this pattern, the somatotopic organization of the medial lemniscus in the medulla resembles a person standing upright. In the pons, the medial lemniscus is located more dorsally than in the medulla and is oriented from medial to lateral (Figure 4–8B); in the midbrain, the medial lemniscus is located more laterally (Figure 4–8A). Axons in the medial lemniscus ascend uninterrupted through the brain stem and synapse in the thalamus.

The caudal brain stem receives blood from perforating branches of the **vertebral-basilar, or posterior, circulation** (see Figure 3–3B). Occlusion of small (unnamed) branches of the vertebral artery can damage axons of the medial lemniscus (Figure 4-8C). As a consequence, touch and limb position senses are disrupted. Vertebral artery infarction produces mechanosensory deficits on the contralateral side of the body, because the internal arcuate fibers decussate at a more caudal level in the medulla (Figure 4–8D). This type of infarction also destroys axons of the corticospinal tract in the pyramid.

Mechanosensory Information Is Processed in the Ventral Posterior Nucleus

The **thalamus** (Figure 4–9) is a nodal point for the transmission of sensory information to the cerebral cortex. Indeed, with the exception of olfaction, information from all sensory systems is processed in the thalamus and then relayed to the cerebral cortex. The dorsal column–medial lemniscal system is no exception. The various aspects of mechanical sensations are processed in the ventral posterior nucleus (Figure 4–9A). The **ventral posterior nucleus** has a lateral division, the **ventral posterior lateral nucleus** (Figures 4–9 and 4–10A), which receives input from the medial lemniscus and projects to the **primary somatic sensory cortex** (Figure 4–9B). The ventral posterior nucleus also has a medial division, the **ventral posterior medial nucleus** (Figures 4–9 and 4–10A), which mediates aspects of somatic sensations from the face and perioral structures (Chapter 6). The ventral posterior nucleus is important in discriminative aspects of the mechanical sensations,

such as being able to precisely localize the stimulation site on the body. The MRI in Figure 4–10B reveals the thalamus, medial to the posterior limb of the internal capsule, but has insufficient resolution to reveal the component nuclei.

The Primary Somatic Sensory Cortex Has a Somatotopic Organization

Mechanoreceptive sensory information is processed primarily by three cortical areas: (1) the primary somatic sensory cortex, (2) the secondary somatic sensory cortex, and (3) the posterior parietal cortex. (The motor cortical areas also receive mechanoreceptive information, but this information is important in controlling movements.) Located in the postcentral gyrus of the parietal lobe (Figure 4–10), the **primary somatic sensory cortex** is the principal region of the parietal lobe to which the ventral posterior nucleus projects. Axons from this nucleus travel to the cerebral cortex through the **posterior limb of the internal capsule** (Figures 4–9A and 4–10; see also Figure 2–14). The primary somatic sensory cortex receives somatotopically organized inputs from the ventral posterior lateral and medial nuclei (Figure 4–9B). This thalamocortical projection forms the basis of a body map on the postcentral gyrus, the **sensory homunculus,** originally described in the human by the Canadian neurosurgeon Wilder Penfield. Local circuit connections, both excitatory and inhibitory, use this information to construct the representations of the various body parts on the sensory map. Remarkably, the representations of different body parts do not have the same proportions as the body itself (Figure 4–9B). Rather, the portions of the body used in common discriminative tactile tasks, such as the fingers, have a disproportionately greater representation on the map than areas that are not as important for touch, such as the elbow. It was once thought that these differences were fixed, established genetically to determine the discriminative capacity of different body parts. We now know that the body map of the brain is not static but is also dynamically controlled by the pattern of use of different body parts in touch exploration.

The Primary Somatic Sensory Cortex Has a Columnar Organization

The cerebral cortex is a laminated structure; most regions have at least six cell layers (Figure 4–11). The thalamus projects primarily to layer IV (and the adjoining portion of layer III), and this incoming information is distributed to neurons in more superficial and deeper layers. Most of the excitatory connections within a local area of cortex remain somewhat confined to a vertical slice of cortex, termed a **cortical column** (Figure 4–11). The cortical column constitutes a functional unit. Neurons within a column in the primary somatic sensory cortex, spanning all cortical layers, receive input from the same peripheral location on the body and from the same class, or classes, of mechanoreceptor. Other cortical regions have a columnar organization. For example, in the primary auditory cortex, neurons within a column are sensitive to the

A

B

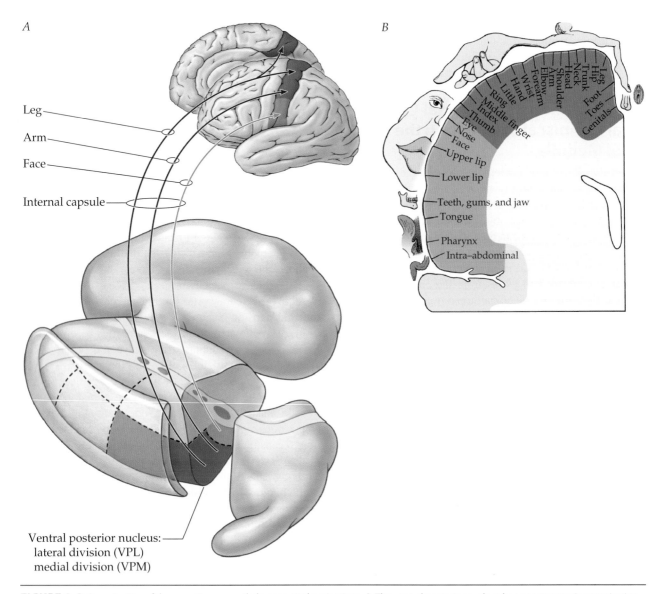

Leg

Arm

Face

Internal capsule

Ventral posterior nucleus:
lateral division (VPL)
medial division (VPM)

Leg
Hip
Trunk
Neck
Head
Shoulder
Arm
Elbow
Forearm
Wrist
Hand
Little
Ring
Middle finger
Index
Thumb
Eye
Nose
Face
Upper lip

Foot
Toes
Genitals

Lower lip

Teeth, gums, and jaw

Tongue

Pharynx

Intra–abdominal

FIGURE 4–9 Organization of the somatic sensory thalamocortical projections. ***A.*** The ventral posterior nucleus has a somatotopic organization: Neurons receiving input from the leg and arm are located in the lateral division of the nucleus (ventral posterior lateral nucleus, VPL; darker shading), whereas neurons receiving input from the face are located in the medial division (ventral posterior medial nucleus, VPM; lighter shading). Axons from the ventral posterior nucleus ascend to the primary somatic sensory cortex in the internal capsule. ***B.*** A schematic slice through the postcentral gyrus, showing the somatotopic organization of the primary somatic sensory cortex. The territory receiving input from the ventral posterior lateral nucleus is shaded darker then the territory receiving input from the ventral posterior medial nucleus.

same frequency of sound, and in the motor cortex, neurons in a column participate in controlling movement of the same joint, or sets of joints.

Efferent projections arise from the primary somatic sensory cortex (Figure 4–11). As discussed in Chapter 2, pyramidal neurons in different layers project to different targets. **Corticocortical association neurons,** located in layers II and III, project to other cortical areas on the same side, including higher-order somatic sensory cortical areas (see next section) for further processing of sensory information, and the primary motor cortex for movement control. **Callosal neurons,** also located in layers II and III, project their axons to the contralateral somatic sensory cortex through the

corpus callosum. One function of these callosal connections may be to join the representations of each half of the body in the primary somatic sensory cortex of each hemisphere. **Descending projection neurons,** located in layers V and VI, send their axons primarily to the thalamus, brain stem, and spinal cord—where somatic sensory information is processed—to act as gatekeepers that regulate the quantity of mechanosensory information that ascends through the central nervous system.

Based on its lamination pattern, the primary somatic sensory cortex consists of four cytoarchitectonic divisions, or **Brodmann's areas** (see Figure 2–19), numbered 1, 2, 3a, and 3b (Figure 4–12). As in other cortical areas, regions of

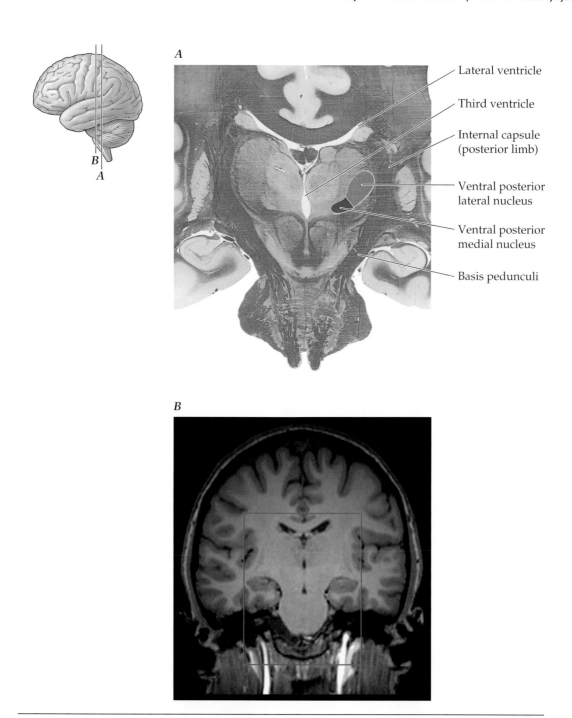

A

Lateral ventricle

Third ventricle

Internal capsule (posterior limb)

Ventral posterior lateral nucleus

Ventral posterior medial nucleus

Basis pedunculi

B

FIGURE 4–10 Myelin-stained transverse sections through the ventral posterior nucleus (*A*) and corresponding MRI (*B*). The boxed region over the MRI corresponds to the myelin-stained section in part A. The shape of the thalamus and brain stem can be discerned, but not the component nuclei. The inset shows the approximate planes of section.

the primary somatic sensory cortex with a different cytoarchitecture have different functions. Area 3a processes information from mechanoreceptors located in deep structures, such as the muscles and joints, and plays an important role in limb position sense. Areas 3b and 1 process information from mechanoreceptors of the skin, and are important in texture discrimination. Area 2 receives information from both deep structures and the skin and is important in discrimination of the shape of grasped objects.

Higher-Order Somatic Sensory Cortical Areas Are Located in the Parietal Lobe, Parietal Operculum, and Insular Cortex

Projections from the primary sensory cortical area distribute the information to multiple cortical regions, although these other areas may also receive direct thalamic inputs. These upstream areas appear to be devoted to processing a specific aspect of the sensory experience. Although sequential pathways from one

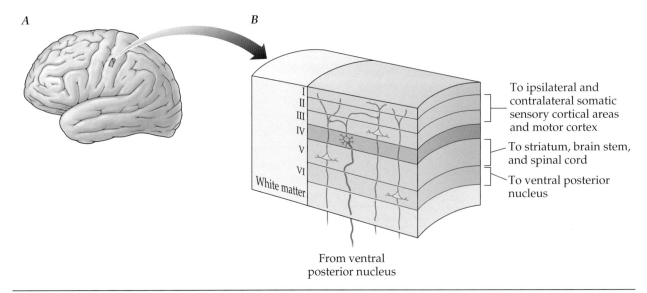

FIGURE 4–11 Three-dimensional schematic of a portion of the postcentral gyrus (**A**). The cortex comprises six layers (**B**) where neuronal cell bodies and their processes are located. Neurons whose cell bodies are located in layers II and III project to other cortical areas, those in layer V project their axons to subcortical regions, and those in layer VI project to the thalamus. Neurons in layer IV receive thalamic input and transmit information to neurons in other cortical layers.

region to the next can be identified, the primary and higher-order sensory areas are also extensively interconnected and the operations of any one set of connections are dependent on the operations of others. The higher-order sensory areas typically project to cortical regions that receive inputs from the multiple sensory modalities and are termed association areas. One such multimodal convergent zone is the large expanse of cortex at the junction of the parietal, temporal, and occipital lobes.

There are three major projection streams from primary somatic sensory cortex: ventral, dorsal, and rostral. The ventral

and dorsal projections comprise the "what" and "where" pathways, respectively. The "what" pathway targets the **secondary somatic sensory cortex,** which is located on the parietal operculum and insular cortex (Figure 4–12A). Similar to the primary area, the secondary somatic sensory cortex is somatotopically organized. This part of the cortex begins a sequence of somatic sensory projections to insular cortical areas and the temporal lobe that are important for recognizing objects by touch alone, without vision, such as distinguishing one coin from another in your pocket.

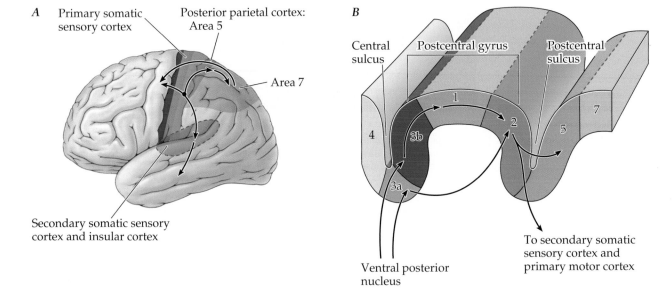

FIGURE 4–12 A. The locations of the primary and higher order somatic sensory areas are indicated on a lateral view of the cerebral cortex. The light green region corresponds to the areas beneath the surface, in the insular cortex and the parietal and temporal operculum. **B.** A schematic section cut perpendicular to the mediolateral axis of the postcentral gyrus. (Adapted from Marshall WH, Woolsey CN, Bard P. Observations on cortical somatic sensory mechanisms of cat and monkey. *J Neurophysiol.* 1941;4:1-24.)

The "where" pathway targets the **posterior parietal cortex** (Figure 4–12A), which includes Brodmann's area 5, sometimes termed the tertiary somatic sensory cortex, and area 7. In addition to the awareness of object location, the projection to the posterior parietal cortex plays two other major functions. First, these areas play an important role in perception of body image. A lesion of this region in the nondominant hemisphere (typically the right hemisphere) produces a complex sensory syndrome in which the individual neglects the contralateral half of the body. For example, a patient may fail to dress one side of her body or comb half of her hair. Second, portions of the posterior parietal cortex receive visual and auditory inputs as well as somatic sensory information. These areas are involved in integrating somatic sensory, visual, and auditory information for perception and attention.

The "where" pathway, together with the rostral projection, targets the motor areas of the frontal lobe, especially the motor cortex. This projection is important for using mechanoreceptive sensory information to guide reaching movements. The motor cortex is essential for production and control of voluntary movements. The "where" pathway is also the "how" pathway for action.

Summary

Sensory Receptor Neurons

The *dorsal column–medial lemniscal system* mediates touch and limb position sense (Figure 4–2; Table 4–1). *Dorsal root ganglion neurons* are *pseudounipolar neurons* (Figure 4–2A). They receive somatic sensory information and transmit it from the periphery to the spinal cord. The distal terminal of dorsal root ganglion neurons is the *sensory receptor.* Neurons sensitive to mechanical stimuli have encapsulated endings and *large-diameter axons* (A-α; A-β). Four major mechanoreceptors innervate glabrous skin and subcutaneous tissue (Figure 4–3): *Meissner's corpuscles, Pacinian corpuscles, Merkel's receptors,* and *Ruffini's corpuscles.* The *muscle spindle* is the key receptor for muscle length and the *Golgi tendon organ,* for force (Figures 4–3B and 4–3C).

Spinal Cord and Brain Stem

The spinal cord has a rostrocaudal segmental organization, with 8 *cervical,* 12 *thoracic,* 5 *lumbar,* 5 *sacral,* and 8 to 10 *coccygeal* somites (Figure 4–4). The axons of mechanoreceptive dorsal root ganglion neurons enter the spinal cord via the *dorsal root.* A *dermatome* is the area of skin innervated by a single dorsal root (Figure 4–5). The afferent information carried by adjacent dorsal roots overlaps nearly completely on the body surface. The principal branching pattern of large-diameter fibers is to ascend to the brain stem in the dorsal columns (Figures 4–6 and 4–7).

The dorsal columns have two fascicles (Figures 4–6 and 4–7). The *gracile fascicle* is a tract that carries axons from the leg and lower trunk, and the *cuneate fascicle* carries axons from the upper trunk, arm, neck, and back of the head. The majority of the axons in the dorsal columns are central branches of dorsal root ganglion neurons. Dorsal column axons terminate in the *dorsal column nuclei* in the caudal medulla (Figure 4–8D). Axons of neurons in the dorsal column nuclei decussate and ascend in the *medial lemniscus* (Figure 4–8A-C) and terminate in the thalamus.

Thalamus and Cerebral Cortex

The axons of the medial lemniscus synapse in the *ventral posterior lateral nucleus* (Figures 4–9 and 4–10), which projects to the *primary somatic sensory cortex* (Figures 4–9, 4–11, and 4–12), via the *posterior limb of the internal capsule* (Figures 4–9 and 4–10). The *secondary somatic sensory cortex* and *posterior parietal cortex* receive input from the primary somatic sensory cortex (Figure 4–12). Each of these cortical areas is somatotopically organized.

Inputs from thalamus arrive at layer IV of the cortex (Figure 4–11). Efferent projections from the somatic sensory cortical areas arise from neurons whose cell bodies are from specific cortical layers. *Corticocortical association connections* with other cortical areas on the same side of the cerebral cortex are made by neurons in layers II and III. *Callosal connections* with the other side of the cerebral cortex are also made by neurons in layers II and III. *Descending projections* to the striatum, brain stem, and spinal cord originate from neurons located in layer V, whereas the projection to the thalamus originates from neurons located in layer VI.

Selected Readings

Gardner E, Johnson K. The bodily senses. In: Kandel ER, Schwartz JH, Jessell TM, Siegelbaum SA, Hudspeth AJ, eds. *Principles of Neural Science.* 5th ed. New York, NY: McGraw-Hill; 2008.

Brust, JCM. *The Practice of Neural Science.* New York, NY: McGraw-Hill; 2000.

References

Beauchamp MS. See me, hear me, touch me: multisensory integration in lateral occipital-temporal cortex. *Curr Opin Neurobiol.* Apr 2005;15(2):145-153.

Brown AG. *Organization in the Spinal Cord: The Anatomy and Physiology of Identified Neurons.* New York, NY: Springer; 1981.

Collins RD. *Illustrated Manual of Neurologic Diagnosis.* Philadelphia, PA:Lippincott; 1962.

Dum RP, Levinthal DJ, Strick PL. The spinothalamic system targets motor and sensory areas in the cerebral cortex of monkeys. *J Neurosci.* Nov 11 2009;29(45):14223-14235.

Friedman DP, Murray EA, O'Neil JB, Mishkin M. Cortical connections of the somatosensory fields of the lateral sulcus of macaques: evidence for a corticolimbic pathway for touch. *J Comp Neurol.* 1986;252:323-347.

Haeberle H, Lumpkin EA. Merkel cells in somatosensation. *Chemosens Percept.* Jun 1 2008;1(2):110-118.

Haggard P. Sensory neuroscience: from skin to object in the somatosensory cortex. *Curr Biol.* Oct 24 2006;16(20):R884-886.

Hayward V. A brief taxonomy of tactile illusions and demonstrations that can be done in a hardware store. *Brain Res Bull.* Apr 15 2008;75(6):742-752.

Jones EG. Organization of the thalamocortical complex and its relation to sensory processes. In: Darian-Smith I, ed. *Handbook of Physiology, Section 1: The Nervous System, Vol. 3: Sensory Processes.* American Physiological Society; 1984:149-212.

Jones EG, Friedman DP. Projection pattern of functional components of thalamic ventrobasal complex on monkey somatosensory cortex. *J Neurophysiol.* 1982;48:521-544.

Kass JH. Somatosensory system. In: Paxinos G, Mai JK, eds. *The Human Nervous System.* London: Elsevier; 2004.

Kung C. A possible unifying principle for mechanosensation. *Nature.* Aug 4 2005;436(7051):647-654.

Lackner JR, DiZio P. Vestibular, proprioceptive, and haptic contributions to spatial orientation. *Annu Rev Psychol.* 2005;56:115-147.

Maricich SM, Wellnitz SA, Nelson AM, et al. Merkel cells are essential for light-touch responses. *Science.* Jun 19 2009;324(5934):1580-1582.

Nicolson T. Fishing for key players in mechanotransduction. *TINS.* Mar 2005;28(3):140-144.

Noble R, Riddell JS. Cutaneous excitatory and inhibitory input to neurones of the postsynaptic dorsal column system in the cat. *J Physiol.* 1988;396:497-513.

Olausson H, Lamarre Y, Backlund H, et al. Unmyelinated tactile afferents signal touch and project to insular cortex. *Nat Neurosci.* Sep 2002;5(9):900-904.

Rustioni A, Weinberg RJ. The somatosensory system. In: Bjumörklund A, Hókfelt T, Swanson LW, eds. *Handbook of Chemical Neuroanatomy, Vol. 7: Integrated Systems of the CNS, Part II: Central Visual, Auditory, Somatosensory, Gustatory.* London: Elsevier; 1989:219-321.

Study Questions

1. A 25-year-old male was in an automobile accident and suffered a severe spinal cord injury. He had multiple somatic sensory and motor signs. Focusing only on mechanosensation, he had no sense of touch on his right leg and lower chest, to the level of the umbilicus. Which of the following statements best describes the side and level of injury?
   A. Right side of spinal cord at the 10th thoracic segment (T10)
   B. Right, T4
   C. Left, T10
   D. Left, T4

2. From which of the listed body regions does the gracile nucleus receive mechanoreceptive input?
   A. Contralateral arm
   B. Contralateral leg
   C. Ipsilateral arm
   D. Ipsilateral leg

3. The medial lemniscus—in the medulla, at the level where there is a fourth ventricle—receives its blood supply from which of the following arteries?

   A. Posterior inferior cerebellar artery
   B. Vertebral artery
   C. Posterior spinal artery
   D. Anterior spinal artery

4. A physician tests vibration sense by touching a tuning fork to the body surface. Which of the following receptors mediates vibration sense?
   A. Thermal receptor
   B. Pacinian corpuscle
   C. Ruffini's corpuscle
   D. Meissner's corpuscle

5. Which of the following statements best describes the organization of dermatomes associated with adjacent dorsal roots?
   A. Dermatomes are adjacent, with minimal overlap, so that loss of one dorsal root gives rise to a loss of somatic sensation within the dermatome boundary, as shown in the dermatome maps.
   B. Dermatomes overlap partially, but loss of one dorsal root does not give rise to a noticeable loss of sensation.

C. Dermatomes overlap partially, so that loss of one dorsal root typically gives rise to a noticeable loss of sensation within the dermatomal boundaries.

D. Dermatomes overlap nearly completely, so that loss of one dorsal root typically does not give rise to a noticeable loss of sensation.

6. Large-diameter afferent fibers do not terminate within which region of the spinal cord gray matter?
   A. Superficial laminae of the dorsal horn
   B. Deep layers of the dorsal horn
   C. Intermediate zone
   D. Ventral horn

7. A patient has a small thalamic stroke that affects mechanosensation on the contralateral foot. Which nucleus is most likely affected?
   A. Medial division of the ipsilateral ventral posterior nucleus
   B. Medial division of the contralateral ventral posterior nucleus
   C. Lateral division of the ipsilateral ventral posterior nucleus
   D. Lateral division of the contralateral ventral posterior nucleus

8. Occlusion of which artery would most likely damage the ventral posterior nucleus?
   A. Branches of the middle cerebral artery
   B. Branches of the anterior cerebral artery
   C. Branches of the posterior cerebral artery
   D. Branches of the basilar cerebral artery

9. Complete the following analogy:
   The face area of the primary somatic sensory cortex is to the leg area, as
   A. the middle cerebral artery is to the posterior cerebral artery
   B. the middle cerebral artery is to the anterior cerebral artery
   C. the posterior cerebral artery is to the anterior cerebral artery
   D. the posterior cerebral artery is to the middle cerebral artery

10. After a traumatic head injury, a 45-year-old female develops a seizure disorder. Initially, she experiences a tingling sensation in her right leg. This is followed by tingling on her right back, then right palm, fingers, and finally the right side of the face. Which of the following best describes the location of the start and end of the seizure?
    A. Start: medial left postcentral gyrus; end: lateral left postcentral gyrus
    B. Start: medial left postcentral gyrus; end: left insular cortex
    C. Start: left ventral posterior medial nucleus; end: left ventral posterior lateral nucleus
    D. Start: left ventral posterior lateral nucleus; end: left ventral posterior medial nucleus

Chapter 5

Somatic Sensation: Spinal Systems for Pain, Temperature, and Itch

CLINICAL CASE | Syringomyelia

Approximately one year earlier, a 41-year-old male sustained a painless burn to his right hand. The patient reported, at the time, that as the cigarette he was holding burned down, he noticed that his right index and middle fingers had sustained a burn, although he felt no pain. He reported that he noticed no other sensory, especially touch, or motor problems at that time. Over the next year, he began experiencing reduced right-hand grip strength in addition to the sensory loss. Then he sought medical care.

Neurological examination revealed an extensive territory, bilaterally, over the upper limbs and neck where there was minimal pain and thermal sensation (see Figure 5–1A). The analgesic region extended from the C5 to the T1 dermatomes. At this time, upper extremity tactile sensation and limb proprioception were now affected. Motor testing revealed denervation of several intrinsic right-hand muscles.

Figure 5–1A shows the classical distribution of pain and temperature loss in cervical syringomyelia. Figure 5–1B is an MRI showing a spinal cord syrinx, a pathological cavity coursing centrally and longitudinally within the central spinal cord. The syrinx produces the same MRI signal as CSF.

Answer the following questions based on your reading of the chapter, inspection of the images, and consideration of the neurological signs.

1. **What are the key differences in the location of axons of the anterolateral system and dorsal column–medial lemniscal pathway that enabled the syrinx initially to interrupt pain but not touch or limb proprioception?**

2. **Why did the syrinx initially disrupt pain sensation but only later affect strength?**

Key neurological signs and corresponding damaged brain structures

Bilateral loss of pain and thermal senses

Initially, the syrinx selectively damages the decussating anterolateral fibers producing the bilateral loss of pain and temperature senses; sparing touch and proprioceptive afferents in the dorsal columns. Figure 5–1C is a schematic illustrating the location of a typical syrinx in relation to decussating second-order axons of the anterolateral pathway. The central darkened region corresponds to the size of the syrinx when the patient first noticed pain loss, without additional neurological signs.

—Continued next page

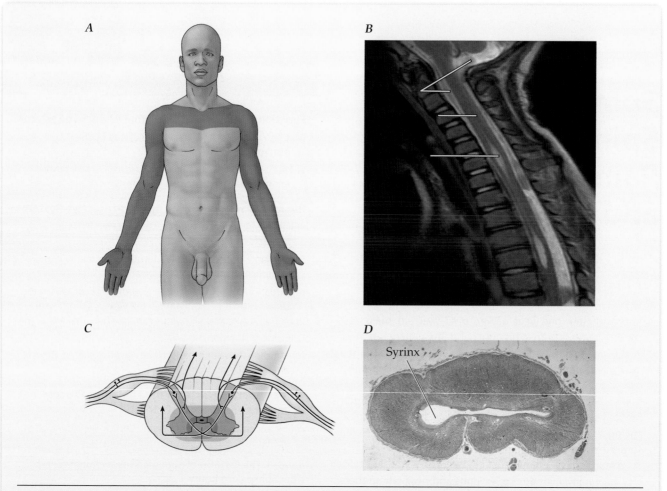

FIGURE 5–1 Syringomyelia. **A.** Distribution of loss of pain and temperature sense over the body. **B.** Midsagittal MRI showing a centrally located cervical spinal cord syrinx. **C.** Spinal cord cross section showing the patterns of terminations of small- and large-diameter axons and how the components of the anterolateral system decussate and ascend. The dorsal column–medial lemniscal system, by contrast, ascends ipsilaterally in the dorsal columns of spinal cord. The darker-tinted region is affected by the formation of a syrinx when the patient first noticed the sensory impairment. The lighter, enlarged, region corresponds to the syrinx when weakness was noticed. **D.** Histological section through a spinal cord syrinx. The central cavity in this spinal cord section is the syrinx. (**B,** Reproduced with permission from Struck AF, Haughton VM. Idiopathic syringomyelia: phase-contrast MR of cerebrospinal fluid flow dynamics at level of foramen magnum. *Radiology.* 2009;253[1]:184-190. **D,** Image courtesy of Dr. D.P. Agamanolis http://neuropathology-web.org.)

Bilateral loss of pain and thermal senses, together with loss of tactile and proprioceptive senses and hand weakness

One year later, because of its enlarged size, the syrinx extends into the dorsal columns, thereby producing tactile and proprioceptive loss. Importantly, the syrinx is large enough also to damage motor neurons, producing hand weakness (Figure 5-1C; lighter region corresponds to the enlarged syrinx). Figure 5–1D is a histological section through the spinal cord of a person who had a syrinx at autopsy. The cavity would have been fluid-filled during life, showing more clearly the damage produced by the syrinx.

Pain, temperature, and itch are our protective senses. Stimuli that evoke these sensations are good predictors of tissue harm. We touch a hot stove and withdraw our hand quickly to prevent a burn. We sense the itch of a mosquito bite and quickly swat at it to prevent further biting. Temperature brings us out of the cold or to seek shade when it is hot outside.

Pain of a more persistent or recurring nature typically brings a patient to visit a physician, who will use this information diagnostically. Persistent itch can signal liver disease.

The stimuli that produce pain, temperature, and itch are sensed by specific sets of sensory receptor neurons that innervate all of our body's tissues—from the skin on the surface to our muscles, bones, and visceral organs, internally—to ensure the best possible protection. These sensory receptor neurons have specific connections with central nervous system structures that, when they become active, orchestrate a complex set of physiological and behavioral events. The evoked perceptions allow us to recognize precisely stimulus modality and where on our body it occurred. The emotions produced by the protective senses help us identify the context in which the stimuli were received, the negative valance of abdominal pain after eating tainted food or the positive side of a cool tropical breeze. The protective senses mobilize our actions, to help ensure removal of the stimulus, to prevent bodily harm. Not surprisingly, the pain, temperature, and itch systems connect directly with diverse brain regions, much more so than for touch. Unique to our protective senses is that they engage areas of the cerebral cortex that are more known for their involvement in emotions than sensation. Unfortunately, our protective senses can be easily fooled; they can be activated into a persistent state of false alarm.

In this chapter, we will examine the neural systems for pain, temperature, and itch. We first examine the systems in overview and then consider the different levels of sensory processing, from the periphery to the cerebral cortex. We will focus on pain because more is known about its anatomical substrates. However, as we learn more about temperature sense and itch, it appears that all three protective senses engage similar spinal cord and brain circuits.

Functional Anatomy of the Spinal Protective Systems

Pain, Temperature, and Itch Are Mediated by the Anterolateral System

The **anterolateral system** (Figure 5–2A, B) is a collection of ascending pathways that travel in the anterior portion of the lateral column of the spinal cord and synapse in different brain regions. Surgical destruction of the anterolateral system spares touch and limb position senses but renders people insensitive or less sensitive to pain. Termed an anterolateral cordotomy, this procedure was commonly used to treat intractable pain before effective analgesics became available. The anterolateral system also mediates a residual, or crude, sense of touch after damage to the dorsal column–medial lemniscal system. Normally, this form of touch is thought to play a role in a sense of well being; it is sometimes termed **sensual touch**.

Sensory receptor neurons sensitive to **noxious** (ie, painful), **pruritic** (ie, itch provoking), and thermal stimuli provide the major sensory inputs to the anterolateral system. The anterolateral system's first relay is in the **dorsal horn** of the spinal cord (Figure 5–2A, B). Here, sensory fibers synapse on ascending projection neurons of the anterolateral systems. The axon of the ascending projection neuron of the anterolateral systems crosses the midline in the spinal cord. Curiously, for both the anterolateral and dorsal column–medial emniscal systems, the axon of the second neuron in the circuit decussates.

The anterolateral system comprises multiple pathways for several distinctive functions. We will focus on the role of these pathways in three aspects of pain but, as indicated above, there are many similarities with temperature and itch: (1) sensory-discriminative aspects of pain, (2) emotional aspects of pain, and (3) arousal and feedback control of pain transmission. Central to the sensory-discriminative aspects of pain—where the stimulus is located and its intensity—is the spinothalamic projection to the **ventral posterior lateral nucleus,** which in turn transmits information to the primary somatic sensory cortex (Figure 5–2A). This projection is somatotopically organized. Functional imaging studies have shown that this projection encodes the physical intensity of the stimulus, not the person's subjective impression of intensity.

Whereas nonpainful stimuli can have emotional overtones, they need not. By contrast, pain seems always to carry a negative emotion. For this reason, much of the pain pathway also targets subcortical and cortical centers for emotions (Figure 5-2B; see Chapter 16). Spinothalamic projections to the **ventromedial posterior nucleus,** which projects to the posterior insular cortex, and the **medial dorsal nucleus** of the thalamus, which transmits information to the **anterior cingulate gyrus,** are important in the emotional aspects of the stimulus (Figure 5–2B). The insular cortex projection is also thought to be important for perception of stimulus quality. The anterior cingulate pain projection is tied closely to the negative valence of pain. Interestingly, the anterior cingulate cortex becomes active both during actual pain (ie, noxious stimulation) and during emotional pain, feeling hurt (see Figure 2-7B).

The **spinoreticular tract** engages a subcortical emotional pathway (Figure 5–2B). This path relays in the **parabrachial nucleus** that, in turn, targets the **amygdala** (see Figure 1-10A). The amygdala has diverse projections to cerebral hemisphere structures, thereby capable of influencing our thoughts, emotions, and behaviors. The amygdala, together with the insular cortex, helps organize our behavioral responses that accompany pain, such as the increase in blood pressure or rubbing the injured site.

Arousal and feedback control of pain transmission center on the brain stem. Nuclei in the brain stem reticular formation in the pons and medulla receive sensory information of various sorts—painful as well as nonpainful somatic stimuli, sounds, and sights—and use this information to regulate arousal. The spinoreticular tract brings information about pain to these nuclei. Many of these reticular formation neurons project to the intralaminar thalamic nuclei that have broad projections to the basal ganglia and cerebral cortex for arousal. The **spinomesencephalic tract** terminates primarily in the midbrain tectum and periaqueductal gray matter. The projection to the tectum integrates somatic sensory information with vision and hearing for orienting the head and body to salient, notably noxious, stimuli (see Chapter 7). Projections to the **periaqueductal gray matter** play a role in the feedback regulation of pain transmission in the spinal cord (see section below on descending control of pain transmission).

A

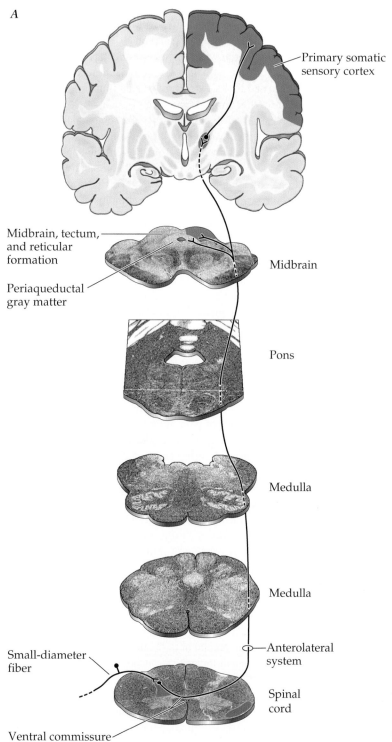

Primary somatic sensory cortex

Midbrain, tectum, and reticular formation

Periaqueductal gray matter

Midbrain

Pons

Medulla

Medulla

Anterolateral system

Small-diameter fiber

Spinal cord

Ventral commissure

FIGURE 5–2 Pain pathways. **A.** The spinothalamic tract is the Path to primary somatic sensory cortex for localizing stimuli and discriminating their intensity.

Visceral Pain Is Mediated by Dorsal Horn Neurons Whose Axons Ascend in the Dorsal Columns

There is a special pathway for pain from caudal visceral structures—such as in the pelvic region and parts of the lower gut—that is different from that of pain originating from other body parts (Figure 5–2C). Rather than synapse on dorsal horn neurons that send their axons into the anterolateral white matter, dorsal horn visceral pain neurons send their axons into the medial portion of the dorsal columns, the gracile column. Recall that most axons in the dorsal columns, approximately 85%, are the central branches of mechanoreceptors (Chapter 4); the remaining 15% receive nociceptive information.

B

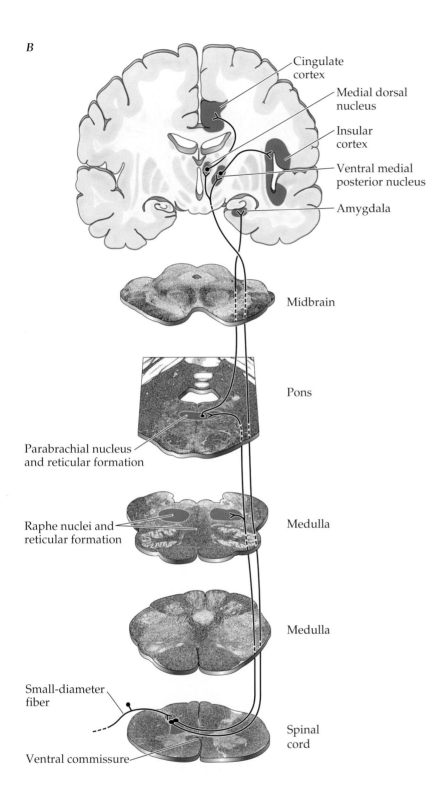

Cingulate cortex

Medial dorsal nucleus

Insular cortex

Ventral medial posterior nucleus

Amygdala

Midbrain

Pons

Parabrachial nucleus and reticular formation

Raphe nuclei and reticular formation

Medulla

Medulla

Small-diameter fiber

Spinal cord

Ventral commissure

Continued— **FIGURE 5–2** The projection to the midbrain, the spinomesencephalic tract, is also shown. *B.* Pathways for the affective aspects of pain. The spinothalamic tract projects to other thalamic nuclei for the emotional aspects of pain. The spinoreticular tract is also important for the affective aspects of pain, thermal senses, and itch.

Surprisingly, the visceral pain pathway follows a course similar to the mechanosensory pathway, synapsing in the dorsal column nuclei, decussating in the medulla, ascending in the brain stem in the medial lemniscus, and synapsing within the thalamus. There is a significant difference; the visceral pain path synapses in separate portions of the dorsal column nuclei and thalamus than the mechanosensory pathway. Much less is known of this potentially very important pathway than the anterolateral pathways.

Regional Anatomy of the Spinal Protective Systems

Small-Diameter Sensory Fibers Mediate Pain, Temperature, and Itch

Nociceptors are sensory receptor neurons that are sensitive to noxious or tissue-damaging stimuli and mediate pain. These receptor neurons respond to chemicals released from traumatized tissue.

C

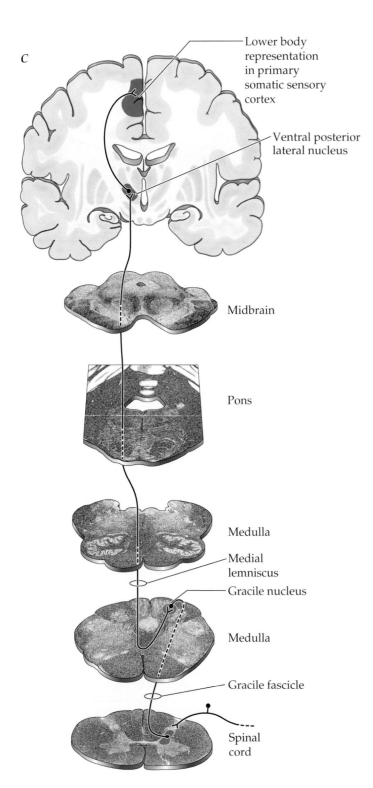

Lower body
representation
in primary
somatic sensory
cortex

Ventral posterior
lateral nucleus

Midbrain

Pons

Medulla

Medial
lemniscus

Gracile nucleus

Medulla

Gracile fascicle

Spinal
cord

Continued— **FIGURE 5–2 C.** Visceral pain pathway.

There are three principal classes of nociceptor: thermal, mechanical, and polymodal. Thermal nociceptors are activated by temperatures less than about 5° and greater than 45°. Mechanical nociceptors are activated by a tissue-damaging mechanical stimulus, such as a needle. Polymodal nociceptors are activated by noxious thermal or mechanical stimuli. **Itch-sensitive receptors,** or **pruriceptors,** respond to histamine. Itch is evoked when histamine is injected intradermally. Receptor neurons sensitive to cold or warmth are termed **thermoreceptors.**

The morphology of these classes of receptor neurons is simple; they are **bare nerve endings** (see Figure 4–3). In contrast to mechanoreceptors, which have a large diameter and thickly myelinated axon (A-α and A-β), nociceptors, thermoreceptors, and pruriceptors have small-diameter axons, which fall into the A-δ and C-fiber categories (see Table 4–1). Nociceptors are both thinly myelinated (A-δ) and unmyelinated (C fibers). A brief noxious stimulus evokes initially a sharp, pricking pain, sometimes termed "fast" pain, mediated by A-δ nociceptors followed by a dull burning pain, sometimes termed "slow" pain, mediated by C-fiber nociceptors. Thermoreceptor axons also conduct action potentials in the A-δ and C-fiber ranges. Pruriceptors are C-fibers only.

There has been much research on the mechanisms of transduction of noxious stimuli into depolarizing sensory potentials. Important among the various membrane receptors that nociceptors have are the diverse members of the transient receptor potential (TRP) receptors. For example, TRPV1, TRPV2, TRPV3, and TRPV4 receptors are responsible for thermal sensitivity in the warm (ie, innocuous) to hot (noxious) range. TRPV1 receptors mediate the hot of capsaicin, and TRPV2 receptors are activated by very high temperatures (TRPV2). By contrast, TRPM8 receptors are activated at very low temperatures and by certain chemical, such as menthol (TRPM8). There are several candidate membrane receptors for mechanotransduction in mechanonociceptors. Pruriceptors are sensitive to histamine.

Pain sensitivity naturally changes, and much of this plasticity occurs at the periphery. Nociceptors can become sensitized—that is, develop a memory of prior injury—and the pain system becomes more responsive. This can be produced by factors that are released at the injury site as a consequence of the tissue damage and ensuing inflammation. **Hyperalgesia** is an exaggerated response to a noxious stimulus. **Allodynia** is feeling pain to a stimulus that normally does not produce pain, such as light touch. Pain also can get out of control, signaling a persistent "false alarm." These chronic pain states can be debilitating. They have both peripheral and central nervous system components, including maladaptive plasticity in the dorsal horn (see next section) and abnormal modulatory signals from the brain.

Small-Diameter Sensory Fibers Terminate Primarily in the Superficial Laminae of the Dorsal Horn

Small-diameter axons—which subserve pain, itch, and temperature senses—enter the spinal cord in **Lissauer tract,** the white matter region that caps the dorsal horn (see Figure 5–4). Note that although Lissauer tract is part of the white matter, it stains lightly because its axons either have a thin myelin sheath or are unmyelinated. Within the tract the fibers bifurcate and ascend and descend before they branch into the gray matter.

Small-diameter fibers have a very specific termination pattern. To better understand the significance of this pattern, we first need to consider the laminar organization of the spinal gray matter (Figure 5–3). Similar to other areas of the central nervous system, spinal cord neurons are clustered. The Swedish neuroanatomist Bror Rexed further recognized that neuron

clusters in the spinal cord often formed flattened sheets, termed **Rexed laminae** (Table 5–1; Figure 5–3), that run parallel to the long axis of the spinal cord. He distinguished 10 laminae. The dorsal horn is now regarded to comprise laminae I through V and the ventral horn, laminae VI through IX. Lamina X comprises the gray matter surrounding the central canal. However, for functional reasons we also distinguish laminae VI, the dorsal part of VII, and X from laminae VIII and IX. Many interneurons important for movement control are located in laminae VI, VII, and X, and this is termed the intermediate zone; motor neurons that innervate axial, proximal, and distal muscles are located ventral to the intermediate zone, in laminae VIII and IX.

Like Brodmann's areas of the cerebral cortex (Figure 1-19), neurons clustered according to Rexed laminae have a functional organization. Laminae I and II receive information from small-diameter myelinated (A-δ) fibers and unmyelinated (C) fibers only, indicating a selective role in pain, temperature, and itch processing. By contrast, laminae III and IV receive only large-diameter (A-α, A-β) fiber terminations. These laminae serve mechanosensory and reflex functions. Lamina V receives information from both small- and large-diameter fibers (Figure 5–3), enabling the neurons there to process a broad range of somatic stimulus intensities, from light touch to pain. The deeper laminae, VI through IX, tend to receive much less afferent fiber information directly. There is one important exception; primary muscle spindle receptors and Golgi tendon organs terminate in the motor regions (laminae VII and IX); and the primary muscle spindle receptors synapse directly on motor neurons.

Anterolateral System Projection Neurons Are Located in the Dorsal Horn and Decussate in the Ventral Commissure

The laminar organization of the dorsal horn is also important for the projections to the brain stem and thalamus. The pathway to thalamic nuclei important for pain, itch, and temperature sensations originates primarily from neurons in lamina I, which receives direct input from small-diameter sensory fibers (Figure 5–3), and lamina V, where neurons receive both small and large fiber inputs and respond to a range of stimuli. The spinal cord neurons whose axons project to the intralaminar nuclei and reticular formation of the pons and medulla, involved primarily in arousal, are located more ventrally in the gray matter, in laminae VI through VIII. The projection to the midbrain, important for orienting to salient stimuli and pain suppression, also originates from neurons in laminae I and V, similar to the projection to the ventral posterior lateral nucleus.

Most axons of the anterolateral system decussate in the spinal cord before ascending to the brain stem or thalamus (Figures 5–2 and 5–3). Decussations occur in **commissures,** in this case in the ventral (anterior) commissure, ventral to the central canal (Figure 5–4A). During early development, this region corresponded to the floor plate, an important site

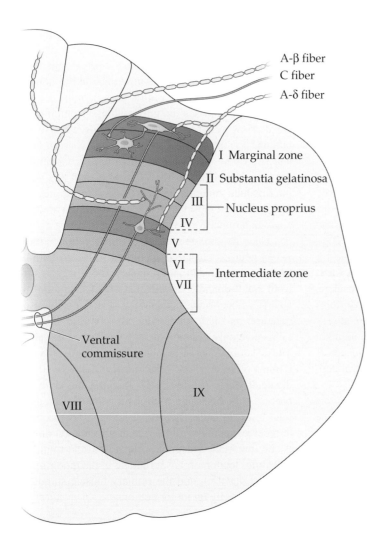

A-β fiber
C fiber
A-δ fiber

I Marginal zone
II Substantia gelatinosa
III — Nucleus proprius
IV
V
VI
VII — Intermediate zone

Ventral commissure

VIII
IX

FIGURE 5–3 Laminar termination patterns of primary sensory axon terminals in the dorsal horn. A-δ and C fibers terminate superficially in the dorsal horn, with a branch of the A-δ fiber also terminating in deeper layers. A-β fibers terminate in the deeper layers of the dorsal horn. However, the major A-β branch ascends in the dorsal column. Projection neurons of the anterolateral system are shown, located in laminae I and V. Their axons decussate in the ventral spinal commissure. Note that while laminae I-VI resemble flattened sheets, laminae VII-IX are more columnar-shaped. (Adapted from Rexed B. A cytoarchitectonic atlas of the spinal cord in the cat. *J Comp Neurol*, 1954;100[2]:297-379.)

for guiding spinal axons across the midline. Developing axons are attracted to the midline at the floor plate. However, once the axons cross the midline, there is a molecular switch. The attraction they had for the midline floor plate is converted to a repulsion that prevents the axons from recrossing. While much is known about how axons cross the midline, why they cross is not known. Once on the opposite side, the developing axons are now attracted to grow toward particular regions of the white

matter, where they ascend to the brain. Less is known about long-distance axon guidance toward the brain than decussation. The location of the ascending axons of the anterolateral system is revealed by examining the degenerated area in the lateral column in Figure 5–4C. Although the anterolateral system is somatotopically organized (Figure 5–4B), it is not as precise as that for the dorsal columns and only a trend is apparent. Axons transmitting sensory information from more caudal segments are located lateral to those from more rostral segments.

Neurons in the dorsal horn in the sacral, lumbar, and thoracic spinal cord receive nociceptive inputs from visceral structures. Rather than projecting their axon to the contralateral white matter, they project to the ipsilateral gracile fascicle and follow a course very similar to the mechanosensory pathway (Figure 5–2C). Many lamina V neurons in the sacral, lumbar, and thoracic spinal cord receive convergent information from visceral nociceptors and cutaneous receptors. This provides the anatomical substrate for "referred pain," whereby pain resulting from visceral tissue damage is perceived as originating from a portion of the body surface. For example, pain associated with a myocardial infarction is felt on the left arm and chest, possibly because sensory fibers from the heart sensing a lack of tissue oxygen converge onto neurons in the upper cervical spinal cord.

Table **5–1** **Correspondence between Rexed laminae and nuclei**

Rexed lamina	Spinal cord nucleus
Lamina I	Marginal zone
Lamina II	Substantia gelatinosa
Laminae III and IV	Nucleus proprius
Lamina V	Base of dorsal horn
Laminae VI and VII	Intermediate zone
Lamina IX	Motor nuclei

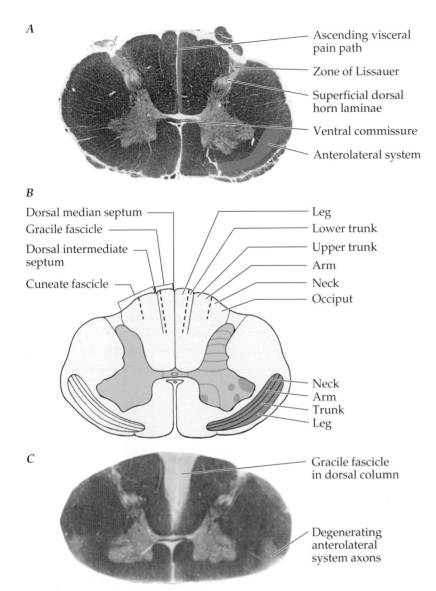

A

Ascending visceral
pain path

Zone of Lissauer

Superficial dorsal
horn laminae

Ventral commissure

Anterolateral system

B

Dorsal median septum

Gracile fascicle

Dorsal intermediate
septum

Cuneate fascicle

Leg

Lower trunk

Upper trunk

Arm

Neck

Occiput

Neck
Arm
Trunk
Leg

C

Gracile fascicle
in dorsal column

Degenerating
anterolateral
system axons

FIGURE 5–4 Spinal cord anatomy. *A.* Myelin-stained section showing key structures of the pain pathway. *B.* Drawing of spinal cord with somatotopy of the anterolateral system. *C.* Location of degenerated somatic sensory paths after a lumbar spinal cord injury.

Box 5–1

The Patterns of Somatic Sensory Impairments After Spinal Cord Injury

Spinal cord injury results in deficits in somatic sensation and in the control of body musculature at the level of, and caudal to, the lesion. Motor deficits that follow such injury are considered in Chapter 10. Here, only somatic sensory deficits are considered. We will integrate our knowledge of the pain, as well as mechanosensory, pathways because traumatic injury to the spinal cord may not distinguish one system from another. In general, somatic sensory deficits after spinal injury have three major characteristics: (1) the sensory **modality** that is affected, for example, whether pain or touch is impaired on a particular body part, (2) the **laterality,** or side of the body where deficits are observed (ie, ipsilateral vs contralateral), and (3) the **body regions** affected. Damage to one half of the spinal cord, or hemisection, illustrates all three of these characteristic deficits (Figure 5–5). Spinal hemisection can occur, for example, when the cord is injured traumatically, such as with a gun-shot wound or when a tumor encroaches on the cord from one side. The sensory and motor deficits that follow spinal cord hemisection are collectively termed the **Brown–Séquard syndrome.**

Axons in the dorsal columns are **ipsilateral** to their origin in the spinal cord; hence, deficits in touch and limb position sense are present ipsilateral to the spinal cord lesion (Figure 5–5). In contrast, the axons of the anterolateral system decussate in the spinal cord. Therefore, **pain and temperature senses** are impaired on the side of the body that is **contralateral** to the lesion. (Note that itch is not usually tested but presumably also is impaired contralaterally.)

The spinal cord level at which injury occurs can be determined by comparing the distribution of sensory loss with the sensory innervation patterns of the dorsal roots (ie, the dermatomal maps; Figure 4–5). Because of the differences in the anatomical organization of the two systems mediating somatic sensations, a single level of spinal injury will result in different levels of sensory impairment for touch and pain sensations. For touch sensation, the most rostral dermatome in which sensation is impaired corresponds to the level of injury in the spinal cord. For pain sensation, the most rostral dermatome in which sensation is impaired is about two

segments lower than the injured spinal cord level. This is because the axons of the anterolateral system decussate over a distance of one to two spinal segments before ascending to the brain stem and diencephalon. This is clinically significant because it gives the injured person more caudal protective sensory awareness, which can help in detecting debilitating events that would otherwise go unnoticed, such as pressure injuries.

Vascular Lesions of the Medulla Differentially Affect Somatic Sensory Function

Axons of the anterolateral system ascend along the antero-lateral margins of the white matter of the spinal cord (Figure 5–4A). When the fibers reach the medulla, they shift dorsally, being displaced by the large inferior olivary nucleus (Figure 5–6A). As we learned in Chapter 3, the medial and dorsolateral medulla receive their arterial supplies from small

direct branches of the vertebral artery and the **posterior inferior cerebellar artery (PICA),** respectively (Figure 5–6A). Occlusion of the PICA damages the ascending pain, temperature, and itch fibers but not the medial lemniscus. A patient who experiences an infarction of the PICA can have diminished pain sensation on the limbs and trunk but unaffected touch sense. The sensory loss is contralateral to the side of the lesion because the axons of the anterolateral system decussate in the spinal cord (Figure 5–5). (Such sensory loss is one of multiple neurological signs that comprise

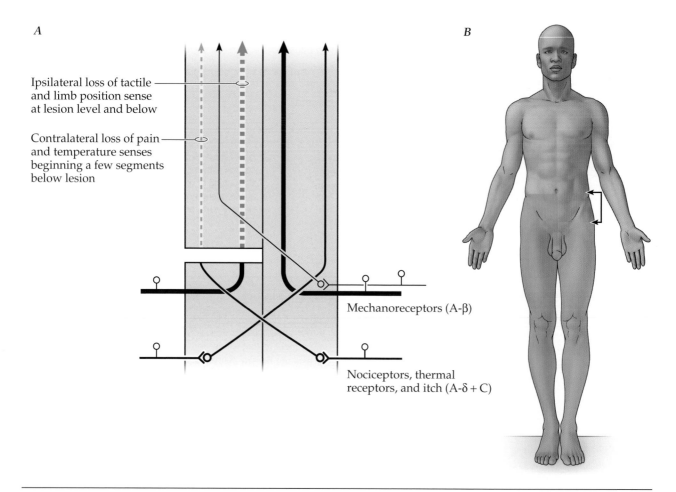

A

Ipsilateral loss of tactile and limb position sense at lesion level and below

Contralateral loss of pain and temperature senses beginning a few segments below lesion

Mechanoreceptors (A-β)

Nociceptors, thermal receptors, and itch (A-δ + C)

B

FIGURE 5–5 *A.* The patterns of decussation of the dorsal column–medial lemniscal and anterolateral systems are illustrated in relation to spinal cord hemisection (Brown-Séquard syndrome). ***B.*** Because projection neurons of the anterolateral system ascend as they decussate, spinal hemisection produces a loss of pain, temperature, and itch one to two segments caudal to the lesion. In contrast, loss of mechanical sensations begins at the level of the lesion.

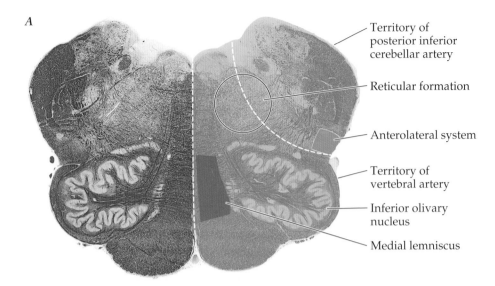

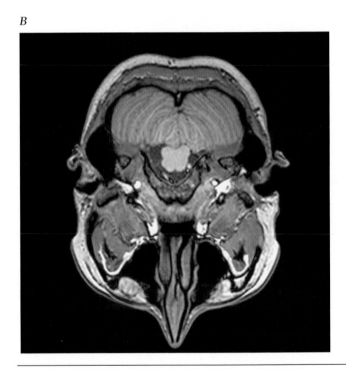

FIGURE 5–6 Myelin-stained section through mid-medulla (**A**) and corresponding MRI (**B**). The pattern of arterial perfusion of the rostral medulla is also shown in part A.

the **lateral medullary,** or **Wallenberg, syndrome,** which is discussed further in Chapters 6 and 15.)

Farther rostrally in the pons and midbrain, the anterolateral system joins the medial lemniscus (Figure 5–7). The **spino-thalamic tract,** like the medial lemniscus, courses through the pons and midbrain en route to the thalamus. The **spinoreticu-lar tract** terminates centrally within the medulla and pons, in a region termed the reticular formation. Once thought to subserve a discrete set of arousal-related functions, what is termed the reticular formation is a heterogeneous collection of nuclei serving many somatic, visceral, and regulatory functions. An important projection of the spinoreticular tract is to the parabrachial nucleus (Figure 5–7B). This is a key relay for visceral afferent information—both nociceptive and innocuous—to the hypo-thalamus and amygdala. One projection of the **spinomesence-phalic tract** that is important for orienting to somatic stimuli is to the superior colliculus (Figure 5–7A; see Chapter 7).

Descending Pain Suppression Pathways Originate From the Brain Stem

While all sensation is mutable, being critically dependent on context and experience, modulation of pain perception is particularly salient and clinically relevant. Consider how pain

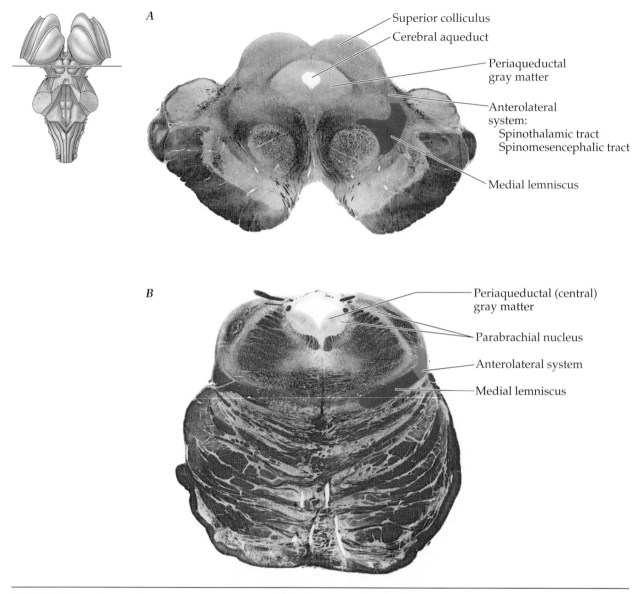

A

Superior colliculus

Cerebral aqueduct

Periaqueductal gray matter

Anterolateral system:
Spinothalamic tract
Spinomesencephalic tract

Medial lemniscus

B

Periaqueductal (central) gray matter

Parabrachial nucleus

Anterolateral system

Medial lemniscus

FIGURE 5–7 Myelin-stained sections through the midbrain (**A**) and pons-midbrain junction (**B**).

becomes diminished during physical combat or in childbirth. Pain suppression may be a survival mechanism that allows people to function better despite sudden pain. The circuit for pain suppression uses serotonergic and noradrenergic mechanisms to inhibit pain transmission in the dorsal horn (Figure 5–8). Beginning in the forebrain, structures involved in emotions as well as pain processing—including the amygdala, hypothalamus, insular cortex, and anterior cingulate cortex—project to excitatory glutamatergic neurons of the **periaqueductal gray matter** (Figures 5–7 and 5–8) that, in turn, regulate a collection of medullary neurons in the **raphe nuclei** that use **serotonin** as their neurotransmitter (5-HT; Figure 5–8, inset). The raphe nuclei give rise to a descending serotonergic pathway to the spinal cord. Similarly, other regions in the brain stem, including the locus ceruleus (see Figure 2–3) and the lateral medullary reticular formation, give rise to descending noradrenergic

projections to the spinal cord (NA; Figure 5–8). Pain transmission in the dorsal horn is suppressed by promoting the inhibitory actions of dorsal horn interneurons, including those using **enkephalin** as their neurotransmitter, decreasing the capacity for nociceptors to activate their postsynaptic targets, and by inhibiting pain ascending projection neurons directly.

Three Separate Nuclei in the Thalamus Process Pain, Temperature, and Itch

The ventral posterior nucleus is an important recipient of both the anterolateral system and the dorsal column system for visceral pain (Figure 5–2C). Although both the mechanosensory and the pain, temperature, and itch projections terminate in the ventral posterior lateral nucleus, their terminal fields hardly overlap, an example of functional localization within the central

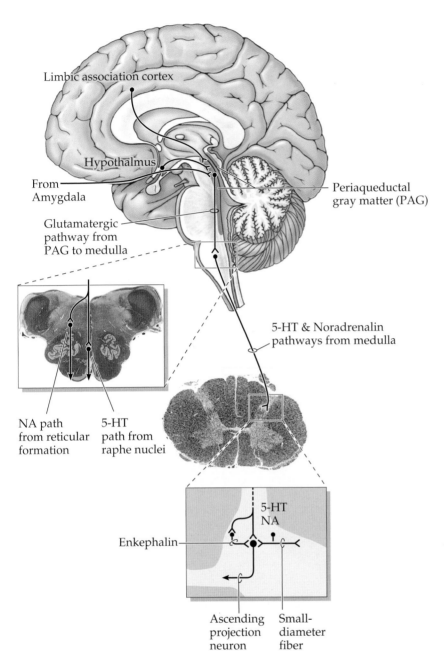

FIGURE 5–8 Pain modulatory system. Information from diverse forebrain regions converge onto the periaqueductal gray matter (PAG). The PAG, in turn, projects to serotonergic (5-HT) nuclei in the medulla, the raphe nuclei, as well as medullary noradrenergic (NA) nuclei in the reticular formation. Descending 5-HT and NA pathways promote inhibition in the spinal cord, thereby suppressing pain transmission.

nervous system. The mechanosensory projections tend to be located rostral to the projections for pain, temperature, and itch.

The **ventromedial posterior nucleus** (Figure 5–9A) is caudal to the ventral posterior nucleus. It projects to the **insular cortex** (Figure 5–10), which, as discussed, is important for perception of the quality and intensity of pain, temperature, and itch, and in mediating behavioral and autonomic responses. The **medial dorsal nucleus** (Figure 5–9B) also receives spinothalamic input and projects to the **anterior cingulate gyrus** (Figure 5–10), which is involved in the emotional aspects of somatic sensory stimulation. The **intralaminar nuclei** (see Figure 2–13) also receive spinothalamic input, visceral pain input from the dorsal column nuclei, as well as information from the reticular formation. However, the pain

functions of the intralaminar nuclei are not understood. The intralaminar nuclei are diffuse-projecting and may participate in arousal and attention (see Table 2–1).

Limbic and Insular Areas Contain the Cortical Representations of Pain, Itch, and Temperature Sensations

The ascending pain, temperature, and itch pathways influence wide areas of the cerebral cortex. For acute pain, which has been studied most thoroughly, a complex set of areas becomes activated: the primary and secondary somatic sensory areas, the insular cortex, the anterior cingulate cortex,

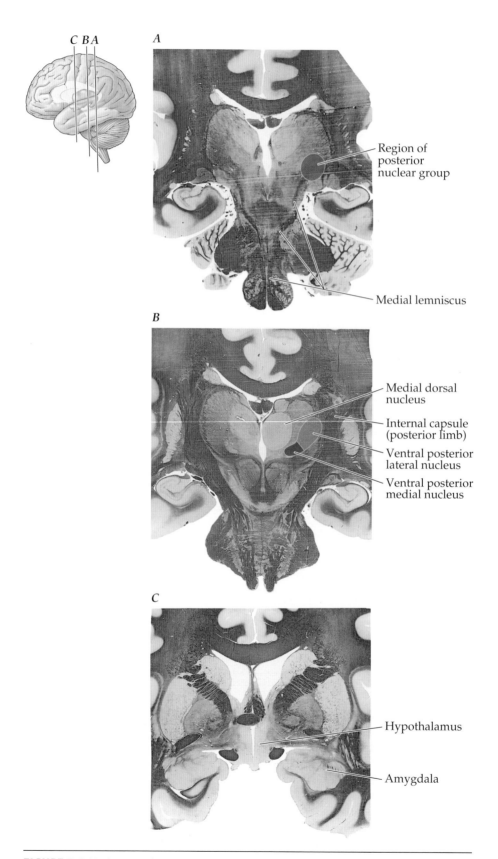

FIGURE 5–9 Myelin-stained sections through the thalamic pain nuclei. **A.** Posterior thalamus, which is the location of the ventral medial posterior nucleus. **B.** Medial dorsal nucleus and the ventral posterior nucleus. Note that the ventral posterior nucleus comprises two nuclear divisions. The ventral posterior lateral nucleus is for spinal somatic sensory processing and the ventral posterior medial nucleus is for the trigeminal system. **C.** Amygdala and hypothalamus.

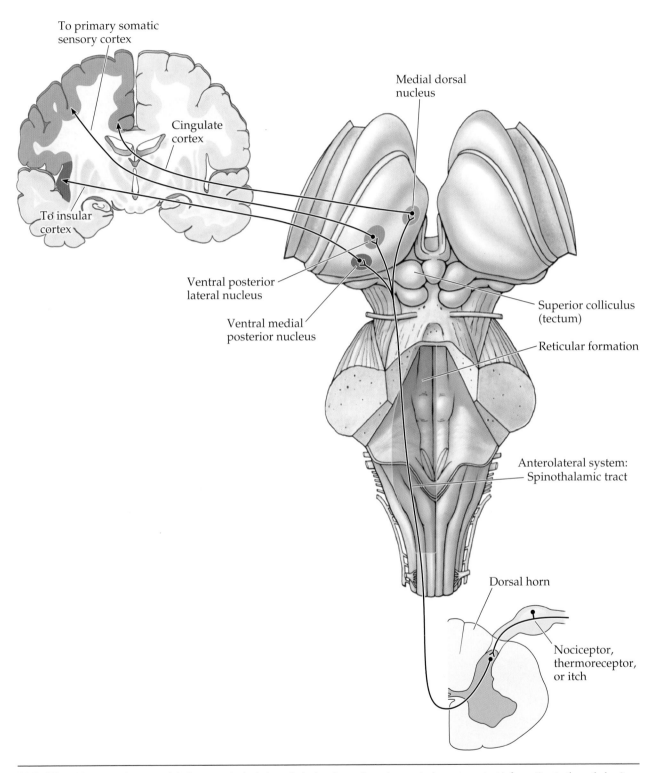

FIGURE 5–10 Pain pathways and thalamo-cortical relations. A single schematic nociceptor is shown to project information to three thalamic nuclei, which in turn, project to three separate cortical areas. The ventral posterior nucleus projects to the primary somatic sensory cortex. The ventral medial posterior nucleus projects to the insular pain cortex. The medial dorsal nucleus, which has diverse frontal lobe projections, transmits pain information to the anterior cingulate cortex.

and the prefrontal cortex. To this, one can add diverse areas of the thalamus and the amygdala. This complex set of brain structures has been termed the "pain matrix." Many of these areas are also activated during thermal stimulation and itch.

Noninvasive imaging studies in humans presented with noxious stimuli, as well as studies in anesthetized animals, are beginning to elucidate the particular contributions of individual components of the pain matrix. The **primary**

somatic sensory cortex is thought to be important in localizing the stimulus and discerning intensity. The **insular cortex** (Figures 5–10 and 5–11) is important in discriminating the quality and intensity of the stimulus, and possible affective aspects of pain. Importantly, the insular cortex is the most consistently activated of all cortical areas during painful stimuli. The pain representation in the insular cortex, together with adjoining representations of taste and internal organs (see Chapters 6 and 9),

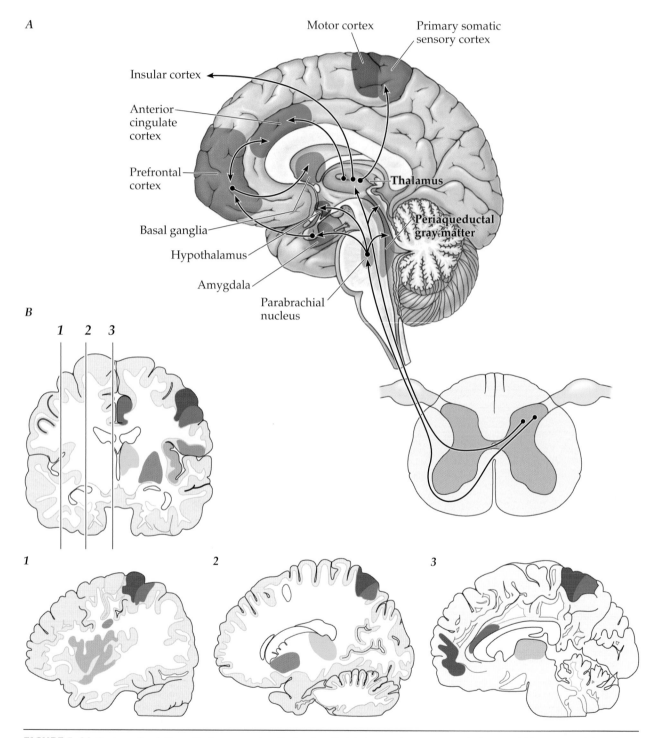

FIGURE 5–11 Noxious stimulation activates many subcortical regions that, in turn, activate many cortical areas, which are termed the pain matrix. **A**. Salient features of the divergence of pain information to the brain stem and cortex are shown on a mid-sagittal brain view. These structures have been identified on the basis of brain imaging studies. The key cortical areas are: somatic sensory cortex, insular cortex, cingulate cortex, and prefrontal cortex. Motor cortex is also shown because it is important in voluntary motor responses evoked by painful stimuli. **B**. Semischematic drawing through the pain matrix structures: coronal slice is shown above three sagittal slices, whose plains are indicated in the coronal slice. (Based on the meta-analysis in Apkarian AV, Bushnell MC, Treede RD, Zubieta JK. Human brain mechanisms of pain perception and regulation in health and disease. *Eur J Pain.* 2005;9[4]:463-484.)

may also be part of a network of cortical regions mediating body homeostasis. These areas also can regulate behavioral and autonomic responses to pain. The **anterior cingulate gyrus** (Brodmann's area 24; see Figure 2–19) is part of the limbic system for emotions. Not surprisingly, the anterior cingulate becomes more activated when painful and thermal stimuli are judged to be more unsettling and unpleasant. Interestingly, the same cingulate area that is important in signaling the emotional aspects of pain is also important for the emotional aspects of somatic sensory stimulation and in the "hurt" of social exclusion (Figure 2-7B).

Summary

Sensory Receptor Neurons

The *anterolateral system* mediates *pain,* temperature, and itch senses and *crude touch* (Figure 5–2A, B). Visceral pain is processed by a small contingent of *dorsal column* axons (Figure 5–2C). *Dorsal root ganglion neurons* sensitive to *noxious stimuli,* warmth, cold, or itch (histamine) have *bare nerve endings* and *small-diameter axons* (A-δ; C; see Table 4–1).

Spinal Cord

The axons of dorsal root ganglion neurons enter the spinal cord via the *dorsal roots.* A *dermatome* is the area of skin innervated by a single dorsal root (see Figure 4–5). Small-diameter fibers enter the spinal cord and ascend and descend in *Lissauer tract* (Figures 5–2 and 5–4); they eventually terminate in the gray matter of the spinal cord (Figure 5–3). The axons of the anterolateral system derive from dorsal horn neurons and decussate in the ventral (anterior) commissure (Figures 5–2, 5–3, and 5–5). The anterolateral system ascends in the lateral column (Figures 5–4). Ascending visceral fibers ascend medially in the dorsal columns, in the *gracile fascicle* (Figure 5–4). Spinal cord hemisection has a differential effect on the somatic sensory modalities caudal to the lesion, producing loss of touch and position senses on the side of the lesion and loss of pain and temperature senses on the opposite side (Figure 5–5).

Brain Stem

Fibers of the anterolateral system terminate in the *reticular formation* (Figure 5–6; spinoreticular tract), *parabrachial nucleus* (Figure 5–7), *midbrain,* including the *periaqueductal gray matter* (Figure 5–7; spinomesencephalic tract), and *thalamus* (spinothalamic tract) (Figures 5–7 and 5–9). Visceral pain fibers synapse in the *gracile nucleus,* in a separate region from mechanosensory fibers, and ascend to the thalamus in the *medial lemniscus* (Figures 5–6 and 5–7). Anterolateral system fibers receive their arterial supply in the medulla by *PICA* (Figure 5–6).

Descending Pain Modulatory Systems

Forebrain structures for emotions and pain processing—including the amygdala, hypothalamus, insular cortex, and anterior cingulate cortex—project to excitatory glutamatergic neurons of the *periaqueductal gray matter* (Figure 5–8). These neurons regulate *serotonergic neurons* in the *raphe nuclei* and noradrenergic neurons in the *reticular formation* that project to the *dorsal horn* (Figure 5–8). Pain transmission in the dorsal horn is suppressed by promoting the inhibitory actions of dorsal horn neurons.

Thalamus and Cerebral Cortex

Axons of the spinothalamic tract, and probably viscerosensory fibers, synapse in the three principal thalamic nuclei that, in turn, project to different cortical areas. The *ventral posterior lateral nucleus* (Figure 5–10), which projects to the primary somatic sensory cortex (Figures 5–10 and 5–11), is important for perception of stimulus intensity and location. The *ventromedial posterior nucleus* (Figure 5–9A), which projects to the insular cortex (Figures 5–10 and 5–11), is also important in stimulus perception as well as affective aspects of pain and thermal stimuli. The third nucleus, the *medial dorsal nucleus* (Figures 5–9 and 5–10), projects to the cingulate cortex (Figure 5–11) for the emotional responses to pain. The insular and anterior cortical regions are also important in the behavioral and autonomic responses to pain, temperature, and itch sensations and the emotions and memories these stimuli evoke.

Selected Readings

Basbaum A, Jessell TM, Foley KM. The perception of pain. In: Kandel ER, Schwartz JH, Jessell TM, Siegelbaum SA, Hudspeth AJ, eds. *Principles of Neural Science.* 5th ed. New York, NY: McGraw-Hill.

Basbaum AI, Bautista DM, Scherrer G, Julius D. Cellular and molecular mechanisms of pain. *Cell.* 2009;139(2): 267-284.

Altschuler SM, Bao XM, Bieger D, Hopkins DA, Miselis RR. Viscerotopic representation of the upper alimentary tract in the rat: sensory ganglia and nuclei of the solitary and spinal trigeminal tracts. *J Comp Neurol.* 1989;283(2):248-268.

Andrew D, Craig AD. Spinothalamic lamina I neurons selectively sensitive to histamine: a central neural pathway for itch. *Nat Neurosci.* 2001;4:72-77.

Apkarian AV, Bushnell MC, Treede RD, Zubieta JK. Human brain mechanisms of pain perception and regulation in health and disease. *Eur J Pain.* 2005;9(4):463-484.

Appelberg AE, Leonard RB, Kenshalo DR Jr., et al. Nuclei in which functionally identified spinothalamic tract neurons terminate. *J Comp Neurol.* 1979;188:575-586.

Augustine JR. The insular lobe in primates including humans. *Neurol Res.* 1985;7:2-10.

Belmonte C, Viana F. Molecular and cellular limits to somatosensory specificity. *Mol Pain.* 2008;4:14.

Berkley KJ, Hubscher CH. Are there separate central nervous system pathways for touch and pain? *Nat Med.* 1995;1(8):766-773.

Blomqvist A, Zhang ET, Craig AD. Cytoarchitectonic and immunohistochemical characterization of a specific pain and temperature relay, the posterior portion of the ventral medial nucleus, in the human thalamus. *Brain.* 2000;123(part 3):601-619.

Bogdanov EI, Heiss JD, Mendelevich EG, Mikhaylov IM, Haass A. Clinical and neuroimaging features of "idiopathic" syringomyelia. *Neurology.* 2004;62(5):791-794.

Bove SE, Flatters SJ, Inglis JJ, Mantyh PW. New advances in musculoskeletal pain. *Brain Res Rev.* Apr 2009;60(1):187-201.

Bushnell MC, Duncan GH, Hofbauer RK, Ha B, Chen JI, Carrier B. Pain perception: is there a role for primary somatosensory cortex? *Proc Natl Acad Sci USA.* 1999;96:7705-7709.

Casey KL. Forebrain mechanisms of nociception and pain: analysis through imaging. *Proc Natl Acad Sci USA.* 1999;96:7668-7674.

Coghill RC, Talbot JD, Evans AC, et al. Distributed processing of pain and vibration by the human brain. *J Neurosci.* 1994;14:4095-4108.

Collins RD. *Illustrated Manual of Neurologic Diagnosis.* Philadelphia, PA: Lippincott; 1962.

Cortright DN, Krause JE, Broom DC. TRP channels and pain. *Biochim Biophys Acta.* 2007;1772(8):978-988.

Craig AD. How do you feel—now? The anterior insula and human awareness. *Nat Rev Neurosci.* 2009;10(1):59-70.

Craig AD. Interoception: the sense of the physiological condition of the body. *Curr Opin Neurobiol.* 2003;13(4):500-505.

Craig AD. Retrograde analyses of spinothalamic projections in the macaque monkey: input to ventral posterior nuclei. *J Comp Neurol.* 2006;499(6):965-978.

Craig AD, Bushnell MC. The thermal grill illusion: unmasking the burn of cold pain. *Science.* 1994;265:252-255.

Craig AD, Bushnell MC, Zhang ET, Blomqvist A. A thalamic nucleus specific for pain and temperature sensation. *Nature.* 1994;372:770-773.

Craig AD, Zhang ET. Retrograde analyses of spinothalamic projections in the macaque monkey: input to posterolateral thalamus. *J Comp Neurol.* 2006;499(6):953-964.

Dubner R. Three decades of pain research and its control. *J Dent Res.* 1997;76:730-733.

Dubner R, Gold M. The neurobiology of pain. *Proc Natl Acad Sci USA.* 1999;96:7627-7630.

Dum RP, Levinthal DJ, Strick PL. The spinothalamic system targets motor and sensory areas in the cerebral cortex of monkeys. *J Neurosci.* 2009;29(45):14223-14235.

Fields H. State-dependent opioid control of pain. *Nat Rev Neurosci.* 2004;5(7):565-575.

Fields HL. *Pain.* New York, NY: McGraw-Hill; 1987.

Fitzgerald M. The development of nociceptive circuits. *Nat Rev Neurosci.* 2005;6(7):507-520.

Gandevia SC, Burke DA. Peripheral motor system. In: Paxinos G, Mai JK, eds. *The Human Nervous System.* London: Elsevier; 2004.

Gebhart GF. Descending modulation of pain. *Neurosci Biobehav Rev.* 2004;27(8):729-737.

Giesler GJ Jr., Nahin RL, Madsen AM. Postsynaptic dorsal column pathway of the rat. I. Anatomical studies. *J Neurophysiol.* 1984;51:260-275.

Hucho T, Levine JD. Signaling pathways in sensitization: toward a nociceptor cell biology. *Neuron.* 2007;55(3):365-376.

Ikoma A, Steinhoff M, Stander S, Yosipovitch G, Schmelz M. The neurobiology of itch. *Nat Rev Neurosci.* Jul 2006;7(7):535-547.

Kass JH. Somatosensory system. In: Paxinos G, Mai JK, eds. *The Human Nervous System.* London: Elsevier; 2004.

Mesulam MM, Mufson EJ. Insula of the old world monkey. Ill: Efferent cortical output and comments on function. *J Comp Neurol.* 1982;212:38-52.

Noble R, Riddell JS. Cutaneous excitatory and inhibitory input to neurones of the postsynaptic dorsal column system in the cat. *J Physiol.* 1988;396:497-513.

Olausson H, Lamarre Y, Backlund H, et al. Unmyelinated tactile afferents signal touch and project to insular cortex. *Nat Neurosci.* 2002;5(9):900-904.

Palecek J. The role of dorsal columns pathway in visceral pain. *Physiol Res.* 2004;53(Suppl 1):S125-130.

Pietrobon D. Migraine: new molecular mechanisms. *Neuroscientist.* 2005;11(4):373-386.

Rinaman L, Schwartz G. Anterograde transneuronal viral tracing of central viscerosensory pathways in rats. *J Neurosci.* 2004;24(11):2782-2786.

Schweinhardt P, Sauro KM, Bushnell MC. Fibromyalgia: a disorder of the brain? *Neuroscientist.* 2008;14(5):415-421.

Struck AF, Haughton VM. Idiopathic syringomyelia: phase-contrast MR of cerebrospinal fluid flow dynamics at level of foramen magnum. *Radiology.* 2009;253(1):184-190.

Suzuki R, Morcuende S, Webber M, Hunt SP, Dickenson AH. Superficial NK1-expressing neurons control spinal excitability through activation of descending pathways. *Nat Neurosci.* 2002;5(12):1319-1326.

Suzuki R, Rygh LJ, Dickenson AH. Bad news from the brain: descending 5-HT pathways that control spinal pain processing. *Trends Pharmacol Sci.* 2004;25(12):613-617.

Talbot JD, Marrett S, Evans AC, et al. Multiple representations of pain in human cerebral cortex. *Science.* 1991;251:1355-1358.

Tracey I. Nociceptive processing in the human brain. *Curr Opin Neurobiol.* 2005;15(4):478-487.

Tracey I, Mantyh PW. The cerebral signature for pain perception and its modulation. *Neuron.* 2007;55(3):377-391.

Treede RD, Apkarian AV, Bromm B, Greenspan JD, Lenz FA. Cortical representation of pain: functional characterization of nociceptive areas near the lateral sulcus. *Pain* 2000;87:113-119.

Wang CC, Willis WD, Westlund KN. Ascending projections from the area around the spinal cord central canal: a Phaseolus vulgaris leucoagglutinin study in rats. *J Comp Neurol.* 1999;415(3):341-367.

Willis WD, Al-Chaer ED, Quast MJ, Westlund KN. A visceral pain pathway in the dorsal column of the spinal cord. *Proc Natl Acad Sci USA.* 1999;96(14):7675-7679.

Willis WD, Kenshalo DR Jr., Leonard RB. The cells of origin of the primate spinothalamic tract. *J Comp Neurol.* 1979;188:543-574.

Willis WD Jr., Westlund KN. The role of the dorsal column pathway in visceral nociception. *Curr Pain Headache Rep.* 2001;5(1):20-26.

Woolf CJ, Ma Q. Nociceptors—noxious stimulus detectors. *Neuron.* 2007;55(3):353-364.

Study Questions

1. A 30-year-old male was driving a motorcycle when he swerved off the road and suffered a severe spinal cord injury. When he was being treated at an emergency room, on neurological examination he was noted to have lost the sense of touch on his right leg and lower chest, to the level of the umbilicus. He also had lost pain sensation. Which of the following statements best describes the side and lowest dermatomal level of remaining pain sensation?
   A. Left side of spinal cord at the 10th thoracic segment (T10)
   B. Left, L1
   C. Right, L1
   D. Right, T10

2. Which of the following best describes a nociceptor?
   A. Pacinian corpusle
   B. Ruffini's corpuscle
   C. Meissner's corpuscle
   D. Unencapsulated receptor

3. Small-diameter afferent fibers terminate within which listed region of the spinal cord gray matter?
   A. Superficial laminae of the dorsal horn
   B. Deep layers of the dorsal horn
   C. Intermediate zone
   D. Ventral horn

4. Pain signals from caudal visceral structures ascend within which spinal pathway?
   A. Cuneate fascicle
   B. Gracile fascicle
   C. Anterolateral column
   D. Ventral column

5. Occlusion of the posterior inferior cerebellar artery results in which of the following patterns of analgesia?
   A. Loss of pain on the ipsilateral arms and legs
   B. Loss of pain on the contralateral arms and legs
   C. Bilateral loss of pain on the arms and legs
   D. There would be no change in pain

6. A soldier was injured in battle. Despite the injury, and the tissue damage that the injury caused, the soldier was able to continue to engage the enemy. Which of the following best explains why the soldier was able to continue engaging the enemy?
   A. Brain stem noradrenergic and serotonergic descending tracts that inhibit dorsal horn pain transmission can be activated by areas of the brain engaged in emotions.
   B. Brain stem cholinergic and serotonergic descending tracts that inhibit dorsal horn pain transmission can be activated by areas of the brain engaged in emotions.
   C. Spinal nociceptive circuits engage local feedback inhibitory mechanisms to limit nociceptive transmission in the dorsal horn.
   D. Cognitive systems of the brain can directly inhibit spinal pain circuits.

7. The raphe nuclei are to the periaqueductal gray matter, as
   A. the spinoreticular tract is to the spinothalamic tract
   B. 5-HT is to glutamate
   C. pain suppression is to pain arousal
   D. burning pain is to sharp pain

8. Which thalamic nucleus does not play a key role in pain and thermal sensations?
    A. Ventral posterior nucleus
    B. Ventral medial posterior nucleus
    C. Medial dorsal nucleus
    D. Lateral geniculate nucleus

9. Which of the following statements best describes how pain signals from the spinal cord reach the amygdala?
    A. Spinoreticular tract, to the parabrachial nucleus, to the amygdala
    B. Spinothalamic tract, to the thalamic reticular nucleus, to the amygdala
    C. Spinothalamic tract, to the ventral posterior lateral nucleus, to the amygdala
    D. Spinomesencephalic tract, to the superior colliculus, to the periaqueductal gray matter, to the amygdala

10. The anterior cingulate gyrus is not important for which of the following pain functions and pain pathway connections?
    A. Localizaing a painful stimulus
    B. Emotional aspects of pain
    C. Emotional hurt
    D. Receives input from the medial dorsal nucleus

Chapter 6

Somatic Sensation: Trigeminal and Viscerosensory Systems

CLINICAL CASE | Lateral Medullary Syndrome and Dissociated Somatic Sensory Loss

A 69-year-old man suddenly developed vertigo and difficulty walking. He went to the emergency room and, upon examination, was found to have several additional sensory and motor deficits. Here we will only consider the somatic sensory deficits. We will revisit this patient in the case in Chapter 15, when we consider his other neurological deficits.

His neurological examination revealed a striking dissociated pattern of mechanosensory and pain/thermal sensory loss. Facial pain and thermal sensation were largely absent on the left side of his face. Remarkably, pain and thermal sensations on the arm, trunk, and leg were absent on the right side. Figure 6–1A (gray tint) shows the approximate distribution of pain and thermal sensory loss. Mechanosensation was spared bilaterally on the face, limbs, and trunk. Jaw and limb proprioception were also spared.

The patient had an MRI of the head. It was normal except for the medulla (Figure 6-1B), which showed a wedge-shaped lesion, dorsolaterally, on the left side. The corresponding myelin-stained section is shown.

You should be able to answer the following questions based on your reading of the chapter, inspection of the images, and consideration of the neurological signs.

1. **What artery supplied the infarcted region in the medulla?**

2. **Explain why pain is lost ipsilaterally on the face and contralaterally on the limbs.**

Key neurological signs and corresponding damaged brain structures

Ipsilateral loss of facial pain and thermal senses

The posterior inferior cerebellar artery (PICA) supplies the dorsolateral medulla. The infarcted region on the MRI in Figure 6-1B was produced by PICA occlusion, which damaged the spinal trigeminal tract and nucleus at the level of the mid-medulla. The locations of these structures are shown in Figure 6-1B, inset. Tract damage results in

—Continued next page

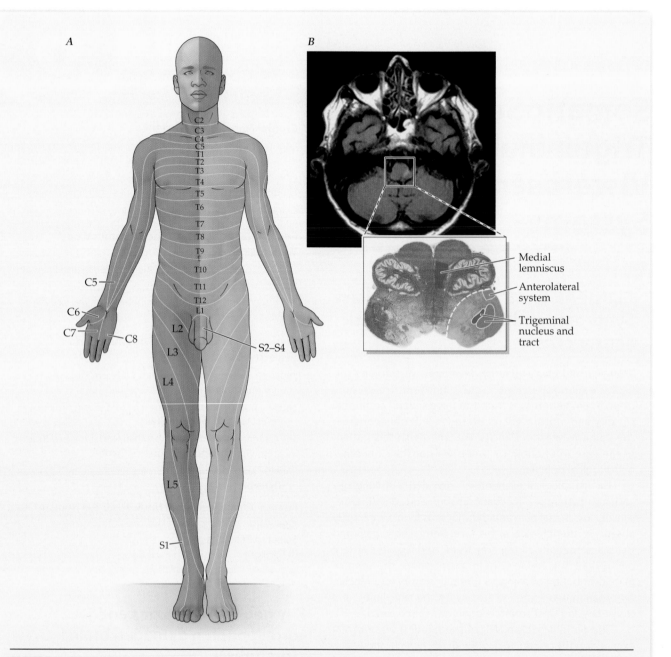

FIGURE 6–1 Dissociated sensory loss after occlusion of posterior inferior cerebellar artery. **A.** Distribution of sensory loss (gray tint). **B.** MRI showing region of occlusion (bright signal). A myelin-stained section at the level of the MRI is shown, indicating the key structures affected by the lesion. (Image in B reproduced with permission from Dr Frank Gaillard, Radiopaedia.org.)

loss of most axons from the level of occlusion, caudally. Because damage occurred before decussation, the nociceptive and thermal innervation of the ipsilateral face was eliminated.

Contralateral loss of pain and thermal senses

There was also loss of pain and temperature sensation on the contralateral limbs and trunk. This is because PICA occlusion damaged the ascending anterolateral pathway, which decussated in the spinal cord (Figure 6–1B, inset; Figure 6-12B).

Sparing of mechanical sensations and limb and jaw proprioception

PICA occlusion spared the medial lemniscus, which carries ascending mechanosensory and limb proprioception information (Figure 6–1B, inset). It also spared trigeminal mechanosensations (touch, vibration sense, jaw proprioception) because the large-diameter fibers that mediate these sensations do not descend within the spinal trigeminal tract. Rather, they synapse on neurons in the main trigeminal sensory nucleus in the pons.

In neuroanatomy, the study of sensation and motor control of cranial structures has traditionally been separate from that of the limbs and trunk. This is because cranial nerves innervate the head, and spinal nerves innervate the limbs and trunk. We can see similarities, however, in the functional organization of the cranial and spinal nerves and of the parts of the central nervous system with which they directly connect. For example, sensory axons in cranial nerves synapse in sensory cranial nerve nuclei in the brain stem. Similarly, sensory axons in spinal nerves synapse on neurons of the dorsal horn of the spinal cord and the dorsal column nuclei. The motor cranial nerve nuclei in the brain stem, like the motor nuclei of the ventral horn, contain the motor neurons whose axons project to the periphery.

This chapter examines the trigeminal system, which mediates somatic sensations—mechanosensations and the protective senses, pain, temperature, and itch—from the face and head. This system is analogous to the dorsal column–medial lemniscal and anterolateral systems of the spinal cord (see Chapters 4 and 5). The chapter also considers the brain stem neural system that processes sensory information from the body's internal organs. Both the peripheral territories innervated and the central nervous system processing centers of the viscerosensory system are closely aligned with those of the trigeminal system. Since the cranial nerves innervate the face and head, we will begin with an overview of the general organization of the cranial nerves and a characteristic feature of the cranial nerve nuclei, their columnar organization. Knowledge of the columnar organization helps explain the functional organization of the cranial nerves and nuclei because the location of the column provides important information about function. Knowledge of the cranial nerves is an essential part of the neurological exam.

Cranial Nerves and Nuclei

Among the 12 pairs of cranial nerves (Figure 6–2; Table 6–1), the first two—olfactory (I) and optic (II)—are purely sensory. The olfactory nerve, which mediates the sense of smell,

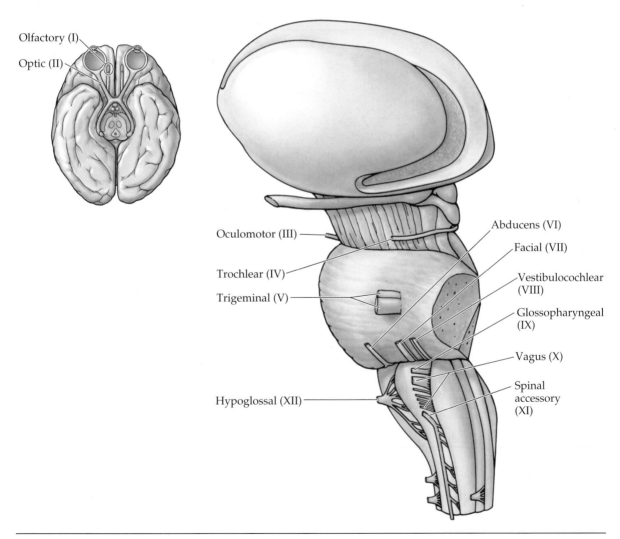

FIGURE 6–2 Lateral view of the brain stem, showing the locations of the cranial nerves that enter and exit the brain stem and diencephalon. The inset shows that the olfactory (I) nerve enters the olfactory bulb, which is part of the telencephalon, and that the optic (II) nerve enters the diencephalon via the optic tract.

Table **6-1** Cranial nerves and nuclei

Cranial nerve and root	Function	Cranial foramina	Peripheral sensory ganglia	CNS nucleus	Peripheral autonomic ganglia	Peripheral structure innervated
I	Olfactory	Smell	Cribriform plate		Olfactory bulb		Olfactory receptors of olfactory epithelium
II	Optic	Vision	Optic		Lateral geniculate nucleus		Retina (ganglion cells)
III	Oculomotor	Somatic skeletal motor	Superior orbital fissure		Oculomotor		Medial, superior, inferior, rectus, inferior oblique, and levator palpebrae muscles
		Autonomic			Edinger-Westphal	Ciliary	Constrictor muscles of iris, ciliary muscle
IV	Trochlear	Somatic skeletal motor	Superior orbital fissure		Trochlear		Superior oblique muscle
V	Trigeminal	Somatic sensory	Superior orbital fissure (Ophthalmic) Rotundum (Maxillary)	Semilunar	Spinal nucleus, main sensory nucleus, mesencephalic nucleus of CN V		Skin and mucous membranes of the head, meninges Muscle receptors in jaw muscles
		Branchiomeric motor	Ovale (Mandibular)		Motor nucleus of CN V		Jaw muscles, tensor tympani, tensor palati, and digastric (anterior belly)
VI	Abducens	Somatic skeletal muscle	Superior orbital fissure		Abducens		Lateral rectus muscle
VII	Intermediate	Taste	Internal auditory meatus	Geniculate	Solitary nucleus		Taste (anterior two thirds of tongue), palate
		Somatic sensory		Geniculate	Spinal nucleus of CN V		Skin of external ear
		Autonomic			Superior salivatory	Pterygopalatine, submandibular	Lacrimal glands, glands of nasal mucosa, salivary glands
	Facial	Branchiomeric motor	Internal auditory meatus		Facial		Muscles of facial expression, digastric (posterior belly), and stapedius
VIII	Vestibulocochlear	Hearing	Internal auditory meatus	Spiral	Cochlear		Hair cells in organ of Corti
		Balance	Internal auditory meatus	Vestibular	Vestibular		Hair cells in vestibular labyrinth

CN	Nerve	Functional component	Ganglion	Nucleus	Peripheral autonomic ganglion	Structures innervated
IX	Glossopharyngeal	Somatic sensory	Jugular (superior)	Spinal nucleus of CN V		Skin of external ear
		Viscerosensory	Petrosal (inferior)	Solitary nucleus (caudal)		Mucous membranes in pharyngeal region, middle ear, carotid body, and sinus
		Taste	Petrosal	Solitary nucleus (rostral)		Taste (posterior one third of tongue)
		Autonomic		Inferior salivatory nucleus	Otic	Parotid gland
		Branchiomeric motor		Ambiguus (rostral)		Striated muscle of pharynx
X	Vagus	Somatic sensory	Jugular (superior)	Spinal nucleus of CN V		Skin of external ear, meninges
		Viscerosensory	Nodose (inferior)	Solitary nucleus (caudal)		Larynx, trachea, gut, aortic arch receptors
		Taste	Nodose (inferior)	Solitary nucleus (rostral)		Taste buds (posterior oral cavity, larynx)
		Autonomic		Dorsal motor nucleus of CN X	Peripheral autonomic	Gut (to splenic flexure of colon), respiratory structures, heart
		Branchiomeric motor		Ambiguus (middle region)		Striated muscles of palate, pharynx, and larynx
XI	Spinal accessory	Branchiomeric motor	Jugular	Ambiguus (caudal)		Striated muscles of larynx (aberrant vagus nerve branches)
		Unclassified[1]	Jugular	Accessory nucleus, pyramidal decussation to C3-C5		Sternocleidomastoid and portion of trapezius muscles
XII	Hypoglossal	Somatic skeletal motor	Hypoglossal	Hypoglossal		Intrinsic muscles of tongue, hyoglossus, genioglossus, and styloglossus muscles

Abbreviation key: CN, cranial nerve.

[1]The accessory nucleus is unclassified because some of the muscles (or compartments of muscles) innervated by this nucleus develop from the occipital somites.

directly enters the **cerebral hemisphere,** and the optic nerve, for vision, enters the **thalamus.** The other 10 cranial nerves enter and leave the **brain stem.** The oculomotor (III) and trochlear (IV) nerves, which are motor nerves, exit from the midbrain. They innervate muscles that move the eyes. The trochlear nerve is further distinguished as the only cranial nerve found on the dorsal brain stem surface.

The pons contains four cranial nerves. The trigeminal (V) nerve is located at the middle of the pons. It is a **mixed nerve;** it has both sensory and motor functions, and it consists of separate sensory and motor roots. This separation is reminiscent of the segregation of function in the dorsal and ventral spinal roots. The sensory root provides the somatic sensory innervation of the facial skin and mucous membranes of parts of the oral and nasal cavities and the teeth. The motor root contains axons that innervate jaw muscles.

The remaining pontine nerves are found at the pontomedullary junction. The abducens (VI) nerve is a motor nerve that, like the oculomotor and trochlear nerves, innervates eye muscles. The facial (VII) nerve is a mixed nerve and has separate motor and sensory roots. The motor root innervates the facial muscles that determine our expressions, whereas the sensory root primarily innervates taste buds and mediates taste. The facial sensory root is sometimes called the intermediate nerve. (The intermediate nerve also contains axons that innervate various cranial autonomic ganglia [Chapter 11].) The vestibulocochlear (VIII) nerve is a sensory nerve and has two separate components. The vestibular component innervates the semicircular canals, saccule, and utricle and mediates balance, whereas the cochlear component innervates the organ of Corti and serves hearing.

The medulla has four cranial nerves, each of which contains numerous roots that leave from different rostrocaudal locations. Although the glossopharyngeal (IX) nerve is a mixed nerve, its major functions are to provide the sensory innervation of the pharynx and to innervate taste buds of the posterior one third of the tongue. The motor function of the glossopharyngeal nerve is to innervate a single pharyngeal muscle and peripheral autonomic ganglion (see Table 6–1). The vagus (X) nerve, a mixed nerve, has myriad sensory and motor functions that include somatic and visceral sensation, innervation of pharyngeal muscles, and much of the visceral autonomic innervation. The spinal accessory (XI) and hypoglossal (XII) nerves subserve motor function, innervating neck and tongue muscles, respectively (see Table 6–1).

Important Differences Exist Between the Sensory and Motor Innervation of Cranial Structures and Those of the Limbs and Trunk

The peripheral organization of sensory (afferent) fibers in cranial nerves is similar to that of spinal nerves. The organization of the primary sensory neurons that innervate the skin and mucous membranes of the head—mediating the somatic senses—is virtually identical to that of the sensory innervation of the limbs and trunk (Figure 6–3). In both cases, the distal portion of the axon of **pseudounipolar** primary sensory neurons is sensitive to stimulus energy, and the cell bodies of these primary sensory neurons are located in **peripheral ganglia.** The proximal portion of the axon projects into the central nervous system to synapse on neurons in the medulla and pons. The peripheral sensory ganglia, which contain the cell bodies of the primary sensory neurons of the different cranial nerves, are listed in Table 6–1.

Despite these similarities, three important differences are evident in the anatomical organization of primary sensory neurons in spinal and cranial nerves:

1. For the senses of taste, vision, hearing, and balance, a separate **receptor cell** transduces stimulus energy (Figure 6–3). The receptor activates synaptically the primary sensory neuron, which transmits information— encoded in the form of action potentials—to the central nervous system. For the spinal and trigeminal somatic sensations, the distal ending of the primary sensory neuron is the sensory receptor for all but one receptor (see Chapter 4; Merkel's receptor). Thus, the primary sensory neuron mediates both stimulus transduction and information transmission.

2. Primary sensory neurons in cranial nerves have either a **pseudounipolar** or a **bipolar** morphology (Figure 6–3). (As is discussed in Chapter 7, a retinal projection neuron is analogous to the primary sensory neurons because it transmits sensory information to the thalamus.)

3. Stretch receptors in jaw muscles, which signal jaw muscle length and thus mediate **jaw proprioception** (or temporal-mandibular joint angle detection), are pseudounipolar primary sensory neurons, but their cell bodies are located within the central nervous system, not in peripheral ganglia. Most primary sensory neurons derive from the neural crest cells, a group of cells that emerge from the dorsal region of the neural tube. Most neural crest cells migrate peripherally and give rise to the neurons whose cell bodies lie outside of the central nervous system. These neurons include most of the primary sensory neurons that innervate body tissues and the peripheral components of the autonomic nervous system (see Chapters 4 and 15). The primary sensory neurons that mediate jaw proprioception derive from a special group of neural crest cells that do not migrate from the central nervous system to the periphery.

The structures innervated by the motor fibers of cranial nerves, similar to motor fibers in spinal nerves, include striated muscle and autonomic postganglionic neurons. In contrast to striated muscle of the limbs and trunk, which develop from body somites, cranial striated muscle develops from

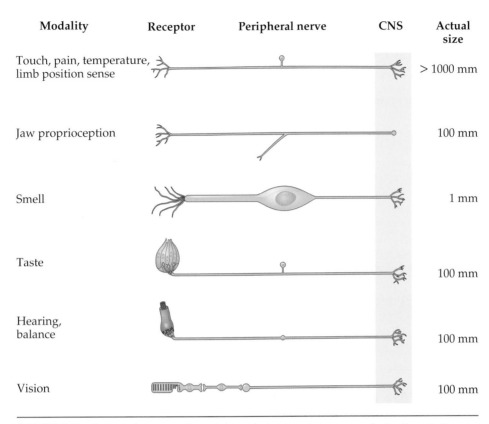

Modality	Receptor	Peripheral nerve	CNS	Actual size
Touch, pain, temperature, limb position sense				> 1000 mm
Jaw proprioception				100 mm
Smell				1 mm
Taste				100 mm
Hearing, balance				100 mm
Vision				100 mm

FIGURE 6–3 Schematic illustration of morphology of primary sensory neurons, the location of cell bodies, and the approximate differences in actual sizes. Whereas primary afferent fibers in the spinal cord have a pseudounipolar morphology, in cranial nerves they have either a pseudounipolar or a bipolar morphology. The primary sensory neuron for jaw proprioception is further distinguished because its cell body is located in the central nervous system. For hearing, balance, and taste, separate receptor cells transduce stimulus information, and primary afferent fiber transmits the resulting signals to the central nervous system. The sensory neurons for hearing, balance, and smell are bipolar. For touch, pain, and temperature senses; jaw proprioception; and taste, the primary sensory neurons are pseudounipolar. For vision, the retina develops from the central nervous system; thus, none of the neural elements are in the periphery.

either the cranial **somites** or the **branchial arches.** The branchial arches correspond to gills that are present early in human development, representing the evolutionary derivatives of aquatic vertebrates. The extraocular and tongue muscles originate from somites, whereas jaw, facial, laryngeal, palatal, and certain neck muscles are of branchiomeric origin.

There Are Seven Functional Categories of Cranial Nerves

Seven functional categories of cranial nerve enter and exit the brain stem. (See Box 6–1.) Four of these categories are similar to those of the spinal nerves:

1. **Somatic sensory fibers** in cranial nerves subserve touch, pain, itch, and temperature senses, as well as jaw and limb proprioception.

2. **Viscerosensory fibers** mediate visceral sensations and chemoreception from body organs and help regulate blood pressure and other bodily functions.

3. **Somatic skeletal motor fibers** are the axons of motor neurons that innervate striated muscle that develops from the somites.

4. **Visceral (autonomic) motor fibers** are the axons of autonomic preganglionic neurons.

Because cranial nerves innervate structures that are more complex than those innervated by spinal nerves—the highly specialized sensory organs of the eye, ear, and tongue, as well as the muscles that develop from the branchial arches—there are three additional categories of cranial nerves:

5. Axons that innervate the eye subserve **vision,** and those that innervate the inner ear mediate **hearing** and **balance.**

6. Fibers that innervate taste buds and the olfactory mucosa mediate **taste** and **smell,** respectively.

7. **Branchiomeric skeletal motor fibers** are the axons of motor neurons that innervate striated muscle that develops from the branchial arches.

Box 6–1

Cranial Nerve and Nuclei Historical Nomenclature

Cranial nerves have historically been classified according to an arcane abbreviated scheme rather than according to their functions. This scheme distinguishes cranial nerves (and their corresponding central nuclei) on the basis of whether the individual component axons provide the **sensory** (afferent) or **motor** (efferent) innervation of the head, whether the innervated structures develop from the somites (and therefore are "**somatic**" structures) or the branchial arches (which are considered "**visceral**"), and whether the structure innervated has simple (**general**) or complex (**special**) morphology:

- General somatic sensory (GSS) corresponds to the somatic sensory innervation, as described in Chapter 11.
- General visceral sensory (GVS) corresponds to the viscerosensory innervation.
- General somatic motor (GSM) corresponds to the somatic motor innervation, such as the innervation of limb muscles.

- General visceral motor (GVM) corresponds to the visceral motor, or autonomic, innervation, such as the innervation of smooth muscle and glands.
- Special somatic sensory (SSS) corresponds to vision and hearing.
- Special visceral sensory (SVS) corresponds to taste and smell.
- Special visceral motor (SVM) corresponds to the innervation of branchiomeric muscles, such as those of the pharynx.

The abbreviated nomenclature is fraught with problems and is not intuitive. For example, special visceral motor (SVM) nerve fibers innervate striated muscles that function just like muscles innervated by the general somatic motor (GSM) fibers. Vision is described as a special somatic sensory (SSS) modality and smell, a visceral modality (SVS), but they have little to do with other somatic or visceral functions. Because of these inconsistencies and the counterintuitive nature of this system, the cranial nerves and their central nuclei are characterized here on the basis of their functions (see Table 6–1).

Cranial Nerve Nuclei Are Organized into Distinctive Columns

As we learned in Chapter 11, the spinal cord has a segmental organization that emerges early in development. Each spinal segment provides the sensory and motor innervation to a corresponding body segment, or somite (see Figure 4-5). The developing caudal brain stem, the pons and medulla, also is segmented. Segmentation may be a mechanism for establishing a basic plan of organization, or "building block," for the various parts of the spinal cord and brain stem. This segmental plan is maintained into maturity for the spinal cord. In the mature brain stem, however, segmentation is obscured by later elaboration of neural interconnections. The developing pons and medulla have eight segments, termed **rhombomeres** (Figure 6–4A), that provide the sensory and motor innervation for most of the head through the cranial nerve peripheral projections. The midbrain and region of midbrain-pons junction may also have an early rhombomeric segmental organization. In contrast to the spinal cord, where each segment contains a pair of dorsal and ventral roots, each rhombomere is not associated with a single pair of sensory and motor cranial nerve roots.

The cranial nerve sensory and motor nuclei are analogous to the dorsal and ventral horns, respectively. Cranial nerve sensory nuclei contain neurons that receive sensory information directly from cranial structures via cranial sensory nerves. Cranial nerve motor nuclei contain the cell bodies of motor neurons, whose axons course through cranial motor nerves to innervate their peripheral targets. Whereas this organization is similar to that of the spinal sensory and motor regions, three important differences exist between the developmental plans of the spinal cord and the brain stem.

First, the sensory and motor nuclear columns in the medulla and pons are aligned roughly from the lateral surface to the midline rather than being oriented in the dorsoventral axis, as in the spinal cord. This is because during development the cavity in the neural tube of the hindbrain expands dorsally ("opens up") to form the fourth ventricle (Figure 6–4B). Compare the dorsoventral organization in Figure 6–4B1, which is before the neural tube expands and therefore is organized like that of the spinal cord, with Figure 6–4B3, where the nuclei are obliquely lateral-to-medial.

Second, in brain stem development, immature neurons migrate more extensively from the ventricular floor to distant sites than in the spinal cord. Cranial nerve nuclei have relatively simple roles in processing afferent information or transmitting motor control signals. However, most other brain stem nuclei have more complex integrative functions. Whereas brain stem integrative nuclei also derive from developing neurons of the sensory and motor plates in the ventricular floor, the immature neurons that give rise to these structures migrate to their destinations in more dorsal or ventral regions (Figure 6–4B3). Most neurons migrate radially (ie, at right angle to the neuraxis) along local paths established by special astrocytes, which are a class of glial cells.

Third, as a consequence of the greater diversity of cranial sensory and motor structures, there is further differentiation of the cranial nerve nuclei. Because there are seven functional categories of cranial nerves, there are also seven categories of cranial nerve nuclei. Nuclei of each of these categories form discontinuous columns that extend rostrocaudally through the brain stem (Figures 6–5A). The seven functional categories are distributed through only six discrete columns, however, because

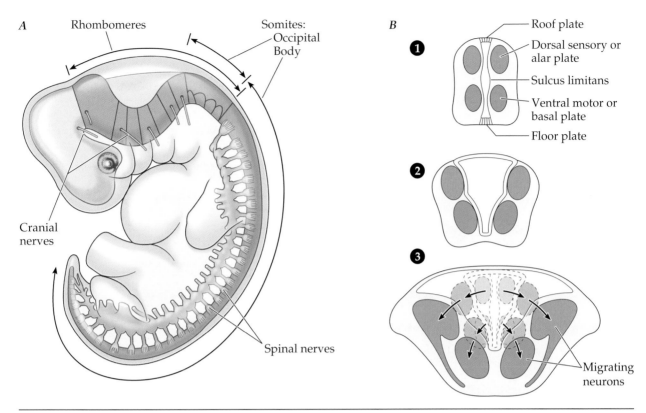

FIGURE 6–4 Development of segmental and columnar organization. **A.** The position of the developing nervous system is illustrated in this lateral view of the embryo. The hindbrain and spinal cord are segmented structures. In the caudal brain stem the segments are called rhombomeres. Four occipital somites form structures of the head. These are located in the caudal medulla. The muscles, bones, and many other structures of the limbs and trunk from the body somites. The cranial nerves that contain the axons of brain stem motor neurons are also shown. From rostral to caudal, the following cranial nerves are illustrated: IV, V, VI, VII, IX, X, and XII. The two mesencephalic segments and the segment between the metacephalon and mesencephalon are not shown. **B.** Schematic sections through the caudal brain stem at three prenatal ages. As neurons and glia in the brain proliferate, the central canal expansds along its dorsal margin. This has the effect of transforming the dorsoventral nuclear organization of the spinal cord into the lateromedial organization of nuclei in the caudal brain stem (the future medulla and pons).

two of the sensory categories synapse on neurons in a single column but at separate rostrocaudal locations. The sensory columns are lateral to the motor columns (Figure 6–5A, B). The somatic sensory, hearing, and balance columns tend to be lateral to the viscerosensory and taste columns. The somatic skeletal motor column is medial to the autonomic motor column. The branchiomeric motor column contains neurons that are located in the region of the reticular formation. The **sulcus limitans,** a shallow grove that separates the sensory and motor columns during development, remains as a landmark on the floor of the fourth ventricle in the adult brain. We will further examine the distinct locations of motor neurons innervating muscles of **somatic** or **branchiomeric** origins in Chapter 11.

Because cranial nerve nuclei that serve similar functions are aligned in the same rostrocaudal columns, knowledge of the locations of these columns aids in understanding their functions. Figure 6–6 shows the longitudinal organization of the cell columns forming the cranial nerve nuclei in the mature brain stem.

Functional Anatomy of the Trigeminal and Viscerosensory Systems

Somatic sensation of the head, including the oral cavity, is carried by four cranial nerves. The **trigeminal nerve** innervates most of the head and oral cavity and is the most important of the four nerves. The **facial, glossopharyngeal,** and **vagus** nerves innervate small areas of the skin around the external ear and the mucous membranes and organs of the body. The facial, glossopharyngeal, and vagus nerves also contain sensory fibers that mediate taste (see Chapter 9).

The sensory fibers that innervate surface skin and oral mucosa project into central **trigeminal nuclei,** whereas the sensory fibers that innervate the mucous membranes of the pharynx and larynx and other internal (visceral) structures project to the caudal portion of the **solitary nucleus** (Figure 6–7). An important exception exists: A small number of sensory fibers that innervate the pharyngeal and

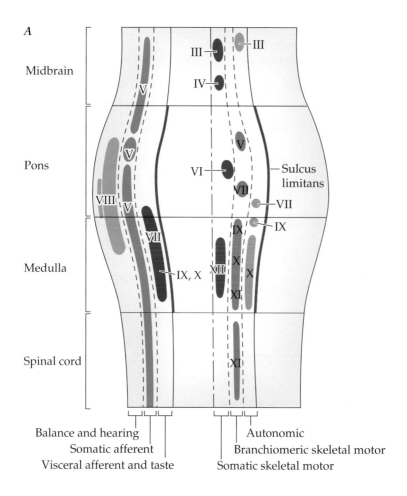

A

Midbrain

Pons

Medulla

Spinal cord

Sulcus limitans

Balance and hearing
Somatic afferent
Visceral afferent and taste

Autonomic
Branchiomeric skeletal motor
Somatic skeletal motor

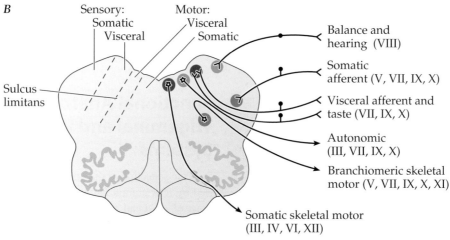

B

Sensory:
Somatic
Visceral

Motor:
Visceral
Somatic

Sulcus limitans

Balance and hearing (VIII)

Somatic afferent (V, VII, IX, X)

Visceral afferent and taste (VII, IX, X)

Autonomic (III, VII, IX, X)

Branchiomeric skeletal motor (V, VII, IX, X, XI)

Somatic skeletal motor (III, IV, VI, XII)

FIGURE 6–5 A. Schematic dorsal view of brain stem, showing that the cranial nerve nuclei are organized into discontinuous columns. The sulcus limitans separates the afferent and motor nuclei. **B.** Schematic cross section through the medulla, showing the locations of cranial nerve nuclear columns.

laryngeal mucosa project information to the trigeminal nuclei. Sensory information transmitted to the trigeminal nuclei is thought to contribute to our conscious awareness of cranial sensations. By contrast, information transmitted to the caudal solitary nucleus may not necessarily reach

consciousness. Although we are aware of visceral pain, we become conscious of other visceral stimuli only under special circumstances, such as when we become nauseated after eating a certain food or when we feel full after eating a large meal. Some internal stimuli are never perceived. For

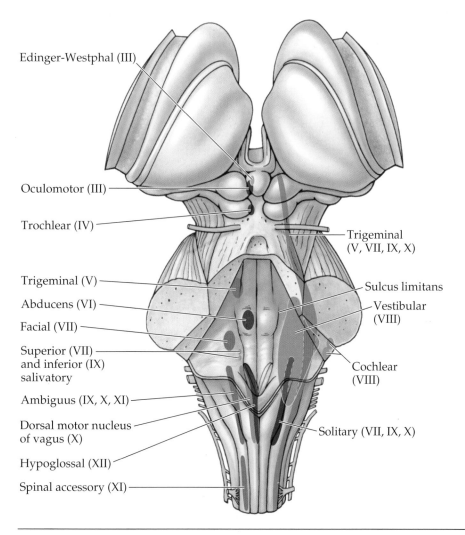

FIGURE 6–6 The cranial nerve nuclei have a longitudinal organization. A dorsal view of the brain stem of the mature central nervous system is illustrated, with the locations of the various cranial nerve nuclei indicated. Colors are as in Figure 6–5.

example, a change in intra-arterial pressure, even a hypertensive episode, can occur unnoticed.

Separate Trigeminal Pathways Mediate Touch and Pain and Temperature Senses

Three trigeminal sensory nuclei serve cranial somatic sensations (eg, from the skin and jaw muscles) from the nerves just described (Figure 6–7). These sensory fibers terminate in two of the trigeminal sensory nuclei, the **main** (or **principal) trigeminal sensory nucleus** and the **spinal trigeminal nucleus.** The third sensory nucleus, the **mesencephalic trigeminal nucleus,** is not a site of termination of primary sensory fibers. Rather, it is equivalent to a peripheral sensory ganglion because it contains the cell bodies of certain trigeminal primary sensory fibers (see below).

The sensory axons of the trigeminal nerve enter the ventral pons (Figure 6–2). Sensory axons from the facial, glossopharyngeal, and vagus nerves enter the brain stem more caudally. Just as in spinal nerves, functional differences distinguish individual sensory axons in these nerves. Large-diameter fibers, which mediate mechanical sensations, terminate mostly in the dorsal pons, in the main trigeminal sensory nucleus. Small-diameter fibers—which mediate pain, temperature sensations, and itch—mostly travel in the **spinal trigeminal tract** and terminate in the spinal trigeminal nucleus. (Some large-diameter mechanoreceptive fibers in the spinal trigeminal tract and nucleus play a role in cranial reflexes; see below.) These differences set the stage for two anatomically and functionally distinct trigeminal ascending sensory systems (Figure 6–8A, B). One system is primarily for cranial touch and dental mechanical senses and is analogous to the dorsal column–medial lemniscal system. The other system is for cranial pain, temperature senses, and itch, and is analogous to the anterolateral system.

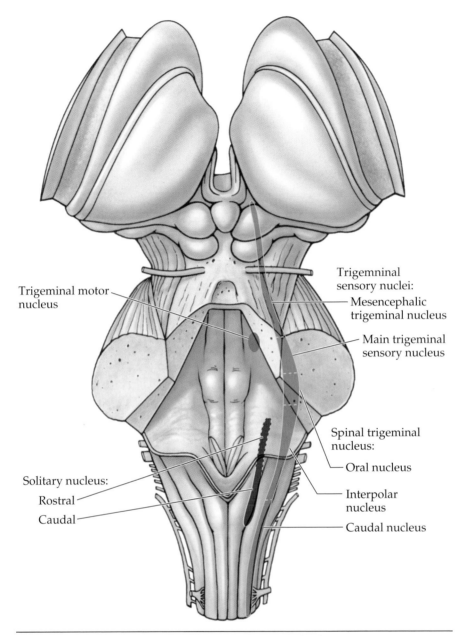

FIGURE 6–7 Dorsal view of the brain stem without the cerebellum, indicating the locations of trigeminal and solitary nuclei.

The main trigeminal sensory nucleus mediates facial mechanical sensations

Most neurons in the **main trigeminal sensory nucleus** receive mechanoreceptive information. Projection neurons in this nucleus give rise to axons that decussate in the pons and ascend dorsomedially to fibers from the dorsal column nuclei in the medial lemniscus. The ascending second-order trigeminal fibers—collectively termed the **trigeminal lemniscus**—synapse in the thalamus, in its **ventral posterior medial nucleus** (Figure 6–8A). (Recall that the ventral posterior lateral nucleus is the thalamic spinal somatic sensory relay nucleus.) From here, the axons of thalamic neurons project, via the posterior limb of the internal capsule, to the lateral part of the **primary somatic sensory cortex,** in the **postcentral gyrus.** The **secondary somatic sensory cortex** and the **posterior parietal cortex** also process cranial mechanosensory information (see Chapter 11). These higher-order somatic sensory areas receive their major input from the primary somatic sensory cortex. Because of similarities in connections, the main trigeminal sensory nucleus is anatomically and functionally similar to the dorsal column nuclei (which comprise the gracile and cuneate nuclei).

A much smaller pathway originates from the dorsal portion of the main trigeminal sensory nucleus (Figure 6–7A), sometimes termed the dorsal trigeminothalamic tract. This pathway ascends ipsilaterally to the ventral posterior medial nucleus and processes mechanical stimuli from the teeth and soft tissues of the oral cavity.

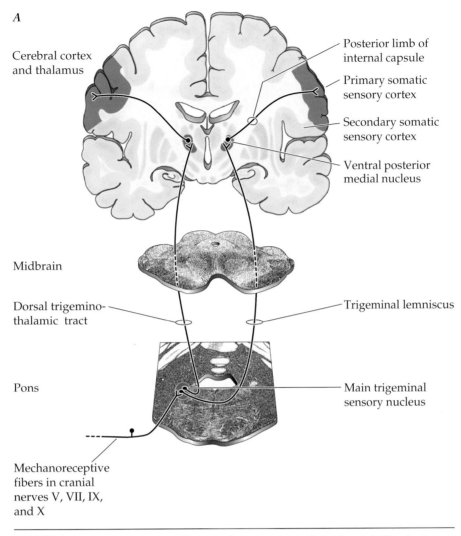

A

Cerebral cortex and thalamus

Posterior limb of internal capsule

Primary somatic sensory cortex

Secondary somatic sensory cortex

Ventral posterior medial nucleus

Midbrain

Dorsal trigemino-thalamic tract

Trigeminal lemniscus

Pons

Main trigeminal sensory nucleus

Mechanoreceptive fibers in cranial nerves V, VII, IX, and X

FIGURE 6–8 General organization of the ascending trigeminal pathways for touch (*A*) and pain, temperature, and itch (*B*) senses.

The pathway for **jaw proprioception,** the conscious awareness of how wide we open our mouth, begins with stretch receptors that encode jaw angle (see Figure 6–14). The cell bodies for these mechanoreceptors are in the **trigeminal mesencephalic nucleus,** and the receptors project to the main trigeminal sensory nucleus and to more rostral portions of the spinal trigeminal nucleus. The projection to the spinal nucleus is analogous to the projection of limb muscle receptor to the deep layers of the dorsal horn. The trigeminal brain stem neurons project to the **ventral posterior medial nucleus** and then to area 3a of the primary somatic sensory cortex. This is the pathway for conscious awareness of temporal-mandibular joint angle. Jaw proprioceptive information also is transmitted to the cerebellum for jaw muscle control (see Chapter 13).

The spinal trigeminal nucleus mediates cranial pain sensation

The spinal trigeminal nucleus has a rostrocaudal anatomical and functional organization with three components (Figures 6–7

and 6–8B): the **oral nucleus,** the **interpolar nucleus,** and the **caudal nucleus.** The functions of the spinal trigeminal nucleus are similar to those of the dorsal horn of the spinal cord, with which it is continuous. Similar to the limb and trunk functions of the dorsal horn, the spinal trigeminal nucleus plays an essential role in facial and dental pain, temperature sensation, and itch and a much lesser role in facial mechanical sensations. In addition, the interpolar and oral nuclei participate in trigeminal reflexes and in transmitting sensory information to jaw motor control structures, such as the cerebellum.

The major ascending trigeminal pathway from the spinal trigeminal nucleus terminates in the contralateral thalamus (Figure 6–8B). The organization of this path, termed the **trigeminothalamic tract,** is similar to that of the **spinothalamic tract,** and it also ascends along with fibers of the **anterolateral system.** Trigeminothalamic axons terminate in three principal locations in the thalamus: the ventral posterior medial nucleus, the ventromedial posterior nucleus, and the medial dorsal nucleus. As discussed in Chapter 5, these thalamic sites have different cortical projections and mediate different

B

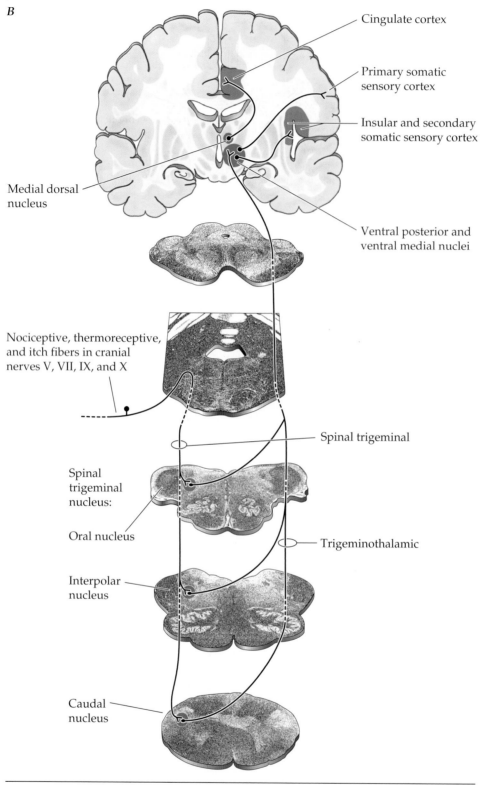

Cingulate cortex

Primary somatic
sensory cortex

Insular and secondary
somatic sensory cortex

Medial dorsal
nucleus

Ventral posterior and
ventral medial nuclei

Nociceptive, thermoreceptive,
and itch fibers in cranial
nerves V, VII, IX, and X

Spinal trigeminal

Spinal
trigeminal
nucleus:

Oral nucleus

Trigeminothalamic

Interpolar
nucleus

Caudal
nucleus

Continued—**FIGURE 6–8**

aspects of pain and temperature senses. The **ventral poste-rior medial nucleus** projects to the primary somatic sensory cortex in the lateral part of the postcentral gyrus, and the **ven-tromedial posterior nucleus** projects to the insular cortex.

These projections are important in perception of pain, tem-perature, and itch. The **medial dorsal nucleus** projects to the anterior cingulate gyrus. Both the insular cortex and the ante-rior cingulate gyrus are thought to participate in the affective and motivational aspects of facial pain, itch, and temperature senses. Like the spinal pain systems, the ascending trigeminal pain system also engages the parabrachial nucleus, which contributes to the affective aspects of pain through projections to the amygdala and hypothalamus.

The Viscerosensory System Originates From the Caudal Solitary Nucleus

The central branches of glossopharyngeal and vagal axons innervate: the pharynx, the larynx, the esophagus, other portions of thoracic and abdominal viscera, and peripheral blood pressure receptive organs. After entering the brain stem, the axons collect into the **solitary tract** of the dorsal medulla and terminate in the surrounding **caudal solitary nucleus.** The solitary nucleus is divided into two functionally distinct parts (Figure 6–7): a rostral portion for taste (considered in Chapter 9) and a caudal portion that serves **viscerosensory functions.** The caudal solitary nucleus projects information to various brain structures for a diversity of functions. For conscious awareness of viscerosensory information, such as a sense of fullness or nausea, there is an ascending projection (Figure 6–9), via the parabrachial nucleus of the pons, to a portion of the ventral posterior nucleus of the thalamus.

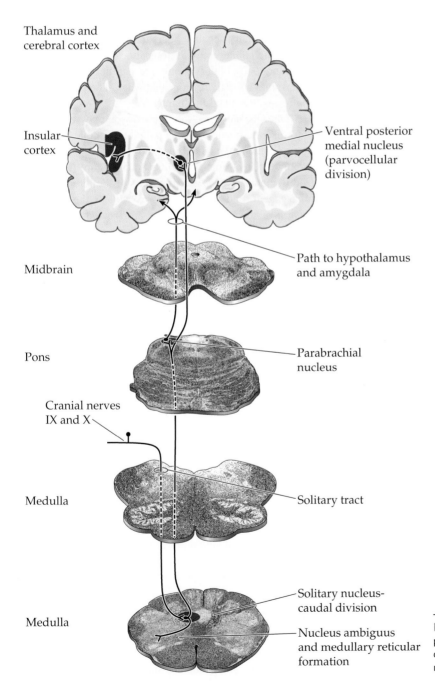

Thalamus and cerebral cortex

Insular cortex

Ventral posterior medial nucleus (parvocellular division)

Midbrain

Path to hypothalamus and amygdala

Pons

Parabrachial nucleus

Cranial nerves IX and X

Medulla

Solitary tract

Medulla

Solitary nucleus-caudal division

Nucleus ambiguus and medullary reticular formation

FIGURE 6–9 General organization of the viscerosensory pathway. Note that neurons in the caudal solitary nucleus contribute to this pathway. Neurons in the rostral solitary nucleus are important in taste (see Chapter 9).

The viscerosensory thalamic neurons, which are distinct from the ones that process mechanical information and those that process taste (see Chapter 11), project to the **insular cortex.** Other projections of the caudal solitary and parabrachial nuclei participate in a variety of visceral reflex and autonomic functions , such as regulation of blood pressure or gastrointestinal motility.

Regional Anatomy of the Trigeminal and Viscerosensory Systems

Separate Sensory Roots Innervate Different Parts of the Face and Mucous Membranes of the Head

The trigeminal nerve consists of three sensory roots that innervate the skin and mucous membranes of separate regions of the head: the **ophthalmic division,** the **maxillary division,** and the **mandibular division** (Figure 6–10A). The maxillary and mandibular divisions also innervate the oral cavity. As in the spinal somatic sensory systems, the cell bodies of the trigeminal sensory fibers that mediate cranial touch, pain, temperature, and itch are found in the **trigeminal** or **semilunar ganglion,** a peripheral sensory ganglion (see Table 6–1). By contrast, the cell bodies of stretch receptors found in jaw muscles are located in the central nervous system, in the **mesencephalic trigeminal nucleus** (Figure 6–7). The trigeminal nerve also innervates stretch receptors in the extraocular muscles, but the cell bodies of these fibers are located in the semilunar ganglion, and their axons course within the ophthalmic division of the trigeminal nerve.

Unlike dorsal roots of adjacent spinal cord segments, where the dermatomes overlap extensively, the trigeminal dermatomes (ie, the area of skin innervated by a single trigeminal sensory nerve division) overlap very little. Thus, a peripheral anesthetic region is more likely to occur after damage to one trigeminal division than after damage to a single dorsal root. Trigeminal neuralgia is an extraordinarily painful neurological condition, often described as a fiery pain that radiates near the border of the ophthalmic and maxillary roots or at the border of the maxillary and mandibular roots.

In addition to the trigeminal nerve, the **intermediate** (a branch of the **facial** nerve), **glossopharyngeal,** and **vagus** nerves innervate portions of the skin of the head. The external ear is innervated by the intermediate and glossopharyngeal nerves, and the external auditory meatus is innervated by the intermediate and vagus nerves (Figure 6–10A). Both the trigeminal and vagus nerves innervate the dura. The cell bodies of the sensory fibers in the facial nerve are located in the **geniculate ganglion,** and those of the glossopharyngeal and vagus nerves are located in the **superior ganglion** of each nerve (see Table 6–1 for nomenclature).

Although the glossopharyngeal and vagus nerves innervate small patches of surface skin, they have a more extensive innervation of the mucous membranes and body organs. The glossopharyngeal nerve innervates the posterior one third of the tongue, the pharynx, portions of the nasal cavity and sinuses, and the eustachian tube. The vagus nerve innervates the hypopharynx, the larynx, the esophagus, and the thoracic and abdominal viscera. The innervation of the pharynx and larynx by the glossopharyngeal and vagus nerves is essential for normal swallowing and for keeping the airway clear of saliva and other liquids during swallowing (see Chapter 11). Branches of the glossopharyngeal and vagus nerves also innervate arterial blood pressure receptors in the **carotid sinus** and **aortic arch,** respectively. These branches are part of the baroreceptor reflex, for blood pressure regulation. For example, they mediate the pressor response to standing. The vagus nerve alone also innervates respiratory structures and the portion of the gut rostral to the splenic flexure. Pelvic visceral organs are innervated by primary sensory fibers that project to the sacral spinal cord. The spinal pathway for pelvic visceral sensation is not well understood but is thought to parallel the organization of the spinal somatic sensory pathways. The pathway for pelvic pain was described in Chapter 5.

After entering the pons, the fibers of each nerve division travel into discrete portions of the spinal trigeminal and solitary tracts en route to the trigeminal and solitary nuclei, where they terminate. The spinal trigeminal tract (Figure 6–10B) is organized like an inverted face: the roots of the intermediate, glossopharyngeal, and vagus nerves as well as the mandibular division of the trigeminal nerve are located dorsal; the ophthalmic division of the trigeminal nerve is located ventral; and the maxillary division of the trigeminal nerve is in between. Axons in the spinal trigeminal tract, in turn, synapse on neurons in the spinal trigeminal nucleus (Figures 6–11A, B and 6–12). The caudal solitary nucleus and tract are located in the caudal medulla (Figure 6–11A); its location is inferred from staining methods that reveal neuronal cell bodies.

The Key Components of the Trigeminal System Are Present at All Levels of the Brain Stem

The three trigeminal nuclei have distinct sensory functions. The **spinal trigeminal nucleus** is primarily important in facial pain, temperature senses, and itch. Despite its name, it is located principally in the medulla and the caudal pons. The **main trigeminal sensory nucleus** mediates facial touch sense and oral mechanosensation and is located in the pons. The **mesencephalic trigeminal nucleus** contains the cell bodies of stretch receptors that signal jaw muscle length, which is the key sensory signal for jaw proprioception. Despite its name, it is located both in the rostral pons and in the midbrain.

The spinal trigeminal nucleus is the rostral extension of the spinal cord dorsal horn

The dorsal horn extends rostrally into the medulla as the spinal trigeminal nucleus. Three nuclear subdivisions comprise the

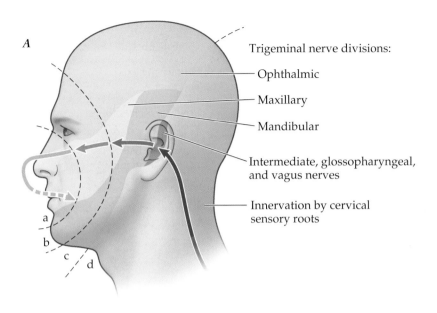

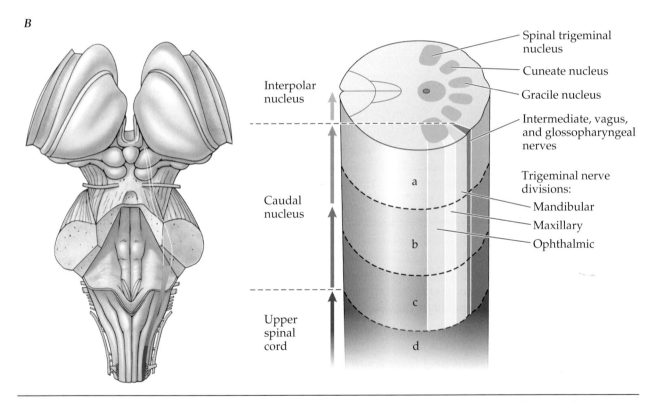

FIGURE 6–10 Somatotopic organization of the trigeminal system. **A.** Peripheral innervation territories of the three divisions of the trigeminal nerve and the intermediate and vagus nerves. **B.** The organization of the spinal trigeminal tract for the portion of the medulla that includes the caudal nucleus. The "onion skin" pattern of representation of trigeminal afferents in the caudal nucleus corresponds to **a, b,** and **c; d** corresponds to the rostral spinal cord representation. Regions marked **a** (located rostrally), **b,** and **c** (located caudally) correspond to the concentric zones on the face indicated in **A**. The intraoral representation is located rostral to region **a** in in the medulla (**B, right**); cervical representation is located caudally (ie, region **d**). (Adapted from Brodal A. *Neurological Anatomy.* 3rd ed. New York, NY: Oxford University Press, 1981.)

spinal trigeminal nucleus, from caudal to rostral: the caudal nucleus, the interpolar nucleus, and the oral nucleus. The **caudal nucleus** and the dorsal horn of the spinal cord are similar structurally and functionally. The laminar terminations of afferent fibers and the origins of trigeminothalamic, trigeminoreticular, and trigeminomesencephalic neurons are like those

of the dorsal horn (see Figure 5–3). In fact, the caudal nucleus is sometimes called the **medullary dorsal horn** because it is so similar to that of the spinal cord dorsal horn. As the nuclear components of the dorsal horn have counterparts in the trigeminal system, so too does the spinal sensory tract. Lissauer's tract extends into the medulla as the **spinal trigeminal tract.** The

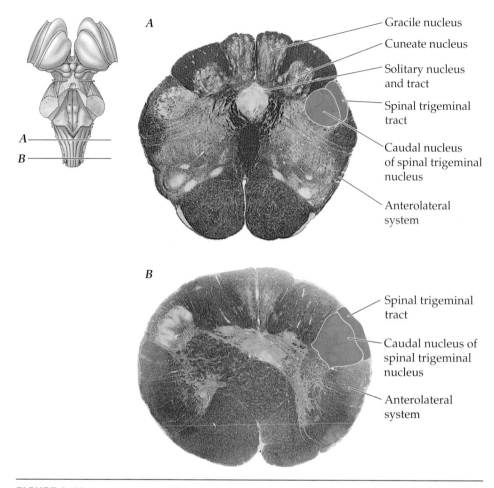

FIGURE 6–11 The organization of the spinal cord–medulla junction and the caudal medulla. Myelin-stained transverse sections through the spinal cord–medulla junction (**B**) and the caudal nucleus—rostral to the pyramidal decussation (**A**). At both levels, the spinal trigeminal tract is located dorsolateral to the nucleus. The inset shows the approximate planes of section.

spinal trigeminal tract is lightly stained (Figure 6–11) because it contains thinly myelinated and unmyelinated axons; this is similar to Lissauer's tract (see Figure 5-4).

The spinal trigeminal nucleus and tract have a rostrocaudal organization

Important insights into the functions of the spinal trigeminal nucleus and tract have been gained from a neurosurgical procedure to relieve intractable facial pain. This operation transects the spinal trigeminal tract and produces selective disruption of such pain and temperature senses with little effect on touch. (Spinal trigeminal tractotomy is rarely done today, however, because analgesic drugs have proved a more effective and consistent therapy.) If the tract is transected rostrally, near the border between the caudal and interpolar nuclei, facial pain and temperature senses over the entire face are disrupted. Transection of the tract between its rostral and caudal borders spares pain and temperature senses over the perioral region and nose.

This clinical finding shows that the spinal trigeminal tract has a rostrocaudal somatotopic organization in addition to a mediolateral organization (Figure 6–10B). Trigeminal fibers that innervate the portion of the head adjacent to the cervical spinal cord representation (Figure 6–10A) project more caudally in the spinal trigeminal tract and terminate in more caudal regions of the caudal nucleus than those that innervate the oral cavity, perioral face, and nose.

The spinal trigeminal nucleus also has a rostrocaudal organization. Proceeding rostrally from the cervical spinal cord, neurons of the spinal dorsal horn process somatic sensory information (predominantly pain, itch, and temperature senses) from the arm, neck, and occiput (ie, region d in Figure 6–10B). Neurons of the trigeminal caudal nucleus, located near the spinal cord–medulla border, process somatic sensory information from the posterior face and ear (ie, regions b and c in Figure 6–10B). These neurons receive input not only from the mandibular trigeminal division but also from the intermediate, glossopharyngeal, and vagus nerves. Farther rostrally, the neurons process information from the perioral region and nose (ie, region a in Figure 6–10B). Finally, neurons in the most rostral part of the trigeminal caudal nucleus, as well as farther rostrally in the trigeminal spinal nucleus (not shown in Figure 6–10B), process pain and temperature information from the oral cavity, particularly from the **teeth.** This organization is termed "onion skin" because of the concentric ring configuration of the peripheral fields processed at a given level by the medullary dorsal horn.

The **caudal nucleus** extends from approximately the first or second cervical segment of the spinal cord to the medullary level at which point the central canal "opens" to form the fourth ventricle (Figures 6–7 and 6–11). The **interpolar nucleus** extends from the rostral boundary of the caudal nucleus to the rostral medulla (Figures 6–7 and 6–12). Finally, the **oral nucleus** extends from the rostral boundary of the interpolar nucleus to the level at which the trigeminal nerve enters the pons (see Figures 6–7 and AII–9).

The **posterior inferior cerebellar artery (PICA)** provides the arterial supply to the dorsolateral portion of the medulla (Figure 6–12; see Chapter 3). The PICA is an end-artery with little collateral flow from other vessels into the territory it serves. As a consequence, the dorsolateral region of the medulla becomes infarcted when the artery is occluded (Figure 6–12). The medial region of the medulla is spared with such an occlusion because of the collateral blood supply to this area from the contralateral vertebral artery and the anterior spinal artery. Occlusion of the PICA produces a complex set of sensory and motor deficits, termed the **lateral medullary,** or **Wallenberg, syndrome.** This syndrome produces a distinctive pattern of somatic sensory signs, which are examined in the case at the beginning of the chapter.

The main trigeminal sensory nucleus is the trigeminal equivalent of the dorsal column nuclei

Rostral to the spinal trigeminal nucleus is the **main trigeminal sensory nucleus** (Figure 6–13C). This part of the trigeminal nuclear complex mediates touch sensation of the face and head and mechanosensation from the teeth. Most of the neurons in this nucleus give rise to axons that decussate and ascend to the **ventral posterior medial nucleus** of the thalamus. Their axons are located in the **trigeminal lemniscus,** dorsomedial to axons of the medial lemniscus. This is another example of segregation of functions. The main trigeminal sensory nucleus is the trigeminal equivalent of the dorsal column nuclei because both nuclei project to the contralateral ventral posterior nucleus (but separately to the medial and lateral subdivisions) and both structures subserve touch sensation (but from different body regions). The trigeminal lemniscus also contains a small number of axons from neurons in the spinal trigeminal nucleus.

A portion of the main trigeminal sensory nucleus receives mechanoreceptive signals from the soft tissues of the oral cavity and the teeth and gives rise to an **ipsilateral pathway** that terminates in the ventral posterior medial nucleus of the thalamus. Apart from transmitting mechanical information

from the oral cavity, the particular function of this ipsilateral path, in relation to the contralateral trigeminal lemniscus, is not known.

The mesencephalic trigeminal nucleus and tract contain the cell bodies and axons of jaw muscle stretch receptors

The mesencephalic trigeminal nucleus, located in the lateral portion of the periventricular and periaqueductal gray matter (Figure 6–13A, B), contains the cell bodies of muscle spindle sensory receptors that innervate jaw muscles. Therefore, this nucleus is equivalent to a peripheral sensory ganglion. The peripheral branch of the primary sensory neuron (Figure 6–3), carrying sensory information to the central nervous system, ascends to the mesencephalic trigeminal nucleus in the **mesencephalic trigeminal tract** (note its myelinated axons lateral to the nucleus in Figure 6–13A). The central branch also projects through the mesencephalic trigeminal tract, to terminate in various brain stem sites important for jaw muscle control and jaw proprioception. For example, a monosynaptic projection to the trigeminal motor nucleus mediates the **jaw-jerk (or closure) reflex** (Figure 6–14), which is analogous to the knee-jerk reflex. Jaw muscle afferents terminate in the main trigeminal and rostral spinal trigeminal nuclei (Figures 6–13A and 6–14). Together these regions play a role in jaw proprioception. In the midbrain, the medial lemniscus and trigeminal lemniscus have migrated laterally (Figure 6–13A). The trigeminal lemniscus terminates in the medial division of the ventral posterior nucleus.

The Caudal Solitary and Parabrachial Nuclei Are Key Brain Stem Viscerosensory Integrative Centers

The **caudal solitary nucleus** (Figures 6–7 and 6–11A) receives input from visceral receptors—chemoreceptors (such as receptors sensitive to blood carbon dioxide), mechanoreceptors (such as mechanoreceptors beneath the mucous membrane of the larynx and arterial pressure receptors), vascular pressure receptors (such as baroreceptors in the carotid body), and nociceptors. Neurons in this nucleus have diverse ascending projections. There are also local projections in the medulla and pons that play important roles in controlling blood pressure and respiration rate and in regulating gastrointestinal motility and secretions. Sensory information processed here, especially mechanical and noxious stimuli from the larynx and pharynx, is important for initiating protective reflexes, such as the **laryngeal closure reflex** to prevent fluid aspiration into the lungs. The caudal solitary nucleus has **descending projections** to the spinal cord for directly controlling portions of the autonomic nervous system.

A

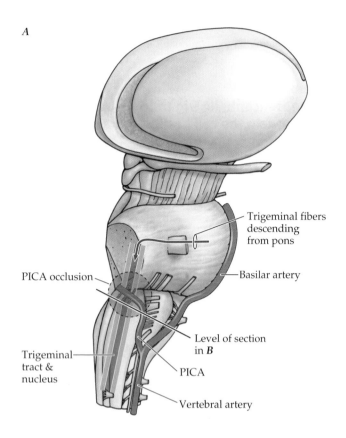

Trigeminal fibers descending from pons

PICA occlusion

Basilar artery

Trigeminal tract & nucleus

Level of section in *B*

PICA

Vertebral artery

B

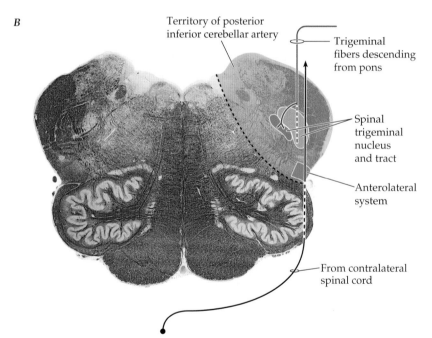

Territory of posterior inferior cerebellar artery

Trigeminal fibers descending from pons

Spinal trigeminal nucleus and tract

Anterolateral system

From contralateral spinal cord

FIGURE 6–12 The arterial supply of the medulla. **A.** The vertebral-basilar arterial system on a portion of the ventral and lateral brain stem. Occlusion of the posterior inferior cerebellar artery (PICA) can lead to infarction of the circled territory. The spinal trigeminal tract (light blue) and nucleus (dark blue) are shown in relation to the infarcted region. PICA occlusion will lead to damage of both the nucleus locally, and the descending trigeminal axons from this level caudally. **B.** Myelin-stained section through the mid-medulla (plane shown in *A*). PICA occlusion (yellow) will: (1) interrupt descending trigeminal fibers and damage the trigeminal nucleus (causing ipsilateral loss of facial pain and temperature senses); and (2) interrupt ascending anterolateral system fibers (causing contralateral loss of pain and temperature senses on limbs and trunk). Other damage caused by PICA occlusion will be considered in later chapters.

The ascending projections of the caudal solitary nucleus are focused on the **parabrachial nucleus** (Figure 6–13B; see Figure AII–12), which, in turn, has diverse forebrain projections. One ascending projection of the parabrachial nucleus is to the parvocellular (small celled) division of the **ventral posterior medial nucleus** of the thalamus, which is the thalamic viscerosensory relay (see next section). The parabrachial nucleus also transmits viscerosensory information rostrally to the **hypothalamus** and the **amygdala** (see Figure 6–9), two brain structures thought to participate in a variety of autonomic and endocrine functions, for example, feeding and reproductive behaviors (see Chapter 15).

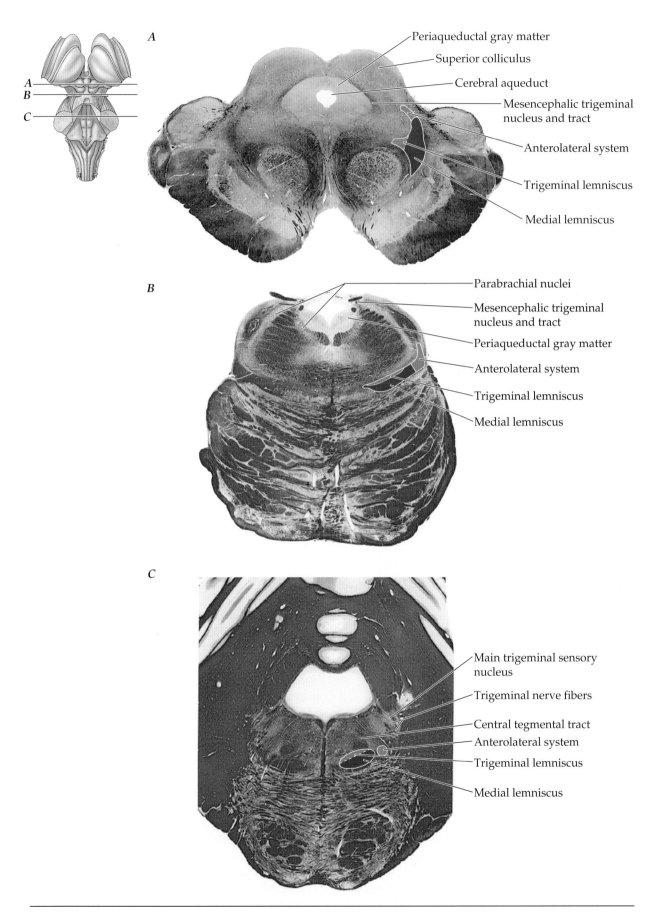

FIGURE 6–13 Myelin-stained sections through the pons at the level of the midbrain (**A**), the parabrachial nucleus (**B**), and the main sensory nucleus of the pons (**C**).

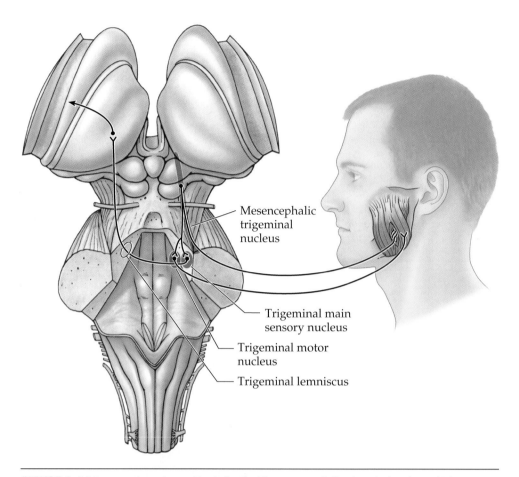

FIGURE 6–14 Jaw proprioception and jaw jerk reflex. The mesencephalic trigeminal nucleus, which contains cell bodies of primary sensory neurons innervating stretch receptors in jaw muscles, and the trigeminal motor nucleus, containing jaw muscle motor neurons, are part of the jaw-jerk reflex circuit. Ascending branch trigeminal sensory nucleus is important in jaw proprioception.

As discussed in Chapter 5, the parabrachial nucleus is also involved in transmitting information about somatic pain to areas of cortex that are important in emotions. Viscerosensory control of bodily functions is considered further in Chapter 15, which covers the hypothalamus and autonomic nervous system.

Somatic and Visceral Sensation Are Processed by Separate Thalamic Nuclei

The ventral posterior medial division of the ventral posterior nucleus, often simply termed **ventral posterior medial nucleus** (Figure 6–15A), processes mechanosensory information from the head. This information, in turn, is projected to the lateral postcentral gyrus, forming the face and head cortical sensory representations (Figure 6–16). The ventral posterior medial nucleus is the trigeminal complement to the spinal mechanosensory nucleus, the ventral posterior lateral nucleus. Similar to the overrepresentation of the hands (see Chapter 4), the representations of the tongue and perioral region in the primary somatic sensory cortex are larger than

the cortical representations of other body parts because they are used more extensively during speech and chewing, for example. In many species of rodents and carnivores, the face representation is more extensive than that of the fingers or tongue and perioral regions, because the large whiskers of these species are their principal tactile discriminative and exploratory organs. The primary somatic sensory cortex, in turn, projects to higher-order somatic sensory areas in the parietal and insular cortex for the further elaboration of the sensory message (see Figure 4–12). The MRI (Figure 6–15B) is through a similar part of the thalamus as in part A, showing the approximate location of the ventral posterior nucleus.

Similar to the systems for spinal somatic sensory information processing, cranial pain, itch, and temperature are transmitted to the **ventral posterior medial** and **ventromedial posterior nuclei.** These thalamic nuclei project to the postcentral gyrus and the insular cortex, respectively. As discussed in Chapter 5, these cortical regions play a role in perception of pain, itch, and temperature senses. In addition, the insular representation may be important in memories of painful experiences and the somatic and autonomic behaviors

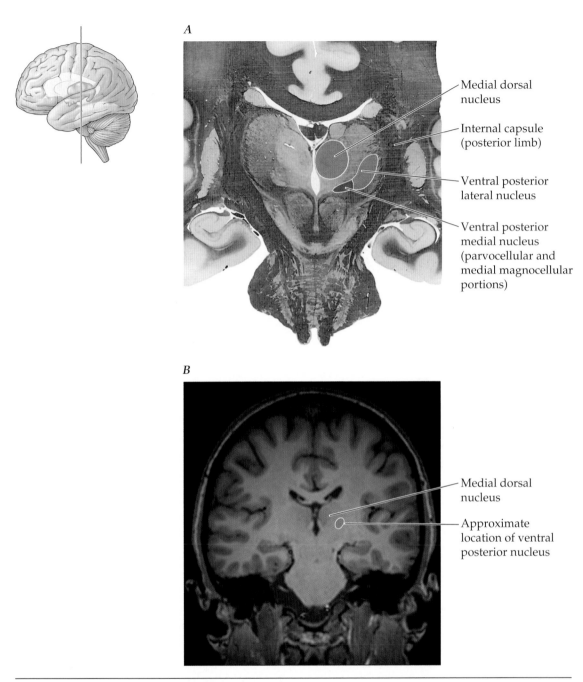

FIGURE 6–15 Thalamus. **A.** Myelin-stained section through ventral posterior nucleus. **B.** MRI. Myelin-stained coronal section through the ventral posterior nucleus of the thalamus. The magnocellular and parvocellular portions of the medial division (ventral posterior medial nucleus) are the trigeminal and taste relay nuclei, whereas the lateral division (ventral posterior lateral nucleus) is the relay nucleus for the medial lemniscus (ie, spinal sensory input).

that pain evokes. The **medial dorsal nucleus** (Figure 6–15) is the third thalamic area to receive information about pain, temperature, and itch. It receives trigeminal thalamic and spinothalamic inputs and projects to the anterior cingulate cortex, which is important in the emotional aspects of pain, itch, and temperature perception.

Viscerosensory information from the pharynx, larynx, esophagus, and other internal organs is processed by a

thalamic region that is located posterior to the ventral posterior medial nucleus and this area projects to the cortex within the lateral sulcus, where the viscera are represented (Figure 6–16B). This nucleus, which is located within an ill-defined posterior thalamic region, may take on one of several names, including ventral posterior medial parvocellular nucleus (which also processes taste; Chapter 9) and the posterior nucleus.

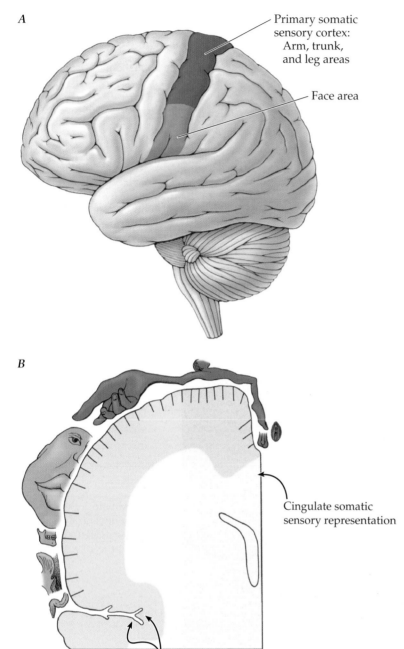

A

Primary somatic
sensory cortex:
Arm, trunk,
and leg areas

Face area

B

Cingulate somatic
sensory representation

Secondary and insular somatic
sensory representations

FIGURE 6–16 *A.* Lateral view of the cerebral hemisphere, showing the locations of the face area laterally and the limbs and trunk area medially. *B.* A coronal slice through the postcentral gyrus showing the somatotopic organization, as represented by the homunculus. (**B,** Adapted from Penfield W, Rasmussen T. *The Cerebral Cortex of Man: a Clinical Study of Localization of Function.* New York, NY: Macmillan; 1950.)

Summary

The Cranial Nerves

Of the 12 cranial nerves (Table 6–1 and Figure 6–2), the first two, the *olfactory* (I) and *optic* (II) nerves, are sensory and enter the telencephalon and diencephalon directly. The 3rd through 12th cranial nerves enter and exit from the brain stem directly. Two cranial nerves, the *oculomotor* (III) and the *trochlear* (IV), are motor nerves located in the midbrain. The pons contains the *trigeminal* (V), a mixed nerve; the *abducens* (VI), a motor nerve; the *facial* (VII), a mixed nerve; and the *vestibulocochlear* (VIII), a sensory nerve. The medulla also contains four cranial nerves: the *glossopharyngeal* (IX) and *vagus* (X) are mixed nerves, whereas the *spinal accessory* (XI) and *hypoglossal* (XII) are motor nerves.

Cranial Nerve Nuclei Columns

Separate columns of cranial nerve nuclei course through the brain stem along its rostrocaudal axis (Figures 6–4 through 6–7). Each column has a separate sensory (afferent) or motor function, and the nomenclature conforms to that for the cranial nerves: (1) *skeletal somatic motor,* (2) *branchiomeric skeletal motor,* (3) *visceral (autonomic) motor,* (4) *viscerosensory and taste,* (5) *somatic sensory,* and (6) *hearing* and *balance* (Table 6–1). Each column has its own mediolateral location (Figures 6–4 and 6–6). The *sulcus limitans* separates the sensory from the motor nuclear columns (Figure 6–4 and 6–5).

Trigeminal Sensory System

Somatic sensation of cranial structures is mediated predominantly by the trigeminal nerve, which has three sensory divisions (Figure 6–10A): *ophthalmic, maxillary,* and *mandibular.* The cell bodies of the primary sensory neurons that innervate the skin and mucous membranes of the head are located in the *semilunar* (or *trigeminal*) *ganglion.* Three other cranial nerves also innervate portions of the head: (1) the *intermediate* (VII) nerve (a branch of the *facial* nerve) innervates the skin of the ear; (2) the *glossopharyngeal* (IX) nerve innervates the posterior tongue and portions of the oral cavity, nasal cavity, pharynx, and middle ear (Figure 6–10A); and (3) the *vagus* (X) nerve innervates the skin of the ear and mucous membranes of the larynx. The cell bodies of the primary afferent fibers in the facial nerve are located in the *geniculate ganglion,* and those of the glossopharyngeal and vagus nerves are located in the *superior ganglion* of each nerve. Afferent fibers in these four cranial nerves enter the brain stem and ascend and descend in the *spinal trigeminal tract* (Figures 6–8 and 6–11). The fibers of the trigeminal nerve, whose cell bodies lie in the semilunar ganglion, terminate in two of the three major components of the trigeminal nuclear complex: the *main (or principal) trigeminal sensory nucleus* (Figures 6–8A and 6–13C) and the *spinal trigeminal nucleus* (Figures 6–7, 6–8B, 6–10, and 6–11). The spinal trigeminal nucleus has three subdivisions: the *oral nucleus, the interpolar nucleus,* and the *caudal nucleus* (Figure 6–7). The afferent fibers of the facial, glossopharyngeal, and vagus nerves terminate in the spinal trigeminal nucleus.

Mechanoreceptive afferent fibers of the trigeminal nerve terminate predominantly in the *main trigeminal sensory nucleus.* The majority of the ascending projection neurons of this nucleus send their axons to the contralateral *ventral posterior medial nucleus* of the thalamus (Figure 6–15). From here, thalamic neurons project, via the posterior limb of the internal capsule, to the face representation of the *primary somatic sensory cortex,* which is located in the lateral portion of the *postcentral gyrus* (Figure 6–16). Projections from the primary cortex engage the secondary somatic sensory cortex and the posterior parietal lobe. A small pathway ascends ipsilaterally to the thalamus and cortex, conveying mechanical information from the mouth, especially the teeth (Figure 6–8A).

Pain, temperature, and *itch* afferents from cranial structures enter and descend in the spinal trigeminal tract. The ascending pathway for pain and temperature sensations originates from the *spinal trigeminal nucleus,* primarily from the *caudal* and *interpolar nuclei* (Figures 6–7 and 6–10). The axons of most ascending projection neurons in these nuclei decussate. The ascending fibers course with the anterolateral system in the lateral medulla and pons en route to the rostral brain stem and thalamus. The thalamic nuclei in which the fibers terminate are the *ventral posterior medial nucleus,* the *ventromedial posterior nucleus,* and the *medial dorsal nucleus* (Figure 6–15).

Afferent fibers carrying proprioceptive information from the jaw muscles form the *mesencephalic trigeminal tract* (Figure 6–14). Their cell bodies are located in the *mesencephalic trigeminal nucleus* and are unique because they are the only primary sensory neurons with cell bodies located in the central nervous system (Figure 6–3). These afferents project to the *main trigeminal nucleus* and rostral parts of the *spinal trigeminal nucleus,* which give rise to a pathway to the *ventral posterior medial nucleus* and *primary somatic sensory cortex.*

Viscerosensory System

Viscerosensory receptors are innervated by the *glossopharyngeal* (IX) and *vagus* (X) nerves, which project into the caudal solitary nucleus (Figures 6–7 and 6–9). Axons ascend ipsilaterally from the solitary nucleus to the *parabrachial nucleus* in the rostral pons (Figure 6–13B). The third-order neurons project to the *hypothalamus* and *limbic systems,* structures for regulating behavior and autonomic responses. Other third-order neurons project to the medial part of the *ventral posterior nucleus* and then to the visceral representation in the *insular cortex* (Figures 6–9 and 6–16). Pelvic visceral organs are innervated by primary sensory fibers that project to the sacral spinal cord. Apart from the dorsal column (Chapter 5), the brain circuits for pelvic visceral sensation are not well understood.

Selected Reading

Saper CB, Lumsden A, Richerson GB. The sensory, motor, and reflex functions of the brain stem. In: Kandel ER, Schwartz JH,

Jessell TM, Siegelbaum SA, Hudspeth AJ, eds. *Principles of Neural Science.* 5th ed. New York, NY: McGraw-Hill; in press.

Al-Chaer ED, Feng Y, Willis WD. Comparative study of viscerosomatic input onto postsynaptic dorsal column and spinothalamic tract neurons in the primate. *J Neurophysiol.* 1999;82:1876-1882.

Altschuler SM, Bao XM, Bieger D, Hopkins DA, Miselis RR. Viscerotopic representation of the upper alimentary tract in the rat: sensory ganglia and nuclei of the solitary and spinal trigeminal tracts. *J Comp Neurol.* 1989;283:248-268.

Altschuler SM, Escardo J, Lynn RB, Miselis RR. The central organization of the vagus nerve innervating the colon of the rat. *Gastroenterology.* 1993;104:502-509.

Arvidsson J, Gobel S. An HRP study of the central projections of primary trigeminal neurons which innervate tooth pulp in the cat. *Brain Res.* 1981;210:1-16.

Arvidsson J, Thomander L. An HRP study of the central course of sensory intermediate and vagal fibers in peripheral facial nerve branches in the cat. *J Comp Neurol.* 1984;223:35-45.

Barnett EM, Evans GD, Sun N, Perlman S, Cassell MD. Anterograde tracing of trigeminal afferent pathways from the murine tooth pulp to cortex using herpes simplex virus type 1. *J Neurosci.* 1995;15:2972-2984.

Beck PD, Kaas JH. Thalamic connections of the dorsomedial visual area in primates. *J Comp Neurol.* 1998;396:381-398.

Blomqvist A, Zhang ET, Craig AD. Cytoarchitectonic and immunohistochemical characterization of a specific pain and temperature relay, the posterior portion of the ventral medial nucleus, in the human thalamus. *Brain.* 2000;123(part 3):601-619.

Broussard DL, Altschuler SM. Brainstem viscerotopic organization of afferents and efferents involved in the control of swallowing. *Am J Med.* 2000;108(suppl 4a):79S-86S.

Bruggemann J, Shi T, Apkarian AV. Viscero-somatic neurons in the primary somatosensory cortex (SI) of the squirrel monkey. *Brain Res.* 1997;756:297-300.

Burton H, Craig AD Jr. Distribution of trigeminothalamic projection cells in cat and monkey. *Brain Res.* 1979;161:515-521.

Capra NF. Mechanisms of oral sensation. *Dysphagia.* 1995;10:235-247.

Capra NF, Ro JY, Wax TD. Physiological identification of jaw-movement-related neurons in the trigeminal nucleus of cats. *Somatosens Mot Res.* 1994;11:77-88.

Chien CH, Shieh JY, Ling EA, Tan CK, Wen CY. The composition and central projections of the internal auricular nerves of the dog. *J Anat.* 1996;189:349-362.

Dubner R, Gold M. The neurobiology of pain. *Proc Natl Acad Sci USA.* 1999;96:7627-7630.

Esaki H, Umezaki T, Takagi S, Shin T. Characteristics of laryngeal receptors analyzed by presynaptic recording from the cat medulla oblongata. *Auris Nasus Larynx.* 1997;24:73-83.

Grelot L, Barillot JC, Bianchi AL. Central distributions of the efferent and afferent components of the pharyngeal branches of the vagus and glossopharyngeal nerves: an HRP study in the cat. *Exp Brain Res.* 1989;78:327-335.

Hanamori T, Smith DV. Gustatory innervation in the rabbit: central distribution of sensory and motor components of the chorda tympani, glossopharyngeal, and superior laryngeal nerves. *J Comp Neurol.* 1989;282:1-14.

Hayakawa T, Takanaga A, Maeda S, Seki M, Yajima Y. Subnuclear distribution of afferents from the oral, pharyngeal and laryngeal regions in the nucleus tractus solitarii of the rat: a study using transganglionic transport of cholera toxin. *Neurosci Res.* 2001;39:221-232.

Hayashi H, Sumino R, Sessle BJ. Functional organization of trigeminal subnucleus interpolaris: nociceptive and innocuous afferent inputs, projections to thalamus, cerebellum, and spinal cord, and descending modulation from periaqueductal gray. *J Neurophysiol.* 1984;51:890-905.

Hu JW, Sessle BJ. Comparison of responses of cutaneous nociceptive and nonnociceptive brain stem neurons in trigeminal subnucleus caudalis (medullary dorsal horn) and subnucleus oralis to natural and electrical stimulation of tooth pulp. *J Neurophysiol.* 1984;52:39-53.

Jones EG, Schwark HD, Callahan PA. Extent of the ipsilateral representation in the ventral posterior medial nucleus of the monkey thalamus. *Exp Brain Res.* 1984;63:310-320.

Kruger L. Functional subdivision of the brainstem sensory trigeminal nuclear complex. In: Bonica JJ, Liebeskind JC, Albe-Fessard DG, eds. *Advances in Pain Research and Therapy,* Vol. 3. New York, NY: Raven Press; 1984:197-209.

Kuo DC, de Groat WC. Primary afferent projections of the major splanchnic nerve to the spinal cord and gracile nucleus of the cat. *J Comp Neurol.* 1985;231:421-434.

Kuo DC, Nadelhaft I, Hisamitsu T, de Groat WC. Segmental distribution and central projections of renal afferent fibers in the cat studied by transganglionic transport of horseradish peroxidase. *J Comp Neurol.* 1983;216:162-174.

Lenz FA, Gracely RH, Zirh TA, Leopold DA, Rowland LH, Dougherty PM. Human thalamic nucleus mediating taste and multiple other sensations related to ingestive behavior. *J Neurophysiol.* 1997;77:3406-3409.

Martin GF, Holstege G, Mehler WR. Reticular formation of the pons and medulla. In: Paxinos G, ed. *The Human Nervous System.* Amsterdam: Academic Press; 1990:203–220.

Menetrey D, Basbaum AI. Spinal and trigeminal projections to the nucleus of the solitary tract: a possible substrate for somatovisceral and viscerovisceral reflex activation. *J Comp Neurol.* 1987;255:439-450.

Mifflin SW. Laryngeal afferent inputs to the nucleus of the solitary tract. *Am J Physiol.* 1993;265:R269-R276.

Nomura S, Mizuno N. Central distribution of primary afferent fibers in the Arnold's nerve (the auricular branch of the vagus nerve): a transganglionic HRP study in the cat. *Brain Res.* 1984;292:199-205.

Paxinos G, Tork I, Halliday G, Mehler WR. Human homologs to brainstem nuclei identified in other animals as revealed by acetylcholinesterase activity. In: Paxinos G, ed. *The Human Nervous System.* Amsterdam: Academic Press; 1990:149-202.

Ro JY, Capra NF. Physiological evidence for caudal brain-stem projections of jaw muscle spindle afferents. *Exp Brain Res.* 1999;128:425-434.

Ropper AH, Samuels MA. *Adams & Victor's Principles of Neurology*. 9th ed. New York, NY: McGraw-Hill; 2009.

Satoda T, Takahashi O, Murakami C, Uchida T, Mizuno N. The sites of origin and termination of afferent and efferent components in the lingual and pharyngeal branches of the glossopharyngeal nerve in the Japanese monkey (Macaca fuscata). *Neurosci Res*. 1996;24:385-392.

Shigenaga Y, Chen IC, Suemune S, et al. Oral and facial representation within the medullary and upper cervical dorsal horns in the cat. *J Comp Neurol*. 1986;243:388-408.

Shigenaga Y, Nishimura M, Suemune S, et al. Somatotopic organization of tooth pulp primary afferent neurons in the cat. *Brain Res*. 1989;477:66-89.

Smith RL. Axonal projections and connections of the principal sensory trigeminal nucleus in the monkey. *J Comp Neurol* 1975;163:347-376.

Sweazey RD, Bradley RM. Central connections of the lingual-tonsillar branch of the glossopharyngeal nerve and the superior laryngeal nerve in lamb. *J Comp Neurol*. 1986;245:471-482.

Sweazey RD, Bradley RM. Response characteristics of lamb pontine neurons to stimulation of the oral cavity and epiglottis with different sensory modalities. *J Neurophysiol*. 1993;70:1168-1180.

Takagi S, Umezaki T, Shin T. Convergence of laryngeal afferents with different natures upon cat NTS neurons. *Brain Res Bull*. 1995;38:261-268.

Takemura M, Nagase Y, Yoshida A, et al. The central projections of the monkey tooth pulp afferent neurons. *Somatosens Mot Res*. 1993;10:217-227.

Topolovec JC, Gati JS, Menon RS, Shoemaker JK, Cechetto DF. Human cardiovascular and gustatory brainstem sites observed by functional magnetic resonance imaging. *J Comp Neurol*. 2004;471(4):446-461.

Treede RD, Apkarian AV, Bromm B, Greenspan JD, Lenz FA. Cortical representation of pain: functional characterization of nociceptive areas near the lateral sulcus. *Pain*. 2000;87:113-119.

Wild JM, Johnston BM, Gluckman PD. Central projections of the nodose ganglion and the origin of vagal efferents in the lamb. *J Anat*. 1991;175:105-129.

Study Questions

1. Which of the following choices does not list the cranial nerves in correct rostral-to-caudal order?
   A. Optic, trochlear, abducens, glossopharyngeal, spinal accessory
   B. Olfactory, oculomotor, facial, trigeminal, glossopharyngeal, vagus
   C. Oculomotor, facial, vagus, spinal accessory
   D. Trochlear, trigeminal, vestibular, glossopharyngeal, spinal accessory

2. Which of the listed statements best describes development of the cranial sensory and motor nerve nuclei?
   A. Cranial nerve sensory nuclei develop from the alar plate, and motor nuclei, the basal plate.
   B. Motor nuclei are displaced dorsally as the fourth ventricle matures.
   C. Sensory nuclei are displaced ventrally as the fourth ventricle matures.
   D. Body somites determine the developmental plan of the brain stem.

3. Which of the following statements best describes the spatial relationships between two cranial nerve nuclear columns?
   A. The branchiomeric motor column is located dorsal to the somatic motor column.
   B. The column for visceral sensations is located lateral to the column for somatic sensation.
   C. The somatic motor column is located medial to the somatic sensory column.
   D. The autonomic nuclei column is located ventral to the somatic sensory column.

4. The caudal nucleus of the spinal trigeminal nucleus is to the parabrachial nucleus, as
   A. mechanosensation is to visceral sensation
   B. visceral sensation is to thermal sensation
   C. visceral sensensation is to pain
   D. pain is to visceral sensation

5. The cell bodies of jaw muscle receptors are located in
   A. dorsal root ganglia
   B. trigeminal ganglion
   C. mesencephalic trigeminal nucleus
   D. interpolar trigeminal nucleus

6. Which of the following statements best describes the somatotopic organization of the caudal and interpolar trigeminal nuclei?
   A. The interpolar nucleus represents the oral cavity, including the teeth, the rostral caudal nucleus represents the perioral face, and the caudal portion of the caudal nucleus represents the back of the face, close to the ear.
   B. The interpolar nucleus represents the oral cavity, including the teeth, the rostral caudal nucleus represents the back of the face, close to the ear, and the caudal portion of the caudal nucleus represents the perioral face.
   C. The interpolar nucleus represents the ophthalamic division of the trigeminal nerve, the rostral caudal nucleus represents the maxillary division, and the caudal portion of the caudal nucleus represents the mandibular division.

D. The interpolar nucleus represents the ophthalmic division of the trigeminal nerve, the rostral caudal nucleus represents the maxillary and mandibular divisions, and the caudal portion of the caudal nucleus represents the intermediate, vagal, and glossopharyngeal nerves.

7. The posterior inferior cerebellar artery (PICA) supplies which of the following structures?
   A. Solitary nucleus
   B. Oral trigeminal nucleus
   C. Medial lemniscus
   D. Pyramid

8. A patient suffers from occlusion of PICA. Which of the following best describes his neurological impairment?
   A. Contralateral loss of facial pain; contralateral loss of limb pain
   B. Ipsilateral loss of facial pain; contralateral loss of limb pain
   C. Contralateral loss of facial pain; ipsilateral loss of facial touch
   D. Contralateral loss of taste; contralateral loss of facial and limb pain

9. A patient has an impaired laryngeal closure reflex. Which of the following nuclei is important in processing mechanosensory information from the mucous membranes near the larynx?
   A. Caudal solitary nucleus
   B. Cuneate nucleus
   C. Main trigeminal sensory nucleus
   D. Gracile nucleus

10. The insular cortex represents
    A. visceral organs
    B. the contralateral face
    C. sensory information from cranial nerves
    D. sensory information from spinal nerves

Chapter 7

The Visual System

CLINICAL CASE | Homonymous Hemianopsia

A 70-year-old woman suddenly developed difficulty seeing on the left side. She was taken to the emergency room. She reported that when she looked directly at her husband, she only saw the right side of his face. On testing in the emergency room, she was found to have a homonymous hemianopsia field defect. The patient did not have left hemineglect or difficulty drawing shapes or in describing the spatial relationships between objects. Figure 7–1A is an MRI showing damage to the right medial occipital lobe and underlying white matter. This was produced by occlusion of the posterior cerebral artery distal to the thalamus.

Answer the following questions based on your reading of the chapter, inspection of the images, and consideration of the neurological signs.

1. **Draw the visual field impairment.**

2. **Explain why the patient does not have macula sparing.**

3. **Why is it that the patient's visual spatial aptitude is not impaired and that she does not have hemineglect?**

Key neurological signs and corresponding damaged brain structures

Homonymous hemianopsia

This is loss of sight in the contralateral visual fields (see Figure 7–3). It can be due to lesion of the visual pathway proximal to the optic chiasm, on one side: along the optic tract, the lateral geniculate nucleus, optic radiations, and occipital lobe. The MRI shows a lesion of the medial occipital lobe. The primary and higher-order visual cortical areas are located here (see Figure 7–15). The basic visual loss is attributed to primary visual cortex damage.

Lack of macular sparing

After occlusion of the occipital branch of the posterior cerebral artery, a distal artery supplying more selectively the visual cortex, the occipital pole may be relatively unaffected. This is because of collateral blood supply from the middle cerebral artery. Figure 7–1B shows this overlap schematically. In the patient, the infarction was not limited to the visual cortex gray matter; there was some involvement of the optic radiations.

—Continued next page

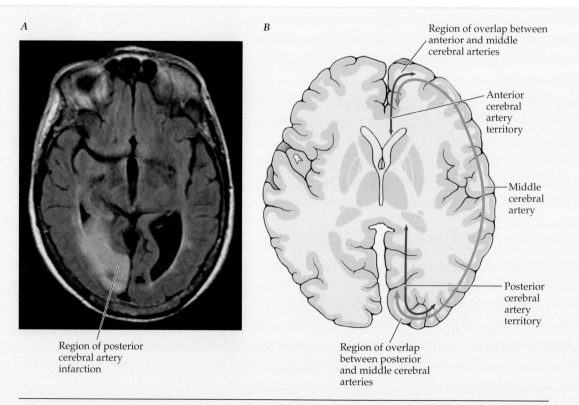

Region of posterior
cerebral artery
infarction

Region of overlap between
anterior and middle
cerebral arteries

Anterior
cerebral
artery
territory

Middle
cerebral
artery

Posterior
cerebral
artery
territory

Region of overlap
between posterior
and middle cerebral
arteries

FIGURE 7–1 Homonymous hemiopsia. **A.** MRI showing right occipital lobe damage. **B.** Schematic drawing of horizontal slice showing the overlapping distributions of the middle and posterior cerebral arteries.

Lack of hemineglect and preservation of visuo spatial aptitude

Damage to the region of the right posterior parietal and occipital lobes can produce hemineglect and disorders of visuospatial aptitude. This could be produced by occlusion/hemorrhage of superficial branches of the middle cerebral artery, which supplies the posterior parietal lobe, or the deep branches of these two arteries, which supply parts of the underlying white matter. These impairments are notably absent in this patient. This is because the lesion spares the posterior parietal lobe and the lateral occipital lobe.

As a species, humans depend more on vision than any other sensory modality. If strength in numbers is an indication of the importance of vision, then a simple axon count and an inventory of brain areas devoted to vision are very telling. The optic nerves, which connect the eyes with the visual processing centers of the brain, each contain about 1 million axons. The cerebral cortex, where visual messages from our eyes are analyzed and perceptions are formed, contains a bewilderingly large number of distinct areas—more than two dozen by some estimates—devoted to one or another aspect of visual processing.

In many ways, the visual system is organized like the somatic sensory systems, considered in Chapters 4 and 5. For instance, the topography of connections in the visual system is determined largely by how the receptive sheet is organized. In fact, these connections are so systematized and

predictable that clinicians can use a visual sensory defect to pinpoint with remarkable precision the location of central nervous system damage. Another similarity is that both systems have a **hierarchical** and **parallel organization.** In a hierarchically organized system, distinct functional levels can be discerned with respect to one another, each with clear anatomical substrates. In vision, as in somatic sensation, multiple hierarchically organized pathways carry information from receptors to structures in the central nervous system. Each pathway processes visual information for a different purpose, such as perception of the shape, motion, and color of objects.

Visual perception, like perception for the other senses, is not a passive process; our eyes do not simply receive visual stimulation. Rather, the position of the eyes is precisely controlled to scan the environment and to attend selectively and orient to specific visual stimuli. In addition to the pathways from the retina to the cortex for perception, there is a separate pathway to the brain stem for controlling eye movements. This chapter begins with an overview of the visual pathways for perception and eye movement control. It then considers the structure and anatomical connections of the components of these pathways. Finally, the chapter examines how the clinician can, with remarkable precision, localize disturbances of brain function by using knowledge of the organization of the visual system. The visual path for eye movement control will be revisited when we consider the circuits for eye movement control (see Chapter 12).

Functional Anatomy of the Visual System

Anatomically Separate Visual Pathways Mediate Perception and Ocular Reflex Function

The visual pathway that mediates perception and the pathway that controls eye movement originate in the retina, a thin sheet of neurons and glial cells that adheres to the posterior inner surface of the eyeball (Figure 7–2A). Also located here are the photoreceptors (Figure 7–2A, inset), which synapse on retinal interneurons that, in turn, synapse on ganglion cells. **Ganglion cells** are the retinal projection neurons, which synapse in the thalamus and brain stem. The axons of ganglion cells travel in the **optic nerve** (cranial nerve II), and ganglion cells from each eye contribute axons to the optic nerve on the same side. Some ganglion cell axons decussate in the **optic chiasm** (Figure 7–2A, B) en route to the thalamus and brain stem, whereas other axons remain uncrossed. Together the crossed and uncrossed ganglion cell axons, reordered according to a precise plan (see below), course in the **optic tract** (Figure 7–2B). Thus, each optic tract contains axons from both eyes.

The Pathway to the Primary Visual Cortex Is Important for Perception of the Form, Color, and Motion of Visual Stimuli

The principal thalamic target for ganglion cells is the **lateral geniculate nucleus.** This thalamic relay nucleus is analogous to the ventral posterior nucleus, the main somatic sensory relay nucleus. The lateral geniculate nucleus projects to the **primary visual cortex** via a pathway called the **optic radiations.** This projection is important for perception. It comprises multiple functional pathways, whose axons intermingle: one that is more important for perceiving the form of visual stimuli, another for color, and a third for the location and speed of motion of stimuli.

The primary visual cortex, or V1, is located in the occipital lobe, along the banks and within the depths of the calcarine fissure (Figure 7–2A). The primary visual cortex is also referred to as the **striate cortex** because myelinated axons (termed the stripe of Gennari) form a prominent striation. Efferent projections from the primary visual cortex follow one of three principal pathways. One pathway projects to the **secondary and higher-order visual cortical areas** in the occipital lobe (see Figure 7–16). The higher-order visual areas partially encircle the primary visual cortex. Each of these visual cortical areas is retinotopically organized. Whereas the primary visual cortex is important in visual signal processing that is fundamental to all aspects of visual perception, many of the higher-order cortical areas are each important in different aspects of vision. For example, the primary visual cortex processes information for stimulus form, color, and motion; one of the higher-order areas (V4) is important for color vision; and a different area is important for discriminating the direction and speed of a moving stimulus (V5; see Figure 7–15). The axons of the second path from the primary visual cortex decussate in the corpus callosum and terminate in the contralateral primary visual cortex. This projection is also for visual perception. It helps to unify images from the two eyes into a perception of a single visual world. Finally, the third path from the primary visual cortex descends to the visuomotor centers of the midbrain for focusing the images of interest on the retina and for moving the eyes to salient objects.

The Pathway to the Midbrain Is Important in Voluntary and Reflexive Control of the Eyes

Certain retinal ganglion cells project to the midbrain directly (Figure 7–2A, C), principally to two structures: the **superior colliculus** and the **pretectal nuclei.** The ganglion cell axons traveling to the midbrain skirt the lateral geniculate nucleus and course in a tract named the **brachium of superior colliculus** (Figure 7–2B; see also Figure 7–9). The superior colliculus, found in the **tectum** of the midbrain (see Figure 2–9), is dorsal to the cerebral aqueduct (Figure 7–2C). In lower vertebrates, such as amphibians and birds, the superior colliculus is termed the **optic tectum** and is the principal brain structure for vision, in lieu of a visual cortex. In mammals and especially humans, the superior colliculus has a minimal role in perception but an important role in the control of **saccades,** rapid eye movements that quickly shift visual gaze from one object to another. The pretectal nuclei are rostral to the tectum, at the midbrain-diencephalic junction (see Figure 7–9). The pretectal nuclei participate in **pupillary reflexes,** which regulate the amount of light reaching the retina, as well as other visual reflexes (see Chapter 12).

Additional brain stem and diencephalic projections of the optic tract serve other functions. For example, one projection reaches midbrain nuclei that are important in the reflexive control of eye position to stabilize images on the retina when the head is moving. These nuclei comprise

A

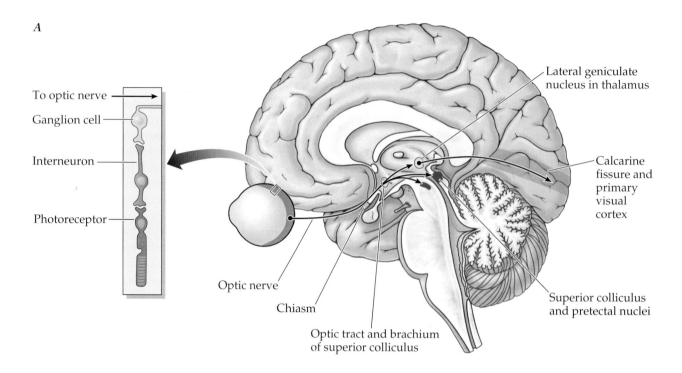

B

C

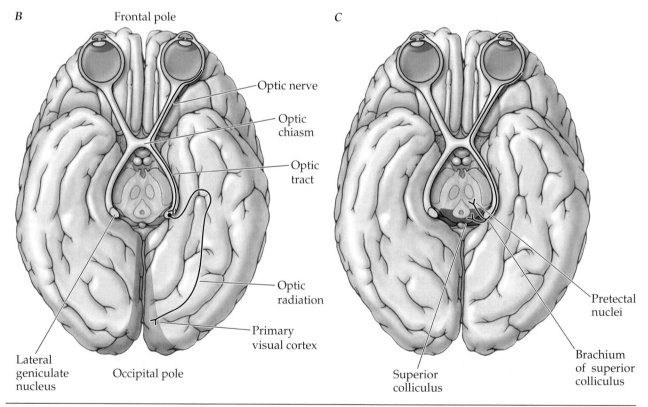

FIGURE 7–2 Organization of the two visual pathways, the retinal-geniculate-calcarine pathway (**A, B**) and the pathway to the midbrain (**A, C**). The inset on the left shows the general organization of the retina. The photoreceptor transduces visual stimuli and transmits the sensory information, encoded in the form of nonpropagated potentials, to retinal interneurons. The interneurons transmit the visual information to the ganglion cells. Ganglion cell axons form the optic nerve once they exit the eyeball. **A.** Midsagittal view of the brain, showing visual paths to the thalamus and cortex and the path to the midbrain. **B.** Inferior brain view, showing the retinal-geniculate-calcarine pathway. **C.** Inferior brain view, showing the pathway to the midbrain.

the **accessory optic system.** As another example, a retinal projection to the hypothalamus is important for circadian rhythms (see Chapter 15).

Regional Anatomy of the Visual System

The Visual Field of Each Eye Partially Overlaps

When the eyes are fixed straight ahead, the total area seen is called the **visual field,** the combined visual fields of each eye (Figure 7–3A). Although the visual field can be divided into right and left hemifields, the visual field of each eye is not simply one hemifield. Similar to when you look through binoculars, the field of view of each eye overlaps extensively. As a result, the visual field includes a central binocular zone (Figure 7–3A, dark shading), where there is stereoscopic vision, and two monocular zones (Figure 7–3A, lighter shading). Each hemifield is therefore seen by parts of the retina of each eye.

Optical Properties of the Eye Transform Visual Stimuli

After light enters the eye through the **cornea,** the transparent avascular portion of the **sclera,** it is focused onto the retinal surface by the **lens** (Figure 7–4A). The lens inverts and reverses the visual image projected on the retina. When you look at an object, you move your eyes so that the object's image falls upon the **fovea,** a specialized high-resolution portion of the retina. The fovea is centered within a morphologically distinct region of the retina called the **macula lutea** (Figure 7–4B). The brain precisely controls the position of the eyes to ensure that the key portion of an image falls on the fovea of each eye. A vertical line passing through the fovea divides the retina into two halves, a **nasal hemiretina** and a **temporal hemiretina.** Each hemiretina includes half of the fovea and the remaining perifoveal and peripheral portions of the retina. The anterior portions of the nasal hemiretinae correspond to the temporal crescents, which are monocular zones receiving visual information from the temporal parts of the visual fields (Figure 7–5).

Consider the relationship between an object being viewed and where its image falls on the retina (Figure 7–5). When you look at someone's face and, for example, fixate on the person's nose, the left side of the face is within the left visual hemifield. The image of the left side falls on the nasal hemiretina of the left eye and the temporal hemiretina of the right eye. Although each eye views the entire face, visual information from the visual hemifield on one side is processed by the visual cortex on the opposite side (see below).

Figure 7–4B also shows the **optic disk,** where retinal axons leave the eyeball and the blood vessels serving a part of the retina enter and leave the eye. This corresponds to the **blind spot** (Figure 7–3B) because the optic disk has no photoreceptors. Interestingly, an individual is not aware of his or her own visual blind spot until it is demonstrated. The fovea and optic disk can be examined clinically using an ophthalmoscope to peer into the back of the eye.

The Retina Contains Three Major Cell Layers

The retina is a laminated structure, as revealed in a section oriented at a right angle to its surface (Figure 7–6). Other components of the visual system also have a laminar organization.

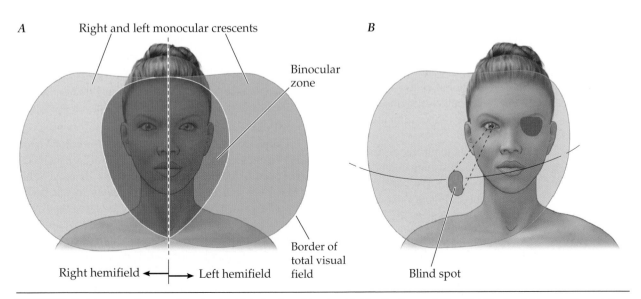

FIGURE 7–3 Schematic diagram of the visual field. **A.** Overlap of the visual fields of both eyes. **B.** Visual field for the right eye (with a patch over the left eye) with the projection of the blind spot indicated.

A

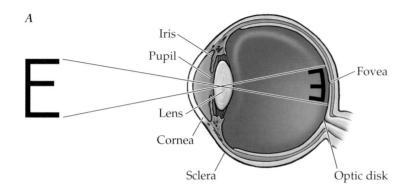

Iris

Pupil

Fovea

Lens

Cornea

Sclera

Optic disk

B

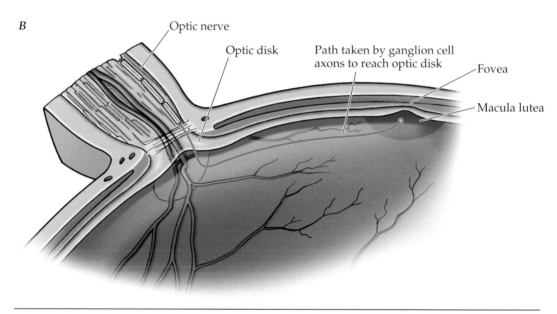

Optic nerve

Optic disk

Path taken by ganglion cell
axons to reach optic disk

Fovea

Macula lutea

FIGURE 7–4   *A.* Sagittal view shows the key features of the optical properties of the eye. *B.* Course of ganglion cell axons along the surface of the retina and into the optic nerve at the optic disk. (*B,* Adapted from Patten H. *Neurological Differential Diagnosis.* 2nd ed. New York, NY: Springer-Verlag; 1998.)

Lamination is one way the nervous system packs together neurons with similar functions and patterns of connections. The spatial reference point for describing the location of the different layers is the **three-dimensional center** of the eye. The **inner,** or proximal, retinal layers are close to the center of the eye; the **outer,** or distal, layers are farther from the center (Figure 7–6, inset).

Although the retina has many anatomically distinct layers (Figure 7–6), the cell bodies of most retinal neurons are located within three layers. This can be best observed in a micrograph of the retina of the mouse (Figure 7–7), in which the various cell types can be identified genetically or immunohistochemically.

1. The cell bodies of the two classes of photoreceptors—rods, for night vision, and cones, for high-acuity daylight vision—are located in the **outer nuclear layer.**

2. The cell bodies and many dendritic processes of retinal interneurons—bipolar, horizontal, and amacrine cells—are located in the **inner nuclear layer.**

3. Ganglion cells, the retinal projection neuron, are located in the innermost retinal cell layer, the **ganglion cell layer.**

Cones contain the photopigments for color vision and come in three different classes according to their absorption spectra: red, green, or blue. Cone density is highest at the fovea and decreases continuously to the peripheral retina. This is why visual acuity is greatest at the foveal and decreases to the peripheral retina. **Rods** contain the photopigment **rhodopsin** and are optimally suited for detecting low levels of illumination, such as at dusk or at night. In fact, a single photon can activate a rod cell. Rods are absent in the fovea and are densest along an elliptical ring in the perifoveal region, which is the location of maximal light

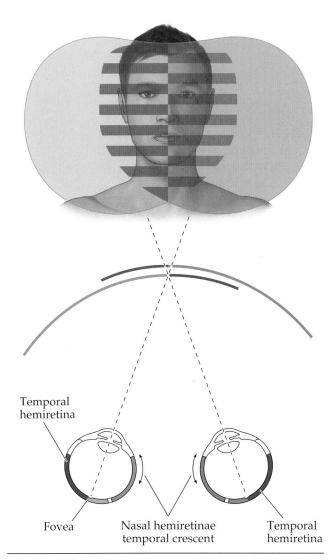

Temporal
hemiretina

Fovea   Nasal hemiretinae   Temporal
                     temporal crescent   hemiretina

FIGURE 7–5 Schematic horizontal view of the eyes looking toward a person, showing the location of the visual fields for each eye and how information projects on the two retinae. The left and right visual fields are shown in blue and green; overlapping regions are striped. For the left eye, visual information from the dark blue region falls on the left temporal hemiretina, and from the light blue region, on the left nasal hemiretina. For the right eye, visual information from the dark green region falls on the right temporal hemiretina, and from the light green region, on the right nasal hemiretina.

sensitivity. This helps to explain why, when discerning a faint object at night, we do best by looking off to one side, rather than directly at it.

Bipolar cells connect photoreceptors directly with the ganglion cells (Figure 7–7). Of the two principal classes of bipolar cells, **cone bipolar cells** and **rod bipolar cells,** the former receive synaptic input from a small number of cone cells to give high visual acuity and color vision. By contrast, rod bipolar cells receive convergent input from many rods for less visual acuity but increased sensitivity to

low levels of illumination. The actions of **horizontal cells** and **amacrine cells** enhance visual contrast through interactions between laterally located photoreceptors and bipolar cells. Horizontal cells are located in the outer part of the inner nuclear layer, whereas amacrine cells are found in the inner portion. Many amacrine cells contain **dopamine,** which plays a role in adapting retinal synaptic activity to the dark.

There are two major classes of **retinal ganglion cells**—M and P cells. The **M (or magnocellular) cell** has a large dendritic arbor, enabling it to integrate visual information from a wide portion of the retina. M cells are thought to play a key role in the analysis of stimulus motion as well as gross spatial features of a stimulus. The **P** (or **parvocellular) cell,** with its small dendritic arbor, processes visual information from a small portion of the retina. These cells are color sensitive and are important for discriminative aspects of vision, such as distinguishing form and color. Ganglion cell axons collect along the inner retinal surface (Figures 7–4B, 7–6, and 7–7) and leave the eye at the optic disk (Figure 7–4B), where they form the **optic nerve.**

Connections between many retinal neurons are also made within specific laminae (Figure 7–7). Connections between photoreceptors and retinal interneurons are in the **outer synaptic (or plexiform) layer.** Bipolar cells synapse on ganglion cells in the **inner synaptic** (or **plexiform) layer.**

The cellular organization of the retina might seem unexpected because light must travel through retinal layers that contain axons, projection neurons, and interneurons to reach the photoreceptors. The consequences of this organization on visual acuity are minimized by an anatomical specialization at the fovea. Here the retinal interneurons and ganglion cells are displaced, exposing the photoreceptors directly to visual stimuli and optimizing the optical quality of the image (Figure 7–7, inset). Moreover, ganglion cell axons are unmyelinated while they are in the retina, which increases the transparency of the retina and facilitates light transmission to the photoreceptor layer. Ganglion cell axons become myelinated once they enter the optic nerve. Since the retina develops from the central nervous system, the myelin sheath surrounding ganglion cell axons is formed by oligodendrocytes (see next section).

There are important nonneural cells in the retina. **Müller cells,** a kind of astrocyte, have important structural and metabolic functions. Their nuclei are located in the inner nuclear layer, and their processes stretch vertically across most of the retina (Figure 7–6). The other nonneural element associated with the retina, the **pigment epithelium,** is external to the photoreceptor layer (Figure 7–5A) and serves metabolic and phagocytic roles. For example, cells in the pigment epithelium help remove rod outer segment disks that are discarded as part of a normal renewal process. Because the retina does not tightly adhere to the pigment epithelium, it can become detached following a blow to the head or eye. This results in a partially **detached retina** and loss of vision in the detached portion.

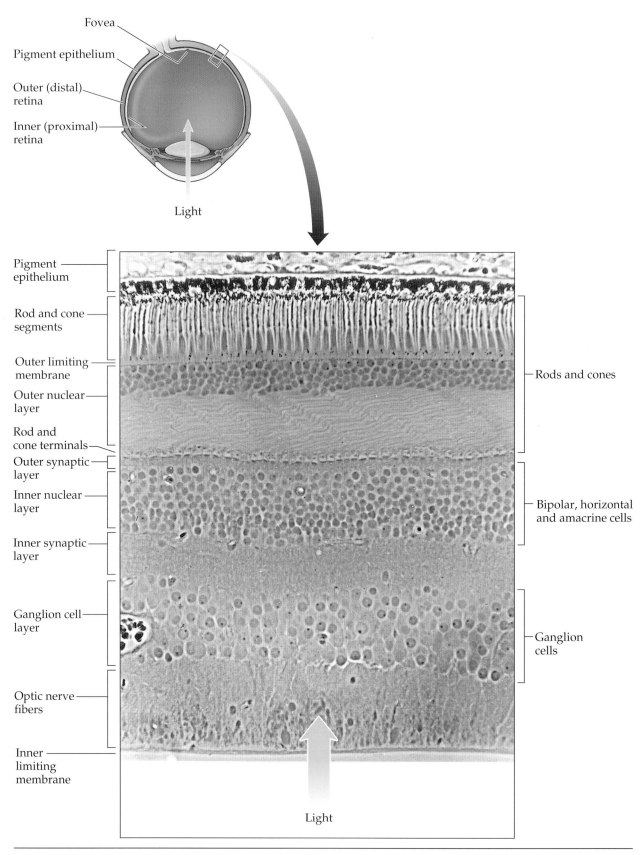

FIGURE 7–6 Transverse section of the retina. Inset shows a schematic diagram of the eyeball, indicating the inner and outer portions of the retina. (Courtesy of Dr. John E. Dowling, Harvard University.)

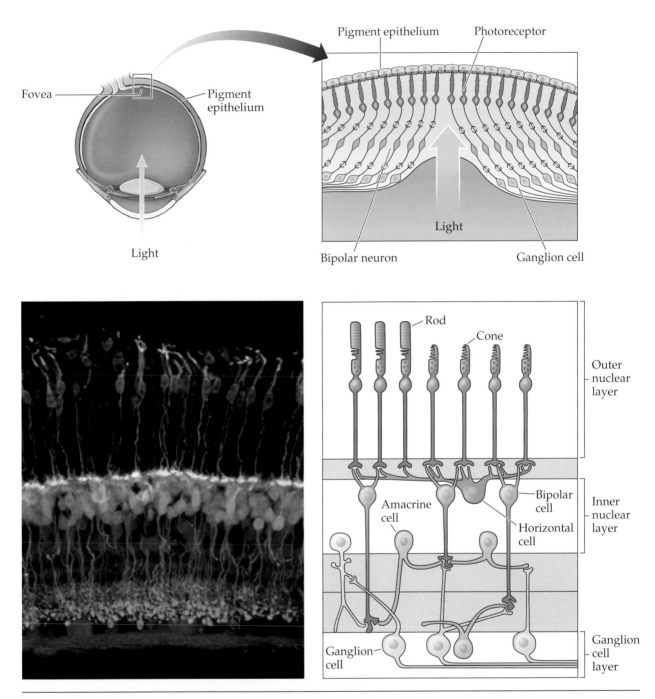

FIGURE 7–7 At the fovea, retinal interneurons and ganglion neurons are displaced so that light falls directly onto the photoreceptors (top). A cross-section through the mouse retina showing lamination of cell bodies and synapses (bottom left). Photoreceptors are stained purple-blue (using an antibody to cone arrestin). Amacrine and ganglion cells are stained red (calcium binding protein calbindin). Bipolar cells are green. (Micrograph courtesy of Dr. Rachel Wong, University of Washington. Schematic diagram showing major cell types and connections in the vertebrate retina. Adapted from Dowling JE, Boycott BB. Organization of the primate retina: electron microscopy. *Proc R Soc Lond B.* 1966;166:80-111.)

The circulation of the retina has a dual organization. The arterial supply of the inner retina is provided by branches of the ophthalmic artery, which is a branch of the internal carotid. The outer retina is devoid of blood vessels. Its nourishment derives from arteries in the choroid, the layer of ocular tissue between the inner retina and the outer sclera. This may be why the photoreceptors are in the outer retina.

Each Optic Nerve Contains All of the Axons of Ganglion Cells in the Ipsilateral Retina

The optic nerve is **cranial nerve II,** but it is actually a central nervous system pathway rather than a peripheral nerve. This is because the retina develops from a displaced portion of the diencephalon, rather than from neural crest cell, as primary somatic sensory neurons. The optic nerves from both eyes converge at the **optic chiasm** (Figure 7–8). The axons of ganglion cells of each **nasal hemiretina** decussate in the optic chiasm and enter the contralateral optic tract, whereas those of each **temporal hemiretina** remain on the same side and enter the ipsilateral optic tract (Figure 7–8). Thus, each optic tract contains axons from the contralateral nasal hemiretina and the ipsilateral temporal hemiretina (Figure 7–8). Despite the incomplete decussation of the optic nerves in the chiasm, there is a complete crossover of visual information: Visual stimuli from one half of the **visual field** are processed within the **contralateral thalamus, cerebral cortex,** and **midbrain.**

The Superior Colliculus Is Important in Ocular Motor Control and Orientation

The optic tract splits on the ventral diencephalic surface. The major contingent of axons terminates in the lateral geniculate nucleus and gives rise to the pathway for visual perception (see next section). A smaller contingent skirts the lateral geniculate nucleus and passes over the surface of the medial geniculate nucleus, which is the thalamic auditory nucleus (see Chapter 8). These axons collectively are termed the **brachium of superior colliculus** (Figure 7–9C) because their major site of termination is the superior colliculus.

The superior colliculus is laminated on microscopic appearance: Incoming visual information is processed by the dorsal layers (Figure 7–9C), whereas somatic sensory, auditory, and other information is processed by neurons in the ventral layers. The ventral layers of the superior colliculus contain part of the neural apparatus for eye and neck muscle control (see Chapter 10). A function of the superior colliculus is to combine visual and other sensory information to generate

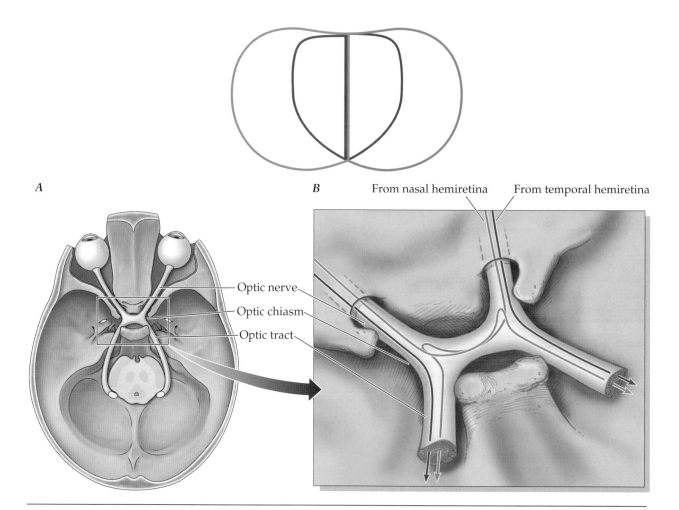

A *B* From nasal hemiretina From temporal hemiretina

Optic nerve
Optic chiasm
Optic tract

FIGURE 7–8 Horizontal view of the visual system, showing the portions of the retina of each eye that receive information from the left visual field. Ganglion neuron axons from the nasal hemiretinae decussate; those from the temporal hemiretinae project to the brain ipsilaterally. **A.** View of the base of the skull showing the regional anatomy of the optic chiasm. **B.** Paths taken by ganglion cell axons from the different parts of the retinae of each eye. (**B,** Adapted from Patten H. *Neurological Differential Diagnosis.* 2nd ed. New York, NY: Springer-Verlag; 1998.)

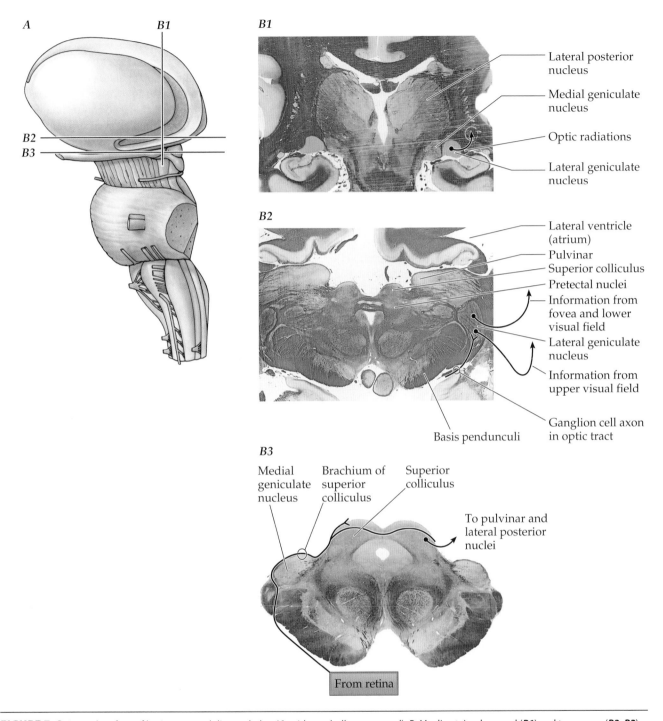

FIGURE 7–9 Lateral surface of brain stem and diencephalon (**A**; with cerebellum removed). **B.** Myelin-stained coronal (**B1**) and transverse (**B2, B3**) sections through the lateral geniculate nucleus and rostral midbrain. The path of a thalamic neuron's axons into the optic radiations is shown in **B1**. The path of a ganglion cell axon from the retina to the lateral geniculate nucleus is shown in **B2**, and to the superior colliculus, in **B3**. The lines in **A** show the planes of section in **B**.

motor control signals to help orient the eyes and head to salient stimuli in the environment.

The neural systems for visuomotor function and visual perception appear to converge in the cerebral cortex. Certain superior colliculus neurons have an axon that ascends to two thalamic nuclei that serve more integrative functions than

sensory relay alone, the **lateral posterior** and **pulvinar nuclei** of the thalamus (see Table 2–1; Figure 2–13). These thalamic nuclei project primarily to **higher-order visual areas** and to the **parietal-temporal-occipital association areas.** One function of this ascending projection from the superior colliculus may be to inform cortical areas important for visual

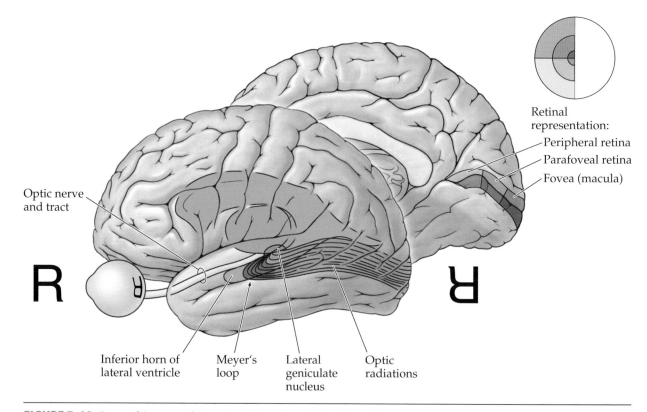

perception about the speed and direction of eye movements. This information is important for distinguishing between movement of a stimulus and movement of the eyes.

The Lateral Geniculate Nucleus Transmits Retinotopic Information to the Primary Visual Cortex

The major retinal projection is to the **lateral geniculate nucleus** of the thalamus. This nucleus forms a surface landmark on the ventral diencephalon that is sometimes called the lateral geniculate body (Figures 7–10 and 7–11). It is located just lateral to the medial geniculate nucleus, the thalamic auditory nucleus (see Chapter 8). The lateral geniculate nucleus is retinotopically organized. The fovea is represented posteriorly in the lateral geniculate nucleus, with progressively more peripheral parts of the retina represented anteriorly. The medial superior part of the lateral geniculate nucleus represents the inferior visual field, and the lateral inferior part, the superior visual field.

The lateral geniculate nucleus sends its axons to the primary visual cortex via the **optic radiations** (Figures 7–10 and also 7–9A, B). The optic radiations take an indirect course around the lateral ventricle to reach their cortical targets. A portion of the optic radiations transmitting visual information from the superior visual field courses rostrally within the

temporal lobe (termed **Meyer's loop),** before heading caudally to the primary visual cortex.

The primary visual cortex, which is located mostly on the medial brain surface, corresponds to Brodmann's cytoarchitectonic area 17 (see Table 2–2; Figure 2–19). The retina and, in consequence, visual space are precisely represented in the primary visual cortex (Figure 7–10) because of the orderly projection from the thalamus to the cortex. The foveal representation, corresponding to central vision, is caudal to the perifoveal and peripheral portions. The inferior retina, receiving information from the upper visual field, is represented in the inferior bank of the calcarine fissure. The superior retina, receiving visual input from the lower visual field, is represented in the superior bank. Although the fovea region is a small portion of the retina, the area of primary visual cortex devoted to it is greatly expanded with respect to the rest of the retina. This organization is similar to the large representation of the fingertips in the primary somatic sensory cortex (see Figure 4-9B).

The Primary Visual Cortex Has a Columnar Organization

Different areas of the cerebral cortex have a similar anatomical organization: They each have six principal cell layers, often with multiple sublaminae, and the thalamic relay nucleus

Retinal
representation:
Peripheral retina
Parafoveal retina
Fovea (macula)

Optic nerve
and tract

R

 Я

Inferior horn of
lateral ventricle

Meyer's
loop

Lateral
geniculate
nucleus

Optic
radiations

FIGURE 7–10 Course of the axons of the optic radiations from the lateral geniculate nucleus, over the lateral ventricle, to reach the primary visual cortex. The primary visual cortex has a retinotopic organization in which the macula is located caudally and the perimacular and peripheral parts of the retina are represented rostrally. The portions of the left visual field (inset) are coded to match the corresponding representations in the right visual cortex.

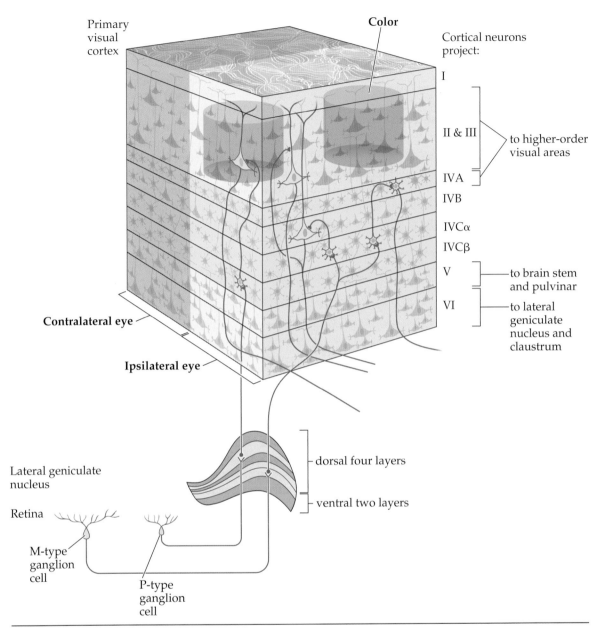

FIGURE 7–11 Magno- and parvocellular systems. Projections of the parvocellular and magnocellular visual systems to the primary visual cortex, represented as a cube with the pial surface on top and the white matter, at the bottom. The magnocellular projection from the lateral geniculate nucleus terminates primarily in layer IVCα, whereas the parvocellular projection terminates primarily in layer IVCβ. In addition, both projections terminate in layer VI, which contains neurons that project back to the thalamus. (Only laminae receiving major thalamic projections are shaded.)

makes most of its synapses within layer IV. Different cortical areas also share a similar functional organization: Neurons located above and below one another—yet in different layers—have similar properties. This is the **columnar organization** of the cerebral cortex. In the primary somatic sensory cortex, neurons in a cortical column all process sensory information from the same **peripheral location** and the same somatic **submodality** (see Chapter 4; Figure 4–11).

The primary visual cortex also has a columnar organization (Figure 7–11). Neurons in a cortical column have similar properties and functions because local connections primarily

distribute the thalamic input vertically, from layer IV to superficial and deeper layers, rather than horizontally within the same layer. Horizontal connections do exist; however, they mediate other kinds of functions, such as enhancing contrast and helping to associate visual information from different parts of a scene to form perceptions. These horizontal connections run in the **stria** (or **stripe**) **of Gennari**.

The primary visual cortex has at least three types of columns (Figure 7–11): (1) **Ocular dominance columns** contain neurons that receive visual input primarily from the ipsilateral or the contralateral eye; (2) **orientation columns** contain neurons that are maximally sensitive to visual stimuli with similar spatial orientations (see Figure 7–13); and (3) **color columns,** termed **blobs,** are vertically oriented aggregates of neurons in layers II and III that are sensitive to the color of visual stimuli.

Ocular dominance columns segregate input from the two eyes

The lateral geniculate nucleus contains six principal cell layers, stacked on top of one another. Each layer receives information exclusively from ganglion cells from the **ipsilateral** or the **contralateral retina.** Neurons in the dorsal four layers have different functions than those in the ventral two layers (see below). In layer IV of primary visual cortex, the axon terminals of lateral geniculate neurons that receive input from the ipsilateral retina remain segregated from the terminals of neurons that receive their input from the contralateral retina (Figures 7–11 and 7–12).

Ocular dominance columns can be shown in human primary visual cortex at autopsy in a person who had one eye removed before death, for example, because of an ocular tumor. When stained for the mitochondrial enzyme cytochrome oxidase, tissue sections show alternating stripes of reduced and normal staining (Figure 7–12A). The stripes with reduced staining correspond to the ocular dominance columns of the removed eye, which were inactive following enucleation. Normal staining corresponds to the columns of the intact eye, active until death. The ocular dominance columns can be analyzed on histological sections and the three-dimensional configuration of the columns drawn on the surface of the primary visual cortex (Figure 7–12B, C).

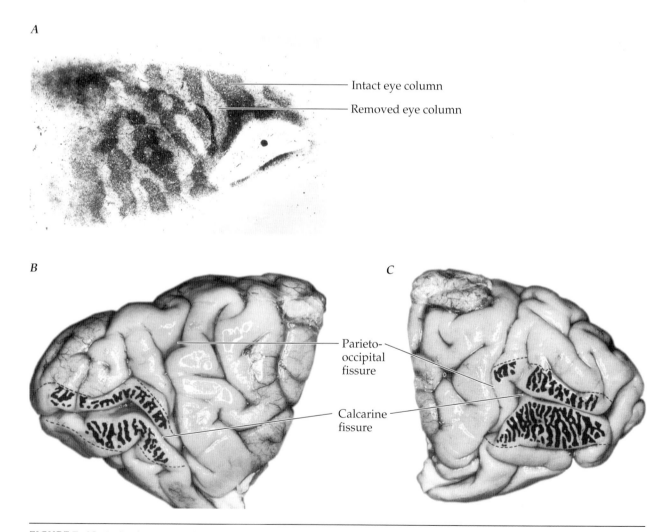

A

———— Intact eye column
———— Removed eye column

B   *C*

Parieto-
occipital
fissure

Calcarine
fissure

FIGURE 7–12 Ocular dominance columns in the human brain from a person who had one eye removed 23 years prior to death. **A.** A section cut approximately parallel to the surface of the cortex stained for the presence of the mitochondrial enzyme cytochrome oxidase. The alternating dark and light bands correspond to the locations of the ocular dominance columns for the intact and removed eyes. Enucleation resulted in very low levels of the enzyme in columns for that eye. **B** and **C.** Photographs of the left (**B**) and right (**C**) occipital lobes, with the ocular dominance columns from the intact eye drawn directly on the surface of the cortex. The intervening spaces correspond to the columns for the removed eye. Calibration bar is 1 cm. (Courtesy of Dr. Jonathan C. Horton. Adapted from Horton JC, Hedley-White ET. Mapping of cytochrome oxidase patches and ocular dominance columns in human visual cortex. *Phil Trans R Soc Lond B.* 1984;304, 255-272.)

Mixing of information from both eyes, giving rise to binocular inputs, occurs in neurons located above and below layer IV. These binocular interactions are mediated largely by cortical interneurons. The binocular neurons receive a stronger synaptic input from the same eye that projected information to the monocular neurons in layer IV, and a weaker input from the other eye. This pattern of lateral geniculate axon terminations in layer IV (Figure 7–11) and blending of connections above and below layer IV forms the anatomical basis of the **ocular dominance columns.** A given retinal location in each eye is represented in the cortex by a pair of adjacent ocular dominance columns. Horizontal connections between neurons in adjacent ocular dominance columns are thought to be important for depth perception.

Orientation columns are revealed by mapping cortical functional organization

Physiological studies have shown that most neurons in the primary visual cortex respond to simple bar-shaped stimuli with a particular orientation. However, unlike ocular dominance, which is an attribute based on anatomical connections from one eye or the other, orientation specificity of neurons in a column in the primary visual cortex is a property produced by synaptic connections between local cortical neurons. Orientation columns can be revealed in experimental animals using methods that provide an image of neuronal function, such as neuronal activity or local blood flow, which correlates with neural activity. Figure 7–13 is an image of a small portion of the surface of the primary visual cortex of a monkey as it viewed contours of different orientations. The figure shows the pattern of activation of cortical neurons in response to stimuli of different orientations. Neurons sensitive to particular stimulus orientations are located within territories of one or another color. Neurons sensitive to all orientations are present within a local area, but they are distributed in a radial pattern resembling a pinwheel. Cells selective for stimulus orientation (and therefore the orientation columns themselves) are located from layer II to layer VI, and spare a portion of layer IV, which contains neurons that are insensitive to stimulus orientation.

Clusters of color-sensitive neurons in layers II and III are distinguished by high levels of cytochrome oxidase activity

Neurons sensitive to the wavelength of the visual stimulus are clustered within the ocular dominance columns in layers II and III. The locations of these color-sensitive cells correspond to regions of primary visual cortex that have high levels of activity of the mitochondrial metabolic enzyme **cytochrome oxidase** (Figure 7–14). The regions of increased enzyme activity, which correspond to the clusters of color-sensitive neurons, are termed **blobs** (Figure 7–14, small dots). The adjoining secondary visual cortex (area 18; V2) has no blobs, but shows alternating stripes of increased (thick and thin stripes)

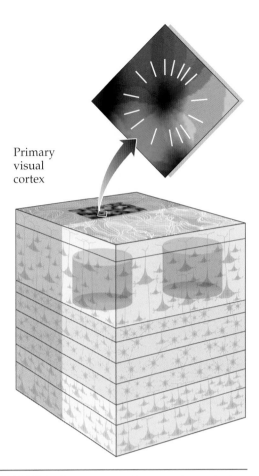

Primary visual cortex

FIGURE 7–13 Orientation columns in primary visual cortex. This is an image of a portion of the primary visual cortex of the monkey, obtained using an optical imaging technique that measures local changes in tissue reflectance, which indicates neuronal activity. Neurons sensitive to a particular stimulus orientation are located in areas with different color (inset, right). Note the swirling pattern of orientation sensitivity, resembling a pinwheel, would correspond to a column in which neurons are sensitive to all orientations within a local area of visual space. (Courtesy of Dr. Aniruddha Das, Columbia University.)

or decreased (pale interstripe) cytochrome oxidase activity (Figure 7–14). The section on higher-order areas addresses how neurons in the thick stripe, thin stripe, and pale interstripe are part of distinct visual processing channels.

The Magnocellular and Parvocellular Systems Have Differential Laminar Projections in the Primary Visual Cortex

The M (**magnocellular**) and P (**parvocellular**) ganglion cells give rise to visual information channels that process distinctive stimulus features. M ganglion cells synapse in the ventral laminae of the lateral geniculate nucleus, whereas P cells synapse in the dorsal laminae; this is in addition to

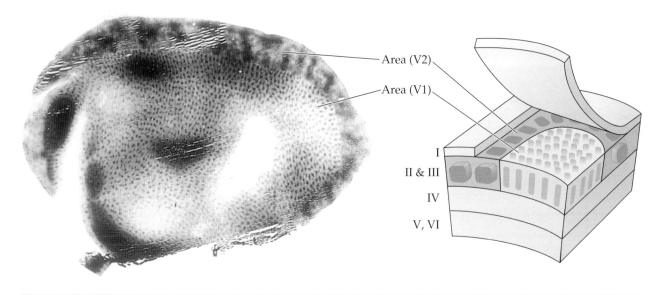

FIGURE 7–14 Clusters of neurons involved in color vision are identified by histochemical localization of cytochrome oxidase. The section was cut parallel to the pial surface and predominantly through layers II and III of the occipital lobe of the visual cortex in a rhesus monkey (inset). Cytochrome oxidase activity is greater in the dark regions than in the light regions. In area 17 (primary visual cortex), regions that have high cytochrome oxidase activity have a spherical shape in cross section and are cylindrical in three dimensions. Cytochrome oxidase staining in area 18 (secondary visual cortex) reveals thick and thin stripes rather than the polka-dot pattern. (Courtesy of Drs. Margaret Livingstone and David Hubel, Harvard University.)

receiving input from ganglion cells from either the ipsilateral or the contralateral halves of the retina (Figure 7–11). Because the thalamocortical neurons located in the ventral layers are larger than those in the dorsal layers, they are also called magnocellular and parvocellular layers, respectively. M cells are the major input to a visual circuit for the analysis of stimulus motion and generalized aspects of form, whereas P cells provide the input for analyzing the color and fine details of stimuli.

Neurons in the magnocellular and parvocellular layers of the lateral geniculate nucleus project to different sublaminae in layer IV of the primary visual cortex. The magnocellular system projects primarily to layer IVCα, whereas the parvocellular system projects primarily to layers IVA and IVCβ. Interneurons in the layer IV sublaminae connect with neurons in superficial and deeper cortical layers, which distribute visual information to other cortical and subcortical regions (Figure 7–11). The differential laminar projections of the magnocellular and parvocellular systems set the stage for distinct visual processing channels that distribute information about different aspects of a stimulus to the secondary and higher-order visual cortical areas.

Higher-Order Visual Cortical Areas Analyze Distinct Aspects of Visual Stimuli

The higher-order visual areas, located in Brodmann's areas 18 and 19, are located in the occipital lobe; they partially encircle area 17 (Figure 7–15). They receive visual information directly or indirectly from the primary visual area as well as from the integrative thalamic nuclei, the pulvinar and lateral posterior nuclei. Each is also retinotopically organized. (Higher-order visual areas are collectively termed the **extrastriate cortex** because they lie outside the primary area, or striate cortex, which contains the stripe of Gennari.) Intracortical connections between the visual areas are bewilderingly complex; they have both a hierarchical and a parallel component. For example, the primary visual cortex projects to the secondary visual cortex (V2), which in turn projects to V5. This is a hierarchically organized projection to V5. The parallel projection to V5 is a direct one, skipping V2. Although it can be deduced that less information processing occurs in the parallel projection, it is not yet clear how the parallel and hierarchical paths differ functionally.

Research analyzing connections of the monkey visual system suggests that out of the myriad cortico-cortical projections among the primary and higher-order visual areas, different pathways are involved in perceiving stimulus motion, color, and form (Figure 7–16A). The secondary visual cortex (V2) plays a key role in all three pathways.

1. The **motion pathway** derives from the M-type ganglion cells. Information passes through the magnocellular layers of the lateral geniculate nucleus, to neurons in layer IVCα of the primary visual cortex (Figure 7–11), and from there to neurons in layer IVB (Figure 7–11). Neurons in layer IVB project directly to V5 and indirectly via neurons in the thick cytochrome oxidase

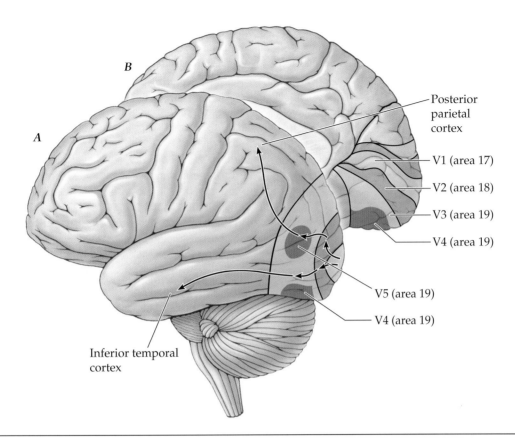

FIGURE 7–15 Visual cortical areas and their major projections. V1 through V5 are shown. Separate pathways projecting dorsally into the parietal lobe and ventrally into the temporal lobe are thought to mediate spatial vision (the analysis of motion and location of visual stimuli) and object vision (the analysis of form and color of visual stimuli), respectively.

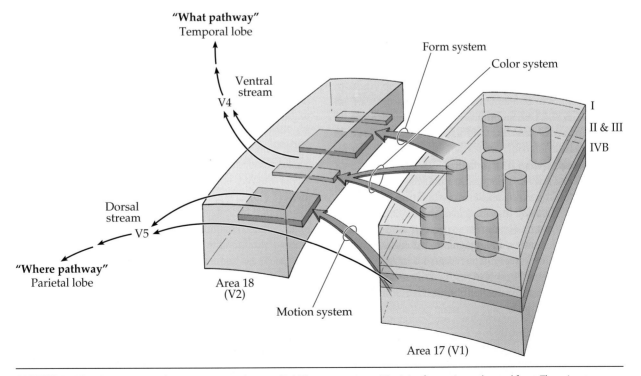

FIGURE 7–16 Efferent streams from primary visual cortex (V1). There are separate VI origins for motion, color, and form. The primary visual cortex (area 17) is shown on the right, and the secondary visual cortex (area 18) is shown on the left. The motion system is also used for generating and controlling limb and eye movements.

stripes of V2 (Figure 7–16). In the rhesus monkey, V5 corresponds to a region named MT, for middle temporal area. This region is important not only for motion detection but also for regulating slow eye movements (see Chapter 12). The pathway from VI (and V2) to V3 may be important for analyzing aspects of **visual form in motion.** A region

thought to be analogous to V5 in the human can be imaged while the subject views moving visual stimuli (Box 7–1).

2. The **color pathway** derives from the P-type ganglion cells, which terminate in the parvocellular layers of the lateral geniculate nucleus. From there the thalamocortical projection is, via neurons in layer IVCβ

Box 7–1

The Functions of the Different Higher-Order Visual Areas Are Revealed by Imaging and Analysis of Deficits Produced by Lesions

The functions of the different higher-order visual areas of the cortex are sufficiently distinct that selective damage to one can impair a remarkably specific aspect of vision. This specificity derives in part from the duality of the parvocellular and magnocellular pathways, as well as the projection from interlaminar lateral geniculate neurons to the color blobs in layers II and III of the primary visual cortex. But, because the different systems do not remain completely separate in the cortex (eg, see Figure 7–11), greater functional specificity appears to be achieved by combining information from the two systems in complex ways, probably by circuits within the various cortical areas.

Functional localization in the visual system can be revealed by imaging techniques such as PET and functional magnetic resonance imaging (fMRI) as well as by considering the deficits in visual perception that occur following localized damage to the different visual cortical areas. Figure 7–17A is an fMRI scan of the first through fourth visual areas of the human brain. The image was created by taking advantage of the retinotopic organization of the different areas.

Whereas the primary and secondary visual areas become active irrespective of whether an individual views a monochromatic scene in motion or a stationary colorful scene, the higher visual areas are driven by particular stimulation patterns. A parallel situation exists with visual system trauma. Damage to the lower-order visual areas (and subcortical centers) produces **scotomas,** or blind spots, of different configurations (see section on visual field changes). By contrast, damage to the higher-order visual areas produces more subtle defects.

Imaging and Lesion of the "Where" Pathway

An area on the lateral surface of the occipital lobe, close to the juncture of the inferior temporal sulcus and one of the lateral occipital gyri, becomes selectively activated by visual motion (Figure 7–18B). This area closely corresponds to V5. Damage to this region can produce a remarkable visual disorder, motion blindness (hemiakinetopsia), in the contralateral visual field. Patients with this disorder do not report seeing an object move. Rather, objects undergo episodic shifts in location. An approaching form is in the distance at one time and close by the next.

Lesions farther along the "where" pathway, in the posterior parietal association cortex (Figure 7–17B), impair spatial vision and orientation. A lesion here alters complex aspects of perception that involve more than vision, because this region receives convergent inputs from the somatic sensory and auditory cortical areas. Patients can experience deficits in pointing and reaching

and in avoiding obstacles. As discussed in Chapter 4, patients with lesion in this parietal lobe area also can neglect a portion of their body and a portion of the external world around them. Deficits are most profound when the right hemisphere becomes damaged, a reflection of lateralization of spatial awareness. This pattern of progressively more complex, and more specific, sensory and behavioral impairment illustrates the hierarchical organization of the higher visual pathways.

Posterior Cerebral Artery Infarction Can Produce a Lesion of the "What" Pathway

A region on the medial brain surface, in the caudal portion of the fusiform gyrus, becomes active when a subject views a colorful scene (Figure 7–18C). This may correspond to area V4 in the human brain. A lesion of this portion of the fusiform gyrus can produce cortical color blindness (hemiachromatopsia) in the contralateral visual field. Individuals with such damage may not experience severe loss of form vision, presumably because of the residual capabilities of the intact lower-order visual areas. Whereas color blindness due to the absence of certain photopigments is a common condition, color blindness due to a cortical lesion is rare because it depends on damage to a localized portion of the cortex. Larger lesions, common with infarction of the posterior cerebral artery territory, would more typically produce some form of contralateral blindness because of damage to the primary visual cortex.

Medial to the color territory, in the posterior fusiform gyrus, is a cortical area activated by viewing faces. Patients with a lesion of this posterior and medial portion of the fusiform gyrus can have the bizarre condition termed **prosopagnosia,** in which they lose the ability to recognize faces, even of persons well known to them. Similar to spatial awareness, which is preferentially organized by the right hemisphere, face recognition is also right-side dominant. However, unilateral lesions produce less marked effects. Unfortunately, bilateral vascular lesions can occur because this region is within the territory of the posterior cerebral artery. Recall that the posterior cerebral artery derives its blood supply from the basilar artery, an unpaired artery. Depending on the effectiveness of collateral circulation, basilar artery occlusion can occlude the posterior cerebral arteries bilaterally (see Chapter 3). Lesions that produce prosopagnosia also commonly produce some degree of color blindness (achromatopsia) as well as generalized object recognition impairment (agnosia). This is because vascular lesions are often large enough to encompass several distinct functional regions.

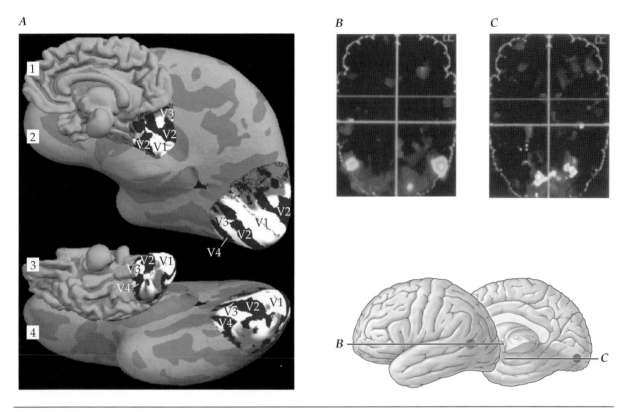

FIGURE 7–17 Visual cortical areas imaged in the human brain. **A.** Functional magnetic resonance imaging scans of human brains showing several visual cortical areas in the occipital lobe. **A1** and **A3** are lateral and ventral views of the brain reconstructed from MR images. **A2** and **A4** are data from "smoothed" brains in which data from within sulci are revealed on an unfolded brain surface. These images were obtained while subjects viewed a checkerboard stimulus that was rotated slowly. **B.** Positron emission tomography (PET) scans through the human brain, showing increased cerebral blood flow in a cortical region thought be V5, while the subject views a monochromatic scene in motion. **C.** PET scan showing increased cerebral blood flow in a cortical region thought be V4, while the subject views a stationary color scene. (**A,** From Sereno MI, Dale AM, Reppas JB, et al. Borders of multiple visual areas in humans revealed by functional magnetic resonance imaging. *Science.* 1995;268:889-893. **B,** Courtesy of Professor S. Zeki, Oxford University.)

(Figure 7–11), to neurons in the color blobs (layers II and III), then to the thin stripes in V2 (Figure 7–16), and next to V4. A region that may be equivalent to V4 in the human cortex has been described using functional imaging (Box 7–1). The color blobs also receive a direct projection from the interlaminar neurons in the lateral geniculate neurons, which are located in the region between the principal magnocellular and parvocellular cell layers.

3. The **form pathway** also derives primarily from the P-type ganglion cells and the parvocellular layers of the lateral geniculate nucleus. In V1, neurons in layer IVCβ (Figure 7–11) project to the interblob regions of layers II and III, and from there to the pale interstripe portion of V2 (Figure 7–16). Next, V2 neurons project to V4. Whereas the motion and form systems are thought to contribute to depth perception, the color system does not.

Object Recognition Is Transmitted by the Ventral Stream and Spatial Localization and Action, by the Dorsal Stream

The notion of functionally distinct pathways for different attributes of a visual stimulus helps to explain the remarkable perceptual defects that occur in humans following damage to the temporal and parietal lobes. Damage to the inferior temporal lobe produces a selective defect in **object recognition.** By contrast, damage to the posterior parietal lobe impairs the patient's capacity for **object localization** in the environment but spares the patient's ability to recognize objects. These findings suggest that there are two streams of visual processing in the cortex (Figures 7–15 and 7–16): The ventral stream to the temporal lobe carries information about specific features of objects and scenes, and the dorsal stream to the parietal lobe carries spatial information. Thus, the ventral stream is concerned with seeing *what,* as opposed to *where,* which is the function of the dorsal stream. Although extensive inter-connections exist, the ventral stream for object recognition may receive a preferential input from the parvocellular, or form and color, system. In contrast, the dorsal stream for localization receives input primarily from the magnocel-lular system. The dorsal stream for stimulus localization is also important using visual information to guide movement. Through connections to the frontal lobe, the where stream is also an action, or *how,* system. The dorsal-ventral pathway distinction is also present in the mechanosensory (Chapter 4) and auditory (Chapter 8) systems.

The Visual Field Changes in Characteristic Ways After Damage to the Visual System

The pattern of projection of retinal ganglion cells to the lateral geniculate nucleus and then to the cerebral cortex is remarkably precise, defined by the retinotopic organization. Damage at specific locations in the visual pathway produces characteristic changes in visual perception. This section examines how clinicians can apply knowledge of the topog-raphy of retinal projections to localize central nervous system damage.

Functional connections in the visual system can be understood by delineating the visual field. Recall that the **visual field** corresponds to the total field of view of both eyes when their position remains fixed (Figure 7–3). The visual fields of the two eyes overlap extensively. A change in the size and shape of the visual field—a **visual field defect**—often points to specific pathological processes in the central nervous system (Table 7–1). Such defects may reflect damage to any of six key visual system components (Figure 7–18).

Optic Nerve: Complete destruction of the optic nerve produces blindness in one eye (Figure 7–18A; Table 7–1); partial damage often produces a **scotoma,** a small blind spot. When a scotoma occurs in the central field of vision, for example, in the fovea, the patient notices reduced visual acuity. Remarkably, a peripheral scotoma is often unnoticed. This emphasizes the importance of foveal vision in our day-to-day activities (see below). Optic nerve damage also produces characteristic changes in the appearance of the optic disk (Figure 7–4B) because the damaged ganglion cell axons degenerate. Tumors and vascular disease commonly cause optic nerve damage.

Optic Chiasm: Ganglion cell axons from the nasal halves of the retina decussate in the optic chiasm (Figure 7–8). These fibers transmit visual information from the temporal visual fields. A common cause for chiasmal damage is a **pituitary tumor.** The pituitary gland is located ventral to the optic chiasm. As the tumor grows it expands dorsally, because the bony floor of the cavity in which the pituitary gland is located (the sella turcica) is ventral to the pituitary gland. The mass encroaches on the optic chiasm from its ventral surface. This results in preferential damage of the decussating fibers and produces a **bilateral temporal visual field defect** (bitemporal heteronymous hemianopia) (Figure 7–18B; Table 7–1). Patients may not notice such a defect because it occurs in their peripheral vision. They commonly come to an emergency room following an accident caused by peripheral visual loss, for example, a traumatic injury incurred from the side, such as being hit by an automobile.

Optic Tract or the Lateral Geniculate Nucleus: Damage to the optic tract or the lateral geniculate nucleus, also due to tumors or a vascular accident, produces a defect in the **contralateral visual field** (homonymous hemianopia) (Figure 7–18C; Table 7–1). If a lesion is due to compression, such as produced by a tumor, the basis pedunculi can become affected (Figure 7–9C), resulting in contralateral limb motor control impairments.

Optic Radiations: Axons of lateral geniculate neurons course around the rostral and lateral surfaces of the lateral ventricle en route to the primary visual cortex at the occipital pole (Figure 7–9B2). Neurons in the lateral geniculate nucleus that mediate vision from the **superior visual fields** have axons that course rostrally into the **temporal lobe** (**Meyer's loop**) before they course caudally to the primary visual cortex. Temporal lobe lesions can produce a visual field defect limited to the **contralateral upper quadrant** of each visual field (quadrantanopia) (Figure 7–18D; Table 7–1). This is sometimes referred to as a "pie in the sky" defect because it is often wedge shaped. Neurons in the lateral geniculate nucleus that serve the macular region and the lower visual field project their axons laterally around the ventricle and caudally through the white matter underlying the parietal cortex. A lesion of the white matter within the parietal lobe can affect the optic radiations and produce visual field defects (homonymous hemianopia) (Figure 7–18E; Table 7–1).

Primary Visual Cortex: Damage to the primary visual cortex, which commonly occurs after an infarction of the **posterior cerebral artery,** produces a **contralateral visual field** defect that can sometimes spare the **macular region** of the visual field (homonymous hemianopia with macular sparing) when the lesion affects visual cortex gray matter not subcortical white matter (Figure 7–18F; Table 7–1). Two factors contribute to **macular sparing.** First, in the case of infarctions, the arterial supply to the cortical area that serves the macular region is provided primarily by the **posterior cerebral artery,**

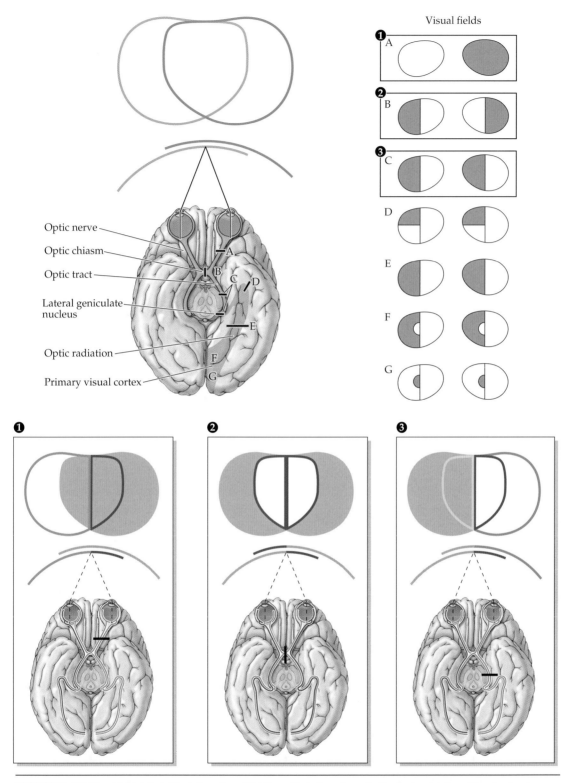

Visual fields

FIGURE 7–18 Visual field defects. The left portion of the figure illustrates schematically a horizontal view of the visual system, as if viewed from top, showing the right visual field on the right side, and the left visual field, on the left. Visual field defects are shown to the right and are listed in Table 7–1. For each defect, the visual fields of the right and left eyes are separated. All defects are presented schematically. Rarely do such defects present as bilaterally symmetrical. *A,* optic nerve; *B,* optic chiasm; *C,* optic tract (which is similar to lateral geniculate nucleus); *D,* Meyer's loop component of optic radiations; *E,* main component of optic radiations; *F* and *G,* primary visual cortex (*F*—infarction producing macular sparing, *G*—direct trauma to the occipital pole). Insets *1–3* show the essential circuit components of the visual pathway that are affected by the injuries shown in parts *A, B,* and *C,* respectively. *1.* With optic nerve damage, the nasal and temporal hemiretinae of the right eye are affected. *2.* With an optic chiasm lesion, the nasal hemiretinae of both eyes are affected. *3.* With optic tract damage, the nasal hemiretina from the left eye and the temporal hemiretina of the right eye are affected.

Table **7-1** Visual field defects[1]

Site of lesion	Location in Figure 7-18	Deficit
Optic nerve	A	Unilateral blindness
Optic chiasm	B	Bitemporal heteronymous hemianopia
Contralateral Defects		
Optic tract	C	Homonymous hemianopia
Lateral geniculate nucleus	C	Homonymous hemianopia
Optic radiations		
Meyer's loop	D	Upper visual quadrant homonymous hemianopia (quadrantanopia)
Main radiations	E	Homonymous hemianopia
Visual cortex		
Rostral	F	Homonymous hemianopia with macular spring
Caudal	G	Homonymous hemianopia of the macular region

[1] Visual field defects are termed *homonymous* (or congruous) if they affect similar locations for the two eyes and are termed *heteronymous* (or incongruous) if they are different. Hemianopia is loss of half of the visual field in each eye.

with a collateral supply coming from the **middle cerebral artery** (see Figure 3–4B). After occlusion of the posterior cerebral artery, the middle cerebral artery can rescue the macular representation. Second, the area of cortex that mediates central vision is so large that a single infarction, or other pathological process, rarely destroys it entirely. Although rare, a traumatic injury to the occipital pole can produce a defect involving only the macular region (Figure 7–18G; Table 7–1).

Summary

Retina

The retina is the peripheral portion of the visual system (Figures 7–6 and 7–7). Retinal neurons are located in three cell layers. The cell bodies of photoreceptors are located in the *outer nuclear layer* (1): *Cones* are the photoreceptors for *color vision* and *high-acuity vision; rods* are for *night vision*. The cell bodies of retinal interneurons—bipolar cells, amacrine cells, and horizontal cells—are located in the *inner nuclear layer* (2). Ganglion cells are located in the *ganglion cell layer* (3) (Figures 7–6 and 7–7). Connections between many retinal neurons are also made within specific laminae (Figure 7–7). Connections between photoreceptors and retinal interneurons are in the *outer synaptic layer*. Bipolar cells synapse on ganglion cells in the *inner synaptic layer*. Light must pass through the ganglion cells and interneurons before reaching the photoreceptors. *Müller cells* are the principal retinal neuroglia.

Visual Field and Optic Nerves

The retina receives a visual image that is transformed by the optical elements of the eye (Figure 7–5): The image becomes inverted and reversed. Images from one half of the *visual field* (Figure 7–3) are projected on the *ipsilateral nasal hemiretina* and the *contralateral temporal hemiretina* (Figure 7–5). The axons from ganglion cells exit from the eye at the optic disk (Figure 7–8B). Axons from ganglion cells in the temporal hemiretina project into the *ipsilateral optic nerve* and *ipsilateral optic tract* (Figure 7–8B). Ganglion cell axons from the nasal hemiretina project into the ipsilateral optic nerve, decussate in the *optic chiasm,* and course through the *contralateral optic tract* (Figure 7–8).

Midbrain Projections for Eye Movement Control

Ganglion cell axons destined for the midbrain leave the optic tract and course in the *brachium of superior colliculus* (Figures 7–2C and 7–9). A key midbrain site for the ganglion cell axon terminals is the *superior colliculus,* a laminated structure (Figure 7–9). The *superficial layers* of the superior colliculus mediate *visuomotor and visual reflex function,* and the *deeper layers* subserve *orientation of the eyes* and *head to salient stimuli.* The *pretectal nuclei,* where interneurons for the pupillary light reflex are located, also receive retinal input (Figure 7–9B; see Chapter 12).

Thalamic and Cortical Projections for Perception

The *lateral geniculate nucleus* (dorsal division) is the thalamic nucleus that receives the principal projection from the retina (Figures 7–9 and 7–10). Like other structures in the visual system, the lateral geniculate nucleus is laminated, and each of the *six layers* receives input from either the *ipsilateral* or *contralateral retina*. Visual information comes from the *contralateral visual hemifield*.

Visual Cortical Areas

The lateral geniculate nucleus projects to the *primary visual cortex* via the *optic radiations* (Figures 7–9 and 7–10), which course through the white matter of the temporal, parietal, and occipital lobes. Thalamic input terminates principally in *layer IV*, in sublaminae A and C, of the primary visual cortex (Figure 7–12). Input from the ipsilateral and contralateral eyes remains segregated in this layer. This is the anatomical substrate of the *ocular dominance columns* (Figures 7–11 and 7–12). Another type of column is the *orientation column* (Figures 7–11 and 7–13). Vertically oriented aggregates of neurons in layers II and III,

centered in the ocular dominance columns, are *color-sensitive columns* (or color blobs) (Figures 7–11 and 7–14), the third column type.

The primary visual cortex is retinotopically organized (Figure 7–10B). The primary area projects to the higher-order visual areas of the occipital, parietal, and temporal lobes (Figures 7–15 and 7–17). There are at least three functional pathways from the primary visual cortex to higher-order visual areas: (1) for perception of stimulus *form,* (2) for perception of stimulus *color,* and (3) for perception of stimulus *motion*. The *ventral stream* comprises the pathway into the temporal lobe for object recognition. The *dorsal stream* is the path for stimulus location and action.

Visual Field Defects

Damage to the visual pathway produces characteristic changes in visual perception (Figure 7–18; Table 7–1): (1) complete transection of the optic nerve, *total blindness in the ipsilateral eye,* (2) optic chiasm, *bitemporal heteronymous hemianopia,* (3) optic tract and lateral geniculate nucleus, *contralateral homonymous hemianopia,* (4) optic radiation in the temporal lobe (Meyer's loop), *contralateral upper quadrant homonymous hemianopia,* (5) optic radiations in parietal and occipital lobes, *contralateral homonymous hemianopia,* and (6) primary visual cortex, *contralateral homonymous hemianopia with macular sparing.*

Selected Readings

Albright T. High-level vision and cognitive influences. In: Kandel ER, Schwartz JH, Jessell TM, Siegelbaum SA, Hudspeth AJ, eds. *Principles of Neural Science*. 5th ed. New York, NY: McGraw-Hill; in press.

Gilbert C. Visual primitives and intermediate-level vision. In: Kandel ER, Schwartz JH, Jessell TM, Siegelbaum SA, Hudspeth AJ, eds. *Principles of Neural Science*. 5th ed. New York, NY: McGraw-Hill; in press.

Meister M, Tessier-Lavigne M. The retina. In: Kandel ER, Schwartz JH, Jessell TM, Siegelbaum SA, Hudspeth AJ,

eds. *Principles of Neural Science*. 5th ed. New York, NY: McGraw-Hill; in press.

Wurtz R, Goldberg M. Vision for action. In: Kandel ER, Schwartz JH, Jessell TM, Siegelbaum SA, Hudspeth AJ, eds. *Principles of Neural Science*. 5th ed. New York, NY: McGraw-Hill; in press.

Patten H. *Neurological Differential Diagnosis*. 2nd ed. London: Springer-Verlag; 1996.

References

Adams MM, Hof PR, Gattass R, Webster MJ, Ungerleider LG. Visual cortical projections and chemoarchitecture of macaque monkey pulvinar. *J Comp Neurol*. 2000;419:377-393.

Bachevalier J, Meunier M, Lu MX, Ungerleider LG. Thalamic and temporal cortex input to medial prefrontal cortex in rhesus monkeys. *Exp Brain Res*. 1997;115:430-444.

Baleydier C, Morel A. Segregated thalamocortical pathways to inferior parietal and inferotemporal cortex in macaque monkey. *Vis Neurosci*. 1992;8:391-405.

Beauchamp MS. See me, hear me, touch me: multisensory integration in lateral occipital-temporal cortex. *Curr Opin Neurobiol*. 2005;15(2):145-153.

Beck PD, Kaas JH. Thalamic connections of the dorsomedial visual area in primates. *J Comp Neurol*. 1998;396:381-398.

Chen W, Zhu XH, Thulborn KR, Ugurbil K. Retinotopic mapping of lateral geniculate nucleus in humans using functional magnetic resonance imaging. *Proc Natl Acad Sci USA*. 1999;96(5): 2430-2434.

Clarke S, Miklossy J. Occipital cortex in man: organization of callosal connections, related myelo and cytoarchitecture, and putative boundaries of functional visual areas. *J Comp Neurol*. 1990;298:188-214.

Curcio CA, Sloan KR, Kalina RE, Hendrickson AE. Human photo-receptor topography. *J Comp Neurol*. 1990;292:497-523.

Das A, Huxlin KR. New approaches to visual rehabilitation for cortical blindness: outcomes and putative mechanisms. *Neuroscientist*. 2010;16(4):374-387.

DeYoe EA, Van Essen DC. Concurrent processing streams in monkey visual cortex. *Trends Neurosci*. 1988;11:219-226.

Dowling JE. *The Retina: An Approachable Part of the Brain*. Cambridge, MA: Harvard University Press; 1987.

Dowling JE, Boycott BB. Organization of the primate retina: electron microscopy. *Proc R Soc Lond B*. 1966;166:80-111.

Fox PT, Miezin FM, Allman JM, et al. Retinotopic organization of human visual cortex mapped with positron emission tomography. *J Neurosci*. 1987;7:913-922.

Gilbert CD, Li W, Piech V. Perceptual learning and adult cortical plasticity. *J Physiol*. 2009;587(Pt 12):2743-2751.

Goebel R, Muckli L, Kim D-S. Visual system. In: Paxinos G, Mai JK, eds. *The Human Nervous System*. 2nd ed. London: Elsevier; 2004.

Gray D, Gutierrez C, Cusick CG. Neurochemical organization of inferior pulvinar complex in squirrel monkeys and macaques revealed by acetylcholinesterase histochemistry, calbindin and Cat-301 immunostaining, and Wisteria floribunda agglutinin binding. *J Comp Neurol*. 1999;409:452-468.

Gutierrez C, Cola MG, Seltzer B, Cusick C. Neurochemical and connectional organization of the dorsal pulvinar complex in monkeys. *J Comp Neurol*. 2000;419:61-86.

Harting JK, Updyke BV, Van Lieshout DP. Corticotectal projections in the cat: anterograde transport studies of twenty-five cortical areas. *J Comp Neurol*. 1992;324(3):379-414.

Hendry SH, Reid RC. The koniocellular pathway in primate vision. *Annu Rev Neurosci*. 2000;23:127-153.

Hendry SH, Yoshioka T. A neurochemically distinct third channel in the macaque dorsal lateral geniculate nucleus. *Science*. 1994;264:575-577.

Horton JC, Hedley-Whyte ET. Mapping of cytochrome oxidase patches and ocular dominance columns in human visual cortex. *Philos Trans R Soc Lond B*. 1984;304:255-272.

Horton JC, Hocking DR. Effect of early monocular enucleation upon ocular dominance columns and cytochrome oxidase activity in monkey and human visual cortex. *Vis Neurosci*. 1998;15:289-303.

Horton JC, Hocking DR. Monocular core zones and binocular border strips in primate striate cortex revealed by the contrasting effects of enucleation, eyelid suture, and retinal laser lesions on cytochrome oxidase activity. *J Neurosci*. 1998;18:5433-5455.

Hubel DH, Wiesel TN. Ferrier lecture: functional architecture of macaque monkey visual cortex. *Proc R Soc Lond B*. 1977;198:l-59.

Huerta MF, Harting JK. Connectional organization of the superior colliculus. *Trends Neurosci*. 1984;7:286-289.

Kosslyn SM, Pascual-Leone A, Felician O, et al. The role of area 17 in visual imagery: convergent evidence from PET and rTMS. *Science*. 1999;284:167-170.

Levitt JB. Function following form. *Science*. 2001;292:232-233.

Livingston CA, Mustari MJ. The anatomical organization of the macaque pregeniculate complex. *Brain Res*. 2000;876: 166-179.

Livingstone MS, Hubel DH. Anatomy and physiology of a color system in the primate visual cortex. *J Neurosci*. 1984;4:309-356.

Markowitsch HJ, Emmans D, Irle E, Streicher M, Preilowski B. Cortical and subcortical afferent connections of the primate's temporal pole: a study of rhesus monkeys, squirrel monkeys, and marmosets. *J Comp Neurol*. 1985;242:425-458.

Merigan WH. Human V4? *Curr Biol*. 1993;3:226-229.

Merigan WH, Maunsell JHR. How parallel are the primate visual pathways? *Annu Rev Neurosci*. 1993;16:369-402.

Mishkin M, Ungerleider LG, Macko KA. Object vision: two cortical pathways. *Trends Neurosci*. 1983;6:414-416.

Nassi JJ, Callaway EM. Parallel processing strategies of the primate visual system. *Nat Rev Neurosci*. 2009;10(5):360-372.

Newman E, Reichenbach A. The Müller cell: a functional element of the retina. *Trends Neurosci*. 1996;19:307-312.

Reppas JB, Niyogi S, Dale AM, Sereno MI, Tootell RB. Representation of motion boundaries in retinotopic human visual cortical areas. *Nature*. 1997;388(6638):175-179.

Robinson DL, Petersen SE. The pulvinar and visual salience. *Trends Neurosci*. 1992;15:127-132.

Ropper AH, Samuels MA. *Disturbances of Vision. Adams & Victor's Principles of Neurology*. 9th ed. McGraw-Hill; 2009.

Scares JG, Gattass R, Souza AP, Rosa MG, Fiorani M Jr., Brandao BL. Connectional and neurochemical subdivisions of the pulvinar in Cebus monkeys. *Vis Neurosci*. 2001;18:25-41.

Schneider KA, Richter MC, Kastner S. Retinotopic organization and functional subdivisions of the human lateral geniculate nucleus: a high-resolution functional magnetic resonance imaging study. *J Neurosci*. 2004;24(41):8975-8985.

Sereno MI, Dale AM, Reppas JB, et al. Borders of multiple visual areas in humans revealed by functional magnetic resonance imaging. *Science*. 1995;268:889-893.

Sereno MI, Pitzalis S, Martinez A. Mapping of contralateral space in retinotopic coordinates by a parietal cortical area in humans. *Science*. 2001;294:1350-1354.

Stepniewska I, Qi HX, Kaas JH. Do superior colliculus projection zones in the inferior pulvinar project to MT in primates? *Eur J Neurosci*. 1999;11:469-480.

Stepniewska I, Qi HX, Kaas JH. Projections of the superior colliculus to subdivisions of the inferior pulvinar in New World and Old World monkeys. *Vis Neurosci*. 2000;17: 529-549.

Tootell RB, Mendola JD, Hadjikhani NK, et al. Functional analysis of V3A and related areas in human visual cortex. *J Neurosci*. 1997;17(18):7060-7078.

Tovée M. *An Introduction to the Visual System.* 2nd ed. New York, NY: Cambridge University Press; 2008.

Tsao DY, Vanduffel W, Sasaki Y, et al. Stereopsis activates V3A and caudal intraparietal areas in macaques and humans. *Neuron.* 2003;39(3):555-568.

Yabuta NH, Sawatari A, Callaway EM. Two functional channels from primary visual cortex to dorsal visual cortical areas. *Science.* 2001;292:297-300.

Yeterian EH, Pandya DN. Corticothalamic connections of extrastriate visual areas in rhesus monkeys. *J Comp Neurol.* 1997;378:562-585.

Yoshioka T, Levitt JB, Lund JS. Independence and merger of thalamocortical channels within macaque monkey primary visual cortex: anatomy of interlaminar projections. *Vis Neurosci.* 1994;11:467-489.

Zeki S. *A Vision of the Brain.* Boston: Blackwell Scientific Publications; 1993.

Zeki S, Watson JDG, Lueck CJ, et al. A direct demonstration of functional specialization in human visual cortex. *J Neurosci.* 1991;11:641-649.

Study Questions

1. Which of the following statements best describes how a visual image is transmitted upon the retinal surface by the lens?
   A. The visual image is projected onto the retina without distortion.
   B. The image is reversed, from right to left only.
   C. The image is reversed from right to left and inverted from top to bottom.
   D. The image is inverted, from top to bottom.

2. Retinal ganglion cell axons leave the eye at the
   A. optic disk
   B. fovea
   C. macula
   D. optic nerve

3. A patient is blind in one eye. Which of the following does not describe the patient's visual fields?
   A. The visual field of the sighted eye corresponds precisely to one hemifield in a normally sighted individual.
   B. The monocular crescent of the sighted eye is not affected by blindness in the other eye.
   C. There is a loss of overlap of the two visual fields.
   D. The visual field of the sighted eye extends beyond the midline.

4. A person with retinitus pigmentosa has a functional impairment in which retinal layer?
   A. Ganglion cell layer
   B. Bipolar layer
   C. Pigment epithelium
   D. Layer of optic nerve fibers

5. Which of the following best describes the retinal location of all ganglion cells that send their axon across the midline in the optic chiasm?
   A. Nasal hemiretina
   B. Temporal hemiretina
   C. Superior retina
   D. Inferior retina

6. The lateral geniculate nucleus receives input from
   A. ipsilateral ganglion cells
   B. contralateral ganglion cells
   C. both ipsilateral and contralateal ganglion cells, sorted into separate layers
   D. both ipsilateral and contralateral ganglion cells, with convergence of both eyes into certain layers

7. The inferior bank of the calcarine fissure at the occipital pole receives information, via the thalamus, from retinal ganglion cells
   A. of the inferior peripheral retina
   B. of the inferior central retina
   C. of the superior peripheral retina
   D. of the superior central retina

8. Which of the following statements best describes the function of the projection of retinal ganglion cells to the midbrain?
   A. Eye movement control and pupilary reflexes
   B. Visual motion detection
   C. Color vision
   D. Form vision

9. A patient has a scotoma, blinding a portion of the upper right visual field. Which of the following statements best describes the location of a lesion that could produce this visual field defect?
   A. Parietal lobe
   B. Occipital lobe
   C. Temporal lobe
   D. Where the fibers exit the lateral geniculate nucleus

10. Which statement best completes the following analogy?
    The magnocellular visual pathway is to the parvocellular pathway, as
    A. color vision is to achromatic vision
    B. daylight vision is to night vision
    C. form and color vision is to visual motion
    D. visual motion is to form and color vision

11. Which statement best completes the following analogy?
    The "what" visual pathway is to the "where" pathway, as
    A. the middle cerebral artery is to the posterior cerebral artery
    B. Brodmann's area 3 is to area 17
    C. temporal lobe is to parietal lobe
    D. object recognition is to object distance

12. Which of the following is not a major visual cortex column type?
    A. Orientation
    B. Ocular dominance
    C. Color
    D. Movement direction

13. A patient is capable of central vision but has impaired peripheral vision. Given this limited information, which of the following locations is the most likely site of damage?
    A. Optic chiasm
    B. Optic tract
    C. Lateral geniculate nucleus
    D. Primary visual cortex

The Auditory System

CLINICAL CASE | Acoustic Neuroma

A 40-year-old woman notes that she has been having difficulty understanding what people are saying when they stand on her left side. She also finds she hears better with the phone over her right, not left, ear. On examination, when a vibrating tuning fork is held at a distance from her left or right ear, she hears better with the right ear. When the tuning fork is placed on the mastoid process, thus eliminating air conduction, the same pattern of hearing ability persists, better on the right than left side. For either side, when placed on either mastoid process, the tuning fork sounds softer than when held near the ear. She is also observed to have a mild gait instability and mild flattening of the left nasolabial fold.

Figure 8–1A1 is an MRI, with gadolinium, showing a lesion in the left internal auditory canal, which is indicative of an acoustic neuroma. Figure 8–1 A2 shows an MRI from approximately the same level from a healthy person.

Based on your reading of this chapter, answer the following questions.

1. **Explain why this patient has the following three signs: unilateral hearing loss, gait instability, and mild flattening of the left nasolabial fold.**

2. **What is the significance of preservation of the left hearing impairment whether the tuning fork is held at a distance from her ear or when it contacts the mastoid process?**

Key neurological signs and corresponding damaged brain structures

Unilateral hearing loss

An acoustic neuroma—typically a Schwann cell tumor, or schwannoma—preferentially impairs the function of the auditory division of the eighth cranial nerve. As the tumor grows, it expands the internal auditory canal, through which the nerve passes en route to the periphery (Figure 8–1B1-3). The eighth nerve peripheral auditory structures, and cochlear nuclei are the only sites where lesions produce a unilateral impairment. Central auditory system lesions do not produce deafness in one ear because of the numerous opportunities for auditory information to decussate.

Flattening of the nasolabial fold

The facial nerve joins with the eighth nerve to exit through the internal auditory canal (Figure 8–1B1). As a consequence, facial nerve function can also be compromised with acoustic neuromas. The facial nerve, as we will see in Chapter 11, innervates the muscles of facial expression, unilaterally. A clear sign of weakness of these facial muscles is the

—Continued next page

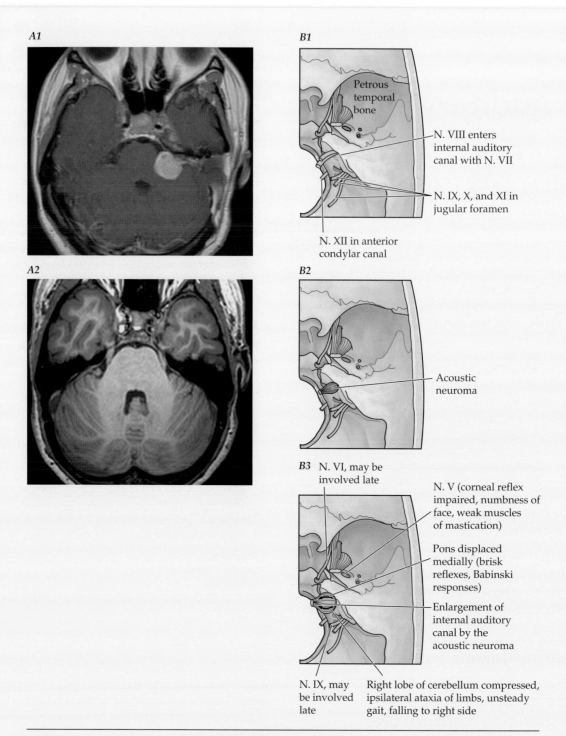

A1

A2

B1

Petrous temporal bone

N. VIII enters internal auditory canal with N. VII

N. IX, X, and XI in jugular foramen

N. XII in anterior condylar canal

B2

Acoustic neuroma

B3 N. VI, may be involved late

N. V (corneal reflex impaired, numbness of face, weak muscles of mastication)

Pons displaced medially (brisk reflexes, Babinski responses)

Enlargement of internal auditory canal by the acoustic neuroma

N. IX, may be involved late

Right lobe of cerebellum compressed, ipsilateral ataxia of limbs, unsteady gait, falling to right side

FIGURE 8–1 Acoustic neuroma. **A.** MRI. **A1.** MRI from a patient, with the contrast material gadolinium, which produces better delineation of the tumor from surrounding tissues showing the tumor. **A2.** MRI from a healthy person. **B.** Inner surface of the skull in the region of the cerebellopontine angle with the brain stem and cerebellum removed to show the cranial nerves and associated foramina through which they exit the cranial cavity. **B1.** Normal. **B2.** Acoustic neuroma at an early stage when it is small and not displacing the brain stem. **B3.** Acoustic neuroma at a later stage when it displaces the pons and cerebellum and can also affect the functions of nearby cranial nerves, as shown in the figure. These include: (1) facial somatic sensation and corneal reflex because of fifth nerve involvement; (2) taste, because of sensory fibers in the seventh nerve; (3) eye muscle control because of the sixth nerve; (4) facial muscle control because of the seventh nerve; and (5) oral-pharyngeal sensory functions of glossopharyngeal nerve. Further, greater expansion into the pons can lead to corticospinal tract impairments, because this motor path is located in the ventral pons, and more severe cerebellar motor impairments. (**A1,** Courtesy of Dr. Frank Gaillard, Radiopaedia.com. **A2,** Courtesy of Dr. Joy Hirsch, Columbia University.)

flattening of the skin fold that extends from the nose to the lateral edge of the mouth; sometimes this is termed a smile line. In addition to the muscles of the lower face, eighth nerve damage also can weaken other facial muscles. Eighth nerve functions are discussed in Chapter 11.

Gait instability

This can be produced either by compromised function of the vestibular division of the eighth nerve or by compression of the pons and cerebellum by the expanding tumor. This patient does not report vertigo, a sign of vestibular dysfunction. Gait instability is a common sign of cerebellar dysfunction (Chapter 13). Ataxia is a form of incoordination associated with cerebellar disease or damage. The gait instability can be due to lower extremity ataxia. Note on the MRI that the tumor is displacing the pons and cerebellum,

making pontocerebellar dysfunction a likely explanation for the instability.

Air versus bone conduction

As discussed in this chapter (also see Figure 8–3A), sound is conducted to the inner ear via the tympanic membrane and middle ear ossicles. This is the optimal conduction route. Alternatively, sound vibrations can activate the inner ear directly (ie, vibrate the basilar membrane) by conduction through the bone. Under normal conditions, air conduction is much better than bone conduction and, in consequence, sounds are heard better through the air, not bone. The patient shows this normal pattern. This is expected because her problem is not impairment of the middle ear ossicles, but rather conduction of neural signals to the brain.

The auditory system mediates hearing, a sensory experience that is as broad as the sound spectrum itself. From signals of impending danger, like a car horn, to the pleasing sounds that fill a concert hall, much of our daily behavior is determined by the sounds around us. The auditory system is also our principal communication portal, allowing us to understand speech. This system, like the somatic sensory and visual systems, has a topographic organization determined by the peripheral receptive sheet. And similar to the other systems, the auditory system consists of multiple parallel pathways that engage multiple cortical regions, either directly or via complex corticocortical networks. Each auditory pathway is hierarchically organized and has the connections and properties to mediate different aspects of hearing.

The complexity of the auditory pathways derives from the particular properties of natural sounds, with their diverse frequency characteristics, multiple sources of origin, and large dynamic ranges. However, an added measure of complexity is imposed on the human auditory system by the demands of producing and understanding speech. Although the physical characteristics of a spoken word may be simpler than many sounds that are not part of our lexicon, the linguistic quality of the stimulus engages unique cortical areas. This chapter first considers the general functional organization of the auditory system. Then it examines key levels through the brain stem and thalamus, where auditory information is processed. Finally, the complex connections of the auditory and speech centers of the cerebral cortex are examined.

Functional Anatomy of the Auditory System

Parallel Ascending Auditory Pathways Are Involved in Different Aspects of Hearing

The process of hearing begins on the body surface, as sounds are conducted by the auricle and external auditory meatus to the tympanic membrane. Mechanical displacement of the tympanic membrane, produced by changes in sound pressure waves, is transmitted to the inner ear by tiny bones termed the middle ear ossicles (see Figure 8–3). The inner ear transductive machinery is located within the temporal bone in a coiled structure called the **cochlea.** This is the location of the auditory receptors, termed **hair cells** because they each have a bundle of hair-like stereocilia on their apical surface. Each auditory receptor is sensitive to a limited frequency range of sounds. Hair cells in the human cochlea are not mitotically replaced, and their numbers decline throughout life. This reduction can be exacerbated by conditions such as ear infections, exposure to loud sounds or drugs with ototoxic properties.

A topographic relationship exists between the location of a hair cell in the cochlea and the sound frequency to which the receptor is most sensitive. As discussed later, from the base of the cochlea to the apex, the frequency to which a hair cell is maximally sensitive changes systematically from high frequencies to low frequencies. This differential frequency sensitivity of hair cells along the length of the cochlea is the basis of the **tonotopic organization** of the auditory receptive sheet.

Many of the components of the auditory system are tonotopically organized. The topographic relationship between the receptor sheet and the central nervous system is similar to that of the somatic sensory and visual systems, where the subcortical nuclei and cortical areas have a somatotopic or retinotopic organization. In each of these cases, the topographic organization of the central representations is determined by the spatial organization of the peripheral receptive sheet. An important difference exists, however. The receptor sheets of the somatic sensory and visual systems are spatial maps representing stimulus location (eg, hand versus foot, central versus peripheral vision). The cochlea represents the frequency of sounds. Localizing where a sound originates is determined by central nervous system auditory neurons, computed on the basis of the timing, loudness, and spectral characteristics of sounds (see below).

Hair cells are innervated by the distal processes of bipolar primary sensory neurons located in the **spiral ganglion.** The central processes of the bipolar neurons form the **cochlear division** of the **vestibulocochlear nerve (cranial nerve VIII).** These axons project to the ipsilateral **cochlear nuclei** (Figure 8–2), which are located in the rostral medulla. The cochlear nuclei consist of the ventral cochlear nucleus, which has anterior and posterior subdivisions, and the dorsal cochlear nucleus. Neurons in these three components have distinct connections with the rest of the auditory system and give rise to parallel auditory pathways that serve different aspects of hearing. A key function of the ventral cochlear nucleus is **horizontal localization of sound.** In addition, some neurons in the posteroventral division contribute to a system of connections that regulate hair cell sensitivity. The ventral cochlear nucleus projects to the **superior olivary complex,** a cluster of nuclei in the caudal pons. Most neurons in the superior olivary complex project via an ascending pathway called the **lateral lemniscus** to the **inferior colliculus,** located in the midbrain. The projection from the ventral cochlear nucleus to the inferior colliculus is bilateral, reflecting the importance of binaural mechanisms for **horizontal (side-to-side) localization of sounds.** The dorsal cochlear nucleus is thought to play a role in identifying sound source elevation as well as identifying complex spectral characteristics of sounds. It projects directly to the contralateral **inferior colliculus,** also via the lateral lemniscus. The inferior colliculus is the site of convergence of all lower brain stem auditory nuclei. It is tonotopically organized and contains a spatial map of the location of sounds.

In sequence, the next segment of the ascending auditory pathway is the **medial geniculate nucleus,** the thalamic auditory relay nucleus. The medial geniculate nucleus projects to the primary auditory cortex, located within the lateral sulcus (also called the Sylvian fissure) on the superior surface of the temporal lobe. The primary auditory cortex contains multiple tonotopically organized territories, all located on **Heschl's gyri** (Figure 8–2B, inset; see Figure 8–8). The primary cortex forms a central core surrounded by multiple **secondary auditory areas** that form a belt around the primary core. Neurons in the primary core are activated by simple tones, whereas those in the surrounding belt of secondary areas are better activated by complex sounds. Several **higher-order auditory areas** adjoin the secondary areas on the superior and lateral surfaces of the temporal lobe in the **superior temporal gyrus** and **sulcus** (Figure 8–2B). This is where several areas are located that are important for understanding speech (see below).

There is logic to the organization of the projections from the primary cortex, much like that of the visual system's what and where (or how) pathways (see Figure 7–15). There is a ventral stream that originates anteriorly and projects to the ventral portion of the frontal lobe, including Broca's area. This path may be analogous to the "what" path and is thought to be important in identifying the source of speech, such as a bark from a dog or meow from a cat. It is also a path involved in analyzing the linguistic meaning of sounds. There is a dorsal stream that originates caudally and projects to the parietal lobe and, from there, preferentially to the dorsolateral prefrontal and premotor cortical areas of the frontal lobe. This path is thought to be more important for spatial localization of the source of sounds and for using sounds for actions.

The auditory pathways contain decussations and commissures—where axons cross the midline—at multiple levels, so that sounds from one ear are processed by both sides of the brain. The bilateral representation of sounds provides a mechanism for sound localization (see below) and enhancing the detection of sounds through summation of converging inputs. Apart from sound localization, what is the clinical significance of this bilateral organization of central auditory connections? Unilateral brain damage does not cause deafness in one ear unless the injury destroys the cochlear nuclei or the entering fascicles of the cochlear nerve. Unilateral deafness is thus a sign of injury to the peripheral auditory organ or the cochlear nerve. As discussed in later sections of the chapter, unilateral damage to central auditory centers produces impairment in localizing and interpreting sounds or linguistic disorders, not deafness.

Regional Anatomy of the Auditory System

The Auditory Sensory Organs Are Located Within the Membranous Labyrinth

The membranous labyrinth is a complex sac within the bony labyrinth, cavities in the petrous portion of the temporal bone (Figure 8–3). The membranous labyrinth consists of the auditory sensory organ, the **cochlea,** and five vestibular sensory organs, the three **semicircular canals,** and the **saccule and utricle** (Figure 8–3A). (Another name for the semicircular canals, utricle, and saccule is the vestibular labyrinth.) The morphological complexity of the auditory and vestibular sensory organs rivals that of the eyeball. Vestibular sensory organs mediate our sense of acceleration, such as during takeoff in

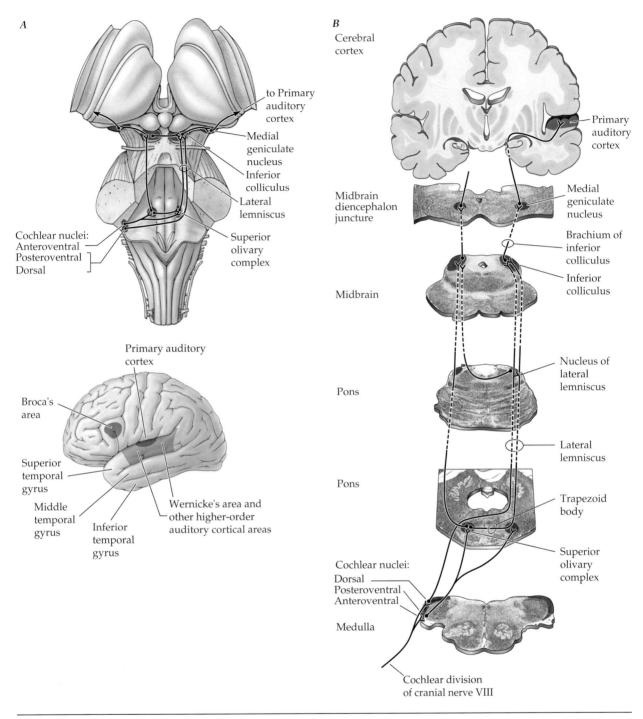

FIGURE 8–2 Organization of the auditory system. **A.** Dorsal view of brain stem, illustrating the organization of major components of the auditory system. **B.** Organization of the auditory system revealed in cross section at different levels through the brain stem and in coronal section through the diencephalon and cerebral hemispheres. The inset shows schematically the locations of the auditory and speech-related areas of the cerebral cortex. Wernicke's area, for understanding speech, is located in the superior temporal gyrus. Broca's area, for articulating speech, is located in the inferior frontal gyrus. Heschl's gyri are located within the lateral sulcus and cannot be seen on the surface.

a jet, and are important in balance and eye movement control. The vestibular system is considered in Chapter 12. Much of the membranous labyrinth is filled with **endolymph,** an extracellular fluid resembling intracellular fluid in its ionic constituents. Endolymph has a high potassium concentration and low sodium concentration. **Perilymph,** a fluid resembling extracellular fluid and cerebrospinal fluid, fills the space between the membranous labyrinth and the temporal bone.

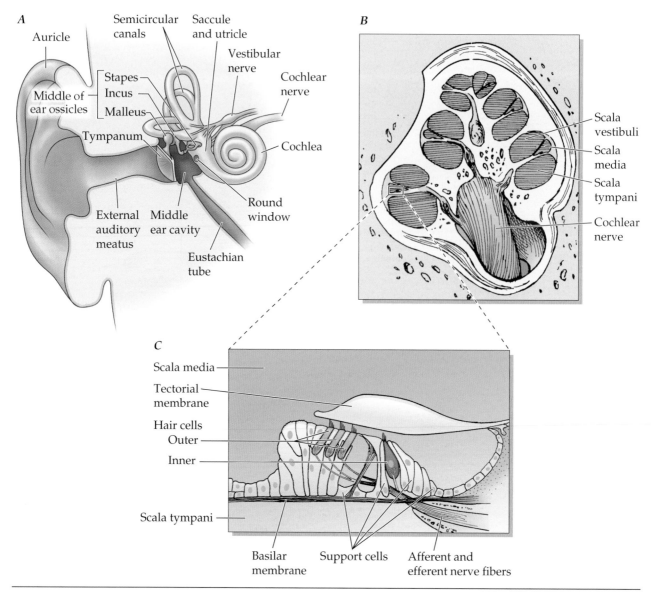

FIGURE 8–3 Structure of the human ear. **A.** The external ear (auricle) focuses sounds into the external auditory meatus. Alternating increasing and decreasing air pressure vibrates the tympanum (ear drum). These vibrations are conducted across the middle ear by the three ear ossicles: malleus, incus, and stapes. Vibration of the stapes stimulates the cochlea. **B.** Cut-away view of the cochlea, showing the three coiled channels: scala vestibuli, scala media, and scala tympani. **C.** Expanded view of a section through the cochlear duct, illustrating the organ of Corti. (**A,** Adapted from Noback CR. *The Human Nervous System: Basic Elements of Structure and Function.* New York, NY: McGraw-Hill; 1967., **C,** Adapted from Dallas P. Peripheral mechanisms of hearing. In: Darian-Smith I, ed. *Handbook of Physiology.* Vol. 3. Sensory Processes. Bethesda, MA: American Physiological Society; 1984:595-637.)

The cochlea is a coiled structure about 30 mm long (Figure 8–3A). The hair cells are located in the **organ of Corti,** a specialized portion of the cochlear duct that rests on the **basilar membrane** (Figure 8–3C). Hair cells of the organ of Corti are covered by the **tectorial membrane** (Figure 8–3C). The basilar membrane, hair cells, and tectorial membrane collectively form the basic auditory transductive apparatus. Two kinds of hair cells are found in the organ of Corti, and their names reflect their position with respect to the axis of the coiled cochlea: **inner** and **outer hair cells.** Inner hair cells are arranged in a single row, whereas outer hair cells are arranged

in three or four rows. Although there are fewer inner than outer hair cells (approximately 3500 vs 12,000), the inner hair cells are responsible for frequency and other fine discriminations in hearing. This is because most of the axons in the cochlear division of cranial nerve VIII innervate the inner hair cells. Each inner hair cell is innervated by as many as 10 auditory nerve fibers, and each auditory fiber contacts only a single, or at most a few, inner hair cells. This is a high-resolution system, like that of the innervation of the fingertips and the fovea. By contrast, only a small fraction of auditory nerve fibers innervates the outer hair cell population. Each fiber branches to contact multiple outer hair cells. Research has shown that outer hair cells are important as **efferent** structures, modulating the sensitivity of the organ of Corti (see the section on the olivocochlear system, below).

The organ of Corti transduces sounds into neural signals. This organ is mechanically coupled to the external environment by the tympanic membrane and the middle ear ossicles (malleus, incus, and stapes), the smallest bones of the body (Figure 8–3A). Pressure changes in the external auditory meatus, resulting from sound waves, cause the **tympanic membrane** to vibrate. The **middle ear ossicles**—the **malleus, incus,** and **stapes**—conduct the external pressure changes from the tympanic membrane to the **scala vestibuli** of the inner ear (Figure 8–3B). These pressure changes are conducted from the scala vestibuli through the fluid to the other compartments of the cochlea, the **scala media** to the **scala tympani** (Figure 8–3B). Pressure changes resulting from sounds set up a traveling wave along the compliant **basilar membrane** (Figure 8–3C), on which the hair cells and their support structures rest. Because the hair cells have hair bundles that are embedded in the less compliant **tectorial membrane,** the traveling wave results in shearing forces between the two membranes. These shearing forces cause the hair bundles to bend, resulting in a membrane conductance change in the hair cells.

Hearing thus depends on movement of the basilar membrane produced by sounds. Outer hair cells can enhance this movement, thereby amplifying the signal generated by the organ of Corti in response to sound. They do so by changing their length in response to sounds (see section on the olivocochlear system, below). This results in a small additional displacement of the basilar membrane that increases the mechanical oscillation produced by changes in sound pressure on the tympanic membrane.

The traveling wave on the basilar membrane, established by changes in sound pressure impinging on the ear resulting from sounds, is extraordinarily complex. High-frequency sounds generate a wave on the basilar membrane with a peak amplitude close to the base of the cochlea; consequently, these sounds preferentially activate the **basal hair cells.** As the frequency of the sound source decreases, the location of the peak amplitude of the wave on the basilar membrane shifts continuously toward the **cochlear apex.** This results in the preferential low-frequency activation of hair cells that are located closer to the cochlear apex. Although the mechanical properties of the basilar membrane are a key determinant of the auditory tuning of hair cells and the tonotopic organization of the organ of Corti, other factors play important roles. For example, the length of the hair bundle varies with position within the cochlea. The bundles act as miniature tuning forks: The shorter bundles are tuned to high frequencies (and are located on hair cells at the cochlear base), whereas the longer bundles are tuned to low frequencies (and are located on hair cells at the apex). The electrical membrane characteristics of hair cells also contribute to frequency tuning. As is discussed in the next section, the tonotopic organization underlies the topography of connections in the central auditory pathways.

The Cochlear Nuclei Are the First Central Nervous System Relays for Auditory Information

The **cochlear nuclei,** located in the rostral medulla, comprise the **ventral cochlear nucleus,** which has anterior and posterior subdivisions, and the **dorsal cochlear nucleus** (Figure 8–4C). The dorsal and ventral cochlear nuclei are each tonotopically organized and have distinctive functions. The ventral cochlear nucleus is important for horizontal sound localization. In addition, some of the neurons in the posteroventral component engage a system for regulating hair cell sensitivity. The ventral cochlear nucleus projects bilaterally to the **superior olivary complex.** Whereas we know much about the physiological characteristics of neurons in the dorsal cochlear nucleus—many process the spectral characteristics of sounds—its perceptional functions are not as well understood. The dorsal cochlear nucleus is thought to be important for vertical sound localization, which depends on spectral information (see next section), and for analyzing complex sounds. It projects directly to the contralateral **inferior colliculus,** bypassing the superior olivary complex.

Most of the axons from each division of the cochlear nucleus decussate and reach the superior olivary complex or the inferior colliculus by one of three paths, all located in the caudal pons. First, the principal auditory decussation is the **trapezoid body** (Figure 8–4B), which contains crossing axons of the ventral cochlear nucleus as they travel to the superior olivary nucleus. Second, the dorsal acoustic stria carries the axons from the dorsal cochlear nucleus, as they cross to project to the inferior colliculus. Third, some axons of the posterior division of the ventral cochlear nucleus decussate in the intermediate acoustic stria. Of the three auditory decussations, only the trapezoid body is shown in Figure 8–4B because it is the only one that can be discerned without using special tracer techniques; it is also the most ventral. The trapezoid body obscures the medial lemniscus at this level.

The cochlear nucleus is the most central site in which a lesion can produce deafness in the **ipsilateral ear.** This is because it receives a projection from only the ipsilateral ear. Lesions of the other central auditory nuclei do not produce deafness, because at each of these sites there is convergence of auditory inputs from both ears. The **anterior inferior cerebellar artery** supplies the cochlear nuclei, and unilateral occlusion can produce deafness in one ear (see Figure 3–2).

The Superior Olivary Complex Processes Stimuli From Both Ears for Horizontal Sound Localization

The **superior olivary complex** (Figure 8–4B) contains three major components: the medial superior olivary nucleus, the lateral superior olivary nucleus, and the nucleus of the trapezoid body. The superior olivary complex should be distinguished from the inferior olivary nucleus (Figure 8–4C), which contains neurons that are important in movement control (see Chapter 13). The superior olivary complex receives input from the ventral

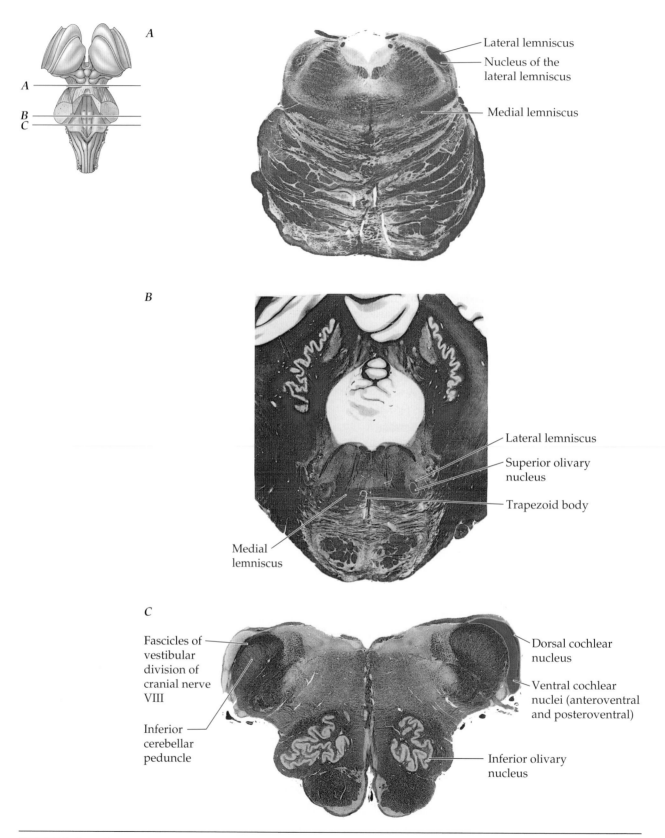

FIGURE 8–4 Myelin-stained transverse sections through the rostral pons (**A**) at the level of the caudal pons (**B**) and cochlear nuclei (**C**). The inset shows the planes of section.

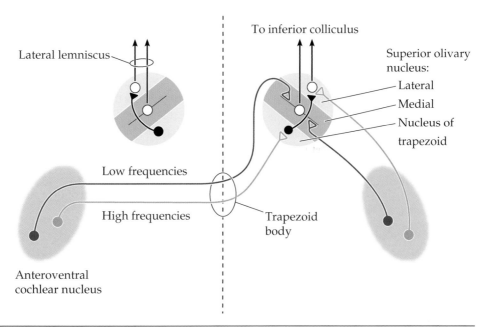

FIGURE 8–5 Key connections between the (antero) ventral cochlear nucleus in the medulla and the superior olivary complex in the pons. Within the superior olivary complex, neurons with open cell bodies and terminals are excitatory, while those with black-filled cell bodies and terminals are inhibitory.

cochlear nucleus, and gives rise to the pathway for **horizontal localization of sounds** (Figure 8–5). To understand how the anatomical connections between the anteroventral cochlear nucleus and the superior olivary complex contribute to this function, consider how sounds in the horizontal plane are localized. A sound is recognized as coming from one side of the head or the other by two means, depending on its frequency. **Low-frequency sounds** activate the two ears at slightly different times, producing a characteristic **interaural time difference.** The farther a sound source is located from the midline, the greater the interaural time difference. For high-frequency sounds, the interaural time difference is very small and is thus an ambiguous cue. However, the head acts as a shield and attenuates these sounds. A high-frequency sound arriving at the distant ear is softer than at the closer ear. This is because sound energy is absorbed by the head, resulting in an **interaural intensity difference.** This is the duplex theory of sound localization because the mechanisms for low and high frequencies differ.

There are distinct neuroanatomical substrates for the localization of low- and high-frequency sounds (Figure 8–5). Neurons in the **medial superior olivary nucleus** are sensitive to **interaural time differences,** and in accord with the duplex theory, they respond selectively to low-frequency tones. Individual neurons in the medial superior olive receive monosynaptic connections from the ventral cochlear nuclei on both sides. Remarkably, these inputs are spatially segregated on the dendrites of medial superior olive neurons (Figure 8–5). This segregation of inputs is thought to underlie the sensitivity to interaural time differences. In contrast, neurons in the **lateral superior olivary nucleus** are sensitive to **interaural intensity differences,** and they are tuned to high-frequency stimuli. Sensitivity to interaural intensity differences is thought to be determined by convergence

of a monosynaptic excitatory input from the ipsilateral ventral cochlear nucleus and a disynaptic inhibitory connection from the contralateral ventral cochlear nucleus, relayed through the **nucleus of the trapezoid body** (Figure 8–5).

Sounds can also be localized along the vertical axis. Here the structure of the external ear is important. The ridges in the auricle reflect sound pressure in complex ways, creating sound spectra that depend on the direction of the source. Specialized neurons within the dorsal cochlear nucleus appear to use this information to determine the elevation of the sound source. Not surprisingly, the ascending projection of the dorsal cochlear nuclei bypasses the superior olivary complex to reach the inferior colliculus directly.

The Olivocochlear System Regulates Auditory Sensitivity in the Periphery

Some neurons in the superior olivary complex are not directly involved in processing the horizontal location of the source of sounds. These neurons receive auditory information from the ventral cochlear nucleus (primarily the posteroventral subdivision) and give rise to axons that project back to the cochlea via the vestibulocochlear nerve. This efferent pathway is called the **olivocochlear bundle.** This **olivocochlear projection** regulates the sensitivity of the peripheral auditory system. This system is thought to improve auditory signal detection, to help the listener attend to particular stimuli in a noisy background, and to protect the peripheral auditory system from damage caused by overly loud sounds.

There are separate medial and lateral efferent control systems; both use acetylcholine as their neurotransmitter but affect sensitivity differently. The medial system originates from neurons near the medial superior olivary nucleus and synapse directly on outer hair cells. This system influences the mechanical properties of the basilar membrane. In vitro studies have shown that outer hair cells contract when acetylcholine is directly applied to the receptor cell. This mechanical change can modulate cochlea sensitivity and frequency tuning by boosting the basilar membrane traveling wave. The other olivocochlear efferent system originates more laterally in the superior olivary nucleus and synapses on the auditory afferent fibers, just beneath the inner hair cells. This system affects auditory afferent activity directly, not through a mechanical action on the basilar membrane.

Auditory Brain Stem Axons Ascend in the Lateral Lemniscus

The **lateral lemniscus** is the ascending brain stem auditory pathway (Figure 8–4A, B). (The lateral lemniscus should be distinguished from the medial lemniscus [Figure 8–4B], which relays somatic sensory information to the thalamus.) The lateral lemniscus carries axons primarily from the contralateral dorsal cochlear nucleus and the superior olivary complex (medial and lateral nuclei) to the inferior colliculus (Figure 8–6). Many of the axons in the lateral lemniscus, especially those from part of the ventral cochlear nucleus, also

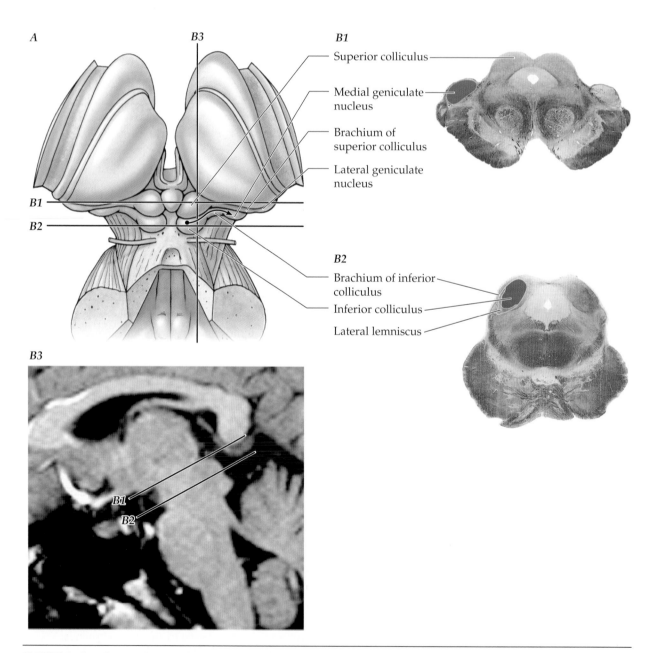

FIGURE 8–6 Midbrain auditory centers. The inferior colliculi and medial geniculate nuclei are shown on the surface view of the brain stem (**A**) and in myelin-stained transverse sections through the rostral (**B1**) and caudal (**B2**) midbrain. The colliculi are also revealed on the midsagittal MRI in **B3**. The planes of section are shown in **A** and **B3**.

send collateral (ie, side) branches into the **nucleus of the lateral lemniscus** (Figure 8–4A). The nucleus of the lateral lemniscus contains mostly inhibitory neurons that project to the inferior colliculus. It is another site in the auditory pathway where information crosses the midline.

The Inferior Colliculus Is Located in the Midbrain Tectum

The inferior colliculus is located on the dorsal surface of the midbrain, caudal to the superior colliculus (Figure 8–6A). The inferior colliculus is an auditory relay nucleus where virtually all ascending fibers in the lateral lemniscus synapse. Recall that the superior colliculus is part of the visual system. It is not a relay nucleus but, rather, participates in visuomotor control (see Chapters 7 and 12). Although the two colliculi look similar on myelin-stained sections, they can be distinguished by the configuration of structures within the center of the midbrain at the two levels (Figure 8–6B1, 2). The superior and inferior colliculi are imaged parasagittally in the MRI in Figure 8–6B3.

Three-component nuclei comprise the inferior colliculus: the central and external nuclei and the dorsal cortex. The **central nucleus** of the inferior colliculus is the principal site of termination of the lateral lemniscus. This nucleus receives convergent input from three major sources: (1) pathways originating from the **superior olivary nuclei,** (2) the direct pathway from the **dorsal cochlear nucleus,** and (3) axons from the **nucleus of the lateral lemniscus.** The central nucleus, receiving convergent information from the ventral and dorsal cochlear nuclei for horizontal and vertical sound source localization, contains a map of auditory space. The central nucleus is **tonotopically organized** and **laminated** (although not apparent on myelin-stained sections): Neurons in a single lamina are maximally sensitive to similar tonal frequencies. As in the somatic sensory and visual systems, lamination is used in the auditory system for packaging neurons with similar functional attributes or connections. The central nucleus gives rise to a tonotopically organized ascending auditory pathway to the thalamus, which continues to the primary auditory cortex.

The functions of the **external nucleus** and **dorsal cortex** are not well understood. Animal studies suggest that the external nucleus may participate in **acousticomotor function,** such as orienting the head and body axis to auditory stimuli. This function of the external nucleus may also use somatic sensory information, which is also projected to this nucleus from the spinal cord and medulla, via the spinotectal and trigeminotectal tracts.

The tract through which the inferior colliculus projects to the thalamus is located just beneath the dorsal surface of the midbrain, the **brachium of inferior colliculus** (Figure 8–6A). As different as the superior and inferior colliculi are, so too are their brachia. The brachium of the superior colliculus brings afferent information to the superior colliculus, whereas that of the inferior colliculus is an efferent pathway carrying axons away from the inferior colliculus to the medial geniculate nucleus (see next section).

The Medial Geniculate Nucleus Is the Thalamic Auditory Relay Nucleus

The **medial geniculate nucleus** is located on the inferior surface of the thalamus, medial to the visual relay, the lateral geniculate nucleus (Figures 8–6A and 8–7). The medial geniculate nucleus comprises several divisions, but only the ventral division is the principal auditory relay nucleus (see Figure AII–15. This component, referred to simply as the medial geniculate nucleus, is the only portion that is tonotopically organized. It receives the major ascending auditory projection from the central nucleus of the inferior colliculus. Although not observable on the myelin-stained section, the ventral division of the medial geniculate nucleus is laminated. Like the central nucleus of the inferior colliculus, individual laminae in the medial geniculate nucleus contain neurons that are maximally sensitive to similar frequencies. The medial geniculate nucleus, like the lateral geniculate nucleus (Figure 7–11), terminates predominantly in layer IV of the primary auditory cortex.

The other divisions of the medial geniculate nucleus (dorsal and medial) receive inputs from the three components of the inferior colliculus as well as somatic sensory and visual information. Rather than relaying auditory information to the cortex, they seem to serve more integrated functions, such as participating in arousal mechanisms. (The dorsal division is shown in Figure AII–15.)

The Primary Auditory Cortex Comprises Several Tonotopically Organized Representations Within Heschl's Gyri

The auditory cortical areas have a concentric, hierarchical organization. The primary cortex is surrounded by the secondary auditory cortex, which is surrounded by higher-order auditory areas (Figure 8–8). The primary auditory cortex (cytoarchitectonic area 41) is located in the temporal lobe within the lateral sulcus, on **Heschl's gyri** (Figures 8–8 and 8–9). These gyri, which vary in number from one to several depending on the side of the brain and the individual, run obliquely from the lateral surface of the cortex medially to the insular region (Figure 8–9). The orientation of Heschl's gyri is nearly orthogonal to the gyri on the lateral surface of the temporal lobe, hence the frequently used term transverse gyri of Heschl. The primary cortex, receiving direct thalamic inputs from the medial geniculate nucleus, processes basic auditory stimulus attributes. The primary auditory cortex is tonotopically organized along the axis of Heschl's gyri, from low frequencies lateral to high frequencies medial. Although not yet well characterized in humans, several tonotopically organized subregions are found within this primary sensory area. This organization of multiple representations of the receptor sheet may be similar to the primary somatic sensory cortex, which

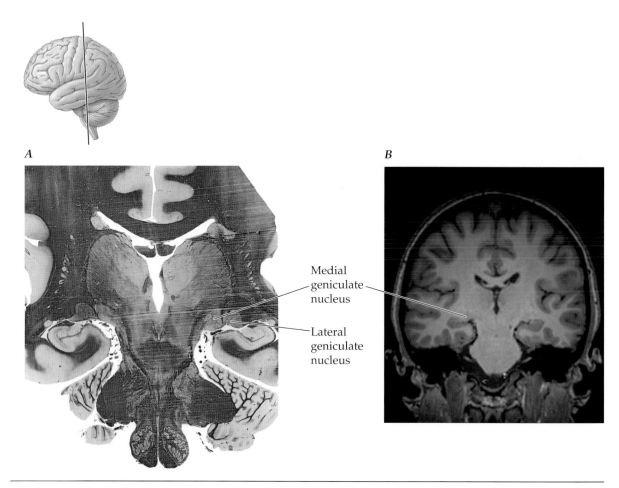

Medial
geniculate
nucleus

Lateral
geniculate
nucleus

FIGURE 8–7   Myelin-stained coronal section through the medial geniculate nucleus (**A**) and closely corresponding MRI (**B**). The inset shows the plane of section.

has multiple somatotopically organized subdivisions (see Figure 4–13). As in other sensory cortical areas, the primary auditory cortex has a columnar (or vertical) organization: Neurons sensitive to similar frequencies are arranged across all six layers, from the pial surface to the white matter. Within the primary cortex, neurons represent other features of auditory stimuli besides frequency, including particular binaural interactions, stimulus timing, and additional tuning characteristics.

Caudal Secondary and Higher-order Auditory Areas Give Rise to Projections for Distinguishing the Location of Sounds

The secondary and higher-order auditory areas form concentric belts surrounding much of the primary core region (Figure 8–8). The secondary areas receive their principal input from the primary areas and, in turn, provide information to higher-order areas. Primary cortex neurons respond to simple stimulus attributes. Not surprisingly, primary cortex neurons respond to simple pure tones as well as the tonal qualities of

more complex sounds. By contrast, neurons in the secondary and higher-order areas respond selectively to more complex aspects of sounds (Figure 8–9). In animals, neurons in the higher-order auditory areas respond to species-specific calls, and in humans, to speech.

There are a myriad of cortical auditory areas, up to 15 by some counts, with at least two major streams of auditory information flow that are strikingly similar to the **"what"** and **"where–how"** paths of the visual system (see Figure 7–15). Research in animals, using anatomical tracing techniques, and in humans, using noninvasive functional imaging techniques, has revealed a dorsal pathway for localizing sound sources and using sounds to guide movements. This **"where–how"** pathway originates from the primary cortex and projects to caudal portions of the secondary and then higher-order areas in the superior temporal gyrus (Figure 8–10). Studies in animals using axon tracing techniques and in humans using diffusion tensor imaging (DTI; see Box 2–2) revealed a long-distance connection between the posterior temporal lobe and the parietal lobe (Figure 8–11A). Receiving converging information from the somatic sensory and visual systems, together with this auditory information, the posterior parietal

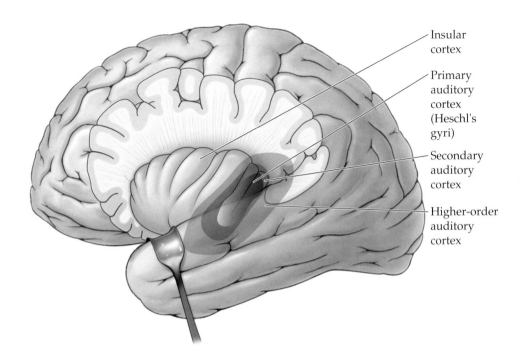

FIGURE 8-8 Auditory cortical areas. The primary auditory cortex is located on Heschl's gyri. It has a tonotopic organization, from high frequencies medially (represented as the less transparent region in the figure) to low frequencies laterally (more transparent region). The secondary auditory cortex surrounds the primary cortex; the higher-order auditory areas surround the secondary areas. The auditory areas are located within the lateral sulcus and extend onto the lateral surface of the superior temporal gyrus.

lobe constructs a representation of extrapersonal space that the brain uses to help establish where we are and where stimuli occur in relation to the world around us. Also using DTI, another connection has been demonstrated between the posterior superior temporal gyrus and two areas of the frontal lobe, the premotor cortex and dorsolateral prefrontal cortex (Figure 8–11B). These frontal areas participate in the planning of movements, receiving information about "where" we

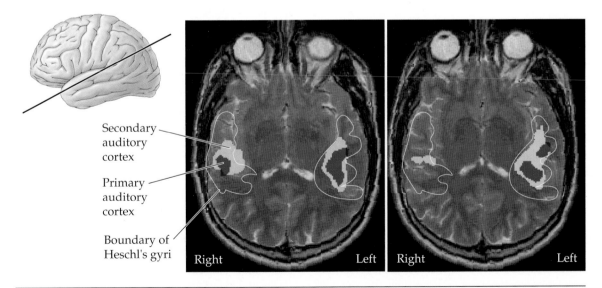

FIGURE 8-9 Functional magnetic resonance images (fMRI) showing activation of the human auditory cortex. The image on the left is slightly more ventral than the one on the right. The green region corresponds approximately to the primary auditory cortex; this area responds to both pure and complex tones (ie, relatively nonselective). The surrounding yellow area corresponds to secondary auditory cortex (ie, surrounding belt), which responds preferentially to complex sounds. (Courtesy of Dr. Josef Rauschecker, Georgetown University. Adapted from Wessinger CM, VanMeter J, Tian B, Van Lare J, Pekar J, Rauschecker JP. Hierarchical organization of the human auditory cortex revealed by functional magnetic resonance imaging. *J Cogn Neurosci.* 2001;13:1–7.)

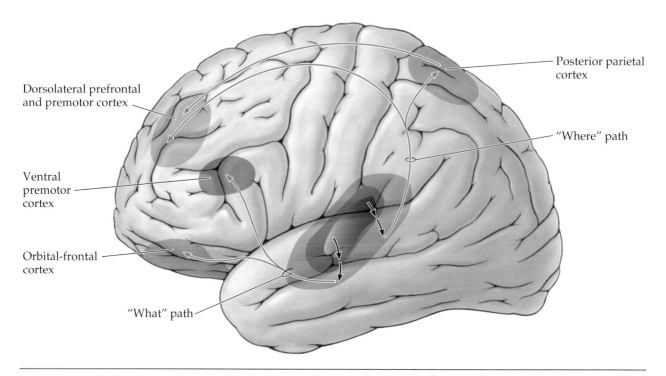

Dorsolateral prefrontal
and premotor cortex

Posterior parietal
cortex

Ventral
premotor
cortex

"Where" path

Orbital-frontal
cortex

"What" path

FIGURE 8–10 Separate "what" and "where" pathways originate from the auditory cortex and project to different regions of the prefrontal cortex and parietal cortex.

wish to move from the parietal lobe (Figure 8–10), and transmitting control signals to the motor cortex about "how" to move. Interestingly, this connection to the frontal lobe travels in the arcuate fasciculus, a C-shaped pathway (Figures 8–10B and 8–11) that curves around the lateral sulcus.

Rostral Secondary and Higher-Order Auditory Areas Give Rise to Projections for Processing the Linguistic Characteristics of Sounds

A second cortical auditory pathway is involved in processing nonspatial characteristics of sounds. This path originates from the primary auditory cortex and projects to rostral portions of the secondary and higher-order areas in the superior temporal gyrus and then to the inferior frontal lobe (Figure 8–10). In monkeys, neurons in this area respond to species-specific calls. Using DTI in humans, a long-distance pathway between the rostral superior temporal gyrus and Broca's area, the motor speech area, has been revealed (Figure 8–11C). In addition to serving a linguistic function, it is thought that the connections between the rostral superior temporal gyrus and ventral frontal lobe are important for identifying the source of speech: who is speaking or "what" is emitting sounds. This pathway may travel within the **uncinate fasciculus** (Figure AII–22). DTI also reveals a link between Broca's area and the inferior parietal lobule (Figure 8–11C), an area long known for its importance in language.

Damage to Frontotemporal Regions in the Left Hemisphere Produces Aphasias

Several higher-order auditory cortical areas on the lateral surface of the left temporal lobe in the human brain (cytoarchitectonic areas 42 and 22) comprise important substrates for understanding speech. Damage to certain areas of the brain can produce a language impairment, or **aphasia.** Damage to the left temporal lobe produces an impairment in understanding speech. Remarkably, words can be spoken well but their positions in sentences are often meaningless. This is sometimes referred to as a "word salad." This kind of impairment has been attributed to an interruption in the function of **Wernicke's area,** and is termed Wernicke's aphasia. Wernicke's area is thought to be located in the posterior superior temporal gyrus, in cytoarchitectonic area 22 (see Table 2–2 and Figure 2–19). However, modern neuropsychological studies point to more significant speech disorders with rostral superior temporal gyrus lesions. Indeed, in Wernicke's original description of the effects of temporal lobe lesion, he placed the critical area along the entire extent rostrocaudal length of the superior temporal gyrus, not just caudally.

Whereas the left temporal lobe is important in understanding or the sensory processing of speech, **Broca's area,** in the left inferior frontal gyrus, is the motor speech area. This region includes the frontal operculum and corresponds approximately to cytoarchitectonic areas 44 and 45 (see Table 2–2 and Figure 2–19). Damage to Broca's area impairs the ability to express language; this is termed Broca's aphasia. Speech is labored; it is slow to start and frequently halted.

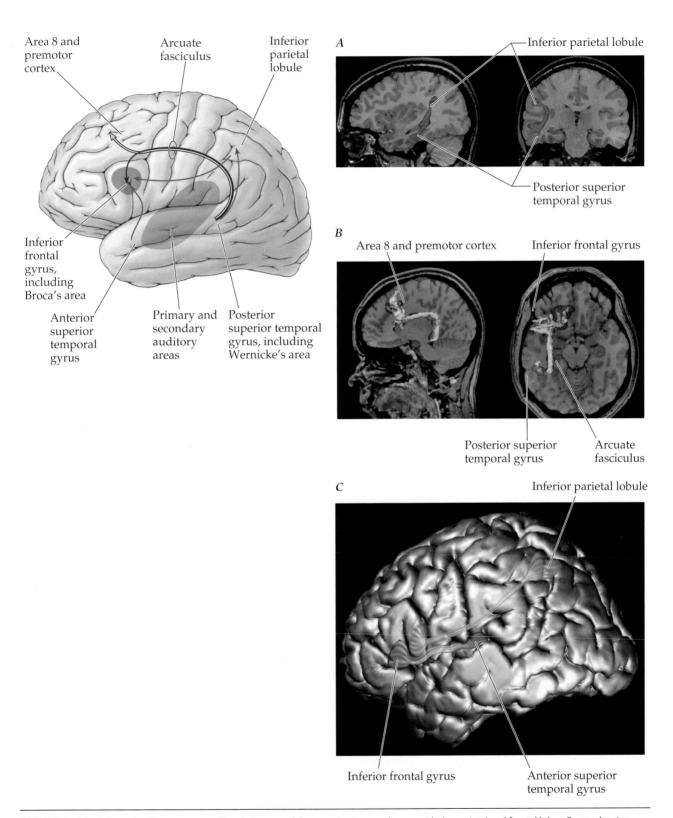

FIGURE 8–11 C-shaped pathways connect linguistic areas of the superior temporal gyrus with the parietal and frontal lobes. Research using DTI is beginning to reveal connections of the language and cognitive centers of the human brain. And some of these connections correspond to known tracts, identified by human brain dissection. The C-shaped arcuate fasciculus interconnects the caudal superior temporal cortex with the inferior parietal lobule (**A**), action centers of the dorsolateral frontal cortex (**B**), and linguistic areas of the inferior frontal cortex (**B**), including Broca's area. A more direct path, possibly corresponding to the uncinate fasciculus (see Figure AII–22), connects the rostral superior temporal gyrus with the inferior frontal lobe (**C**; red). There is also a connection from the parietal lobe to inferior frontal lobe (**C**; green) that is thought to inform frontal linguistic areas about about a person's state of attention. (Reproduced from Frey S, Campbell JS, Pike GB, Petrides M. Dissociating the human language pathways with high angular resolution diffusion fiber tractography. *J Neurosci.* 2008;28(45):11435-11444.)

Homotopic areas in the right hemisphere are important for the rhythm, intonation, and emphasis of speech, not for choosing the correct words or for structuring proper sentences. These areas are especially important in emotional intonation in speech. For example, damage to the right superior temporal gyrus can impair understanding intonation and emotional content, whereas damage to the right inferior frontal gyrus impairs the ability to convey emotion in speech. Interestingly, damage to the linguistic areas of both hemispheres impairs the understanding and production of sign language.

Summary

Peripheral Auditory Apparatus

The auditory transductive apparatus, the *organ of Corti,* is located in the *cochlea,* a coiled structure within the temporal bone (Figure 8–3A, B). The *hair cells* (Figure 8–3C) are the auditory receptors. They are organized into a receptive sheet within the cochlea. This sheet has a precise *tonotopic organization:* Receptors sensitive to high frequencies are located near the cochlear base, and those sensitive to low frequencies are located near the apex. The hair cells are innervated by the peripheral processes of *bipolar cells,* whose cell bodies are located in the *spiral ganglion.* The central processes of the bipolar cells collect into the *cochlear division* of the *vestibulocochlear (VIII) nerve* (Figure 8–2).

Medulla and Pons

The cochlear division of the vestibulocochlear nerve synapses in the *cochlear nuclei.* The cochlear nuclei, which are located in the rostral medulla, have three main divisions (Figures 8–2A and 8–4C): the *anteroventral cochlear nucleus,* the *posteroventral cochlear nucleus,* and the *dorsal cochlear nucleus.* Many neurons in the anteroventral cochlear nucleus project to the *superior olivary complex* in the pons (Figures 8–4B and 8–5), on either the ipsilateral or the contralateral side. Neurons in the superior olivary complex project to either the ipsilateral or the contralateral inferior colliculus via the lateral lemniscus. Some of these decussating axons form a discrete commissure, the *trapezoid body* (Figures 8–4B and 8–5). The function of this pathway is in the *horizontal localization of sounds.* The posteroventral nucleus is involved in regulating hair cell sensitivity, together with the olivary cochlear system. Most of the neurons in the dorsal cochlear nucleus give rise to axons that decussate and then ascend in the *lateral lemniscus* (Figure 8–4A, B) to terminate in the *inferior colliculus* (Figures 8–6 and 8–7).

Midbrain and Thalamus

The inferior colliculus contains three main nuclei (Figure 8–6). The *central nucleus,* the principal auditory relay nucleus in the inferior colliculus, has a precise *tonotopic organization.* It projects to the medial geniculate nucleus (Figures 8–6A and 8–7), which in turn projects to the *primary auditory cortex* (cytoarchitectonic area 41) (Figure 8–8). The other two nuclei, the *external nucleus* and the *dorsal cortex* of the inferior colliculus, give rise to diffuse thalamocortical projections, primarily to *higher-order auditory areas* (Figure 8–8).

Cerebral Cortex

The primary auditory cortex is located largely on the superior surface of the temporal lobe, in *Heschl's gyri* (Figures 8–8 and 8–9). It has a tonotopic organization. The higher-order auditory areas, which encircle the primary area (Figures 8–8 and 8–9), receive their principal input from the primary auditory cortex. At least two projections emerge from higher-order areas. One projection, important in sound localization (ie, where), targets the posterior parietal cortex and the dorsolateral prefrontal cortex (Figures 8–10 and 8–11). A second projection—which is thought to be important in processing of complex sounds, including linguistic functions in humans—terminates in the ventral and medial prefrontal cortex. *Wernicke's area* is a part of the higher-order auditory cortex on the left side that is important in interpreting speech (Figures 8–2B, inset, and 8–11).

Selected Readings

Oertel D, Doupe A. The auditory central nervous system. In: Kandel ER, Schwartz JH, Jessell TM, Siegelbaum SA, Hudspeth AJ, eds. *Principles of Neural Science.* 5th ed. New York, NY: McGraw-Hill; in press.

References

Augustine JR. The insular lobe in primates including humans. *Neurol Res.* 1985;7:2-10.

Bachevalier J, Meunier M, Lu MX, Ungerleider LG. Thalamic and temporal cortex input to medial prefrontal cortex in rhesus monkeys. *Exp Brain Res.* 1997;115:430-444.

Bernal B, Ardila A. The role of the arcuate fasciculus in conduction aphasia. *Brain.* 2009;132(Pt 9):2309-2316.

Brugge JF. An overview of central auditory processing. In: Popper AN, Fay RR, eds. *The Mammalian Auditory Pathway: Neurophysiology.* New York, NY: Springer-Verlag; 1994:1-33.

Bushara KO, Weeks RA, Ishii K, et al. Modality-specific frontal and parietal areas for auditory and visual spatial localization in humans. *Nat Neurosci.* 1999;2:759-766.

Cant NB, Benson CG. Parallel auditory pathways: projection patterns of the different neuronal populations in the dorsal and ventral cochlear nuclei. *Brain Res Bull.* 2003;60 (5-6): 457-474.

Cooper NP, Guinan JJ, Jr. Efferent-mediated control of basilar membrane motion. *J Physiol.* 2006;576(Pt 1):49-54.

Dronkers NF, Wilkins DP, Van Valin RD, Jr., Redfern BB, Jaeger JJ. Lesion analysis of the brain areas involved in language comprehension. *Cognition.* 2004;92(1-2):145-177.

Frey S, Campbell JS, Pike GB, Petrides M. Dissociating the human language pathways with high angular resolution diffusion fiber tractography. *J Neurosci.* 2008;28(45): 11435-11444.

Galaburda A, Sanides F. Cytoarchitectonic organization of the human auditory cortex. *J Comp Neurol.* 1980;190: 597-610.

Galuske RA, Schlote W, Bratzke H, Singer W. Interhemispheric asymmetries of the modular structure in human temporal cortex. *Science.* 2000;289:1946-1949.

Geniec P, Merest DK. The neuronal architecture of the human posterior colliculus. *Acta Otolaryngol Suppl.* 1971;295:1-33.

Geschwind N, Levitsky W. Human brain: left-right asymmetries in temporal speech region. *Science.* 1968;161:186-187.

Guinan JJ, Jr., Warr WB, Norris BE. Differential olivocochlear projections from lateral versus medial zones of the superior olivary complex. *J Comp Neurol.* 1983;221(3): 358-370.

Hackett TA, Stepniewska I, Kaas JH. Subdivisions of auditory cortex and ipsilateral cortical connections of the parabelt auditory cortex in macaque monkeys. *J Comp Neurol.* 1998;394:475-495.

Hackett TA, Stepniewska I, Kaas JH. Thalamocortical connections of the parabelt auditory cortex in macaque monkeys. *J Comp Neurol.* 1998;400:271-286.

Hackett TA, Stepniewska I, Kaas JH. Prefrontal connections of the parabelt auditory cortex in macaque monkeys. *Brain Res.* 1999;817:45-58.

Hickok G, Poeppel D. The cortical organization of speech processing. *Nat Rev Neurosci.* 2007;8(5):393-402.

Kaas JH, Hackett TA. "What" and "where" processing in auditory cortex. *Nat Neurosci.* 1999;2:1045-1047.

Kaas JH, Hackett TA. Subdivisions of auditory cortex and processing streams in primates. *Proc Natl Acad Sci USA.* 2000;97:11793-11799.

Kaas JH, Hackett TA, Tramo MJ. Auditory processing in primate cerebral cortex. *Curr Opin Neurobiol.* 1999;9:164-170.

Kandler K, Clause A, Noh J. Tonotopic reorganization of developing auditory brainstem circuits. *Nat Neurosci.* 2009;12(6):711-717.

King AJ, Nelken I. Unraveling the principles of auditory cortical processing: can we learn from the visual system? *Nat Neurosci.* 2009;12(6):698-701.

Lim HH, Lenarz T, Joseph G, et al. Electrical stimulation of the midbrain for hearing restoration: insight into the functional organization of the human central auditory system. *J Neurosci.* 2007;27(49):13541-13551.

Markowitsch HJ, Emmans D, Irle E, Streicher M, Preilowski B. Cortical and subcortical afferent connections of the primate's temporal pole: a study of rhesus monkeys, squirrel monkeys, and marmosets. *J Comp Neurol.* 1985;242:425-458.

May BJ. Role of the dorsal cochlear nucleus in the sound localization behavior of cats. *Hear Res.* 2000;148(1-2):74-87.

Merabet LB, Rizzo JF, Amedi A, Somers DC, Pascual-Leone A. What blindness can tell us about seeing again: merging neuroplasticity and neuroprostheses. *Nat Rev Neurosci.* 2005;6(1):71-77.

Merzenich MM, Brugge JF. Representation of the cochlear partition on the superior temporal plane of the macaque monkey. *Brain Res.* 1973;50:275-296.

Mesulam MM, Mufson EJ. Insula of the old world monkey. Ill: Efferent cortical output and comments on function. *J Comp Neurol.* 1982;212:38-52.

Moore JK, Linthicum FH. Auditory system. In: Paxinos G, Mai JK, eds. *The Human Nervous System.* 2nd ed. London: Elsevier; 2004:1242-1279.

Moore JK, Osen KK. The human cochlear nuclei. In: Creutzfeldt O, Scheich H, Schreiner C, eds. *Hearing Mechanisms and Speech.* New York, NY: Springer-Verlag; 1979:36-44.

Moore DR, Shannon RV. Beyond cochlear implants: awakening the deafened brain. *Nat Neurosci.* 2009;12(6):686-691.

Oertel D, Bal R, Gardner SM, Smith PH, Joris PX. Detection of synchrony in the activity of auditory nerve fibers by octopus cells of the mammalian cochlear nucleus. *Proc Natl Acad Sci USA.* 2000;97:11773-11779.

Owen AM, Coleman MR. Functional neuroimaging of the vegetative state. *Nat Rev Neurosci.* 2008;9(3):235-243.

Peretz I, Zatorre RJ. Brain organization for music processing. *Annu Rev Psychol.* 2005;56:89-114.

Pollak GD, Burger RM, Klug A. Dissecting the circuitry of the auditory system. *TINS.* 2003;26(1):33-39.

Pulvermuller F. Brain mechanisms linking language and action. *Nat Rev Neurosci.* 2005;6(7):576-582.

Rauschecker JP. An expanded role for the dorsal auditory pathway in sensorimotor control and integration. *Hear Res.* 2010; 271:16-25.

Rauschecker JP. Processing of complex sounds in the auditory cortex of cat, monkey, and man. *Acta Otolaryngol Suppl.* 1997:532:34-38.

Rauschecker JP, Scott SK. Maps and streams in the auditory cortex: nonhuman primates illuminate human speech processing. *Nat Neurosci.* 2009;12(6):718-724.

Rauschecker JP, Tian B. Mechanisms and streams for processing of "what" and "where" in auditory cortex. *Proc Natl Acad Sci USA.* 2000;97:11800-11806.

Recanzone GH, Schreiner CE, Sutter ML, Beitel RE, Merzenich MM. Functional organization of spectral receptive fields in the primary auditory cortex of the owl monkey. *J Comp Neurol.* 1999;415:460-481.

Recanzone GH, Sutter ML. The biological basis of audition. *Annu Rev Psychol.* 2008;59:119-142.

Romanski LM, Tian B, Fritz J, Mishkin M, Goldman-Rakic PS, Rauschecker JP. Dual streams of auditory afferents target multiple domains in the primate prefrontal cortex. *Nat Neurosci.* 1999;2:1131-1136.

Schreiner CE, Read HL, Sutter ML. Modular organization of frequency integration in primary auditory cortex. *Annu Rev Neurosci.* 2000;23:501-529.

Schwartz IR. The superior olivary complex and lateral lemniscal nuclei. In: Webster DB, Popper AN, Fay RR, eds. *The Mammalian Auditory Pathway: Neuroanatomy.* New York, NY: Springer-Verlag; 1992:117-167.

Scott SK, Blank CC, Rosen S, Wise RJ. Identification of a pathway for intelligible speech in the left temporal lobe. *Brain.* 2000;123(part 12):2400-2406.

Scott SK, Johnsrude IS. The neuroanatomical and functional organization of speech perception. *TINS.* 2003;26(2):100-107.

Scott SK, McGettigan C, Eisner F. A little more conversation, a little less action—candidate roles for the motor cortex in speech perception. *Nat Rev Neurosci.* 2009;10(4):295-302.

Spirou GA, Davis KA, Nelken I, Young ED. Spectral integration by type II interneurons in dorsal cochlear nucleus. *J Neurophysiol.* 1999;82:648-663.

Stone JA, Chakeres DW, Schmalbrock P. High-resolution MR imaging of the auditory pathway. *Magn Reson Imaging Clin N Am.* 1998;6:195-217.

Strominger NL, Nelson LR, Dougherty WJ. Second order auditory pathways in the chimpanzee. *J Comp Neurol.* 1977;172:349-366.

Tollin DJ. The lateral superior olive: a functional role in sound source localization. *Neuroscientist.* 2003;9(2):127-143.

Vargha-Khadem F, Gadian DG, Copp A, Mishkin M. FOXP2 and the neuroanatomy of speech and language. *Nat Rev Neurosci.* 2005;6(2):131-138.

von Economo C, Horn J. Über windungsrelief, masse und rinderarchitektonik der supratemporalflache, ihre indi-viduellen und ihre seitenunterschiede. *Z Ges Neurol Psychiat.* 1930;130:678-757.

Webster DB. An overview of mammalian auditory pathways with an emphasis on humans. In: Webster DB, Popper AN, Fay RR, eds. *The Mammalian Auditory Pathway: Neuroanatomy.* New York, NY: Springer-Verlag; 1992:1-22.

Weeks RA, Aziz-Sultan A, Bushara KO, et al. A PET study of human auditory spatial processing. *Neurosci Lett.* 1999;262:155-158.

Wessinger CM, VanMeter J, Tian B, Van Lare J, Pekar J, Rauschecker JP. Hierarchical organization of the human auditory cortex revealed by functional magnetic resonance imaging. *J Cogn Neurosci.* 2001;13:1-7.

Yu JJ, Young ED. Linear and nonlinear pathways of spectral information transmission in the cochlear nucleus. *Proc Natl Acad Sci USA.* 2000;97:11780-11786.

Zatorre RJ, Penhune VB. Spatial localization after excision of human auditory cortex. *J Neurosci.* 2001;21:6321-6328.

Study Questions

1. A person has unilateral hearing loss. Based only on this limited amount of information, which of the following statements best indicates a likely site of lesion?
   A. Acoustic division of the eighth cranial nerve
   B. Superior olivary complex
   C. Lateral lemniscus
   D. Primary auditory cortex

2. Preferential loss of perception of high-frequency sounds is best explained by which of the following conditions?
   A. Degeneration of hair cells at the apex of the cochlear
   B. Degeneration of hair cells at the base of the cochlear
   C. Damage to the lateral superior olivary nucleus
   D. Damage to the inferior colliculus

3. Which of the following contributes most of the axons in the trapezoid body?
   A. Inferior colliculus
   B. Superior olivary nucleus
   C. Dorsal cochlear nucleus
   D. Anteroventral cochlear nucleus

4. Which is not a property of the medial superior olivary nucleus?
   A. Important for processing low-frequency sounds
   B. Receives an inhibitory input from the nucleus of the trapezoid body
   C. Receives monosynaptic input from the ipsilateral and contralateral anteroventral nucleus
   D. Projects to the inferior colliculus

5. Which of the following statements best describes the connections/functions of the brachia of the two colliculi?
   A. The brachia of the two colliculi are both afferent structures because they carry sensory information.
   B. The brachia of the two colliculi are both efferent structures because they carry information from each of the colliculi to other brain structures.
   C. The brachium of the inferior colliculus is an afferent structure because it transmits auditory information, and the brachium of the superior colliculus is an efferent structure because it transmits information about eye movement control.
   D. The brachium of the inferior colliculus is an efferent structure because it transmits information away from the inferior colliculus, and the brachium of the superior colliculus is an afferent structure because it brings information into the superior colliculus.

6. Which of the following best completes this sentence: The inferior colliculus
   A. receives convergent auditory information from all of the lower auditory brain stem nuclei.
   B. receives information only from the dorsal cochlear nucleus.
   C. recieves information only from the anteroventral cochlear nucleus.
   D. receives convergent information from the medial and lateral superior olivary nuclei.

7. The medial geniculate nucleus projects tonotopically to which of the following cortical areas?
   A. Primary auditory cortex
   B. Secondary auditory cortex
   C. Tertiary auditory cortex
   D. Auditory association cortex

8. Which of the following best describes the location of the various cortical auditory areas?
   A. The areas are organized in strips from primary cortex rostrally, to higher-order areas caudally.
   B. The areas are organized in strips from primary cortex caudally, to higher-order areas rostrally.
   C. The areas are largely organized in a concentric scheme, with the primary area peripheral and the higher-order area central.
   D. The areas are largely organized in a concentric scheme, with the primary area central and the higher-order area peripheral.

9. The auditory "what" and "where" pathways
   A. are for sound identification and localization.
   B. engage temporal and parietal cortical areas, respectively.
   C. engage cortical areas supplied by the middle and anterior cerebral arteries, respectively.
   D. are preferentially localized to the arcuate and uncinate fasciculi.

10. Diffusion tensor imaging (DTI) can be used to identify brain pathways in humans noninvasively. Using this approach, which of the following best describes the arcuate fasciculus?
    A. This is a relatively straight path between the temporal and frontal lobes.
    B. This is a C-shaped structure connecting the temporal and parietal lobes.
    C. This is C-shaped tract linking the temporal lobe with the frontal lobe.
    D. This is a relatively straight path that connects temporal with occipital lobes.

Chapter 9

Chemical Senses: Taste and Smell

CLINICAL CASE | Central Tegmental Tract Lesion and Unilateral Taste Loss

A 25-year-old woman suddenly complained of diplopia (double vision) and impaired sense of taste. On examination, taste was probed carefully by applying solutions of different qualities (salty, sweet, acidic, and bitter) to the tongue. The results indicated a loss of all tested qualities of taste on the right side of the tongue. A taste researcher in the Otolaryngology Department was contacted, and the patient was subsequently examined using an electronic device to examine taste thresholds. This confirmed loss of taste on the right half of the tongue and soft palate.

A T1-weighted MRI with gadolinium enhancement (Figure 9–1A) revealed a focal lesion in pontine tegmentum. Figure 9–1B is a closely corresponding myelin-stained section. An MRI from a healthy person (Figure 9–1C) shows the location of the pons in parts A and B, in relation to the brain in the skull. Note that the dorsal brain surface is down in all of these images. The lesion in A corresponds to the region of the central tegmental tract. The lesion also includes parts of the superior cerebellar peduncle, which transmits mostly the output of part of the cerebellum for movement control, and the medial longitudinal fasciculus, which contains axons that coordinate eye movements. Here we will only consider the loss of taste and the central tegmental tract lesion. The ocular control impairments will be considered in another case in Chapter 12. On the basis of the MRI and additional tests, the patient was diagnosed with multiple sclerosis, a demyelinating disease.

Answer the following questions.

1. **Why is unilateral taste loss more likely a result of a peripheral than central lesion?**
2. **Why is loss of taste ipsilateral to the lesion?**
3. **What key pontine gustatory structure is likely to be damaged in the patient?**

Key neurological signs and corresponding damaged brain structures

Peripheral versus central

First consider that the three nerves that supply taste buds each have a limited distribution on the tongue (see Figure 9–4). Damage to a single nerve likely would result in partial taste

—Continued next page

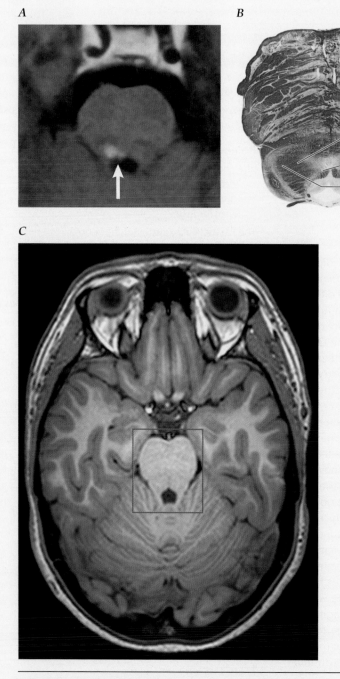

A

B

Central tegmental
tract

Medial longitudinal
fasciculus

Superior cerebellar
peduncle

C

FIGURE 9–1 Lesion of the gustatory pathway. ***A.*** MRI of patient with multiple sclerosis showing a region of demyelination (or plaque) in the pontine tegmentum. The arrow points to the plaque. ***B.*** Myelin-stained section through the rostral pons, close to the levels of the MRIs in ***A*** and ***C***. ***C.*** MRI from a healthy person showing the location of the regions in ***A*** and ***B***. (***A,*** Reproduced with permission from Uesaka Y, Nose H, Ida M. The pathway of gustatory fibers in the human ascends ipsilaterally. *Neurology*. 1998;50:827. ***B,*** Courtesy of Dr. Joy Hirsch, Columbia University.)

loss, such as only on the anterior two thirds of the tongue with damage to a branch of the facial nerve. Thus, a peripheral lesion is unlikely. Next consider that central sensory systems receive convergent input from their various peripheral components, so that a system on each side will represent completely the peripheral receptive sheet from which it receives information (eg, the homunculus, Figure 4–9; indicates a complete contralateral body representation for mechanosensations). The three nerves supplying taste buds converge upon the rostral solitary nucleus.

Ipsilateral taste loss

The gustatory pathway, unlike the other sensory pathways, is ipsilateral. Thus, the loss of taste likely involves lesion somewhere along this central path.

Critical structures

The projection from the solitary nucleus ascends in the central tegmental tract, and terminates in the parvocellular division of the ipsilateral ventral posterior medial nucleus of the thalamus. The pontine lesion is also likely to damage the parabrachial nucleus, which could contribute to the impairment. However, we learned in Chapter 6 that the parabrachial nucleus is more important for visceral sensations. Further, other studies in the human reveal taste loss with small vascular lesions that are more selective to the central tegmental tract, demonstrating, at least, the importance of the tract.

References

Shikama Y, Kato T, Nagaoka U, et al. Localization of the gustatory pathway in the human midbrain. *Neurosci Lett.* 1996;218(3):198-200.

Uesaka Y, Nose H, Ida M. The pathway of gustatory fibers in the human ascends ipsilaterally. *Neurology.* 1998;50:827.

Two distinct neural systems are used to sense the molecular environment of the world around us: the gustatory system, which mediates taste, and the olfactory system, which serves smell. These systems are among the phylogenetically oldest neural systems of the brain. Compared with those of the other sensory systems, the neural systems for processing chemical stimuli are remarkably different. For example, both taste and smell have ipsilateral ascending projections, whereas those of the other sensory systems are either contralateral or bilateral. Moreover, the primary cortical areas for taste and smell are within limbic system regions, where emotions and their associated behaviors are formed. Information from the other sensory modalities reaches the limbic system only after additional processing stages. Smells and tastes have a particular knack for evocative recall of our dearest memories. Recall Marcel Proust's vivid description of how a spoonful of tea-soaked madeleine brought back childhood memories.

The gustatory and olfactory systems work jointly in perceiving chemicals in the oral and nasal cavities, a more essential collaboration than that which occurs between the other sensory modalities. For example, even though the gustatory system is concerned with the primary taste sensations—such as sweet or sour—the perception of richer and more complex flavors such as those present in wine or chocolate is dependent on a properly functioning sense of smell. Chewing and swallowing cause chemicals to be released from food that waft into the nasal cavity from the orapharynx, where they stimulate the olfactory system. Damage to the olfactory system, as a result of head trauma—or even the common cold, which temporarily impairs conduction of airborne molecules in the nasal passages—can dull the perception of flavor even though basic taste sensations are preserved. Although taste and smell work together and share similarities in their neural substrates, the anatomical organization of these systems is sufficiently different to be considered separately.

The Gustatory System: Taste

There are classically four taste qualities—sweet, sour, bitter, and salty—and there are corresponding taste receptor cells for each of these modalities. A fifth quality has been proposed, termed savory, which is best associated with a meaty broth because a fifth class of taste receptor cell has been identified, umami (Japanese, flavor). Whereas we may think our gustatory system's primary function is to identify foods, this is more a role of sights and smells. Rather, the system is exquisitely organized to identify nutrients or harmful agents in what we ingest, in relation to particular physiological processes: sweet and savory are key to maintaining proper energy stores, salty for electrolyte balance, bitter and sour for maintaining pH, and bitter also for avoiding toxins.

Taste is mediated by three cranial nerves, through their innervation of oral structures: **facial** (VII), **glossopharyngeal** (IX), and **vagus** (X). As discussed in Chapter 6, the glossopharyngeal and vagus nerves also provide much of the afferent innervation of the gut, cardiovascular system, and lungs. This visceral afferent innervation provides the central nervous system with information about the internal state of the body.

The Ascending Gustatory Pathway Projects to the Ipsilateral Insular Cortex

Taste receptor cells are clustered in the **taste buds,** located on the tongue and at various intraoral sites. Chemicals from food, termed **tastants,** either bind to surface membrane receptors or pass directly through membrane channels, depending on the particular chemical, to activate taste cells. Taste cells are innervated by the distal branches of the primary afferent fibers in the facial, glossopharyngeal, and vagus nerves (Figure 9–2). These afferent fibers have a pseudounipolar morphology, similar to that of the dorsal root ganglion neurons. In contrast to the nerves of the skin and mucous membranes, where generally the terminal portion of the afferent fiber is sensitive to stimulus energy, taste receptor cells are separate from the primary afferent fibers. For taste, the role of the primary afferent fiber is to receive information from particular classes of taste receptor cells and to transmit this sensory information to the central nervous system, encoded as action potentials. For touch, the role of the primary afferent fiber is both to transduce stimulus energy into action potentials and to transmit this information to the central nervous system.

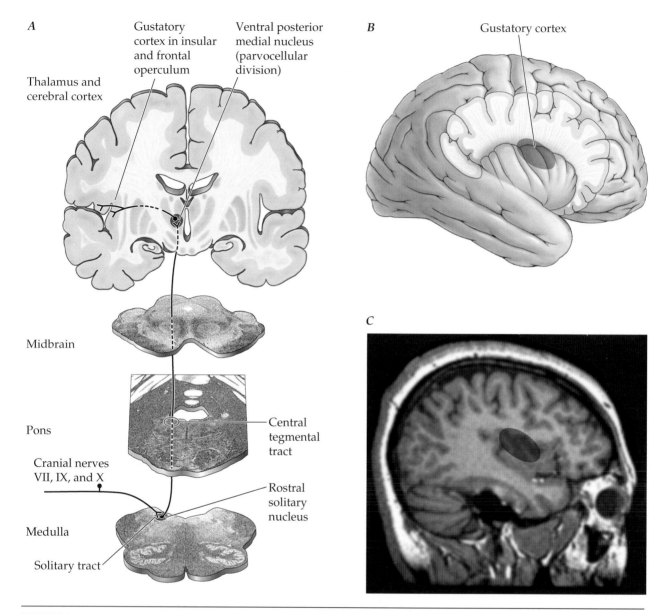

FIGURE 9–2 General organization of the gustatory system. **A.** Ascending gustatory pathway. **B.** Approximate location of the gustatory cortex in the insular cortex. The frontal operculum has been removed to show the insular cortex. **C.** MRI showing insular cortex and approximate region of the gustatory cortex in the insular cortex.

The central branches of the afferent fibers, after entering the brain stem, collect into the **solitary tract** (Figure 9–2) of the dorsal medulla and terminate in the rostral portion of the **solitary nucleus** (Figure 9–2, lower inset). Recall that the caudal solitary nucleus is a viscerosensory nucleus, critically involved in regulating body functions and transmitting information to the cortex for perception of visceral information as well as the emotional and behavioral aspects of visceral sensations.

The axons of second-order neurons in the rostral solitary nucleus ascend ipsilaterally in the brain stem, in the **central tegmental tract,** and terminate in the **parvocellular division** of the **ventral posterior medial nucleus** (Figure 9–2). From the thalamus, third-order neurons project to the **insular cortex** and the nearby **operculum,** where the primary

gustatory cortical areas are located (Figure 9–2). This pathway is thought to mediate the discriminative aspects of taste, which enable us to distinguish one quality from another. The insular cortex projects to several brain structures for further processing of taste stimuli. Projections to the **orbitofrontal cortex** (see Figure 9-11), as well as the insular and cingulate cortical areas, are thought to be integrated with olfactory information, for the awareness of flavors. In addition, these cortical areas may be important for the behavioral and affective significance of tastes, such as the pleasure experienced with a fine meal or the dissatisfaction after one poorly prepared. A component of the processing of painful stimuli also involves the limbic system cortex, and pain in humans is not without emotional significance.

Although taste and visceral afferent information (see Chapter 6) are distinct modalities and have separate central pathways, the two modalities interact. In fact, linking information about the taste of a food and its effect on body functions upon ingestion is key to an individual's survival. One of the most robust forms of learning, called **conditioned taste aversion,** associates the taste of spoiled food with the nausea that it causes when eaten. Another name for this learning is bait shyness, referring to a method used by ranchers to discourage predators from attacking their livestock. In this technique, ranchers contaminate livestock meat with an emetic, such as lithium chloride, which causes nausea and vomiting after ingestion. After eating the bait, the predator develops an aversion for the contaminated meat and will not attack the livestock. People can experience a phenomenon related to conditioned taste aversion, in which they develop an intense aversion to food they ate before becoming nauseated and vomiting, even if the food was not spoiled and the illness resulted from a viral infection. Experimental studies in rats have shown that such interactions between the gustatory and viscerosensory systems, leading to conditioned taste aversion, may occur in the insular cortex.

Regional Anatomy of the Gustatory System

Branches of the Facial, Glossopharyngeal, and Vagus Nerves Innervate Different Parts of the Oral Cavity

Taste receptor cells are epithelial cells that transduce soluble chemical stimuli within the oral cavity into neural signals. They are present in complex microscopic sensory organs, called **taste buds** (Figure 9–3A). Taste receptor cells are short lived; they are regenerated approximately every 10 days. Taste receptor cells are responsive to a single taste quality. In addition to the taste receptor cells, taste buds contain two additional types of cells: **basal cells,** which are thought to be **stem cells** that differentiate to become receptor cells, and **supporting cells,** which provide structural and possibly trophic support (Figure 9–3A). Taste receptor cells have a synaptic contact with the distal processes of primary afferent fibers.

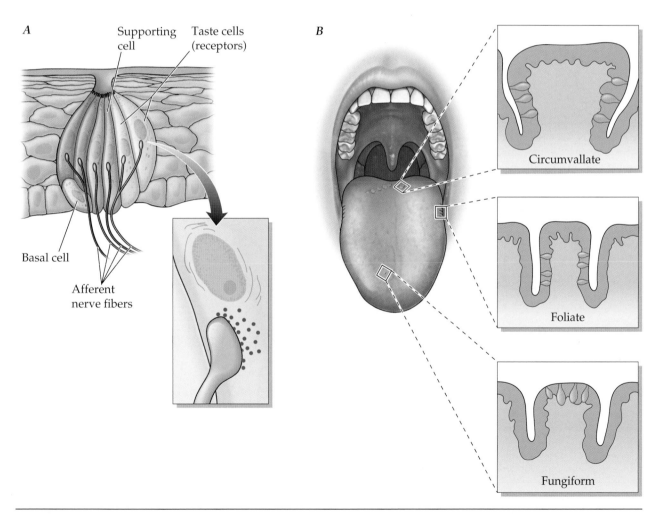

FIGURE 9–3 Taste receptors (**A**) and tongue (**B**). Taste buds (**A**) consist of taste receptor cells, supporting cells, and basal cells. The colors show particular afferent nerve fibers innervating corresponding taste receptor cells. The three types of papillae—circumvallate, foliate, and fungiform—are shown in **B.** Taste buds in papillae are shown in light purple.

A single afferent fiber terminal branches many times, both within a single taste bud and between different taste buds, so that it forms synapses with many taste cells. However, each sensory fiber will contact taste receptor cells that are responsive to a single taste modality.

Taste buds are present on the tongue, soft palate, epiglottis, pharynx, and larynx. Taste buds on the tongue are clustered on papillae (Figure 9–3B), whereas those at the other sites are located in pseudostratified columnar epithelium or stratified squamous epithelium rather than distinct papillae.

Taste receptor cells that are located on the anterior two thirds of the tongue are innervated by the **chorda tympani nerve,** a branch of the facial (VII) nerve. (The facial nerve consists of two separate roots [Figure 9–4], a motor root commonly known as the **facial nerve** and a combined sensory and autonomic root called the **intermediate nerve.**)

Taste buds on the posterior third of the tongue, which are located primarily in the circumvallate and foliate papillae (Figure 9–3B), are innervated by the **glossopharyngeal (IX) nerve** (Figure 9–4). Taste buds on the palate are innervated by

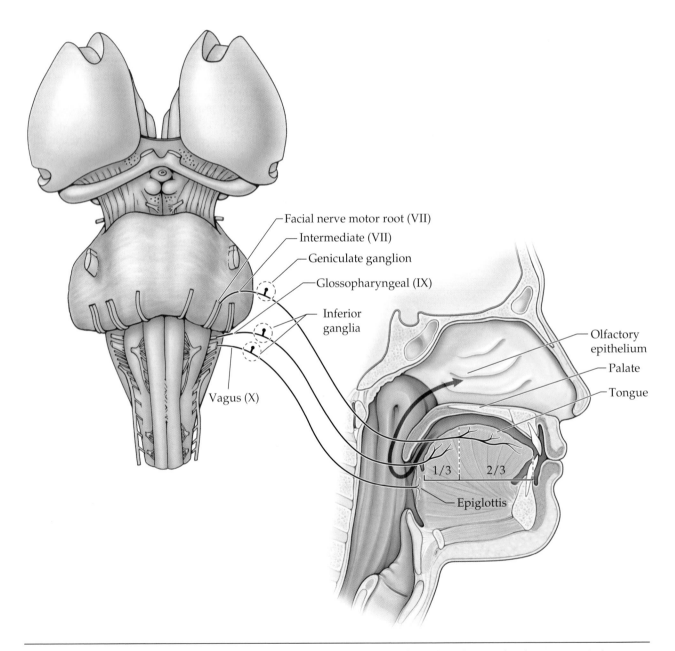

FIGURE 9–4 Oropharynx and brain stem. Gustatory innervation of the oral cavity by the facial, glossopharyngeal, and vagus nerves. In the periphery the chorda tympani nerve (a branch of cranial nerve VII) supplies taste buds on the anterior two thirds of the tongue, the lingual branches of the glossopharyngeal (IX) nerve supply taste buds on the posterior third, and the superior laryngeal (X) nerve supplies taste buds on the epiglottis. The greater petrosal nerve (another branch of cranial nerve VII) supplies taste buds on the palate. The olfactory epithelium in the nasal cavity is also shown. Volatile molecules from the oral cavity waft into the nasal cavity during chewing to activate olfactory receptors by retronasal olfaction (arrow).

a branch of the intermediate nerve. Taste buds on the epiglottis and larynx are innervated by the vagus (X) nerve, whereas those on the pharynx are innervated by the glossopharyngeal nerve. The familiar taste map of the tongue—showing that sweet and salty are sensed in the front of the tongue, sour laterally, and bitter at the back of the tongue—is wrong. Taste buds in all regions are sensitive to the five basic taste attributes.

The cell bodies of the afferent fibers innervating taste cells are located in peripheral sensory ganglia. The cell bodies of afferent fibers in the intermediate branch of the facial nerve are found in the **geniculate ganglion.** Those of the vagus and glossopharyngeal nerves are located in their respective **inferior ganglia.** As discussed in Chapter 6, the glossopharyngeal and vagus nerves also contain afferent fibers that innervate cranial skin and mucous membranes; the cell bodies of these afferent fibers are found in the **superior ganglia.** The afferent fibers of the intermediate branch of the facial nerve enter the brain stem at the **pontomedullary junction,** immediately lateral to the root that contains somatic motor axons

(Figure 9–4). The taste fibers of the glossopharyngeal and vagus nerves enter the brain stem in the rostral medulla.

The Solitary Nucleus Is the First Central Nervous System Relay for Taste

Gustatory fibers innervating the taste buds enter the brain stem and collect in the **solitary tract,** located in the dorsal medulla. The axons of the facial nerve enter the tract rostral to those of the glossopharyngeal and vagus nerves. After entering, however, the fibers send branches that ascend and descend within the tract, similar to the terminals of afferent fibers in Lissauer's tract of the spinal cord. The axon terminals leave the tract and synapse on neurons in the surrounding rostral solitary nucleus where second-order neurons (Figures 9–2, 9–5A, and 9–6B) project their axons into the ipsilateral **central tegmental tract** (Figures 9–5A and 9–6A) and ascend to the thalamus. The trigeminal and medial lemnisci, which carry the ascending somatic sensory projection from the

A

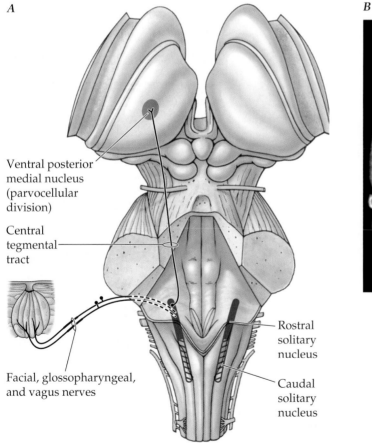

Ventral posterior medial nucleus (parvocellular division)

Central tegmental tract

Facial, glossopharyngeal, and vagus nerves

Rostral solitary nucleus

Caudal solitary nucleus

B

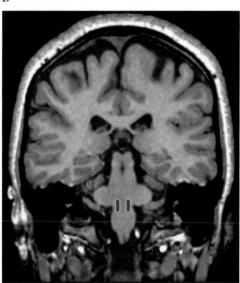

FIGURE 9–5 Brain stem and thalamic components of the gustatory system. ***A.*** Dorsal view of the brain stem, illustrating the rostral solitary nucleus receiving input from the taste buds (unilaterally) and the ascending projection of the rostral, or gustatory division, of the nucleus to the ipsilateral ventral posterior medial nucleus (parvocellular division). This path travels within the central tegmental tract. The caudal solitary nucleus is shown by the hatched lines. ***B.*** Coronal MRI, slicing the brain stem along its long axis, showing the approximate locations of the rostral solitary nuclei (blue).

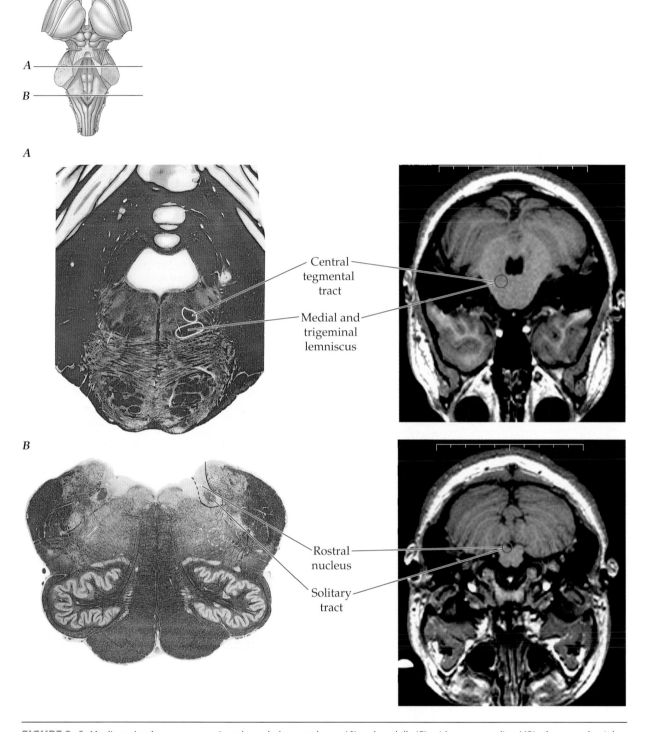

FIGURE 9–6 Myelin-stained transverse sections through the rostral pons (**A**) and medulla (**B**), with corresponding MRIs shown to the right. Note, the dorsal surfaces of both the sections and the MRIs are up. The locations of the structures indicated can only be approximated to the circled areas on the MRIs. Note that dorsal is up and ventral is down in the sections and images in this figure. The inset shows the planes of section.

main trigeminal and dorsal column nuclei, are ventral to the central tegmental tract (Figure 9–6A). Recall that the caudal solitary nucleus is important for visceral sensory function. It has a projection to the parabrachial nucleus, a pontine nucleus that is critical for relaying interoceptive information to the hypothalamus and amygdala for controlling various bodily functions, such as autonomic nervous system regulation. Brain stem centers that respond to tastants can be imaged using fMRI. The active region is the rostral pons, where the rostral solitary nucleus is located.

The Parvocellular Portion of the Ventral Posterior Medial Nucleus Relays Gustatory Information to the Insular Cortex and Operculum

Similar to somatic sensations, vision, and hearing, a thalamic relay nucleus receives taste information and projects this information to a circumscribed area of the cerebral cortex. The ascending projection from the rostral solitary nucleus terminates in the **parvocellular division** of the **ventral posterior medial nucleus.** This nucleus has a characteristic pale appearance on myelin-stained sections (Figure 9–7A). The axons of thalamocortical projection neurons in the thalamic gustatory nucleus project into the **posterior limb of the internal capsule** (Figure 9–7A, B) and ascend to the **insular cortex** and the nearby **operculum** (Figure 9–8B, C). These are the locations of the primary gustatory cortex. A PET scan of the human brain when sucrose is used as a tastant (Figure 9–8D) reveals activation in the insular and opercular regions. Different nuclei in the ventromedial thalamus receive different inputs and project to different cortical areas. Viscerosensory inputs are processed in adjacent but slightly separated thalamic regions and project to adjoining areas of the insular cortex. Touch and pain also engage different thalamic nuclei and nearby cortical areas in the postcentral gyrus and parietal operculum.

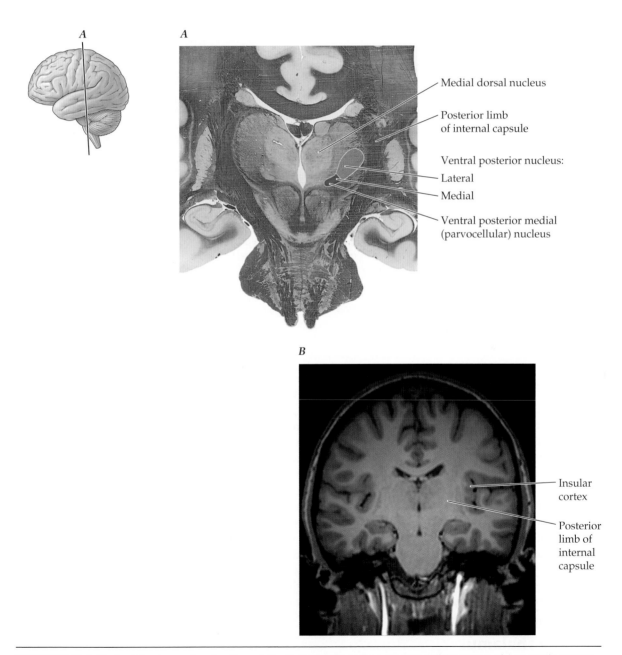

FIGURE 9–7 A. Myelin-stained coronal section through the thalamic taste nucleus, the parvocellular portion of the ventral posterior medial nucleus. The medial dorsal nucleus is also shown on this section; a portion of this nucleus may play a role in olfactory perception. **B.** MRI at a level close to that of the myelin-stained section in **A.** The inset shows the plane of section.

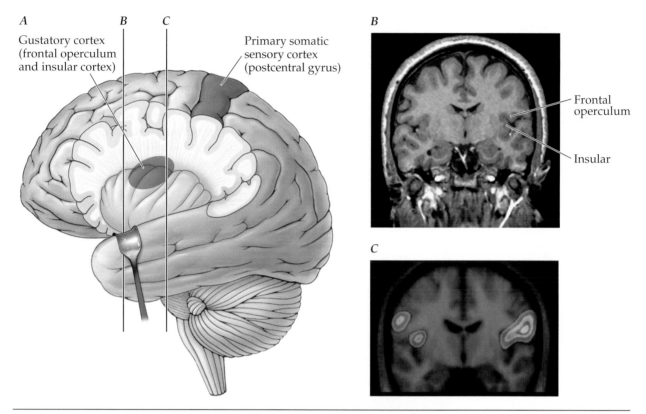

FIGURE 9-8 Cortical taste areas (**A**) and structural and functional MRIs (**B, C**). Cortical gustatory areax. **A.** Lateral view of human cerebral hemisphere; the blue-tinted field on the insular cortex corresponds approximately to insular gustatory area. In addition, there is a region of the frontal operculum, shown on the MRI in **B**, that represents taste. The primary somatic sensory cortex is also highlighted. **B.** MRI through the frontal operculum. **C.** $H_2^{15}O$ positron emission tomography scan shows bilateral areas of cortical activation in response to tasting a 5% sucrose solution. The color scale indicates that intensity of activation, measured as cerebral blood flow, which correlates with neural activity. White indicates maximal blood flow (or high neural activity), whereas blue indicates low blood flow (or activity). Note that two distinct taste areas are distinguished in the subject's right cortex (left side of image). The single zone on the other side is probably due to blurring of the PET signal. The planes of section are shown in **A.** (**C,** Courtesy of Dr. Stephen Trey, McGill University; Frey S, Petrides M. Re-examination of the human taste region: a positron emission tomography study. *Eur J Neurosci.* 1999;11:2985-2988.)

The Olfactory System: Smell

The sense of smell is mediated by the **olfactory (I) nerve.** There are two major differences between smell and the other sensory modalities, including taste. First, information about airborne chemicals impinging on the nasal mucosa is relayed directly to a part of the cerebral cortex without first relaying in the thalamus. The thalamic nucleus that processes olfactory information receives input from the cortical olfactory areas. Second, these cortical olfactory areas are phylogenetically older (allocortex) than the primary cortical regions (neocortex) that process other stimuli (see Chapter 16).

The Olfactory Projection to the Cerebral Cortex Does Not Relay Through the Thalamus

Primary olfactory neurons are found in the olfactory epithelium, a portion of the nasal cavity (Figure 9–9A). The primary olfactory neurons have a bipolar morphology (see Figure 6–3). The peripheral portion of the primary olfactory neuron is chemosensitive, and the central process is an **unmyelinated axon** that projects to the central nervous system. Recall that taste receptor cells, which transduce chemical stimuli on the tongue, and the primary taste fibers, which transmit information to the brain stem, are separate cells. Primary olfactory neurons are sensitive to airborne chemicals, or **odorants**; they have transmembrane olfactory receptors on their chemosensitive membranes in the olfactory epithelium. Each primary olfactory neuron has one type of olfactory receptor, which determines the spectrum of odorants to which the neuron is sensitive. Although most odorant molecules are carried into the olfactory epithelium with inhaled air, some travel from the oral cavity during chewing and swallowing.

The unmyelinated axons of the primary olfactory neurons collect into numerous small fascicles, which together form the **olfactory nerve.** Olfactory nerve fascicles pass through foramina in a portion of the **ethmoid bone** termed the **cribriform plate** (Figure 9–9A) and synapse on second-order

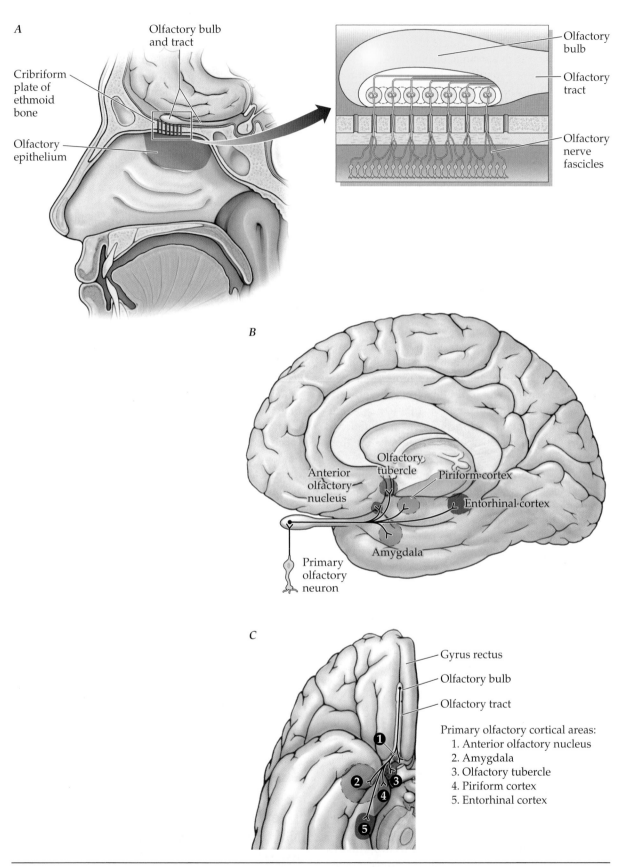

FIGURE 9–9 Organization of the olfactory system. **A.** Olfactory epithelium (red shading) on the superior nasal concha. The nasal septum is not shown. The inset shows a cutaway view of the cribriform plate, through which the olfactory nerve fibers course, the olfactory epithelium, and olfactory bulb. **B.** Schematic of medial surface of cerebral hemisphere, illustrating the five main termination sites of olfactory tract fibers. **C.** Similar to **B,** but showing the main olfactory tract termination sites on the inferior brain surface.

neurons in the **olfactory bulb** (Figures 9–9A, inset and 9–10). Head trauma can shear off these delicate fascicles as they traverse the bone, resulting in **anosmia,** the inability to.

Neurons that have a particular olfactory receptor are scattered randomly within a portion of the olfactory epithelium. The axons of these olfactory neurons all converge onto a **glomerulus** (Figure 9–9A, inset), which contains projection neurons and interneurons. The glomerulus is the basic processing unit of the olfactory bulb. The next link in the olfactory pathway is the projection of second-order neurons in the olfactory bulb through the **olfactory tract,** directly to the primitive allocortex (see Figure 16–16) on the ventral surface of the cerebral hemispheres. Five separate areas of the cerebral hemisphere receive a direct projection from the olfactory bulb (Figure 9–9B, C): (1) the **anterior olfactory nucleus,** which modulates information processing in the olfactory bulb, (2) the **amygdala** and (3) the **olfactory tubercle,** which together are thought to be important in the emotional, endocrine, and visceral consequences of odors, (4) the adjacent **piriform cortex,** which may be important for olfactory perception, and (5) the **rostral entorhinal cortex,** which is thought to be important in olfactory memories. Several higher-order projections arise from the primary areas. The projection from the piriform cortex to the **orbitofrontal cortex** is thought to be particularly critical for perception. Surprisingly, the medial dorsal nucleus of the thalamus receives olfactory information from the primary areas.

Animals, and likely humans, have additional olfactory organs in and around the nose that complement the principal olfactory organ that originates from the main portion of the olfactory epithelium, which was discussed earlier. One of these is the **vomeronasal organ,** which is discussed later. The various olfactory organs—together with the targets of their cortical projections—form a network that is the basis of olfactory discriminations, memory, emotions, and the diversity of olfactory-regulated behaviors, such as feeding and mating and sexual behaviors in animals. The trigeminal nerve also innervates the nasal mucosa and has a protective function. These trigeminal sensory fibers respond to the inhalation of noxious or irritating chemical stimuli and trigger protective reflexes, such as apnea or sneezing.

Regional Anatomy of the Olfactory System

The Primary Olfactory Neurons Are Located in the Nasal Mucosa

Most of the lining of the nasal cavity is part of the respiratory epithelium, which warms and humidifies inspired air. The **olfactory epithelium** is a specialized portion of the nasal epithelial surface that contains the primary olfactory neurons. It is located on the superior nasal concha on each side as well as the midline septum and roof. Primary

olfactory neurons, of which there are approximately several million, are short lived, similar to taste cells. Regenerated olfactory neurons also must regenerate their axon and form synaptic connections with their appropriate target neurons in the olfactory bulb. These bipolar sensory neurons have an apical portion with hairlike structures (olfactory cilia) that contain the molecular machinery for receiving chemical stimuli (Figure 9–10A). In addition to the olfactory neurons, the olfactory epithelium contains two other cell types: (1) glial-like **supporting cells** and (2) **basal cells,** which are stem cells that differentiate into primary olfactory neurons as the mature sensory neurons die.

The initial step in olfactory perception is the interaction of an odorant molecule with an **olfactory receptor protein,** a complex transmembrane protein located in the apical membrane of primary olfactory neurons. Olfactory receptor proteins are encoded by a large family of olfactory genes, which number up to approximately 1000 in many animals. Remarkably, individual primary olfactory sensory neurons each contain only one olfactory receptor protein type. How a neuron comes to express one particular olfactory receptor is not known. Olfactory sensory neurons that express the same receptor are scattered about within the olfactory epithelium. Olfactory receptors bind multiple odorants, indicating that individual primary olfactory neurons are sensitive to multiple odorants. Different odorants therefore appear to be initially processed by sensory neurons that are distributed widely and randomly throughout the olfactory epithelium. The scattering of olfactory receptor types within the olfactory epithelium is similar to the distribution of taste cells in the oral cavity. There are fewer olfactory receptor genes in primates, including humans. Despite having fewer olfactory genes, primates have a well-developed sense of smell. It is thought that the decline in olfactory genes is compensated by having larger and more complex brains.

Another component of the olfactory system, the **vomeronasal organ,** comprises a portion of the olfactory epithelium separate from the main olfactory epithelium (Figure 9–9). Whereas olfactory sensory neurons in the main olfactory epithelium can sense **pheromones,** in animals the vomeronasal organ is also important in detecting pheromones that have important effects on the individual animal's social and sexual behavior. Rather than project to the olfactory bulb, virtually all the neurons of the vomeronasal organ project to a different structure, the accessory olfactory bulb, which projects only to the amygdala. Whereas humans have a vomeronasal organ, whether it is a functioning olfactory sensing organ is in dispute.

The Olfactory Bulb Is the First Central Nervous System Relay for Olfactory Input

Primary olfactory neurons synapse on neurons in the **olfactory bulb** (Figure 9–10), which is actually a portion of the

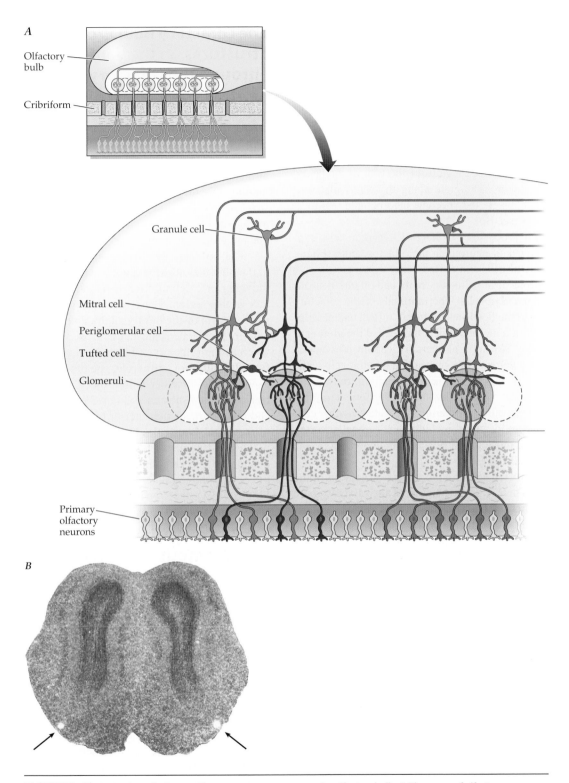

FIGURE 9–10 Projection of primary olfactory sensory neurons to the olfactory bulb. **A.** The axons of olfactory bipolar cells synapse on the projection neurons of the olfactory bulb, the mitral cells and the tufted cells, as well as the periglomerular cells, a type of inhibitory interneuron. **B.** In situ hybridization of olfactory receptor mRNA in the axon terminals of primary olfactory sensory neurons in a single glomerulus in the olfactory bulb of the rat. The two bright spots on the ventral surface of the bulb (arrows) correspond to the two labeled glomeruli. (**A,** Reproduced with permission from Yoshihara Y. Basic principles and molecular mechanisms of olfactory axon pathfinding. *Cell & Tissue Research.* Oct:290(2):457-463, 1997. **B,** Courtesy of Dr. Robert Vassar, Columbia University; Vassar R, Chao SK, Sticheran R, Nuñez JM, Vosshall LB, Axel R. Topographic organization of sensory projections to the olfactory bulb. *Cell.* 1994;79:981-991.)

cerebral hemispheres. This is because the olfactory bulb develops as a small outpouching on the ventral surface of the telencephalon. The olfactory bulb has a very small, vestigial, ventricular space (see Figure 9–13B). Compared with rodents and carnivores, the olfactory bulb is reduced in size in monkeys, apes, and humans. Similar to most other components of the cerebral hemisphere, neurons in the olfactory bulb are organized into discrete laminae. Surprisingly, the olfactory bulb is the recipient of migrating neurons that are born in maturity within specialized regions of the wall of the lateral ventricle. These neurons migrate along the ventricular wall and into the bulb, where they become incorporated into local olfactory circuits (see Box 9–1).

The central processes of olfactory receptor cells synapse on three types of neurons in the olfactory bulb (Figure 9–10A): on **mitral cells** and **tufted cells,** which are the two projection neurons of the olfactory bulb, and on interneurons called **periglomerular cells.** The terminals of the olfactory receptor cells and the dendrites of mitral, tufted, and periglomerular cells form a morphological unit called the **glomerulus** (Figure 9–10). Within a glomerulus, certain presynaptic and postsynaptic elements are ensheathed by **glial cells.** This sheath ensures specificity of action, limiting the spread of neurotransmitter released by the presynaptic terminal. Whereas structures called glomeruli are located in other central nervous system locations, including the cerebellar cortex (see Chapter 13), those in the olfactory bulb are among the largest and most distinct.

Mitral and **tufted cells** are the projection neurons of the olfactory bulb. Their axons project from the olfactory bulb through the **olfactory tract** to the primary olfactory cortical areas (Figures 9–11 and 9–12). The **granule cell** (Figure 9–10A) is an inhibitory interneuron that receives excitatory synaptic input from mitral cells to which it feeds back inhibition. Another inhibitory interneuron in the olfactory bulb is the **periglomerular cell,** which receives a direct input from the primary olfactory neurons. This neuron inhibits mitral cells in the same and adjacent glomeruli. One function of these inhibitory interneurons is to make the neural responses to different odorants more distinct, thereby facilitating discrimination.

A remarkable specificity exists in the projections of olfactory sensory neurons to the glomeruli. Even though primary olfactory neurons that contain a particular type of olfactory receptor are widely distributed throughout part of the olfactory epithelium, they project to one or a small number of glomeruli in the olfactory bulb (Figure 9–10B). Because there are up to about 1000 different olfactory receptor genes, and double the number of glomeruli on each side, researchers have suggested that each glomerulus may receive projections from olfactory sensory neurons that have a single type of receptor. This finding suggests that the neuronal processes within the glomerulus—the dendrites of mitral, tufted, and periglomerular cells—comprise a functional unit for processing a particular set of odorants.

The Olfactory Bulb Projects to Structures on the Ventral Brain Surface Through the Olfactory Tract

The olfactory bulb and tract lie in the **olfactory sulcus** on the ventral surface of the frontal lobe (Figure 9–11). The **gyrus rectus** (or straight gyrus) is located medial to the olfactory bulb and tract (Figure 9–11). As the olfactory tract approaches the region where it fuses with the cerebral hemispheres, it bifurcates into a prominent **lateral olfactory stria** and a small **medial olfactory stria** (Figure 9–11). The lateral olfactory stria contains the axons from the olfactory bulb, whereas the medial olfactory stria contains axons from other brain regions that are projecting to the olfactory bulb.

The **anterior perforated substance** is located caudal to the olfactory striae (Figure 9–11, inset). Tiny branches of the anterior cerebral artery perforate the ventral brain surface in this region. These branches provide the arterial supply for parts of the basal ganglia and internal capsule. The anterior perforated substance is gray matter (see below), whereas the olfactory striae are pathways on the brain surface. The **olfactory tubercle,** one of the gray matter regions to which the olfactory bulb projects, is located in the anterior perforated substance (Figure 9–11, inset). The tubercle and other parts of the anterior perforated substance are part of the **basal forebrain.** One nucleus of the basal forebrain is the basal nucleus of Meynert, which comprises neurons containing acetylcholine that project diffusely throughout the cortex and regulate cortical excitability (see Chapter 2; Figure 2–3A).

The Primary Olfactory Cortex Receives a Direct Input From the Olfactory Bulb

The projection neurons of the olfactory bulb (tufted and mitral cells) send their axons directly to five spatially disparate regions on the ventral and medial surfaces of the cerebral hemispheres. These areas are collectively termed the **primary olfactory cortex** (Figure 9–9B): (1) anterior olfactory nucleus, (2) amygdala, (3) olfactory tubercle, (4) piriform cortex, and (5) rostral entorhinal cortex.

Primary olfactory areas are allocortex

Most of the primary olfactory areas on the ventral and medial surfaces of the cerebral hemispheres (Figure 9–9B, C) have a cytoarchitecture that is characteristically different from the nonolfactory cortical regions located lateral to them. Recall that most of the cerebral cortex is **neocortex,** with at least six cell layers (see Chapter 2, Figure 2-19; also Figure 16–16). Somatic sensory, visual, auditory, and gustatory cortical areas are all part of the neocortex. In contrast, the olfactory cortex has fewer than six layers, termed **allocortex** (see Figure 16–16). With fewer layers, allocortex is more limited than neocortex in its processing capabilities.

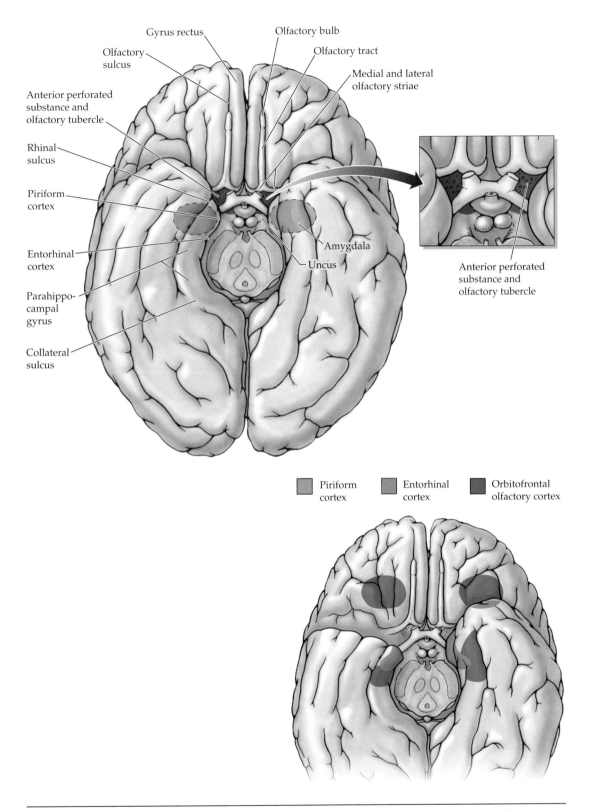

FIGURE 9–11 Ventral surface of the cerebral hemisphere showing regional anatomy and key olfactory areas. The parahippocampal gyrus contains numerous anatomical and functional divisions, two of which are the entorhinal cortex and piriform cortex. Allocortex is located medial to the collateral sulcus and rhinal fissure. The approximate location of the amygdala is indicated. The inset shows the location of the olfactory tubercle within the region of the anterior perforated substance (red). Primary olfactory regions of the temporal lobe and the medial orbital surfaces of the frontal lobe (bottom) are shown. The orbitofrontal cortex receives a projection from the primary olfactory areas, as well as the medial dorsal nucleus of the thalamus.

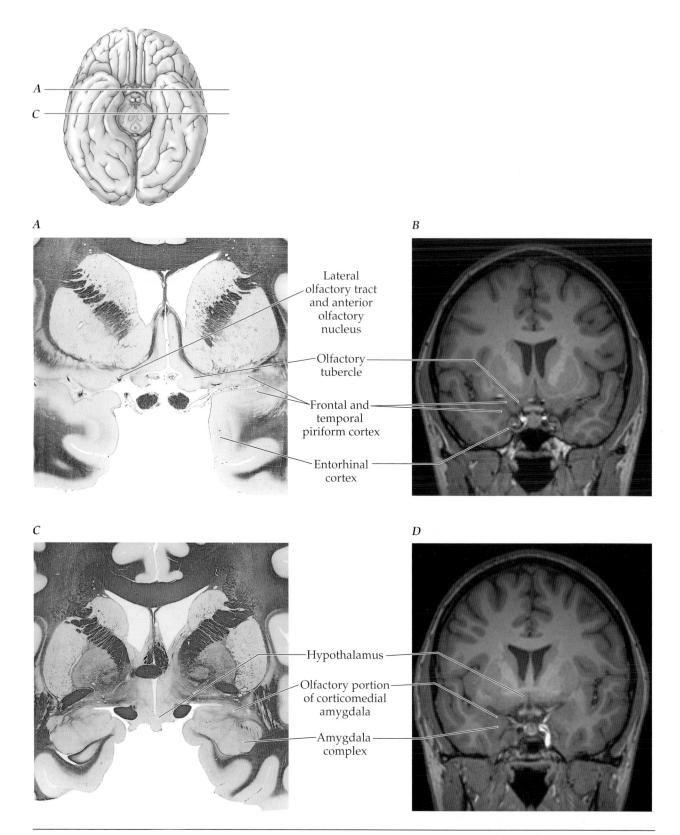

FIGURE 9–12 Olfactory areas shown on myelin-stained coronal sections (**A, C**) and corresponding MRIs (**B, D**). The inset shows the approximate planes of section.

Allocortical areas also receive little direct input from the thalamus. There are two major kinds of allocortex: archicortex and paleocortex. **Archicortex** is located primarily in the hippocampal formation (see Chapter 16). **Paleocortex** is located on the basal surface of the cerebral hemispheres, in part of the insular cortex, and caudally along the parahippocampal gyrus and retrosplenial cortex (the area of cortex located caudal to the splenium of the corpus callosum; see Figure AI–4). In addition to archicortex and paleocortex, there are various forms of transitional cortex with characteristics of both neocortex and allocortex. On the ventral brain surface, allocortex and transitional cortex remain medial to the **rhinal sulcus** and its caudal extension, the **collateral sulcus** (Figure 9–11). The paleocortical olfactory areas each have three morphologically distinct layers. Axons of the olfactory tract course in the most superficial layer before synapsing on neurons in the deeper layers.

Neurons in the anterior olfactory nucleus modulate information transmission in the olfactory bulb bilaterally

The anterior olfactory nucleus is located caudal to the olfactory bulb, near where the olfactory tract fuses with the cerebral hemispheres (Figure 9–11A). It contains many neurons that use acetylcholine as their neurotransmitter. Neurons of the anterior olfactory nucleus are also scattered along the olfactory tract. Many neurons in this nucleus project their axons back to the olfactory bulb, both ipsilaterally and contralaterally. Because of these connections, the anterior olfactory nucleus is well positioned to regulate early olfactory processing. In Alzheimer disease, a progressive neurological degenerative disease in which individuals become severely demented, the anterior olfactory nucleus undergoes characteristic structural changes. Early in Alzheimer's patients, there is a loss of cholinergic neurons in the anterior olfactory nucleus, as well as another cholinergic cell group, the basal nucleus of Meynert. Interestingly, there is also a reduction in adult neurogenesis in Alzheimer's patients. Damage of the anterior olfactory nucleus, and possibly the reduction in neurogenesis, may underlie the impaired sense of smell in Alzheimer's patients.

Projections of the olfactory bulb to the amygdala and olfactory tubercle play a role in olfactory regulation of behavior

A major projection of the olfactory bulb is to the **amygdala,** a heterogeneous structure located in the anterior temporal lobe (Figures 9–11 and 9–12C, D). The amygdala has three major nuclear divisions: the corticomedial nuclear group, the basolateral nuclear group, and the central nucleus. The olfactory bulb projects to a portion of the **corticomedial** nuclear group (Figure 9–12C). This olfactory projection is thought to be important in behavior regulation rather than in odor perception and discrimination. For example, neurons in the corticomedial nuclear group are part of a circuit transmitting

olfactory information to the hypothalamus (Figure 9–12C), for the regulation of food intake. Also, in certain animals the corticomedial nuclear group plays an essential role in the olfactory regulation of reproductive behaviors. The organization of the amygdala is considered in detail in Chapter 16.

The **olfactory tubercle** is a part of the basal forebrain located medial to the olfactory tract (Figure 9–12A). Compared with the amygdala, which receives a major olfactory projection in most animal species, the olfactory projections to the olfactory tubercle are fewer in number in primates. Neurons in the olfactory tubercle receive input from and project their axons to brain regions that play a role in emotions (see Chapter 16).

The olfactory areas of the temporal and frontal lobes may be important in olfactory perceptions and discriminations

The olfactory bulb also projects directly to the caudolateral frontal lobe and the rostromedial temporal lobe. These areas consist of the piriform cortex and the rostral entorhinal cortex (Figures 9–11 and 9–12). Receiving the largest projection from the olfactory bulb, the piriform cortex—named for its appearance in certain mammals, where the rostral temporal lobe is shaped like a pear (*pirum* is Latin for "pear")—is important in the initial processing of odors leading to perception. The piriform cortex projects directly, and indirectly via the **medial dorsal nucleus** (Figure 9–7), to the **orbitofrontal cortex** (Figure 9–13). When humans are engaged in olfactory discriminations, functional imaging studies indicate consistent activation within a consistent area near the intersection of the medial and transverse orbital sulci (Figure 9–13). Damage to the orbitofrontal cortex in humans and monkeys impairs **olfactory discrimination.**

The **rostral entorhinal cortex** is located on the parahippocampal gyrus (Figure 9–13). This area is thought to be important in allowing a particular smell to evoke memories of a place or event. This cortex projects to the hippocampal formation, which has been shown to be essential for consolidation of short-term memories into long-term memories (see Chapter 16).

Olfactory and Gustatory Information Interacts in the Insular and Orbitofrontal Cortex for Sensing Flavors

Perception of the flavor of foods and beverages we ingest not only reflects the combined sensing of the five primary taste qualities, but depends on our sense of smell; without smell, flavors become flat. Smell is actively integrated with tastes to achieve our sense of flavors. Human brain imaging studies show, not surprisingly, odors alone activate the olfactory cortical areas in the temporal and orbitofrontal cortical regions. And tastes alone activate the primary taste cortical areas in the insular and opercular regions. Interestingly,

Box 9–1

Adult Neurogenesis in the Olfactory Bulb

Surprisingly, neurons are continuously born, a process termed **neurogenesis,** and incorporated into local neural circuits in the mature mammalian brain. Whereas there is evidence for and against neurogenesis in multiple brain regions, including the cerebral neocortex, there is clear and well-documented evidence for adult neurogenesis in only two locations: a specialized region of the wall of the lateral ventricle, the subventricular zone (SVZ), and a portion of the hippocampal formation, the dentate gyrus. Neurogenesis in other brain regions is controversial.

Adult neurogenesis occurs anteriorly in the SVZ, just under the walls of the lateral ventricle, and posteriorly in the dentate gyrus of the hippocampal formation, in a region termed the subgranular zone (SGZ) (Figure 9–13A). Neurons born in the SVZ migrate a long distance farther anteriorly to reach the olfactory bulb. There, they become one of two classes of inhibitory interneuron: periglomerular cells and granule cells (Figures 9–10 and 9–13A). Neurons born in the posterior region migrate only a short distance to become granule cells within the dentate gyrus of the hippocampal formation. This will be discussed in Chapter 16. Here we focus on the SVZ and olfactory bulb.

Along the ventricular wall, embryonic stem cells divide to generate an intermediate cell type (termed transit amplifying cell) that, in turn, gives rise to neuroblasts, which are cells that develop into neurons (Figure 9–13A3). These adult-born neuroblasts migrate along a predefined path, termed the rostral migratory stream (RMS), to reach the olfactory bulb (Figure 9–13A). The rostral migratory stream has recently been described in the human brain (Figure 9–13C). The parasagittal myelin-stained section (C1) shows the general location of the rostral migratory stream (red line). On the Nissl-stained sagittal section (C2), a line of cells can be seen that can be stained for a protein that marks proliferating cells (C3), proliferating cell nuclear antigen (PCNA). It is estimated that about 100,000 cells comprise the RMS in the human brain. Once neuroblasts from the RMS arrive at the olfactory bulb, they migrate into their appropriate layers (Figure 9–13A1). Interestingly, animal studies reveal that only about 50% of the migrating neuroblasts that arrive at the olfactory bulb and mature to become neurons survive for more than a month. We think that there is a balance between potential benefits of adult-born neurons and the disadvantages to adding more cells to the brain; which, of course, is located within the confined cranial cavity.

Not surprisingly, the process of adult neurogenesis has a complex regulation. Intrinsic factors local to the sites of neurogenesis (A3) and migration (A2) are important, including neurotransmitters, guidance molecules, and signaling molecules. Extrinsic factors, such as the animal's physical activity level and environmental enrichments, are also important. Much ongoing research is aimed at determining the extent to which these adult-born neurons, which incorporate into the correct locations in the olfactory bulb, form functioning circuits and what role these neurons serve in olfaction. The minority of long-term surviving adult-born neurons is apt to be playing an important role, but exactly what that role is, is not yet understood. We do know that reduced neurogenesis in the olfactory bulb can impair discrimination and other olfactory-related behaviors. Why are we so fascinated by adult neurogenesis? In addition to the continued mystery of their function, further knowledge of adult neurogenesis may lead to devising cell-replacement therapies for such degenerative neurological disorders as Alzheimer and Parkinson disease.

combined presentation of odorants and tastants coactivated many of these regions as well as activated new, neighboring, regions. This shows how our brain is exquisitely sensitive to combinations of chemical stimuli necessary for flavor perception.

Physical interactions between odorants and tastants occur largely through an unexpected route. As shown in Figure 9–4, the oropharynx communicates with the nasal cavity. Volatile molecules during chewing and swallowing can activate olfactory sensory neurons in the olfactory epithelium through **retronasal olfaction** (Figure 9–4, arrow), as opposed to **orthonasal olfaction** where molecules travel from the external environment through the nostrils (nares). Retronasal olfaction, when studied in the laboratory, is sensed as taste, whereas orthonasal olfaction is sensed as a smell originating in the external environment. Imaging studies have revealed different patterns of brain activation dependent on the route a molecule takes to reach the olfactory epithelium. When the same molecule, such as a component of chocolate, is delivered via the ortho- and retronasal routes, a different pattern of activated brain regions occurs. Interestingly, one difference is that the retronasal route leads to activation of the tongue area of the primary somatic sensory cortex activation. This further emphasizes how sensing the flavor of what we ingest is a multisensory experience, with intraoral texture and temperature also playing an important role.

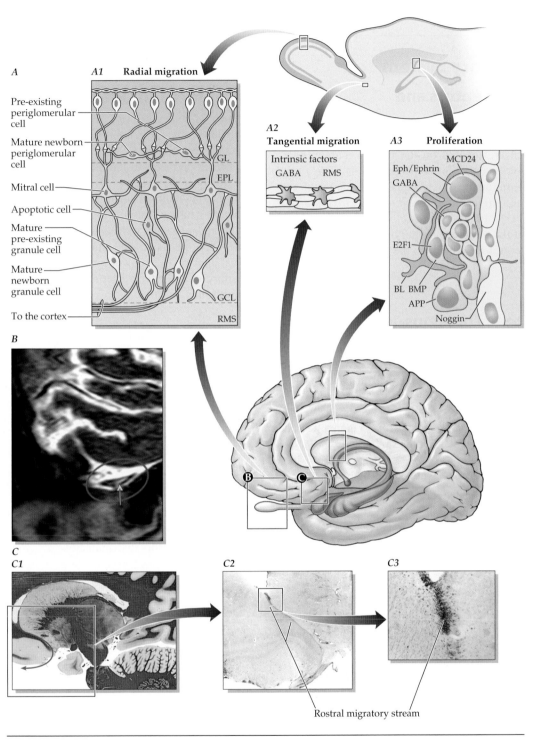

FIGURE 9-13 Sites of adult neurogenesis in the rat brain (**A**, top) and corresponding regions in the human brain (**B**, bottom). In the rat brain, the site of neurogenesis is within the wall of the lateral ventricle (**A3**). Cells migrate anteriorly (**A2**) to become incorporated into olfactory bulb circuitry (**A1**). Neurogenesis in the human brain and the migratory path for neuroblasts from the subventricular zone to the olfactory bulb. **B** shows the olfactory bulb on T2-weighted MRI; the arrow points to a cavity within the olfactory bulb that is the extension of the lateral ventricle. **C** shows the path likely taken by newly born neurons in the human brain. The migration path is shown in **C**; **C1** gives an overview of the migratory path (red line); **C2** and **C3**, (expanded) show the region in a Nissl (**C2**) and are stained using a primary antibody to a marker of the newborn cells (proliferating cell nuclear antigen; PCNA). Adult neurogenesis is regulated by many local molecules, such as: the neurotransmitter GABA; guidance molecules and receptors, such as ephrin and Eph receptors; growth factors, such as bone morphogenic protein (BMP); and many other signaling molecules and proteins (eg, MCD24, E2F1, amyloid precursor protein [APP]). (**B, C2,** and **C3,** Reproduced with permission from Curtis MA, Kam M, Nannmark U, et al. Human neuroblasts migrate to the olfactory bulb via a lateral ventricular extension. *Science.* 2007;315[5816]:1243-1249.)

The Gustatory System

Sensory Receptors and Peripheral Nerves

Gustatory receptors are clustered in *taste buds* (Figure 9–3), which are located on the tongue, palate, pharynx, larynx, and epiglottis (Figure 9–4). The *facial (VII) nerve* innervates taste buds on the anterior two thirds of the tongue and the *palate; the glossopharyngeal (IX) nerve* innervates taste buds on the posterior one third of the tongue and pharynx; and the *vagus (X) nerve* innervates taste buds on the epiglottis and larynx (Figure 9–4).

Brain Stem, Thalamus, and Cerebral Cortex

Afferent fibers of the three cranial nerves serving taste enter the solitary tract and terminate principally in the rostral portion of the *solitary nucleus* (Figures 9–2, 9–5, and 9–6B). Projection neurons from the solitary nucleus ascend ipsilaterally, in the *central tegmental tract* (Figures 9–5 and 9–6A), to the parvocellular portion of the *ventral posterior medial nucleus* (Figure 9–7). The cortical areas to which the thalamic neurons project are located in the *insular cortex* and nearby *operculum* (Figure 9–8). These areas are separate from the representation of tactile sensation on the tongue.

The Olfactory System

Receptors and Olfactory Nerve

Primary olfactory neurons, located in the *olfactory epithelium,* are *bipolar neurons* (Figures 9–9 and 9–10). The distal process is sensitive to chemical stimuli, and the central process projects to the olfactory bulb (Figures 9–9C and 9–10) as the *olfactory (I) nerve.* The olfactory nerve is formed by multiple small fascicles of axons of primary olfactory neurons that pass through foramina in a portion of the *ethmoid bone* termed the *cribriform plate* (Figure 9–9). There are about 1000 olfactory receptors, but an individual olfactory neuron contains one type of receptor. The olfactory receptor type determines the odorants to which the neuron is sensitive.

Cerebral Cortex

Olfactory nerve fibers synapse on neurons in the glomeruli of the olfactory bulb (Figure 9–10). Primary olfactory neurons with a particular olfactory receptor send their axons to one or just a few glomeruli (Figure 9–10). Projection neurons in glomeruli send their axons, via the *olfactory tract,* to five regions of the cerebral hemisphere (Figures 9–11 and 9–12): (1) the *anterior olfactory nucleus,* (2) the *olfactory tubercle* (a portion of the *anterior perforated substance*), (3) the *amygdala,* (4) the *piriform* and *periamygdaloid cortical areas,* and (5) the *rostral entorhinal cortex.* The piriform cortex projects, via the *medial dorsal nucleus* (Figure 9–7), to the *orbitofrontal cortex* (Figure 9–11), which is thought to be important in olfactory discrimination.

Buck LB, Bargmann C. Smell and taste: the chemical senses. In: Kandel ER, Schwartz JH, Jessell TM, Siegelbaum SA, Hudspeth AJ, eds. *Principles of Neural Science.* 5th ed. New York, NY: McGraw-Hill; in press.

Beckstead RM, Morse JR, Norgren R. The nucleus of the solitary tract in the monkey: projections to the thalamus and brain stem nuclei. *J Comp Neurol.* 1980;190:259-282.

Bermudez-Rattoni F. Molecular mechanisms of taste-recognition memory. *Nat Rev Neurosci.* 2004;5(3):209-217.

Bhutta MF. Sex and the nose: human pheromonal responses. *J R Soc Med.* 2007;100(6):268-274.

Bourque CW. Central mechanisms of osmosensation and systemic osmoregulation. *Nat Rev Neurosci.* 2008;9(7):519-531.

Braak H. *Architectonics of the Human Telencephalic Cortex.* New York, NY: Springer-Verlag; 1980:147.

Buck LB, Axel R. A novel multigene family may encode odorant receptors: a molecular basis for odor recognition. *Cell.* 1991;65:175-187.

Buck LB. The molecular architecture of odor and pheromone sensing in mammals. *Cell.* 2000;100:611-618.

Carmichael ST, Price JL. Limbic connections of the orbital and medial prefrontal cortex in macaque monkeys. *J Comp Neurol.* 1995;363:615-641.

Cavada C, Company T, Tejedor J, Cruz-Rizzolo RJ, Reinoso-Suarez F. The anatomical connections of the macaque monkey orbitofrontal cortex. A review. *Cereb Cortex* 2000;10: 220-242.

Cechetto DF, Saper CB. Evidence for a viscerotopic sensory representation in the cortex and thalamus in the rat. *J Comp Neurol.* 1987;262:27-45.

Chiavaras MM, Petrides M. Orbitofrontal sulci of the human and macaque monkey brain. *J Comp Neurol.* 2000;422:35-54.

Craig AD. How do you feel—-now? The anterior insula and human awareness. *Nat Rev Neurosci.* 2009;10(1):59-70.

Curtis MA, Kam M, Nannmark U, et al. Human neuroblasts migrate to the olfactory bulb via a lateral ventricular extension. *Science.* 2007;315(5816):1243-1249.

de Araujo IE, Kringelbach ML, Rolls ET, McGlone F. Human cortical responses to water in the mouth, and the effects of thirst. *J Neurophysiol.* 2003;90(3):1865-1876.

Doetsch F, Caille I, Lim DA, Garcia-Verdugo JM, Alvarez-Buylla A. Subventricular zone astrocytes are neural stem cells in the adult mammalian brain. *Cell.* 1999;97(6):703-716.

Doty RL. Olfaction. *Annu Rev Psychol.* 2001;52:423-452.

Dulac C. How does the brain smell? *Neuron.* 1997;19:477-480.

Dulac C. The physiology of taste, vintage 2000. *Cell.* 2000;100: 607-610.

Finger TE. Gustatory nuclei and pathways in the central nervous system. In: Finger TE, Silver WL, eds. *Neurobiology of Taste and Smell.* New York, NY: John Wiley and Sons; 1987:331-353.

Frey S, Petrides M. Re-examination of the human taste region: a positron emission tomography study. *Eur J Neurosci.* 1999;11(8):2985-2988.

Gottfried JA, Smith AP, Rugg MD, Dolan RJ. Remembrance of odors past: human olfactory cortex in cross-modal recognition memory. *Neuron.* 2004;42(4):687-695.

Gottfried JA, Zald DH. On the scent of human olfactory orbitofrontal cortex: meta-analysis and comparison to non-human primates. *Brain Res Brain Res Rev.* 2005;50(2): 287-304.

Gould E. How widespread is adult neurogenesis in mammals? *Nat Rev Neurosci.* 2007;8(6):481-488.

Haberly LB. Olfactory cortex. In: Shepherd GM, ed. *The Synaptic Organization of the Brain.* New York, NY: Oxford University Press; 1990:317-345.

Herness MS, Gilbertson TA. Cellular mechanisms of taste transduction. *Annu Rev Physiol.* 1999;61:873-900.

Horowitz LF, Montmayeur JP, Echelard Y, Buck LB. A genetic approach to trace neural circuits. *Proc Natl Acad Sci USA.* 1999;96:3194-3199.

Kaye WH, Fudge JL, Paulus M. New insights into symptoms and neurocircuit function of anorexia nervosa. *Nat Rev Neurosci.* 2009;10(8):573-584.

Lazarini F, Lledo PM. Is adult neurogenesis essential for olfaction? *TINS.* 2011;34:20-30.

Lenz FA, Gracely RH, Zirh TA, Leopold DA, Rowland LH, Dougherty PM. Human thalamic nucleus mediating taste and multiple other sensations related to ingestive behavior. *J Neurophysiol.* 1997;77:3406-3409.

Lledo PM, Alonso M, Grubb MS. Adult neurogenesis and functional plasticity in neuronal circuits. *Nat Rev Neurosci.* 2006;7(3):179-193.

Markowitsch HJ, Emmans D, Irle E, Streicher M, Preilowski B. Cortical and subcortical afferent connections of the primate's temporal pole: a study of rhesus monkeys, squirrel monkeys, and marmosets. *J Comp Neurol.* 1985;242:425-458.

Mast TG, Samuelsen CL. Human pheromone detection by the vomeronasal organ: unnecessary for mate selection? *Chem Senses.* 2009;34(6):529-531.

Meredith M. Human vomeronasal organ function: a critical review of best and worst cases. *Chem Senses.* 2001;26(4):433-445.

Mombaerts P. Genes and ligands for odorant, vomeronasal and taste receptors. *Nat Rev Neurosci.* 2004;5(4): 263-278.

Mori K, Nagao H, Yoshihara Y. The olfactory bulb: coding and processing of odor molecule information. *Science.* 1999;286:711-715.

Mori K, von Campenhause H, Yoshihara Y. Zonal organization of the mammalian main and accessory olfactory systems. *Philos Trans R Soc Lond B Biol Sci.* 2000;355:1801-1812.

Munger SD, Leinders-Zufall T, Zufall F. Subsystem organization of the mammalian sense of smell. *Annu Rev Physiol.* 2009;71:115-140.

Pritchard TC, Hamilton RB, Morse JR, et al. Projections of thalamic gustatory and lingual areas in the monkey, *Macaca fascicularis. J Comp Neurol.* 1986;244:213-228.

Pritchard TC, Norgren R. Gustatory system. In: Paxinos G, Mai JK, eds. *The Human Nervous System.* 2nd ed. London: Elsevier; 2004:1171-1197.

Price JL. Olfaction. In: Paxinos G, Mai JK, eds. *The Human Nervous System.* 2nd ed. London: Elsevier; 2004.

Porter J, Anand T, Johnson B, Khan RM, Sobel N. Brain mechanisms for extracting spatial information from smell. *Neuron.* 2005;47(4):581-592.

Qureshy A, Kawashima R, Imran MB, et al. Functional mapping of human brain in olfactory processing: a PET study. *J Neurophysiol.* 2000;84:1656-1666.

Reilly S. The role of the gustatory thalamus in taste-guided behavior. *Neurosci Biobehav Rev.* 1998;22:883-901.

Ressler KJ, Sullivan SL, Buck LB. A molecular dissection of spatial patterning in the olfactory system. *Curr Opin Neurobiol.* 1994;4:588-596.

Ressler KJ, Sullivan SL, Buck LB. Information coding in the olfactory system: evidence for a stereotyped and highly organized epitope map in the olfactory bulb. *Cell.* 1994;79: 1245-1255.

Rolls ET. The orbitofrontal cortex. *Philos Trans R Soc Lond B Biol Sci.* 1996;351:1433-1443; discussion 1443-1434.

Scott K. Taste recognition: food for thought. *Neuron.* 2005;48(3):455-464.

Scott TR, Plata-Salaman CR. Taste in the monkey cortex. *Physiol Behav.* 1999;67:489-511.

Scott TR, Small DM. The role of the parabrachial nucleus in taste processing and feeding. *Ann N Y Acad Sci.* 2009;1170: 372-377.

Shepherd GM. Smell images and the flavour system in the human brain. *Nature.* 2006;444(7117):316-321.

Shepherd GM, Greer CA. Olfactory bulb. In: Shepherd GM, ed. *The Synaptic Organization of the Brain.* New York, NY: Oxford University Press; 1990:133-169.

Shikama Y, Kato T, Nagaoka U, et al. Localization of the gustatory pathway in the human midbrain. *Neurosci Lett.* 1996;218:198-200.

Small DM. Central gustatory processing in humans. *Adv Otorhinolaryngol.* 2006;63:191-220.

Small DM. Taste representation in the human insula. *Brain Struct Funct.* 2010;214(5-6):551-561.

Small DM, Gerber JC, Mak YE, Hummel T. Differential neural responses evoked by orthonasal versus retronasal odorant perception in humans. *Neuron.* 2005;47(4):593-605.

Small DM, Prescott J. Odor/taste integration and the perception of flavor. *Exp Brain Res.* 2005;166(3-4):345-357.

Small DM, Scott TR. Symposium overview: what happens to the pontine processing? Repercussions of interspecies differences in pontine taste Representation for tasting and feeding. *Ann NY Acad Sci.* 2009;1170:343-346.

Small DM, Zald DH, Jones-Gotman M, et al. Human cortical gustatory areas: a review of functional neuroimaging data. *NeuroReport.* 1999;10(1):7-14.

Small DM, Zatorre RJ, Dagher A, Evans AC, Jones-Gotman M. Changes in brain activity related to eating chocolate: from pleasure to aversion. *Brain.* 2001;124:1720-1733.

Smith DV, Margolskee RF. Making sense of taste. *Sci Am.* 2001;284:32-39.

Stettler DD, Axel R. Representations of odor in the piriform cortex. *Neuron.* 2009;63(6):854-864.

Steward WB, Kauer JS, Shepherd GM. Functional organization of rat olfactory bulb, analyzed by the 2-deoxyglu-cose method. *J Comp Neurol.* 1979;185:715-734.

Su CY, Menuz K, Carlson JR. Olfactory perception: receptors, cells, and circuits. *Cell.* 2009;139(1):45-59.

Sweazey RD, Bradley RM. Response characteristics of lamb pontine neurons to stimulation of the oral cavity and epiglottis with different sensory modalities. *J Neurophysiol.* 1993;70:1168-1180.

Topolovec JC, Gati JS, Menon RS, Shoemaker JK, Cechetto DF. Human cardiovascular and gustatory brainstem sites observed by functional magnetic resonance imaging. *J Comp Neurol.* 2004;471(4):446-461.

Uesaka Y, Nose H, Ida M, Takagi A. The pathway of gustatory fibers of the human ascends ipsilaterally in the pons. *Neurology.* 1998;50:827-828.

Vassar R, Chao SK, Sticheran R, Nuñez JM, Vosshall LB, Axel R. Topographic organization of sensory projections to the olfactory bulb. *Cell.* 1994;79:981-991.

Vassar R, Ngai J, Axel R. Spatial organization of odorant receptor expression in the mammalian olfactory epithelium. *Cell.* 1993;74:309-318.

Vogt BA, Pandya DN, Rosene DL. Cingulate cortex of the rhesus monkey: I. Cytoarchitecture and thalamic afferents. *J Comp Neurol.* 1987;262:256-270.

Zou Z, Horowitz LF, Montmayeur JP, Snapper S, Buck LB. Genetic tracing reveals a stereotyped sensory map in the olfactory cortex. *Nature* 2001;414:173-179.

Zou DJ, Chesler A, Firestein S. How the olfactory bulb got its glomeruli: a just so story? *Nat Rev Neurosci.* 2009;10(8):611-618.

Study Questions

1. A patient with multiple sclerosis suddenly developed impaired taste sensation. An MRI revealed a lesion in the left pontine tegmentum. Which of the following statements best describes the distribution of taste loss on the tongue produced by the lesion?
   A. Left and right sides of tongue; anterior two thirds of each side
   B. Left and right sides of tongue; posterior one third of each side
   C. Left side of tongue, both anterior and posterior parts
   D. Right side of tongue, both anterior and posterior parts

2. Which of the following cranial nerves does not provide any gustatory innervation of the tongue and oral cavity?
   A. XII
   B. X
   C. IX
   D. VIII

3. The rostral solitary nucleus is to the caudal solitary nucleus, as
   A. taste is to smell
   B. taste is to touch
   C. taste is to pain
   D. taste is to visceral sensations

4. A patient with multiple sclerosis has focal demyelination in the pontine tegmentum that damages the ascending gustatory pathway. Which of the thalamic nuclei listed below would be most directly influenced by this demyelination?
   A. Ventral posterior lateral nucleus
   B. Ventral posterior medial nucleus
   C. Medial dorsal nucleus
   D. Ventral medial posterior nucleus

5. A patient has a seizure disorder and has gustatory hallucinations. Which of the following brain regions is most likely to be directly involved in these hallucinations?
   A. Parietal lobe
   B. Occipital lobe
   C. Frontal lobe
   D. Insular cortex

6. A 17-year-old man received a concussion playing football, as a result of a blow to his head. He noticed greatly diminished sense of smell after the incident. Progressively, over the next year, his sense of smell improved. Which of the following is a plausible explanation for the loss and subsequent partial recovery of olfaction?
   A. The axons in the olfactory tracts became damaged as they traveled through the cribriform plate when the concussion displaced the brain transiently. Over the next year, these axons regenerated, thereby restoring function.
   B. The axons of the primary olfactory neuron became damaged as they traveled through the cribriform plate when the concussion displaced the brain transiently. During the next year, these axons regenerated, thereby restoring function.

C. The concussion disrupted neurogenesis, and it takes many months for neurogenesis to return to normal.
   D. The concussion produced inflammation of the olfactory mucosa, thereby damaging primary olfactory neurons, which takes time to repair.

7. Which of the following is not a primary olfactory area?
   A. Piriform cortex
   B. Entorhinal cortex
   C. Insular cortex
   D. Amygdala

8. Which of the following provides the best estimate of the number of glomeruli that would express the gene for a particular olfactory receptor?
   A. 1
   B. 10
   C. 100
   D. 1000

9. Which of the listed components of the olfactory system is the target of migrating newborn neurons from the lateral ventricle wall?
   A. Olfactory cortical areas
   B. Anterior olfactory nucleus
   C. Olfactory tracts
   D. Olfactory bulb

10. Which of the following statements best describes how olfactory information is projected to the orbitofrontal cortex?
    A. Directly from the olfactory tract
    B. Directly from the anterior olfactory nucleus
    C. Directly from the piriform cortex
    D. Directly from the ventral posterior medial thalamic nucleus

MOTOR SYSTEMS

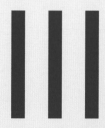

Chapter 10

Descending Motor Pathways and the Motor Function of the Spinal Cord

CLINICAL CASE | Spinal Cord Hemisection

A 21-year-old man suffered a gunshot injury. He was walking home from work with friends when he was hit by a stray bullet. He was unconscious when the ambulance arrived. When he regained consciousness in the emergency room, he reported that he was unable to move his right foot and that his right leg felt numb.

Neurological and radiological examination revealed that the bullet entered at about the mid-thoracic level. There was complete loss of right lower limb motor function and loss of tactile sensation (as well as other mechanosensations, including position sense and vibration sense), also on the right, at T10 and below. Pain sensation was examined with pin prick, and testing revealed an absence of pain on the left leg only, extending rostrally to T11. Figure 10–1A shows the distribution of sensory loss.

Answer the following questions based on your reading of this chapter, as well as review of Chapters 4 and 5 on mechanosensations and pain.

1. **Why are pain and tactile sensations impaired on opposite sides of the body?**

2. **Why does the patient have preserved pain but not touch sensation over the T11 dermatome?**

3. **Explain why the leg on the side with the tactile sensation impairment is paralyzed, but not paralyzed on the side without pain?**

—Continued next page

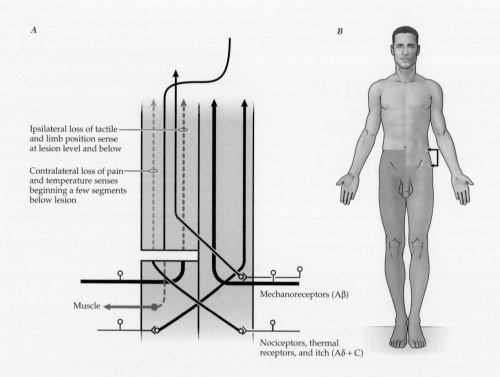

Ipsilateral loss of tactile and limb position sense at lesion level and below

Contralateral loss of pain and temperature senses beginning a few segments below lesion

Muscle

Mechanoreceptors (Aβ)

Nociceptors, thermal receptors, and itch (Aδ + C)

FIGURE 10–1 Spinal hemisection produces paralysis and a loss of mechanosensations caudal to, and on the same side as, the lesion. This injury produces a loss of pain, temperature, and itch caudal to, and on the opposite side as, the lesion **A.** Circuit changes associated with spinal cord hemisection. **B.** Pattern of somatic sensory loss in the patient. Pain is lost on his left side (orange); tactile sensations are lost on the right side (green). Three key pathways are affected. (1) The mechanoreceptive pathway, the dorsal columns, is interrupted ipsilateral to its origin. (2) The pain pathway, the anterolateral system, is interrupted contralateral to its origin. (3) The motor pathway, the corticospinal tract, is interrupted ipsilateral to its target motor neurons and muscle.

Key neurological signs and corresponding damaged structures

Alternate distributions for pain and tactile sensory loss

The lesion damages two distinct populations of ascending somatic sensory fibers. Damaged ascending pain fibers ascend to the lesion site after crossing the midline caudal to the lesion. Damaged ascending tactile fibers ascend to the lesion site without decussating; they cross the midline rostral to the lesion, in the medulla. By following the pain and tactile circuits back to their origins in the periphery, the different sides of sensory loss are revealed.

Preserved pain sense one to two segments caudal to tactile loss

Pain is perceived down to a more caudal level than tactile stimuli. Pain fibers cross the midline over multiple spinal

levels (ie, they cross as they ascend). The first pain fibers to become damaged have entered the spinal cord one to two segments below the lesion (Figure 10–1A; see also Figure 5–1). Pain fibers entering at the level of the injury will bypass the lesion. It should be noted that the spinal injury can damage entering primary afferents themselves, and the nearby dorsal horn, and would be expected to produce a small amount of sensory loss just at the dermatomal level on the side of the lesion. However, because of dermatomal overlap (see Figure 4–5), this will be minimized and may even go unnoticed.

Ipsilateral motor and tactile loss

The corticospinal tract decussates in the medulla (see Figure 10–4A). For this reason, the lesion interrupts the descending pathway controlling muscles on the same side (Figure 10–1A).

The motor systems of the brain and spinal cord work together to control body movements. These systems must fulfill diverse tasks because the functions of the muscles of the body differ markedly. Consider, for instance, the fine control required of hand muscles when grasping a china cup, in contrast to the gross strength required of back and leg muscles in lifting a box full of books. The muscles that move the eyes have an entirely different set of tasks, such as positioning the eyes to capture information from the visual world. The principal function of facial muscles is not movement but rather creating facial expressions as well as assisting in speech articulation. These jobs are so varied that it is not surprising that the motor systems have many specific components devoted to the control of different motor functions.

The motor systems are clinically very important because damage, depending on the location and severity, produces wide-ranging impairments in strength, volition, and coordination. Profound weakness or paralysis after a stroke or a traumatic spinal cord injury limits an injured person's capacity for independence. Disordered coordination can make control of simple daily activities, such as tying a knot or eating, impossible, requiring assistance by a care giver. Defective eye movement control can impair cognitive functions, such as a reduced capacity to read text or discern the locations of objects.

The first three motor system chapters examine the components that connect higher control centers with motor neurons; these motor systems are essential for contracting muscle. This chapter focuses on the neuroanatomy of descending spinal cord pathways and spinal cord circuits for limb control and posture. Next, the pathways that control facial and other head muscles are discussed in Chapter 11. Because eye movement and balance share many neural circuits, and a strong interrelationship with the vestibular system, these topics are covered jointly in Chapter 12. The last two motor system chapters focus on important behavioral integrative centers: the cerebellum (Chapter 13) and basal ganglia (Chapter 14).

Functional Anatomy of the Motor Systems for Limb Control and Posture

Diverse Central Nervous System Structures Comprise the Motor Systems

Four separate components of the central nervous system together control skeletal muscles of the limbs and trunk muscles for posture (Figure 10–2): (1) descending motor pathways, together with their associated origins in the cerebral cortex and brain stem, (2) spinal motor circuits, including motor neurons and interneurons, (3) basal ganglia (yellow), and (4) the cerebellum.

The regions of the cerebral cortex and brain stem that contribute to the **descending motor pathways** are organized much like the ascending sensory pathways but in reverse: from the cerebral cortex or brain stem to the muscles of our limbs and trunk. The brain stem motor pathways engage in relatively automatic control, such as rapid postural adjustments and in-flight correction of misdirected movements. By contrast, the cortical motor pathways participate in more refined, flexible, and adaptive control, such as reaching to objects, grasping, and tool use.

Motor neurons and **interneurons** comprise the spinal motor circuits, the second component of the limb and posture control systems. The motor pathways synapse directly on motor neurons as well as on interneurons that in turn synapse on motor neurons (Figure 10–2). For muscles of the limbs and trunk, motor neurons and most interneurons are found in the **ventral horn** and **intermediate zone** of the spinal cord (Figure 10–3). The intermediate zone corresponds primarily to the spinal gray matter lateral to the central canal. It is sometimes included within the ventral horn. For muscles of the head, including facial muscles, the motor neurons and interneurons are located in the **cranial nerve motor nuclei** and the **reticular formation** (see Chapter 11). The spinal motor circuits are not only the target of the descending motor pathways but also can function relatively independently through their reflexive and intrinsic motor actions. The simplest reflex is the monosynaptic stretch reflex (see Figure 2–6). More complex, polysynaptic, reflexes produce automatic limb withdrawal from a noxious stimulus as well as postural reflexes. Stepping patterns are organized by spinal circuits within the lumbar and sacral segments. When motor pathways synapse directly on motor neurons, they are able to activate individual muscles and even groups of muscle fibers within a muscle. This is because a single motor neuron connects to a limited set of fibers within one muscle, termed the *motor unit*. By connecting to interneurons in spinal circuits, a motor pathway is able to regulate motor reflex actions. For example, if you grasp an unexpectedly hot teacup that is a family heirloom, you may not want to reflexively release your grip, for risk of breaking the cup. Activating muscles through interneurons, rather than more directly through motor neurons, may also enable a motor pathway to select a group of muscles that have a complex behavioral action, such as stepping.

The third and fourth components of the motor systems, the **cerebellum** and the **basal ganglia** (Figure 10–2; see Chapters 13 and 14), do not contain neurons that project directly to spinal motor circuits. Nevertheless, these structures have a powerful regulatory influence over motor behavior. They act indirectly in controlling motor behavior through their effects on the descending brain stem pathways and, via the thalamus, cortical pathways (Figure 10–2). The specific contributions of the cerebellum and basal ganglia to movement control are surprisingly elusive despite centuries of study. The cerebellum is part of a set of neural circuits for ensuring that movements are precise and accurate. However, this description only captures a small part of cerebellar function; the cerebellum has additional nonmotor functions. The specific contributions of the basal ganglia to normal motor action are largely unknown. However, we are well aware of how movements become disordered when the basal ganglia are damaged. For example, in patients with Parkinson disease, a neurodegenerative disease that primarily affects the basal ganglia, movements are slow or fail to be initiated and patients have significant tremor. Like the cerebellum, the basal ganglia have many nonmotor functions.

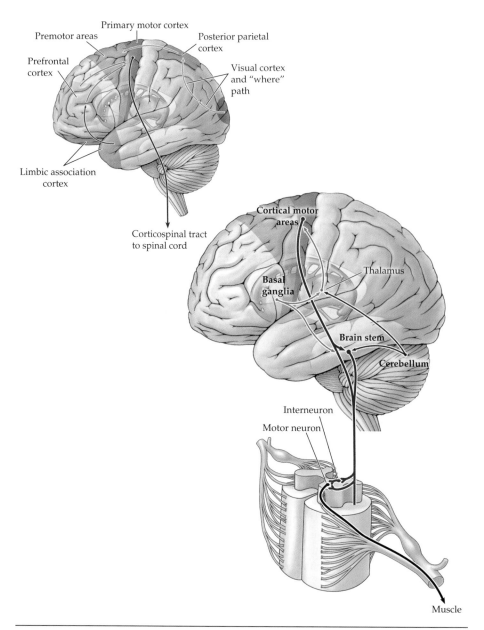

FIGURE 10–2 General organization of the motor systems. **Center.** General organization of the motor systems. There are four major components to the motor systems: descending cortical and brain stem pathways, motor neurons and interneurons of the spinal cord, basal ganglia, and cerebellum. Both the basal ganglia and cerebellum influence movements through connections to the cortical and brain stem motor pathways. **Upper inset.** Key cortical regions for controlling movement. The limbic and prefrontal association areas are involved in the initial decision to move, in relation to motivational and emotional factors. In reaching to grasp an object, the visual areas process information about the location and shape of the object. This information is transmitted, via the "where" or "action" path first to the posterior parietal lobe, and then to the premotor areas, which are important in movement planning. From there, information is transmitted to the primary motor cortex, from which descending control signals are sent to the motor neurons.

Many Cortical Regions Are Recruited Into Action During Visually Guided Movements

Myriad areas of the cerebral cortex provide the motor systems with information essential for making accurate movements. For example, during visually guided movements—such as reaching to grasp a cup—the process of translating thoughts and sensations into action begins with the initial decision to move. This process is dependent on the cortical **limbic** and **prefrontal association areas** (Figure 10–2; brain inset upper left), which are involved in emotions, motivation, and cognition. The **magnocellular visual system** processes visual information about the locations of objects for guiding movements.

It provides the major visual input to the "where" or "action" pathway (Figure 10-2, inset; see Figures 7–15 and 7–16). The magnocellular visual system projects to the **posterior parietal cortex,** an area important for identifying the location of salient objects in the environment and for directing our attention to these objects (Figure 10–2). Visual information next is distributed to certain **premotor areas** of the frontal lobe, where the plan of action to reach for the cup is formed, a plan that specifies the path the hand takes to reach the object and prepares the hand for grasping or manipulation once contact occurs. The next step in translating into action the decision to reach is directing muscles to contract. This step primarily involves the **corticospinal tract,** which originates from both the premotor areas and the **primary motor cortex.** The corticospinal tract transmits control signals to motor neurons and to interneurons (Figure 10–2). The cortical motor pathways also recruit brain stem pathways for coordinating voluntary movements with postural adjustments (Figure 10–2), such as maintaining balance when lifting a heavy object.

Functional Anatomy of the Descending Motor Pathways

Descending pathways serve a diversity of functions. We recognize their principal function in controlling movements because when they become damaged, people become weak or paralyzed. However, in addition to movement control, the descending pathways regulate somatic sensory processing and the autonomic nervous system. Whereas the motor control functions are mediated by synaptic connections with motor neurons and interneurons, the somatic sensory functions are associated with connections on dorsal horn neurons and somatic sensory relay nuclei in the brain stem. We have already learned about one somatic sensory regulatory function: the pain suppression function of the raphespinal pathway (see Chapter 5). The descending pathways synapse on preganglionic autonomic neurons in the brain stem and spinal cord to regulate autonomic nervous system functions. The autonomic control pathways are examined in Chapter 15 with the autonomic nervous system. Finally, the descending pathways also can influence plasticity of spinal circuits during motor learning and have important trophic functions during development. The pathways from the cerebral cortex serve all of these functions. It is not known if the same applies to all of the brain stem pathways. Here we will focus on the motor control functions of the descending pathways.

Multiple Parallel Motor Control Pathways Originate From the Cortex and Brain Stem

Seven major descending motor control pathways terminate in motor centers of the brain stem and spinal cord (Table 10–1). Three of these pathways originate in layer V of the cerebral cortex, primarily in the frontal lobe: (1) the **lateral corticospinal tract,** (2) the **ventral** (or **anterior**) **corticospinal tract,** and (3) the **corticobulbar tract.** The corticobulbar tract terminates primarily in cranial motor nuclei in the pons and medulla and is the cranial equivalent of the corticospinal tracts; it will be considered in Chapter 11. Collectively, these cortical pathways participate in controlling the most adaptive and flexible movements, such as finger control during tool use, regulating posture during limb movements, and during speech. The remaining four pathways originate from brain stem nuclei: (4) the **rubrospinal tract,** involved in automatic limb control; (5) the **reticulospinal tracts,** which participate in automatic control of proximal muscles and locomotion; (6) the **tectospinal tract,** involved in coordinating head movements with eye movements; and (7) the **vestibulospinal tracts,** critical for maintaining balance. There are also neurotransmitter-specific descending pathways (see Chapter 2) that originate from the serotonergic raphe nuclei, noradrenergic locus ceruleus, and dopaminergic neurons of the midbrain and diencephalon, all of which have extensive spinal cord terminations. In addition to pain regulation, the actions of these descending pathways can rapidly regulate both the strength of muscle contraction and reflexes.

Three Rules Govern the Logic of the Organization of the Descending Motor Pathways

How are the actions of the myriad descending motor pathways coordinated during movement? What is the logic of their organization? By taking a combined clinical, anatomical, and physiological perspective, three principles governing the organization of the motor pathways emerge.

The functional organization of the descending pathways parallels the somatotopic organization of the motor nuclei in the ventral horn

The motor neurons innervating **limb muscles,** and the interneurons from which they receive input, are located in the **lateral ventral horn** and **intermediate zone.** In contrast, motor neurons innervating **axial and girdle muscles** (ie, neck and shoulder muscles), and their associated interneurons, are located in the **medial ventral horn** and **intermediate zone.** The mediolateral somatotopic organization of the intermediate zone and ventral horn is easy to remember because it mimics the form of the body (Figure 10–3). This mediolateral somatotopic organization also applies to the location of the descending motor pathways in the spinal cord white matter (discussed in detail below). The pathways that descend in the lateral portion of the spinal cord white matter control limb muscles. In contrast, the pathways that descend in the medial portion of the white matter control axial and girdle muscles.

Movements are controlled by direct cortical projections to the spinal cord and indirect cortical projections via brain stem nuclei

The lateral and ventral corticospinal tracts can control spinal circuits through their direct spinal projections. In addition, the cortical motor regions project to brain stem nuclei that give

Table **10–1** Descending pathways for controlling movement

Tract	Site of origin	Decussation	Spinal cord column	Site of termination	Spinal/brain stem level of termination	Function
Cerebral Cortex Corticospinal						
Lateral	Areas 6, 4, 1, 2, 3, 5, 7, 23	Crossed—pyramidal Decussation	Lateral	Dorsal horn, intermediate zone, ventral horn	All levels	Sensory control, voluntary movement (limb muscles)
Ventral	Areas 6, 4	Uncrossed[1]	Ventral	Intermediate zone, ventral horn	Upper cervical	Voluntary movement (axial muscles)
Corticobulbar	Areas 6, 4, 1, 2, 3, 5, 7, 23	Crossed and uncrossed[2]	Brain stem only	Cranial nerve sensory and motor nuclei, reticular formation	Midbrain, pons, medulla	Sensory control, voluntary movement (cranial muscles)
Brain Stem						
Rubrospinal	Red nucleus (magnocellular)	Ventral tegmentum	Lateral	Lateral intermediate zone, ventral horn	All levels	Voluntary movement, limb muscles
Vestibulospinal						
Lateral	Lateral vestibular nucleus	Ipsilateral[1]	Ventral	Medial intermediate zone, ventral horn	All levels	Balance
Medial	Medial vestibular nucleus	Bilateral	Ventral	Medial intermediate zone, ventral horn	Upper cervical	Head position/neck muscles
Reticulospinal						
Pontine	Pontine reticular formation	Ipsilateral[1]	Ventral	Medial intermediate horn, ventral horn	All levels	Automatic movement, axial, and limb muscles
Medullary	Medullary reticular formation	Ipsilateral[1]	Ventrolateral	Medial intermediate zone, ventral horn	All levels	Automatic movement, axial, and limb muscles
Tectospinal	Deep superior colliculus	Dorsal tegmentum	Ventral	Medial intermediate zone, ventral horn	Upper cervical	Coordinates neck with eye movements
Indirect Cortical Pathways						
Coritcorubrospinal	Frontal lobe → red nucleus					
Corticoreticular	Frontal lobe → reticular formation					
Corticovestibular	Parietal lobe → vestibular nuclei					

[1]Whereas these tracts descend ipsilaterally, they terminate on interneurons whose axons decussate in the ventral commissure and thus influence axial musculature bilaterally.

[2]Most of the projections to the cranial nerve motor nuclei are bilateral; those to the part of the facial nucleus that innervates upper facial muscles are bilateral, and those to the lower facial muscles are contralateral (see Chapter 11).

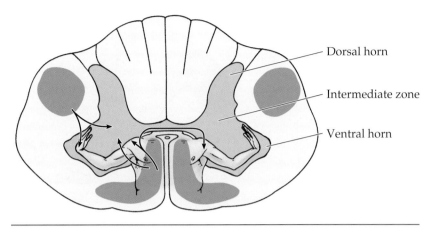

FIGURE 10-3 Somatotopic organization of the ventral horn and motor pathways. Schematic diagram of the spinal cord, showing the somatotopic organization of the ventral horn and indicating the general locations of motor neurons innervating limb and axial muscles and flexor and extensor muscles. A partial homunculus is superimposed on the ventral horns. (Adapted from Crosby EC, Humphrey T, Lauer EW. *Correlative Anatomy of the Nervous System.* New York, NY: Macmillan; 1962.)

rise to motor pathways: the red nucleus, superior colliculus, reticular formation, and vestibular nuclei. This is shown in Figure 10–2 (center) as an arrow connecting the cortical pathway with the brain stem. Thus, the cerebral cortex can also influence movements through indirect brain stem connections. For example, the two components of the **corticoreticulo-spinal pathway** are the cortical projection to particular nuclei of the reticular formation and then the reticulospinal tract's projection to the spinal cord. Considering all combinations of pathways, the projection neurons of the cerebral cortex constitute the highest level in the hierarchy, the brain stem projection neurons comprise the next lower level, and spinal interneurons and the motor neurons are the two lowest levels. Study of patients with motor pathway damage suggests that direct spinal connections mediate more precise joint control, such as our ability to move one finger independent of the others (termed fractionated control), whereas the indirect connections serve coarser control functions, such as moving all fingers together during a powerful grasp. Can brain stem motor pathways work independent of the cortical pathways? The answer is probably yes, based on laboratory animal studies. Both the cerebellum and basal ganglia have direct connections with brain stem motor pathways (Figure 10–2), which could influence brain stem motor pathway function without cortex involvement. A challenge for promoting recovery of motor function after cortical damage, such as a stroke, is to foster a more effective independent brain stem control.

There are monosynaptic and polysynaptic connections between the motor pathways and motor neurons

Typically the axon of a descending projection neuron, in addition to making monosynaptic connections with motoneurons, makes monosynaptic connections with spinal cord interneurons (Figure 10–2, bottom). Depending on the particular

interneuron type (see Figure 10–16A), the interneurons have different functions. Some interneurons receive input from somatic sensory receptors for the reflex control of movement. For example, particular interneurons receive input from nociceptors and mediate limb withdrawal reflexes in response to painful stimuli, such as when you jerk your hand away from a hot stove. Other interneurons coordinate the left-right limb motor actions during walking, while others still are important for upper limb-lower limb coordination.

Two Laterally Descending Pathways Control Limb Muscles

The lateral corticospinal tract and the rubrospinal tract (Table 10–1) are the two lateral motor pathways. The neurons that give rise to these pathways have a **somatotopic** organization. Moreover, the lateral corticospinal and rubrospinal tracts control muscles on the **contralateral** side of the body. The **lateral corticospinal tract** is the principal motor control pathway in humans. A lesion of this pathway anywhere along its path to the motor neuron, such as after a stroke in the subcortical white matter, produces devastating and persistent limb use impairments. Box 10–1 discusses the major changes in motor and reflex function after damage to the corticospinal system. There is a loss of voluntary control and weakness, termed paresis, that can make standing impossible without assistance. There is also a loss of the ability to move one finger independent of the others, which is termed **fractionation.** Manual dexterity depends on fractionation, without which hand movements are clumsy and imprecise. Loss of corticospinal tract control after stroke is the most common cause of paralysis.

The major site of origin of the lateral corticospinal tract is the primary motor cortex (Figure 10–4A, inset), although axons also originate from the premotor cortical regions (supplementary motor area, cingulate motor area, and premotor

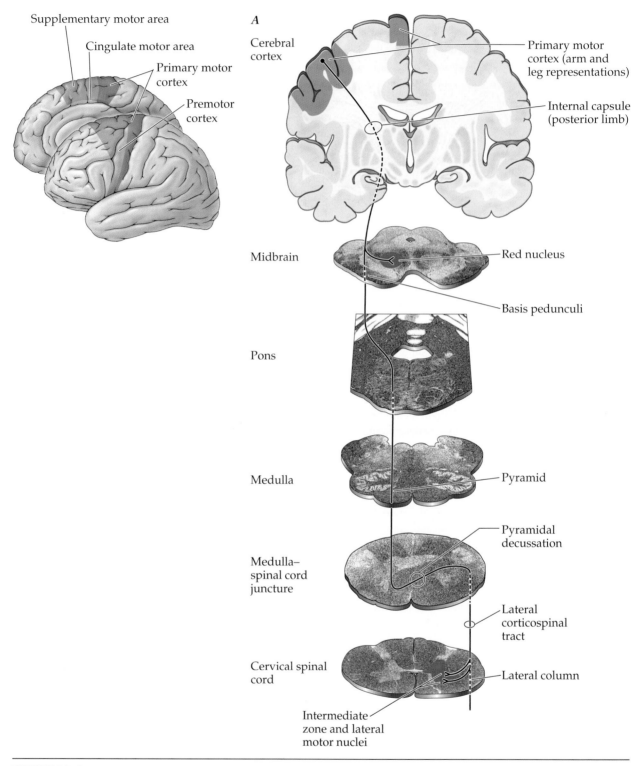

FIGURE 10–4 Laterally descending pathways. **A**. Lateral corticospinal tract. The inset shows the locations of the primary motor cortex and three premotor areas: the supplementary motor area, the cingulate motor areas, and the premotor cortex. The lateral corticospinal tract also originates from neurons located in area 6 and the parietal lobe. Note the branch into the red nucleus; this is the corticorubro component of the indirect corticorubrospinal path.

B

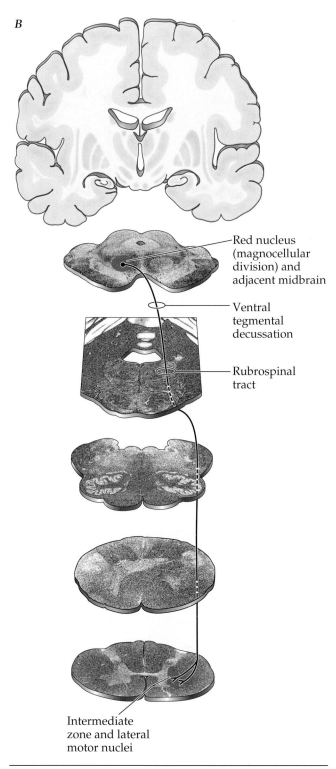

Red nucleus (magnocellular division) and adjacent midbrain

Ventral tegmental decussation

Rubrospinal tract

Intermediate zone and lateral motor nuclei

*Continued—*FIGURE 10–4 *B*. Rubrospinal tract.

cortex) and the somatic sensory cortical areas. Descending axons in the tract that originate in the primary motor cortex course within the cerebral hemisphere in the **posterior limb of the internal capsule** and, in the midbrain, in the **basis pedunculi** (Figure 10–4A). Next on its descending course, the tract disappears beneath the ventral surface of the pons

only to reappear on the ventral surface of the medulla as the **pyramid.** At the junction of the spinal cord and medulla, most of the axons **decussate** (pyramidal decussation) and descend in the dorsolateral portion of the lateral column of the spinal cord white matter; hence the name lateral corticospinal tract (see Figure 10–6). This pathway terminates primarily in the lateral portions of the intermediate zone and ventral horn of the cervical and lumbosacral cord, the locations of neurons that control the arm and leg. There is a contingent of axons that terminate on the ipsilateral side. Some of these axons descend ipsilaterally; many descend contralaterally and re-cross the midline within the gray matter in lamina 10. The function of these ipsilateral axons is not well understood. After unilateral damage to the lateral corticospinal tract, the ipsilaterally terminating axons may contribute to recovery of some motor functions.

The **rubrospinal tract** (Figure 10–4B), which has fewer axons overall than the corticospinal tract, originates from neurons in the **red nucleus,** primarily from the caudal part. This portion is termed the **magnocellular division** because many rubrospinal tract neurons are large. The rubrospinal tract decussates in the midbrain and descends in the dorsolateral portion of the brain stem. Similar to the lateral corticospinal tract, the rubrospinal tract is found in the dorsal portion of the lateral column (see Figure 10–6) and terminates primarily in the lateral portions of the intermediate zone and ventral horn of the cervical cord. In humans, the rubrospinal tract does not descend into the lumbosacral cord, suggesting that it functions in arm but not leg control.

Four Medially Descending Pathways Control Axial and Girdle Muscles to Regulate Posture

Axial and girdle muscles are controlled primarily by the four medially descending pathways: the ventral corticospinal tract, the reticulospinal tracts, the tectospinal tract, and the vestibulospinal tracts (Table 10–1). The medial descending pathways exert **bilateral control** over axial and girdle muscles. Even though individual pathways may project unilaterally (either ipsilaterally or contralaterally), they synapse on commissural interneurons whose axons decussate in the spinal cord. Bilateral control provides a measure of redundancy: Unilateral lesion of a bilateral pathway typically does not have a profound effect on proximal muscle control because the same pathway from the undamaged side of the brain has the same bilateral spinal termination pattern.

The **ventral corticospinal tract** originates from the **primary motor cortex** and the various **premotor areas** (including supplementary motor area, cingulate motor area, and premotor cortex) and descends to the medulla along with the lateral corticospinal tract (Figure 10–5A). However, the ventral corticospinal tract remains uncrossed and descends in the ipsilateral ventral column of the spinal cord (Figures 10–5 and 10–6). Many ventral corticospinal tract axons have branches that decussate in the spinal cord, similar to the re-crossed lateral

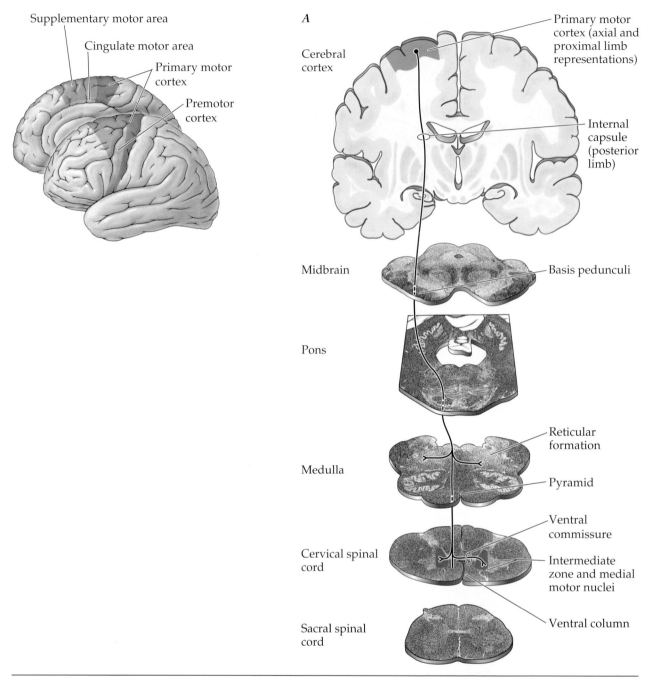

Supplementary motor area

Cingulate motor area

Primary motor cortex

Premotor cortex

A

Cerebral cortex

Primary motor cortex (axial and proximal limb representations)

Internal capsule (posterior limb)

Midbrain

Basis pedunculi

Pons

Medulla

Reticular formation

Pyramid

Cervical spinal cord

Ventral commissure

Intermediate zone and medial motor nuclei

Sacral spinal cord

Ventral column

FIGURE 10–5 Medially descending pathways. **A**. Ventral corticospinal tract. The inset shows the locations of the primary motor cortex and three premotor areas: the supplementary motor area, the cingulate motor areas, and the premotor cortex.

corticospinal tract axons described earlier. This tract terminates in the medial gray matter, synapsing on motor neurons in the medial ventral horn and on interneurons in the intermediate zone. The ventral corticospinal tract projects only to the cervical and upper thoracic spinal cord; thus, it is preferentially involved in the control of the neck, shoulder, and upper trunk muscles.

The **reticulospinal tracts** (Figure 10–5B) originate from different regions of the **pontine and medullary reticular formation.** The pontine reticulospinal tract descends in the ventral column of the spinal cord, whereas the medullary reticulospinal tract descends in the ventrolateral quadrant of the lateral column (Figure 10–6). The reticulospinal tracts descend predominantly in the ipsilateral spinal cord but exert bilateral motor control effects. Laboratory animal studies show that the reticulospinal tracts control relatively automatic movements, such as maintaining posture or walking over even terrain.

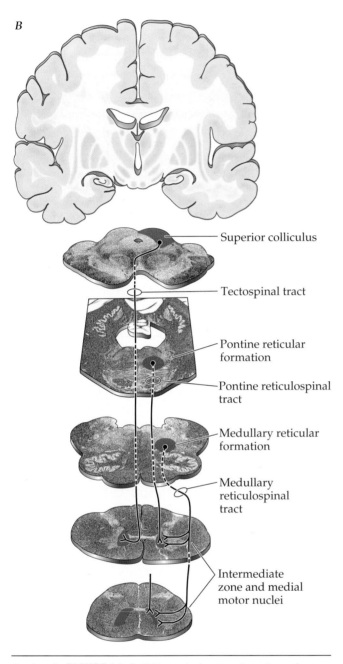

*Continued—***FIGURE 10–5** *B*. Tectospinal tract and pontine and medullary reticulospinal tracts.

The **vestibulospinal tracts** (see Figure 12–3) are essential for maintaining balance. They receive their principal input from the vestibular organs (see Figures 12–2 and 12–8). Originating in the vestibular nuclei of the medulla and pons, the vestibulospinal tracts descend in the ventromedial spinal white matter. There are separate medial and lateral vestibulospinal tracts. The medial vestibulospinal tract only projects to the upper cervical spinal cord and is important in coordinating head movements with eye movements. By contrast, the lateral vestibulospinal tract projects throughout the full length of the spinal cord to control all axial and proximal muscles.

Note that despite its name, the lateral vestibulospinal tract is a medial descending motor pathway. These paths are considered in Chapter 12, along with eye and head movement control.

The **tectospinal tract** (Figure 10–5B) originates primarily from neurons located in the deeper layers of the superior colliculus, which is also termed the **tectum,** the portion of the midbrain dorsal to the cerebral aqueduct (see Figure 10–11A). The tectospinal tract also has a limited rostrocaudal distribution, projecting only to the cervical spinal segments. It therefore participates primarily in the control of neck, shoulder, and upper trunk muscles. Because the superior colliculus also plays a key role in controlling eye movements (see Chapter 12), the tectospinal tract contributes to coordinating head movements with eye movements.

The various descending pathways in the spinal cord are illustrated on the right side of Figure 10–6; the ascending somatic sensory pathways (see Chapters 4 and 5) are illustrated on the left side. The two spinocerebellar pathways, which transmit somatic sensory information to the cerebellum for controlling movement not perception (see Chapter 13), also are illustrated.

Regional Anatomy of the Motor Systems and the Descending Motor Pathways

The rest of this chapter examines the brain and spinal cord with the aim of understanding the motor pathways and their spinal terminations. This discussion begins with the cerebral cortex—the highest level of the movement control hierarchy—and proceeds caudally to the spinal cord, following the natural flow of information processing in the motor systems.

The Cortical Motor Areas Are Located in the Frontal Lobe

Similar to each sensory modality, multiple cortical areas serve motor control functions (Figure 10–7). Four separate motor areas have been identified in the frontal lobe: the primary motor cortex and three premotor areas—the supplementary motor area, the premotor cortex, and the cingulate motor area. These areas are anatomically and functionally different. Each has several distinct subregions. All together, there are more than one dozen distinct cortical motor areas. These frontal motor areas all receive input from the **ventral lateral** and **ventral anterior thalamic nuclei** (see Figure 2–14), but to varying extents. The ventral lateral nucleus is the principal thalamic relay nucleus for the cerebellum and the ventral anterior nucleus, for the basal ganglia. These nuclei have complex subdivisions and the nomenclature used for animal studies—where connections are defined precisely—differs from that used to describe the human thalamus, where neurosurgical procedures are done.

Box 10–1

Lesions of the Descending Cortical Pathway in the Brain and Spinal Cord Produce Flaccid Paralysis Followed by Changes in Spinal Reflex Function

Lesions involving the posterior limb of the internal capsule, ventral brain stem, and spinal cord isolate motor neurons from voluntary motor control signals transmitted by the descending motor pathways. This produces a common set of motor signs. Initially these signs include **flaccid paralysis** and **reduced muscle reflexes** (eg, knee-jerk reflex). Clinical examination also reveals **decreased muscle tone,** signaled by the marked reduction in resistance felt by the examiner to passive movement of the limb. These are the classic signs of weakness and, if sufficiently severe, paralysis. These signs are attributable largely to interruption of the corticospinal fibers even though the corticoreticular and corticopontine fibers are damaged. The laterality of the signs depends on whether the lesion occurs in the brain or the spinal cord. Spinal cord injury is particularly devastating because all muscles of the body caudal to the level of injury can become affected.

With time after the lesion, a similar examination often reveals **increased muscle tone** and exaggerated muscle stretch (or myotatic) reflexes, termed **hyperreflexia.** The increased muscle tone is due to increased reflex activity when the examiner passively stretches the limb. It is not known what causes hyperreflexia; the cause may not be the same after all types of injury. It has been suggested that damage of the indirect corticoreticular pathway may lead to a loss of inhibitory signals to reflex centers in the

spinal cord. This could lead to an increase in reflexes, through disinhibition. Long-term synaptic plasticity of spinal reflex circuits may also play an important role in the delayed time course of this effect. After spinal cord injury, or damage to descending pathways, motor neurons change their intrinsic properties and become more excitable.

In addition to producing hyperreflexia, lesions of the corticospinal tract result in the emergence of abnormal reflexes, the most notable of which is **Babinski's sign.** This sign involves extension (also termed dorsiflexion) of the big toe in response to scratching the lateral margin and then the ball of the foot (but not the toes). Babinski's sign is thought to be a withdrawal reflex. Normally such withdrawal of the big toe is produced by scratching the toe's ventral surface. After damage to the descending cortical fibers, the reflex can be evoked from a much larger area than normal. Interestingly, the Babinski's sign is normally present in young children, before maturation of the corticospinal tract. **Hoffmann's sign,** which is thumb adduction in response to flexion of the distal phalanx of the third digit, is an example of an abnormal upper limb reflex caused by damage to the descending cortical fibers. Vascular lesions are a common cause of damage to the descending motor pathways, thereby affecting both direct and indirect corticospinal projections (see Clinical Case, Chapter 11).

Until specific functions can be ascribed to the various nuclei, it is best to consider them simply and collectively as the motor thalamus. Additionally, some of the premotor areas receive information from the medial dorsal nucleus, which serves more integrative and cognitive functions.

The premotor cortical regions integrate information from diverse sources

The premotor cortical areas receive information from parietal, prefrontal, and other motor areas and, in turn, use this information to help plan movements. Whereas damage to the

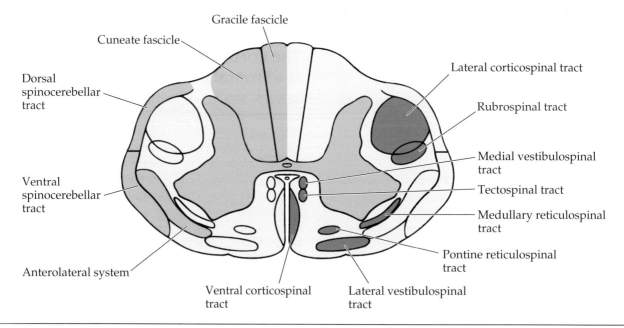

FIGURE 10–6 Schematic diagram of the spinal cord, indicating the locations of the ascending (***left***) and descending (***right***) pathways.

primary motor cortex produces weakness and incoordination, premotor damage produces **apraxias,** a motor planning disorder in which there is a loss of the ability to produce learned purposeful movements, even though the person is physically capable of making the movement. The **supplementary motor area** is located primarily on the medial surface of the cerebral hemisphere, in area 6 (Figure 10–7). Its specific contribution to movement control has not been identified, although research shows it may be important in planning bimanual movements. The **premotor cortex** is located laterally in area 6 (Figure 10–7A). The premotor cortex has at least two distinct motor fields with separate sets of connections and distinctive functions: the dorsal and ventral premotor cortices; each area is further functionally subdivided. The dorsal premotor cortex uses visual information from the external world around us to help control reaching. By contrast, the ventral premotor cortex uses visual information about objects of interest for grasping. Surprisingly, this ventral subregion becomes active not only when we move, but also when we watch others move. Animal studies show that it contains **mirror neurons,** which discharge action potentials when an animal makes a movement and when the animal watches someone else perform the same movement. The ventral premotor cortex may also be important in understanding the meaning of movements and in learning by imitation. The **cingulate motor areas** are found on the medial surface of the cerebral hemisphere, in cytoarchitectonic areas 6, 23, and 24, deep within the cingulate sulcus (Figure 10–7B). Curiously, the cingulate motor areas are located in a cortical region that is considered part of the **limbic system,** which is important for emotions. Although its function is not yet elucidated, this motor area may play a role in motor behaviors that occur in response to emotions and drives.

The primary motor cortex gives rise to most of the fibers of the corticospinal tract

The primary motor cortex, cytoarchitectonic area 4, receives input from three major sources: the premotor cortical regions, the somatic sensory areas (in the parietal lobe), and the motor thalamic nuclei. The cytoarchitecture of the primary motor cortex is different from that of sensory areas in the parietal, temporal, and occipital lobes (see Figure 2–19). Whereas the sensory areas have a thick layer IV and a thin layer V, the primary motor cortex has a thin layer IV and a thick layer V. Recall that layer IV is the principal input layer of the cerebral cortex, where most of the axons from the thalamic relay nuclei terminate, and that layer V is the layer from which descending projections originate (see Figure 2–17). In the primary motor cortex, thalamic axons terminate in most of the cortical layers.

The primary motor cortex, like the somatic sensory cortex (see Chapters 4 and 5), is somatotopically organized (Figure 10–8A). Somatotopy in the primary motor cortex can be revealed by **transcranial magnetic stimulation,** a noninvasive method for activating cortical neurons, or by functional imaging, such as functional magnetic resonance imaging (fMRI) (see Chapter 2). Regions controlling facial muscles (through projections to the cranial nerve motor nuclei; see Chapter 11) are located in the lateral portion of the precentral gyrus, close to the lateral sulcus. Regions controlling other body parts are—from the lateral side of the cerebral cortex to the medial side—neck, arm, and trunk areas. The leg and foot areas are found primarily on the medial surface of the brain. The motor representation in the precentral gyrus forms the **motor homunculus;** it is distorted in a similar way as the **sensory homunculus** of the postcentral gyrus (see Figure 4–9). Arm and leg areas contribute preferentially to the lateral corticospinal tract, and neck, shoulder, and trunk regions to the ventral corticospinal tract (Figure 10–8B). The face area of the primary motor cortex projects to the cranial nerve motor nuclei and thus contributes axons to the corticobulbar projection (see Chapter 11). Interestingly, stimulation of premotor cortical areas rarely produces a movement. Rather, it disrupts the production of an ongoing movement, suggesting that the stimulus altered ongoing firing of neurons important for movement planning.

The Projection From Cortical Motor Regions Passes Through the Internal Capsule En Route to the Brain Stem and Spinal Cord

The **corona radiata** is the portion of the subcortical white matter that contains descending cortical axons and ascending thalamocortical axons (Figure 10–9A). The corona radiata is superficial to the **internal capsule,** which contains approximately the same set of axons but is flanked by the deep nuclei of the basal ganglia and thalamus (see Figure 2–15). The internal capsule is shaped like a curved fan (Figure 10–9A), with three main parts: (1) the rostral component, termed the **anterior limb,** (2) the caudal component, termed the **posterior limb,** and (3) the **genu** (Latin for "knee"), which joins the two limbs (Figures 10–9A). The anterior limb is rostral to the thalamus, and the posterior limb is lateral to the thalamus (Figure 10–9C).

Each cortical motor area sends its axons into a slightly different part of the corona radiata and internal capsule. Within the internal capsule, the descending motor projection from the primary motor cortex to the spinal cord courses in the posterior part of the posterior limb. The location of this projection is revealed in an MRI scan from a patient with a small lesion confined to the posterior limb of the internal capsule (Figure 10–9B). The pathway can be seen in this scan because degenerating axons produce a different magnetic resonance signal from that of normal axons. Retrograde degeneration can be followed back toward the cortex, and anterograde degeneration can be followed into the brain stem. The approximate location of the corticospinal projection in the posterior limb is shown in Figure 10–9C (labeled A, T, and L, for projections controlling muscles of the arm, trunk, and leg). The projection to the caudal brain stem, via the corticobulbar tract, descends rostral to the corticospinal fibers in the genu and posterior limb. Clinically, sufficient numbers

A

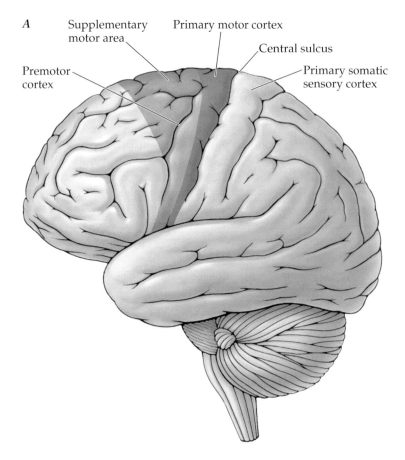

B

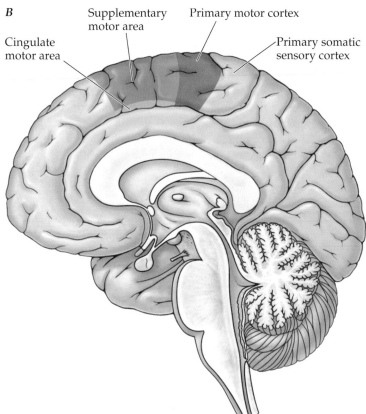

FIGURE 10–7 Lateral (***A***) and medial (***B***) views of the human brain, indicating the locations of the primary motor cortex, premotor cortex, supplementary motor area, and cingulate motor area. The primary somatic sensory cortex is also shown.

A

Lateral corticospinal tract (lumbar and sacral segments)

Ventral corticospinal tract (thoracic segments)

Lateral corticospinal tract (cervical segments)

Ventral corticospinal tract (upper cervical segments)

Corticobulbar tract (pons and medulla)

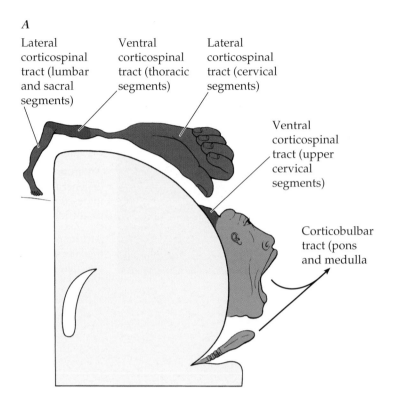

B

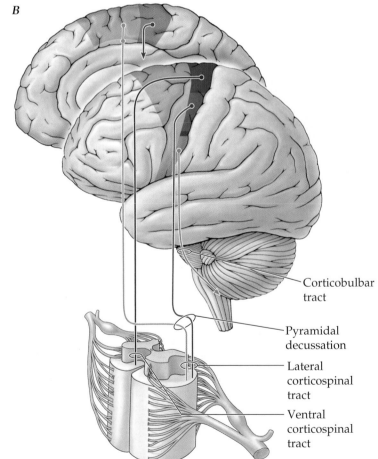

Corticobulbar tract

Pyramidal decussation

Lateral corticospinal tract

Ventral corticospinal tract

FIGURE 10–8 Somatotopic organization of the primary motor cortex (*A*). *B.* The descending pathways by which these areas of primary motor cortex influence motor neurons are indicated. (**A,** Adapted from Penfield W, Rasmussen T. *The Cerebral Cortex of Man: A Clinical Study of Localization.* New York, NY: Macmillan; 1950.)

A

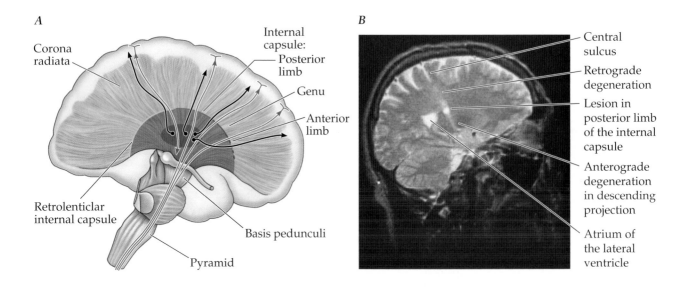

Corona radiata

Internal capsule:
- Posterior limb
- Genu
- Anterior limb

Retrolenticlar internal capsule

Basis pedunculi

Pyramid

B

Central sulcus

Retrograde degeneration

Lesion in posterior limb of the internal capsule

Anterograde degeneration in descending projection

Atrium of the lateral ventricle

C

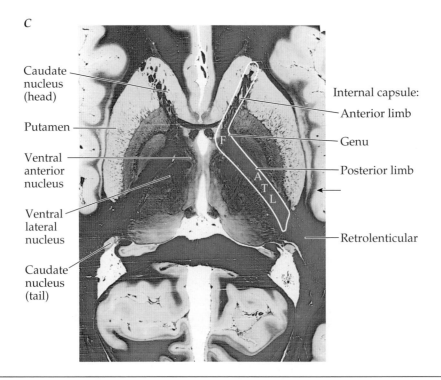

Caudate nucleus (head)

Putamen

Ventral anterior nucleus

Ventral lateral nucleus

Caudate nucleus (tail)

Internal capsule:
- Anterior limb
- Genu
- Posterior limb

Retrolenticular

FIGURE 10–9 *A.* Three-dimensional view of fibers in the white matter of the cerebral cortex. The regions corresponding to the internal capsule, basis pedunculi, and pyramid are indicated. The corona radiata is the portion of the white matter beneath the gray matter of the cerebral cortex. *B.* MRI from a patient with a stroke in the posterior limb of the internal capsule. Degeneration can be followed back (or retrograde) toward the precentral gyrus and forward (or anterograde) toward the brain stem. *C.* Myelin-stained horizontal section through the internal capsule. Note that the thalamus extends rostrally as far as the genu. The head of the caudate nucleus and the putamen are separated by the anterior limb of the internal capsule. The fiber constituents and somatotopic organization of the internal capsule are indicated. F, face; A, arm; T, trunk; L, leg. (**A,** Adapted with permission from Parent A. *Carpenter's Human Neuroanatomy,* 9th ed. Williams & Wilkins; 1996. **B,** Courtesy of Dr. Adrian Danek, Ludwig Maximilians University, Munich, Germany; Danek A, Bauer M, Fries W. Tracing of neuronal connections in the human brain by magnetic resonance imaging in vivo. *Eur J Neurosci.* 1990;2:112-115.)

of corticobulbar fibers are located in the genu, so that lesion of that structure disrupts facial muscle control (fibers labeled F for face in Figure 10–9C). Most of the path of the descending motor projection within the brain can be followed in a coronal section through the cerebral hemispheres, diencephalon, and brain stem (Figure 10–10A), and in an MRI from another patient who had a stroke in the posterior limb of the internal capsule (Figure 10–10C). The diffusion tensor image from a healthy person (Figure 10–10C) shows the white matter course of descending cortical fibers from the arm and leg areas of motor cortex.

The descending projections from the premotor areas also course within the internal capsule but rostral to those from the primary motor cortex. This separation of the projections from primary and premotor cortical areas is clinically significant, especially for the supplemental motor area, which courses most rostral. Because of the high density of corticospinal axons, patients with a small posterior limb stroke can exhibit severe signs because of damage to these axons. Typically, however, they can recover some function, such as strength. This recovery is mediated in part by the spinal projections from the premotor cortical regions that are rostral to the injury. Corticopontine axons, which carry information to the cerebellum for controlling movements, and corticoreticular axons, which affect the reticular formation and reticulospinal tracts, are also located in the internal capsule. The internal capsule also contains ascending axons as well as other descending axons. The **thalamic radiations** are the ascending thalamocortical projections located in the internal capsule (Figure 10–9A). The ascending projections from the ventral anterior and ventral lateral nuclei of the thalamus course here, as do those from many of the other thalamic nuclei that project to the frontal and parietal lobes.

Small strokes tend to damage one or another contingent of internal capsule axons because of the particular vascular distributions in the region of the internal capsule (see Figure 3–6). The **anterior choroidal artery** supplies the posterior limb, where the projections from the primary motor cortex are located. Branches from the **anterior cerebral artery** or the **lenticulostriate branches** (anterior and middle cerebral artery) supply the anterior limb and genu.

The Corticospinal Tract Courses in the Base of the Midbrain

The entire internal capsule appears to condense to form the **basis pedunculi** of the midbrain (Figures 10–9A and 10–11A). The basis pedunculi contains only descending fibers and therefore is smaller than the internal capsule. Each division of the brain stem contains three regions from its dorsal to ventral surfaces: **tectum, tegmentum, and base** (Figure 10–11A). In the rostral midbrain, the tectum consists of the **superior colliculus.** The midbrain base is termed the basis pedunculi. Together, the tegmentum and basis pedunculi constitute the **cerebral peduncle.**

Corticospinal tract axons course within the middle of the basis pedunculi, flanked medially and laterally by corticopontine axons (see Chapter 13) and other descending cortical

axons (Figure 10–11A). The location of these axons can be seen on an MRI scan from a patient with a lesion of the posterior limb of the internal capsule (Figure 10–12B). Figure 10–12C shows atrophy in the cerebral peduncle on the side in which the patient, an 8-year-old child, suffered from **hemiplegic cerebral palsy** produced by damage to the motor cortex and the underlying white matter earlier during childhood.

The rostral midbrain is a key level in the motor system because three nuclei that subserve motor function are located here: the superior colliculus, the red nucleus, and the substantia nigra. Neurons from the deeper layers of the **superior colliculus** (Figure 10–11) give rise to the **tectospinal tract,** a medial descending pathway. The **red nucleus** (Figure 10–11; also Figure 10–10B, dark oval structures medial to the degenerating cortical fibers), the origin of the **rubrospinal tract,** is a lateral descending pathway that begins primarily in the **magnocellular division** of this nucleus. The other major component of the red nucleus, the **parvocellular (or small-celled) division,** is part of a multisynaptic pathway from the cerebral cortex to the cerebellum (see Chapter 13). The tectospinal and rubrospinal tracts decussate in the midbrain. The **substantia nigra** is a part of the basal ganglia (see Chapter 14). Substantia nigra neurons that contain the neurotransmitter dopamine degenerate in patients with Parkinson disease.

The Pontine and Medullary Reticular Formation Gives Rise to the Reticulospinal Tracts

In the pons, the descending cortical fibers no longer occupy the ventral brain stem surface but rather are located deep within the base (Figure 10–12A, B). The pontine nuclei receive their principal input from the cerebral cortex via the **corticopontine pathway.** The corticopontine pathway is an important route by which information from all cerebral cortex lobes influences the cerebellum (see Chapter 13).

The **reticular formation** comprises a diffuse collection of nuclei in the central brain stem (see Figures 2–8 to 2–12). Neurons in the pontine and medullary reticular formation (Figures 10–12A and 10–13A, B) give rise to the **reticulospinal tracts.** (Few reticulospinal neurons originate from the midbrain.) Experiments in laboratory animals suggest that the reticulospinal tracts control relatively automatic motor responses, such as simple postural adjustments, stepping when walking, and rapid corrections of movement errors. When these automatic responses must occur during voluntary movements, such as maintaining an upright posture when reaching to lift something heavy, the corticoreticulo-spinal pathway is engaged.

The Lateral Corticospinal Tract Decussates in the Caudal Medulla

The path of the descending cortical fibers into the medulla can be followed in the sagittal section shown in Figure 10–14. The numerous fascicles of the caudal pons collect on the ventral surface of the medulla to form the **pyramids** (Figures 10–13 and 10–14).

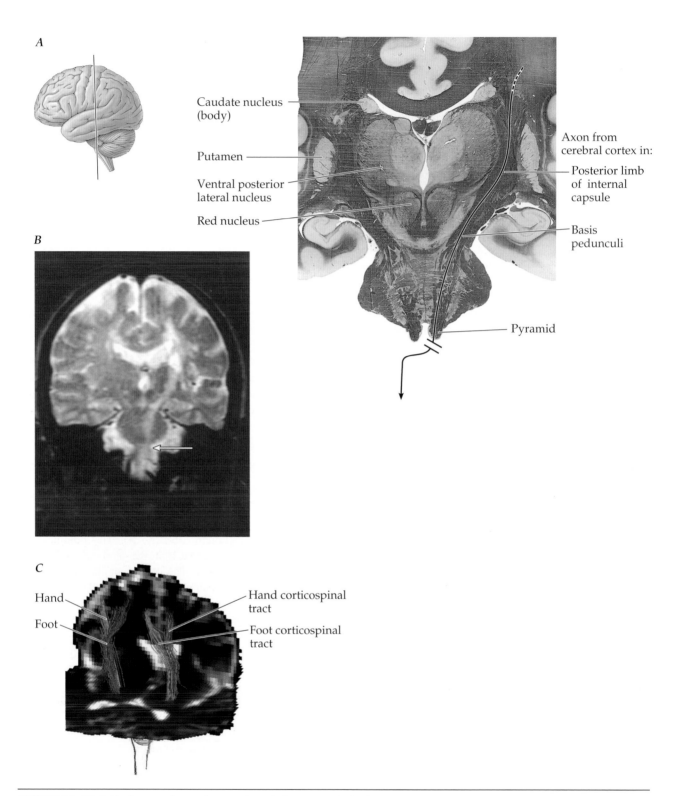

A

Caudate nucleus (body)

Putamen

Ventral posterior lateral nucleus

Red nucleus

Axon from cerebral cortex in:

Posterior limb of internal capsule

Basis pedunculi

Pyramid

B

C

Hand

Foot

Hand corticospinal tract

Foot corticospinal tract

FIGURE 10–10 *A*. Myelin-stained coronal section through the posterior limb of the internal capsule. Note that the component of the internal capsule is identified as the posterior limb in this section because the thalamus is medial to the internal capsule. ***B*.** Magnetic resonance imaging scan from a patient with an internal capsule lesion. Coronal slice through the posterior limb of the internal capsule showing bright vertically oriented band extending from the lesion caudally into the pons. This band corresponds to degenerated axons in the internal capsule, basis pedunculi, and pons. **C.** Diffusion tensor image of the corticospinal tracts from the arm and lege regions of a healthy person. (**B,** Courtesy of Dr. Jesús Pujol; from Pujol J, Martí-Vilalta JL, Junqué C, Vendrell P, Fernández J, Capdevila A. Wallerian degeneration of the pyramidal tract in capsular infarction studied by magnetic resonance imaging. *Stroke.* 1990;21:404-409.)

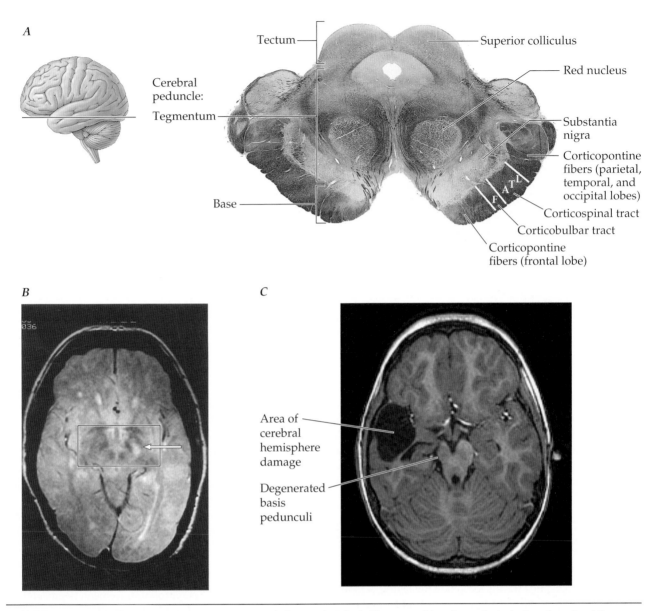

FIGURE 10–11 **A**. Myelin-stained transverse section through the rostral midbrain. The composition of axons in the basis pedunculi and the somatotopic organization of the corticospinal fibers are shown on the right. **B**. Transverse slice through the midbrain (horizontal slice through central hemispheres) showing site of degeneration. **C**. Transverse magnetic resonance imaging (MRI) scan through the midbrain of an 8-year-old child with cerebral palsy, produced by a perinatal lesion of the cerebral hemisphere. The MRI scan shows damage to the right cerebral cortex and underlying white matter and degeneration of the basis pedunculi. The area of the degenerated basis pedunculi in this patient was about half that of the other side. She had severe motor impairments of the right arm, especially for highly skilled hand movements. (**B**, Courtesy of Dr. Jesús Pujol; from Pujol J, Martí-Vilalta JL, Junqué C, Vendrell P, Fernández J, Capdevila A. Wallerian degeneration of the pyramidal tract in capsular infarction studied by magnetic resonance imaging. *Stroke*. 1990; 21:404-409. **C**, Courtesy of Dr. Etienne Olivier, University of Louvain; Duqué J, Thonnard JL, Vandermeeren Y, et al. Correlation between impaired dexterity and corticospinal tract dysgenesis in congenital hemiplegia. *Brain*. 2003; 126:1-16.)

The axons of the lateral and ventral corticospinal tracts, which originate primarily from the ipsilateral frontal lobe, are located in each pyramid. This is why the terms **corticospinal tract** and **pyramidal tract** are often—but inaccurately—used interchangeably. These terms are *not* synonymous because the pyramids also contain **corticobulbar** and **corticoreticular fibers** that terminate in the medulla. Damage to the corticospinal system produces a characteristic set of motor control and muscle impairments (see section below on brain stem and spinal lesions) that are sometimes called **pyramidal signs.**

Lateral corticospinal tract axons descend in the pyramid and most decussate in the caudal medulla, within fascicles. One fascicle of decussating axons is cut in the section shown in Figure 10–13C (solid line). Another group from the other side (located just rostrally or caudally) would likely decussate along the path shown by the dotted line. The rubrospinal tract, which had crossed in the midbrain, maintains its dorsolateral position. Here, at the medulla–spinal cord junction, the crossed lateral corticospinal tract axons join the rubrospinal axons and descend in the lateral column (Figures 10–6 and 10–13C). These are the two lateral

A

B

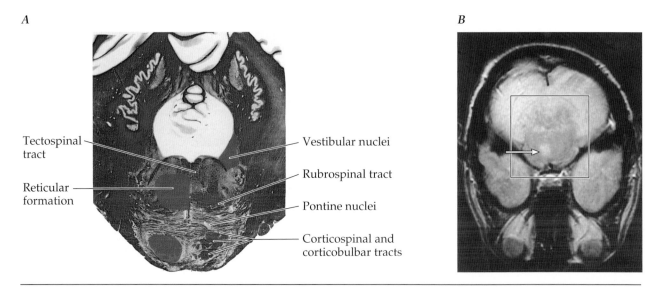

Tectospinal tract

Reticular formation

Vestibular nuclei

Rubrospinal tract

Pontine nuclei

Corticospinal and corticobulbar tracts

FIGURE 10–12 Myelin-stained section through the pons (*A*) and MRI through approximately the same level from a person with unilateral internal capsule lesion (*B*). Note, ventral is down in both images. *A*. Myelin-stained section through the pons, showing the locations of the motor pathways. *B*. Transverse slice through the pons and cerebellum (horizontal slice through central hemispheres) showing site of degeneration. (*B*, Courtesy of Dr. Jesús Pujol; from Pujol J, Martí-Vilalta JL, Junqué C, Vendrell P, Fernández J, Capdevila A. Wallerian degeneration of the pyramidal tract in capsular infarction studied by magnetic resonance imaging. *Stroke.* 1990;21:404-409.)

motor pathways. The reticulospinal, vestibulospinal, and tectospinal tracts remain medially located and assume a more ventral position as they descend in the spinal cord. Note that ventral corticospinal tract axons remain ipsilateral within, traveling to the spinal cord along with the vestibulospinal tract and the tectospinal tract.

The Intermediate Zone and Ventral Horn of the Spinal Cord Receive Input From the Descending Pathways

The lateral corticospinal tract is located in the lateral column, revealed by the zone of degeneration in the lumbar cord from an individual who had a lesions of the internal capsule prior to death (Figure 10–15). (Note that the ventral corticospinal tract descends only as far as the cervical spinal cord. Thus, there are no degenerating fibers in the ventral column.) The brain stem pathways are located in both the lateral and ventral columns (Figure 10–6). The motor pathways terminate within the spinal gray matter. As discussed in Chapter 4, the dorsal horn corresponds to Rexed's laminae I through V, and the ventral horn corresponds to laminae VI and IX (Figure 10–16A). From the perspective of the motor systems, we further distinguish the intermediate zone, which corresponds to laminae VI and VII, from the remaining portions of the ventral horn proper, corresponding to laminae VIII-IX. The intermediate zone contains many important interneurons for movement control. The motor nuclei are located in lamina IX. Lamina X surrounds the spinal cord central canal. We focus on the terminations of the corticospinal tract, because its functions are the clearest. The premotor, primary motor, and primary somatic sensory cortical regions

all have spinal projections in the corticospinal tract, but their target laminae differ in complex ways. Corticospinal tract axons, as well as the other motor pathways, synapse on interneurons and motor neurons.

There are three kinds of spinal cord interneurons: segmental interneurons, commissural interneurons, and propriospinal neurons. **Segmental interneurons** have a short axon that distributes branches ipsilaterally within a single spinal cord segment to synapse on motor neurons and other interneurons (Figure 10–16A). In addition to receiving input from the descending motor pathways, segmental interneurons receive convergent input from different classes of somatic sensory receptors for the reflex control of movement. Segmental interneurons are located primarily in the intermediate zone and the ventral horn. **Commissural interneurons** have axons that distribute bilaterally for coordinating the actions of muscles on both sides of the body during walking and for maintaining balance. **Propriospinal neurons** have an axon that projects for multiple spinal segments before synapsing on motor neurons (Figure 10–16A), and are important for upper-lower limb coordination.

The lateral and medial motor nuclei have different rostrocaudal distributions

The motor neurons that innervate a particular muscle are located within a column-shaped nucleus that runs rostrocaudally over several spinal segments. These column-shaped nuclei of motor neurons collectively form lamina IX (Figures 10–16B and 10–17, inset). Nuclei innervating distal limb muscles are located laterally in the gray matter, whereas those innervating proximal limb and axial muscles

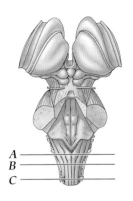

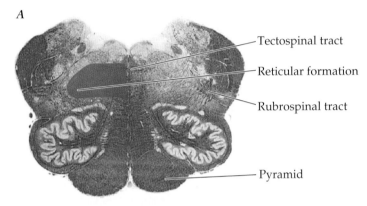

A

Tectospinal tract

Reticular formation

Rubrospinal tract

Pyramid

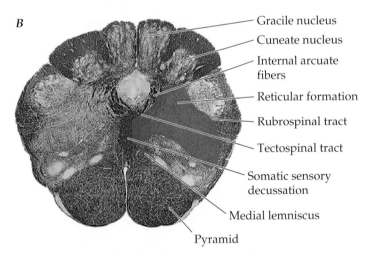

B

Gracile nucleus

Cuneate nucleus

Internal arcuate fibers

Reticular formation

Rubrospinal tract

Tectospinal tract

Somatic sensory decussation

Medial lemniscus

Pyramid

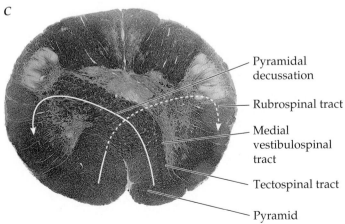

C

Pyramidal decussation

Rubrospinal tract

Medial vestibulospinal tract

Tectospinal tract

Pyramid

FIGURE 10–13   A. Myelin-stained section through the medulla, showing the locations of the motor pathways. **B** and **C**. Myelin-stained transverse sections through the decussation of the internal arcuate fibers, or mechanosensory decussation (**B**), and the pyramidal, or motor, decussation (**C**). Arrows in **C** indicate the pattern of decussating corticospinal fibers. The solid arrow indicates an axon coursing within the portion of the tract shown in the section. The dashed arrow corresponds to a decussating axon a bit rostral or caudal to this level.

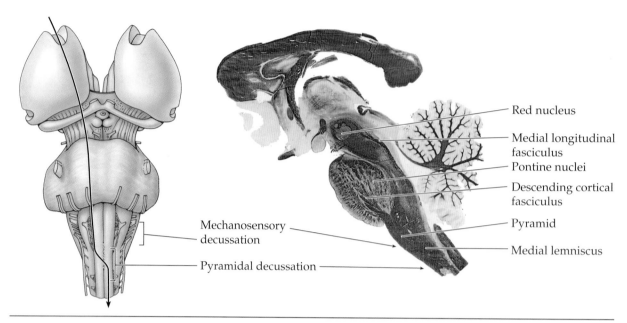

Red nucleus

Medial longitudinal fasciculus

Pontine nuclei

Descending cortical fasciculus

Pyramid

Medial lemniscus

Mechanosensory decussation

Pyramidal decussation

FIGURE 10–14 **A.** Ventral view of the brain stem showing the path of the corticospinal tract. Brackets show the rostrocaudal levels of the somatic sensory and motor decussations. **B.** Myelin-stained sagittal section (close to the midline) through the brain stem.

are located medially (Figure 10–3). The medial motor nuclei are present at all spinal levels (illustrated schematically as a continuous column of nuclei in Figure 10–17, inset), whereas the lateral nuclei are present only in the cervical enlargement (C5-T1) and the lumbosacral enlargement (L1-S2). A single motor neuron innervates multiple muscle fibers within a single muscle. Collectively, all fibers innervated by a single motor neuron are termed a **motor unit.**

In the spinal cord, autonomic preganglionic motor neurons are also arranged in a column (see Chapter 15) and, together with the motor nuclei, have a three-dimensional organization similar to that of the brain stem cranial nerve nuclei columns (see Chapter 6). The longitudinal organization of the somatic and autonomic motor nuclei and the cranial nerve nuclei underscores the common architecture of the spinal cord and brain stem.

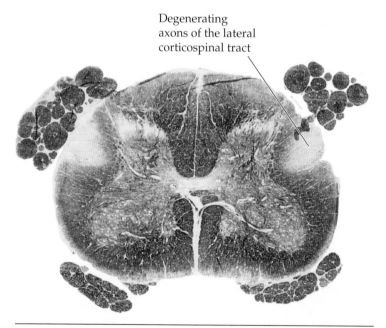

Degenerating axons of the lateral corticospinal tract

FIGURE 10–15 Myelin-stained section through the lumbar spinal cord from an individual who had an internal capsule stroke before death. Region showing degeneration in the lateral column (lightly stained) corresponds to the location of the lateral corticospinal tract. Note that the ventral corticospinal is not present at this level.

A

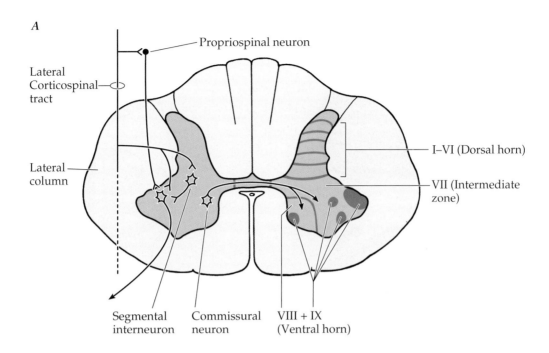

Lateral
Corticospinal
tract

Propriospinal neuron

Lateral
column

I–VI (Dorsal horn)

VII (Intermediate
zone)

Segmental
interneuron

Commissural
neuron

VIII + IX
(Ventral horn)

B

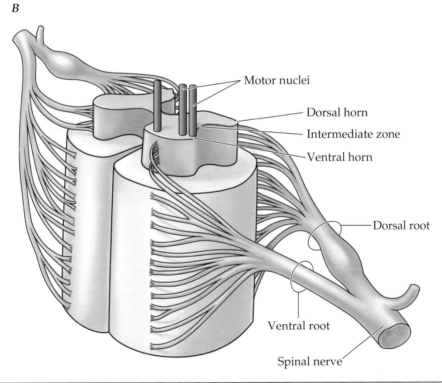

Motor nuclei

Dorsal horn

Intermediate zone

Ventral horn

Dorsal root

Ventral root

Spinal nerve

FIGURE 10–16 **A.** Schematic drawing of the general organization of the spinal cord gray matter and white matter.
Note the three classes of interneuron: propriospinal neuron, segmental interneuron, and commissural neuron.
B. Drawing of a single spinal segment, showing columns of motor nuclei, running rostrocaudally within the ventral horn.

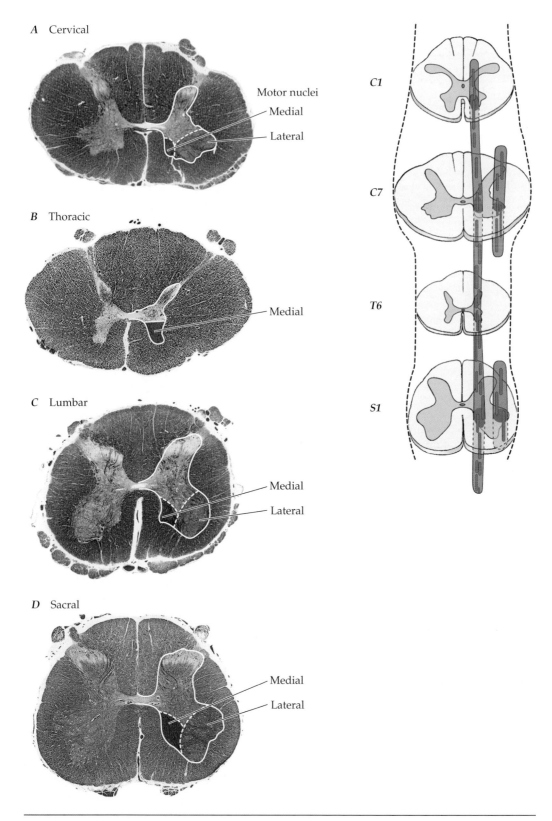

A   Cervical

Motor nuclei
Medial
Lateral

B   Thoracic

Medial

C   Lumbar

Medial
Lateral

D   Sacral

Medial
Lateral

C1

C7

T6

S1

FIGURE 10–17 Approximate locations of the medial and lateral motor nuclei are shown at four spinal cord levels: cervical (*A*), thoracic (*B*), lumbar (*C*), and sacral (*D*). The inset shows the columnar organization of the medial and lateral motor nuclei. The medial column, which contains motor neurons that innervate proximal and axial muscles, runs throughout the entire spinal cord. Motor nuclei that contain the motor neurons that innervate individual muscles also have a columnar shape but are narrower and course for a shorter rostrocaudal distance. The lateral column contains motor neurons that innervate lateral (distal) muscles. This column is present in the cervical and lumbosacral enlargements only. As for the medial column, motor neurons that innervate individual muscles form narrower and shorter columns.

Descending Pathways

Seven descending motor pathways course in the white matter of the brain stem and spinal cord (Figures 10–4 through 10–6; Table 10–1): the *lateral corticospinal tract,* the *rubrospinal tract,* the *ventral corticospinal tract,* the *reticulospinal tract* (which is further subdivided into separate medullary and pontine components), the *vestibulospinal* **tract** (which is subdivided into separate medial and lateral components), and the *tectospinal tract.* These pathways project directly on spinal motor neurons through monosynaptic connections and indirectly by synapsing first on interneurons. The corticobulbar tract projects only to the brain stem (see Chapter 11).

Lateral Descending Pathways

The locations of the descending axons in the spinal cord provide insight into their functions (Figure 10–3). Those that control limb muscles descend in the *lateral column* of the spinal cord and terminate in the *intermediate zone* and *lateral ventral horn* (Figures 10–3, 10–4, and 10–6). The *lateral corticospinal tract* and the *rubrospinal tract* are the two laterally descending pathways. The lateral corticospinal tract is the larger of the two and plays an essential role in movement control. The *primary motor cortex* (area 4), located on the precentral gyrus (Figures 10–7 and 10–8), contributes most of the fibers of the lateral corticospinal tract. The other major contributors to the lateral corticospinal tract are the premotor cortical regions (Figure 10–7), located rostral to the primary motor cortex, mainly in cytoarchitectonic areas 6 and 24, and the somatic sensory areas of the parietal lobe. The descending projection neurons of the cortex are located in layer V, and their axons course through the *posterior limb of the internal capsule* (Figures 10–9 and 10–10) and then along the ventral brain stem surface (Figures 10–11 through 10–14). The lateral corticospinal tract decussates in the ventral medulla in the *pyramidal decussation,* at the junction of the medulla and the spinal cord (Figures 10–8, 10–13, and 10–14). In the spinal cord,

the lateral corticospinal tract courses in the dorsal portion of the *lateral column* (Figures 10–6 and 10–16) and terminates primarily in cervical and lumbosacral segments. The other laterally descending pathway, the *rubrospinal tract,* originates from the *magnocellular division* of the *red nucleus* (Figures 10–10 and 10–14). The axons decussate in the midbrain, descend in the dorsolateral portion of the brain stem and spinal cord (Figures 10–4B and 10–6), and terminate in the cervical cord. The other division of the red nucleus, the *parvocellular division,* is part of a circuit that involves the cerebellum.

Medial Descending Pathways

The remaining four pathways course in the medial portion of the spinal cord white matter, the *ventral column,* and influence axial and girdle muscles. These medially descending pathways terminate in the medial ventral horn—where axial and girdle motor neurons are located—and the intermediate zone (Figure 10–3). These pathways influence motor neurons bilaterally: After descending into the cord, either the axon of the projection neuron decussates in the ventral commissure or lamina X, or its terminals synapse on interneurons whose axons decussate. The *ventral corticospinal tract,* which originates mostly in the primary motor cortex and area 6, descends in the brain stem along with the lateral corticospinal tract but does not decussate in the medulla and courses in the ventral column of the spinal cord (Figures 10–5A and 10–18). The *reticulospinal tracts* (pontine and medullary; Figure 10–5B) originate in the *reticular formation* (Figures 10–12 and 10–13) and descend ipsilaterally for the entire length of the spinal cord and function in posture and automatic responses, such as locomotion. The *tectospinal tract* (Figure 10–5B) originates from the deeper layers of the *superior colliculus* (Figure 10–11), decussates in the midbrain, and descends medially in the caudal brain stem and spinal cord. This pathway descends only to the cervical spinal cord and plays a role in coordination of head and eye movements. (See Chapter 12 for the vestibulospinal tracts.)

Rizzolatti G, Kalaska J. The organization of voluntary movement. In: Kandel ER, Schwartz JH, Jessell TM, Siegelbaum SA, Hudspeth AJ, eds. *Principles of Neural Science.* 5th ed. New York, NY: McGraw-Hill; in press.

Wolpert D, Pearson K, Ghez C. The organization and planning of movement. In: Kandel ER, Schwartz JH, Jessell TM, Siegelbaum SA, Hudspeth AJ, eds. *Principles of Neural Science.* 5th ed. New York, NY: McGraw-Hill; in press.

Asanuma H. The pyramidal tract. In: Brooks VB, ed. *Handbook of Physiology, Section 1: The Nervous System, Vol. 2, Motor Control.* Bethesda, MD: American Physiological Society; 1981:703-733.

Boulenguez P, Liabeuf S, Bos R, et al. Down-regulation of the potassium-chloride cotransporter KCC2 contributes to spasticity after spinal cord injury. *Nat Med.* 2010;16(3): 302-307.

Brösamle C, Huber AB, Fiedler M, Skerra A, Schwab ME. Regeneration of lesioned corticospinal tract fibers in the adult rat induced by a recombinant, humanized IN–1 antibody fragment. *J Neurosci.* 2000;20:8061-8068.

Burman K, Darian-Smith C, Darian-Smith I. Geometry of rubrospinal, rubroolivary and local circuit neurons in the macaque red nucleus. *J Comp Neurol.* 2000;423:197-219.

Burman K, Darian-Smith C, Darian-Smith I. Macaque red nucleus: origins of spinal and olivary projections and terminations of cortical inputs. *J Comp Neurol.* 2000; 423:179–196.

Chakrabarty S, Shulman B, Martin JH. Activity-dependent codevelopment of the corticospinal system and target interneurons in the cervical spinal cord. *J Neurosci.* 2009;29(27): 8816-8827.

Chung CS, Caplan LR, Yamamoto Y, et al. Striatocapsular haemorrhage. *Brain.* 2000;123:1850-1862.

Crosby EC, Humphrey T, Lauer EW. *Correlative Anatomy of the Nervous System.* New York, NY: Macmillan; 1962.

Danek A, Bauer M, Fries W. Tracing of neuronal connections in the human brain by magnetic resonance imaging in vivo. *Eur J Neurosci.* 1990;2:112-115.

Dum RP, Strick PL. Medial wall motor areas and skeletomotor control. *Curr Opin Neurobiol.* 1992;2:836-839.

Dum RP, Strick PL. The origin of corticospinal projections from the premotor areas in the frontal lobe. *J Neurosci.* 1991;11:667-689.

Fries W, Danek A, Scheidtmann K, Hamburger C. Motor recovery following capsular stroke: role of descending pathways from multiple motor areas. *Brain.* 1993;116:369-382.

Fries W, Danek A, Witt TN. Motor responses after transcranial electrical stimulation of cerebral hemispheres with a degenerated pyramidal tract. *Ann Neurol.* 1991;29:646-650.

Gandevia SC, Burke DA. Peripheral motor system. In: Paxinos G, Mai JK, eds. *The Human Nervous System.* London: Elsevier; 2004.

Geyer S, Matelli M, Luppino G, Zilles K. Functional neuroanatomy of the primate isocortical motor system. *Anat Embryol (Berl).* 2000;202(6):443-474.

Habas C, Cabanis EA. Cortical projections to the human red nucleus: a diffusion tensor tractography study with a 1.5-T MRI machine. *Neuroradiology.* 2006;48(10):755-762.

Han BS, Hong JH, Hong C, et al. Location of the corticospinal tract at the corona radiata in human brain. *Brain Res.* 2010;1326:75-80.

He SQ, Dum RP, Strick PL. Topographic organization of corticospinal projections from the frontal lobe: motor areas on the

medial surface of the hemisphere. *J Neurosci.* 1995;15(5 Pt 1): 3284-3306.

Holodny AI, Watts R, Korneinko VN, et al. Diffusion tensor tractography of the motor white matter tracts in man: current controversies and future directions. *Ann N Y Acad Sci.* 2005;1064:88-97.

Holodny AI, Gor DM, Watts R, Gutin PH, Ulug AM. Diffusion-tensor MR tractography of somatotopic organization of corticospinal tracts in the internal capsule: initial anatomic results in contradistinction to prior reports. *Radiology.* 2005;234(3):649-653.

Hong JH, Son SM, Jang SH. Somatotopic location of corticospinal tract at pons in human brain: a diffusion tensor tractography study. *Neuroimage.* 2010;51(3):952-955.

Huang DW, McKerracher L, Braun PE, David S. A therapeutic vaccine approach to stimulate axon regeneration in the adult mammalian spinal cord. *Neuron.* 1999;24:639-647.

Jackson SR, Husain M. Visuomotor functions of the lateral premotor cortex. *Curr Opin Neurobiol.* 1996;6:788-795.

Jang SH. A review of corticospinal tract location at corona radiata and posterior limb of the internal capsule in human brain. *NeuroRehabilitation.* 2009;24(3):279-283.

Jankowska E, Lundberg A. Interneurons in the spinal cord. *Trends Neurosci.* 1981;4:230-233.

Jenny AB, Saper CB. Organization of the facial nucleus and corticofacial projection in the monkey: a reconsideration of the upper motor neuron facial palsy. *Neurology.* 1987;37: 930-939.

Juenger H, Kumar V, Grodd W, Staudt M, Krageloh-Mann I. Preserved crossed corticospinal tract and hand function despite extensive brain maldevelopment. *Pediatr Neurol.* 2009;41(5):388-389.

Kim SG, Ashe J, Georgopoulos AP, et al. Functional imaging of human motor cortex at high magnetic field. *J Neurophysiol.* 1993;69:297-302.

Kim DG, Kim SH, Kim OL, Cho YW, Son SM, Jang SH. Long-term recovery of motor function in a quadriplegic patient with diffuse axonal injury and traumatic hemorrhage: a case report. *NeuroRehabilitation.* 2009;25(2):117-122.

Kumar A, Juhasz C, Asano E, et al. Diffusion tensor imaging study of the cortical origin and course of the corticospinal tract in healthy children. *AJNR Am J Neuroradiol.* 2009;30(10):1963-1970.

Kuypers HGJM. Anatomy of the descending pathways. In: Brooks VB, ed. *Handbook of Physiology, Section 1: The Nervous System, Vol. 2, Motor Control.* Bethesda, MD: American Physiological Society; 1981:597-666.

Kuypers HGJM, Brinkman J. Precentral projections to different parts of the spinal intermediate zone in the rhesus monkey. *Brain Res.* 1970;24:151-188.

Lu M-T, Present JB, Strick PL. Interconnections between the prefrontal cortex and the premotor areas in the frontal lobe. *J Comp Neurol.* 1994;341:375-392.

Luppino G, Rizzolatti G. The organization of the frontal motor cortex. *News physiol sci.* 2000;15:219-224.

Martin JH. Differential spinal projections from the forelimb areas of rostral and caudal subregions of primary motor cortex in the cat. *Exp Brain Res.* 1996;108:191-205.

Matelli M, Luppino G, Geyer S, Zilles K. Motor cortex. In: Paxinos G, Mai JK, eds. *The Human Nervous System.* London: Elsevier; 2004:975-996.

Matsuyama K, Drew T. Organization of the projections from the pericruciate cortex to the pontomedullary brain stem of the cat: a study using the anterograde tracer Phaseolous vulgaris leucoagglutinin. *J Comp Neurol.* 1997;389: 617-641.

Molenaar I, Kuypers HGJM. Cells of origin of propriospinal fibers and of fibers ascending to supraspinal levels: an HRP study in cat and rhesus monkey. *Brain Res.* 1978;152:429-450.

Morecraft RJ, Herrick JL, Stilwell-Morecraft KS, et al. Localization of arm representation in the corona radiata and internal capsule in the non-human primate. *Brain.* 2002;125:176-198.

Morecraft RJ, Louie JL, Herrick JL, Stilwell-Morecraft KS. Cortical innervation of the facial nucleus in the non-human primate: a new interpretation of the effects of stroke and related subtotal brain trauma on the muscles of facial expression. *Brain.* 2001;124:176-208.

Murray EA, Coulter JD. Organization of corticospinal neurons in the monkey. *J Comp Neurol.* 1981;195:339-365.

Nathan PW, Smith MC. The rubrospinal and central tegmental tracts in man. *Brain.* 1982;105:223-269.

Newton JM, Ward NS, Parker GJ, et al. Non-invasive mapping of corticofugal fibres from multiple motor areas—-relevance to stroke recovery. *Brain.* 2006;129(Pt 7):1844-1858.

Penfield W, Rasmussen T. *The Cerebral Cortex of Man: A Clinical Study of Localization of Function.* New York, NY: Macmillan; 1950.

Percheron G. Thalamus. In: Paxinos G, Mai JK, eds. *The Human Nervous System.* London, UK: Elsevier; 2004:592-676.

Picard N, Strick PL. Imaging the premotor areas. *Curr Opin Neurobiol.* 2001;11:663-672.

Pierrot-Deseilligny E, Burke D. *The Circuitry of the Human Spinal Cord.* Cambridge, UK: Cambridge University Press; 2005.

Puig J, Pedraza S, Blasco G, et al. Wallerian degeneration in the corticospinal tract evaluated by diffusion tensor imaging correlates with motor deficit 30 days after middle cerebral artery ischemic stroke. *AJNR Am J Neuroradiol.* 2010; 31:1324-1330.

Pujol J, Martí-Vilalta JL, Junqué C, Vendrell P, Fernández J, Capdevila A. Wallerian degeneration of the pyramidal tract in capsular infarction studied by magnetic resonance imaging. *Stroke.* 1990;21:404-409.

Ramnani N, Behrens TE, Johansen-Berg H, et al. The evolution of prefrontal inputs to the cortico-pontine system: diffusion imaging evidence from Macaque monkeys and humans. *Cereb Cortex.* 2006;16(6):811-818.

Rizzolatti G, Sinigaglia C. The functional role of the parieto-frontal mirror circuit: interpretations and misinterpretations. *Nat Rev Neurosci.* 2010;11(4):264-274.

Roland PE, Zilles K. Functions and structures of the motor cortices in humans. *Curr Opin Neurobiol.* 1996;6:773-781.

Ross ED. Localization of the pyramidal tract in the internal capsule by whole brain dissection. *Neurology.* 1980;30:59-64.

Schell GR, Strick PL. The origin of thalamic inputs to the arcuate premotor and supplementary motor areas. *J Neurosci.* 1984;4:539-560.

Staudt M. Reorganization after pre- and perinatal brain lesions. *J Anat.* 2010;217(4):469-474.

Sterling P, Kuypers HGJM. Anatomical organization of the brachial spinal cord of the cat. III. The propriospinal connections. *Brain Res.* 1967;4:419-443.

Vogt BA, Pandya DN, Rosene DL. Cingulate cortex of the rhesus monkey. I. Cytoarchitecture and thalamic afferents. *J Comp Neurol.* 1987;262:256-270.

Wiesendanger M. Organization of secondary motor areas of cerebral cortex. In: Brooks VB, ed. *Handbook of Physiology, Section 1: The Nervous System, Vol. 2, Motor Control.* Bethesda, MD: American Physiological Society; 1981:1121-1147.

Wrigley PJ, Gustin SM, Macey PM, et al. Anatomical changes in human motor cortex and motor pathways following complete thoracic spinal cord injury. *Cereb Cortex.* 2009;19(1):224-232.

Yarrow K, Brown P, Krakauer JW. Inside the brain of an elite athlete: the neural processes that support high achievement in sports. *Nat Rev Neurosci.* 2009;10(8):585-596.

Study Questions

1. A patient suddenly developed weakness of his left arm. Damage to which of the following brain regions is the most likely site of injury?
   A. Ventral spinal cord white matter
   B. Lateral spinal cord white matter
   C. Ventral pons
   D. Precentral gyrus

2. Complete the following analogy. Limb control is to trunk control, as
   A. the lateral corticospinal tract is to the ventral corticospinal tract.
   B. the reticulospinal tract is to the rubrospinal tract.
   C. the motor cortex on the medial brain surface is to the motor cortex on the lateral brain surface.
   D. the middle cerebral artery is to the basilar artery.

3. Which of the following statements best describes why unilateral damage to the descending cortical pathway in the basis pedunculi results only in weakness/paralysis of contralateral lower facial, arm, and leg muscles?
   A. Upper facial and trunk muscles are not controlled by the corticospinal and corticobulbar tracts.
   B. Upper facial and trunk muscles are controlled by the ventral corticospinal tract only.
   C. Upper facial and trunk muscles receive bilateral corticospinal and corticobulbar tract control.
   D. Upper facial and trunk muscles are not controlled by the corticospinal and corticobulbar tracts.

4. Which of the following statements does not describe a feature of the ventral corticospinal tract?
   A. It descends primarily to the cervical spinal cord only
   B. It controls distal muscles only
   C. It descends in the ipsilateral ventral column
   D. It terminates bilaterally in the spinal cord

5. The rubrospinal tract
   A. is similar in function to the lateral corticospinal tract
   B. decussates in the spinal cord
   C. synapses only on motor neurons
   D. descends in the medial brain stem and spinal cord

6. Which of the following statements best describes a key feature of the reticulospinal tracts?
   A. They are components of the lateral descending pathways.
   B. They descend to the cervical spinal cord only.
   C. They originate from the medulla.
   D. They regulate relatively automatic behaviors.

7. Occlusion of cortical branches of the anterior cerebral artery would disrupt control of which of the following muscle groups?
   A. Foot
   B. Arm
   C. Neck
   D. Face

8. The genu of the internal capsule contains which of the following fibers?
   A. Corticospinal fibers from primary motor cortex
   B. Corticobulbar fibers from primary motor cortex
   C. Corticospinal and corticobulbar fibers from primary motor cortex
   D. Corticospinal and corticobulbar fibers from premotor cortical areas

9. Occlusion of paramedian branches of the basilar artery will most likely infarct which of the following motor system components?
   A. Pyramids
   B. Rubrospinal tract
   C. Corticospinal and corticobulbar tracts
   D. Reticulospinal tract

10. The enlargement segments correspond to which of the following?
    A. Thoracic segments
    B. Segments innervating the limbs
    C. Segments innervating the trunk
    D. Segments with a greater number of motor neurons

Chapter 11

Cranial Nerve Motor Nuclei and Brain Stem Motor Functions

CLINICAL CASE | Hemiparesis and Lower Facial Droop

A 69-year-old man, with a history of hypertension and cigarette smoking, suddenly developed difficulty walking as he was returning home from shopping. Upon reaching his apartment, he was unable to raise a cup of coffee with his right hand. He called his daughter for assistance, who later noted that his speech was slurred. She brought him to the emergency room.

On neurological examination, somatic sensations on his limbs and trunk were normal. His cranial nerve functions were also found to be normal except for a flattening of the right nasolabial fold. The patient understood verbal commands, and speech was intact but slurred (disarthric). He was able to extend his tongue fully at the midline. On further testing, the patient's right arm and leg strength were found to be 3 out of 5. (Note, strength is qualitatively assessed according to a 0 to 5 scale, where 0 is complete paralysis and 5 is normal. In between, 1 is the presence of a small muscle contraction but no movement; 2, movement, but not against gravity; and 3, movement against gravity but not against resistance.) Left arm and leg strength were normal (ie, 5/5). His gait required support. Reflex testing revealed a stronger knee jerk and other tendon reflexes on the right side compared with the left.

Figure 11–1A is a MRI that shows brain structure well. The image in part B, at the same level as A, shows more clearly an intense signal in the ventral pons, on the patient's left side. This corresponds to the site of an infarction. Note that the bright signals in the temporal poles are artifacts. Part C shows the level of the MRIs in relation to brain stem vasculature. The site of infarction is represented on the ventral pontine surface.

Unfortunately, the patient died several years later, due to complications related to the stroke he suffered.

Figure 11–1D shows a myelin-stained cervical spinal section after supraspinal stroke. Two prominent regions of demyelination, and accompanying axon degeneration, are noted (arrows); one on the right side (contralateral to infarction) in the dorsolateral white matter and the other in the left (ipsilateral) ventromedial white matter.

—Continued next page

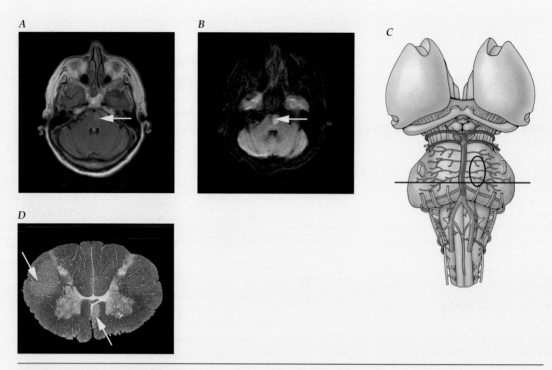

FIGURE 11–1 Hemiparesis after unilateral ventral pontine stroke. **A.** MRI through the pons showing a lesion in the left ventral pons. This is a FLAIR image. Arrow points to the infarcted region. **B.** MRI through the same level showing more clearly the infarction (arrow). Note that the bright signals in the temporal poles are artifacts. **C.** Ventral brain stem showing site of infarction (ellipse) and approximate plane of section of MRIs. **D.** Myelin-stained section from deceased stroke patient showing demyelination (and accompanying axon degeneration) in the left lateral and right ventral columns (arrows). (MR images in are courtesy of Dr. Blair Ford, Dept. of Neurology, Columbia University College of Physicians and Surgeons.)

Answer the following questions based on your reading of this and the previous chapter.

1. **Occlusion of what artery likely produced the infarction?**

2. **Why are the only somatic motor signs a flattening of the contralateral nasolabial fold and contralateral limb muscle weakness?**

3. **Why is the knee jerk reflex stronger (hyperreflexia) on the paretic (weakened) side?**

Key neurological signs and corresponding damaged brain structures

Selective flattening of nasolabial fold

The nasolabial fold is produced by tone in facial musculature; flattening signifies a loss of tone, and associated weakness or paralysis of facial musculature. There is no loss of capacity to contract upper facial muscles. In this patient's case, where the lesion is in the descending cortical fibers in the pons, sparing of upper facial control is likely due to control by both the contralateral and ipsilateral cortical motor areas. Since the lesion is limited to the contralateral pathway, spared ipsilateral descending fibers could mediate control. There is no loss of other cranial motor functions; these, like the upper face, are under more bilateral cortical control. Thus, unilateral lesion will not seriously weaken or paralyze muscle groups under bilateral control (see Figure 11–5). Nevertheless, there can be marked control impairments.

Contralateral limb muscle weakness

Limb muscles, as well as lower facial muscles, receive a predominant contralateral control by the corticospinal and corticobulbar systems. Upper face (and other cranial muscles) and trunk muscles receive predominant bilateral control. Unilateral lesion of these systems will therefore disrupt contralateral limb and lower facial muscle control.

Hyperreflexia concurrent with muscle weakness

Hyperreflexia is a characteristic of lesion of the corticospinal, as well as brain stem, descending motor pathways. The precise mechanism is not well understood, but likely involves maladaptive plasticity in the spinal cord after the lesion (see

Box 10–1). The hyperreflexia after the lesion is typically paralleled by progressively increasing muscle tone.

Disproportionate complex motor control impairment

The lesion produced mild facial muscle weakness; tongue protrusion at the midline was intact indicating significant spared control. Despite relatively modest cranial motor signs, the patient's speech is slurred. This reflects disproportionate impairment in the complex coordination of perioral muscles needed for clear speech. Similarly, with such a lesion, limb muscles are weak and there is also disproportionate incoordination and slowing of movements. This is common with corticospinal and corticobulbar lesions. Spared brain stem pathways—such as the rubrospinal, vestibulospinal, and reticulospinal pathways—may help the patient to regain strength and balance, but the cortical pathways are essential for fine control.

Reference

Brust JCM. *The Practice of Neural Science.* New York, NY: McGraw-Hill; 2000.

Striking parallels exist between the functional and anatomical organization of the spinal and cranial somatic sensory systems. In fact, the principles governing the organization of one are nearly identical to those of the other. A similar comparison can be made between motor control of cranial structures and that of the limbs and trunk: Cranial muscles are innervated by motor neurons found in the cranial nerve motor nuclei, whereas limb and axial muscles are innervated by motor neurons in the motor nuclei of the ventral horn. A similar parallel exists with the control of body organs. Control of the glands and smooth muscle of the head, as well as the pupil, is mediated by parasympathetic preganglionic neurons located in cranial nerve autonomic nuclei. Abdominal visceral organs are controlled by parasympathetic neurons in the sacral cord.

This chapter examines in detail the cranial nerve motor nuclei innervating facial, jaw, and tongue muscles, as well as the muscles for swallowing. It also examines the cortical control of these nuclei, which is accomplished by the corticobulbar tract. This pathway is the cranial equivalent of the corticospinal tract, and the two pathways share numerous organizational principles. Knowing the patterns of corticobulbar connections with the cranial motor nuclei has important diagnostic value because it helps clinicians to understand the cranial motor signs produced by brain stem damage. This knowledge also helps clinicians to plan the proper therapy for the patient to avert potentially life-threatening sequelae. The autonomic and extraocular motor nuclei of the brain stem are also examined to achieve greater knowledge of regional anatomy. Such knowledge is essential for localizing central nervous system damage after trauma.

Organization of Cranial Motor Nuclei

There Are Three Columns of Cranial Nerve Motor Nuclei

As we saw in Chapter 6, the cranial nerve sensory and motor nuclei are organized into columns that course rostrocaudally throughout the brain stem (Figure 11–2). The sensory columns are located laterally and the motor columns, medially. The sensory nuclei derive from a portion of the developing neural ectoderm, the alar plate, of the brain stem and the motor nuclei, from the basal plate (Figure 11–3). The two collections of developing neurons undergo migration and further subdivision to give rise to the various columns of sensory and motor nuclei.

The cranial nerve motor nuclei are organized into three columns (Figure 11–2): somatic skeletal, branchiomeric, and autonomic. Nuclei in the **somatic skeletal motor column** contain motor neurons that innervate striated muscle derived from the **occipital somites** (see Figure 6-4): the extraocular and tongue muscles. This column is close to the midline. Nuclei of the **branchiomeric motor column** contain motor neurons innervating striated muscle derived from the **branchial arches** (ie, branchiomeric or visceral, opposed to somatic, origin): facial, jaw, palatal, pharyngeal, and laryngeal muscles. This column is lateral to the somatic skeletal motor column (Figure 11–2) and is displaced ventrally from the ventricular floor (Figure 11–2, bottom inset). Nuclei of the **autonomic motor column** contain the parasympathetic preganglionic neurons that regulate the functions of cranial exocrine glands, smooth muscle, and many body organs. The autonomic motor column is lateral to the somatic skeletal motor column (Figure 11–2). Sometimes these three columns are termed general somatic motor, special visceral motor, and general visceral motor columns, respectively (see Box 6–1).

Neurons in the Somatic Skeletal Motor Column Innervate Tongue and Extraocular Muscles

Four nuclei comprise the somatic skeletal motor column (Figure 11–2). Three of these nuclei contain motor neurons that innervate the extraocular muscles: the **oculomotor nucleus,** the **trochlear nucleus,** and the **abducens nucleus.** The oculomotor nucleus is located in the rostral midbrain and innervates the **medial rectus, inferior rectus, superior rectus,** and **inferior oblique muscles,** which move the eyes (see Figure 12–4), as well as the **levator palpebrae superioris**

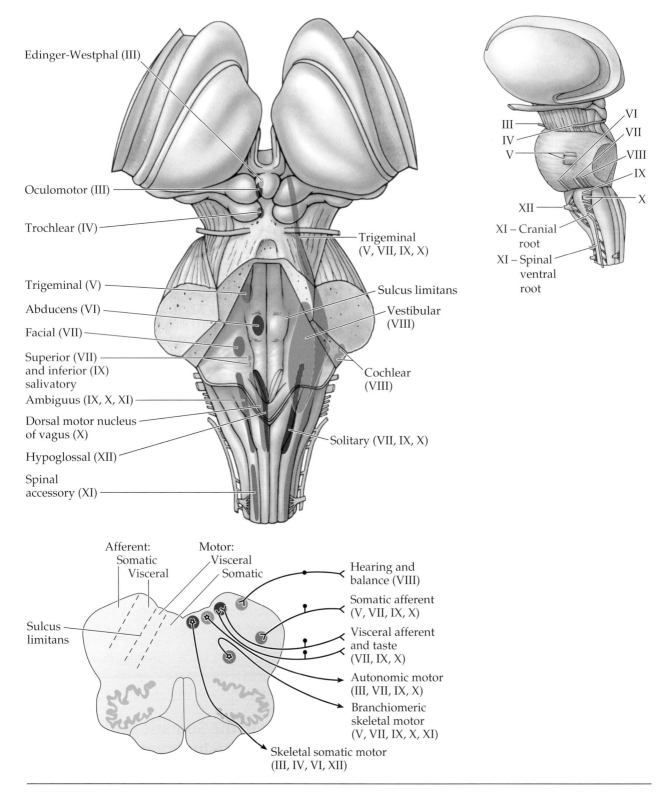

FIGURE 11–2 Dorsal view of the brain stem (without the cerebellum), showing the locations of cranial nerve nuclei. The top left inset, which is a lateral view of the diencephalon and basal ganglia, shows the various cranial nerves, the spinal accessory nerve, and a ventral root. The bottom inset is a schematic cross section through the medulla, showing the location of cranial nerve nuclear columns. (Adapted from Nieuwenhuys R, Voogd J, van Huijzen C. *The Human Central Nervous System: A Synopsis and Atlas.* 4th ed. London: Springer-Verlag; 2007.)

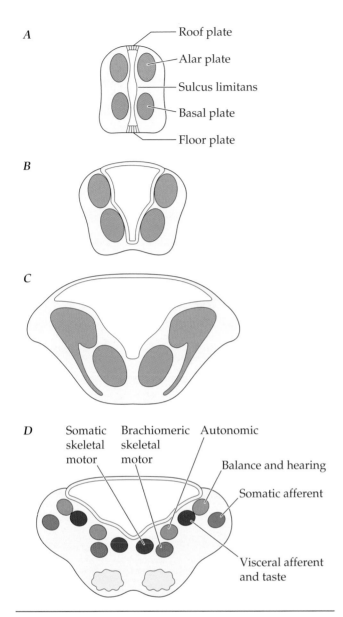

FIGURE 11–3 Development of the cranial nuclei. **A–D.** Schematic section through the hind brain at three developmental time points (**A–C**) and maturity (**D**). The space within the sections is the fourth ventricle. During development the fourth ventricle, initially flattened dorsoventrally just like the spinal cord, expands dorsally. This has the effect of transforming the dorsoventral sensory-motor nuclear organization characteristic of the spinal cord, into the lateromedial organization of sensory and motor nuclei in the caudal brain stem (the future medulla and pons). Developing neurons in the alar plate will become sensory cranial nuclei near the ventricular floor and, in the basal plate, cranial motor nuclei. Additionally, neurons from the plates migrate to more distant locations to serve more integrative functions.

muscle, an eyelid elevator. The motor axons course within the **oculomotor (III) nerve.** Motor neurons in the trochlear nucleus course in the **trochlear (IV) nerve** and innervate the **superior oblique muscle.** The **abducens nucleus** contains the motor neurons that project their axons to the periphery through the **abducens (VI) nerve** and innervate

the **lateral rectus muscle.** The neuroanatomy of eye muscle control is the focus of Chapter 12. The **hypoglossal nucleus** is the fourth member of the somatic skeletal motor column (Figure 11–2). The axons of motor neurons in the hypoglossal nucleus course in the **hypoglossal (XII) nerve** and innervate intrinsic tongue muscles, including the genioglossus, hypoglossus, and styloglossus.

The Branchiomeric Motor Column Innervates Skeletal Muscles That Develop From the Branchial Arches

Three cranial nerve nuclei constitute this nuclear column: the **facial motor nucleus,** the **trigeminal motor nucleus,** and the **nucleus ambiguus.** The facial motor nucleus contains the motor neurons that innervate the muscles of **facial expression.** These axons course in the **facial (VII) nerve.** The axons of motor neurons of the trigeminal motor nucleus course in the **trigeminal (V) nerve** and innervate principally the muscles of **mastication:** masseter, temporalis, and external and internal pterygoid muscles. The nucleus ambiguus contains motor neurons that innervate striated muscles of the **pharynx** and **larynx.** This nucleus and its efferent projections through cranial nerves are organized rostrocaudally. A small number of motor neurons in the most rostral portion of the nucleus ambiguus course in the **glossopharyngeal (IX) nerve** and innervate one pharyngeal muscle, the stylopharyngeus. Most motor neurons in the nucleus send their axons through the **vagus (X) nerve** to innervate the pharynx and larynx. Because the pharyngeal muscles are innervated by the vagus nerve, a lesion of the nucleus ambiguus produces difficulty in swallowing. The vagus nerve is the efferent component of the **gag reflex.** In this reflex, mechanical stimulation of the pharynx, using a cotton swab for example, produces reflex contraction of the pharyngeal muscles. The **glossopharyngeal nerve** contains the afferent fibers that innervate mechanoreceptors of the pharynx that comprise the afferent limb of the gag reflex (see Chapter 6). The most caudal portion of the nucleus ambiguus contains laryngeal motor neurons whose axons course in a portion of the **accessory (XI) nerve.** This cranial nerve consists of distinct **cranial and spinal roots,** and only axons in the cranial root have their cell bodies in the **nucleus ambiguus.** These axons are probably displaced vagal fibers. They join the vagus nerve as they exit from the cranium and innervate the same structures as the vagus; accordingly, they are sometimes considered to be part of the vagus nerve.

Cell bodies of axons in the spinal root of the spinal accessory nerve are located in the **spinal accessory nucleus** (Figure 11–2). This nucleus is a part of the ventral horn of the upper cervical spinal cord—from the pyramidal decussation to about the fourth or fifth cervical segments—not the branchiomeric motor column. Axons in the spinal root of the spinal accessory nerve innervate the **sternocleidomastoid muscle** and the upper part of the **trapezius muscle,** which develop from the somites and not the branchial arches.

The Autonomic Motor Column Contains Parasympathetic Preganglionic Neurons

The autonomic motor column contains neurons that regulate the function of various body organs, smooth muscles, and exocrine glands. These neurons are part of the **parasympathetic nervous system,** a division of the **autonomic nervous system** (see Chapters 1 and 15). In contrast to the innervation of skeletal muscle, which is mediated by a single motor neuron (Figure 11–4A), the innervation of smooth muscle and glands is accomplished by two

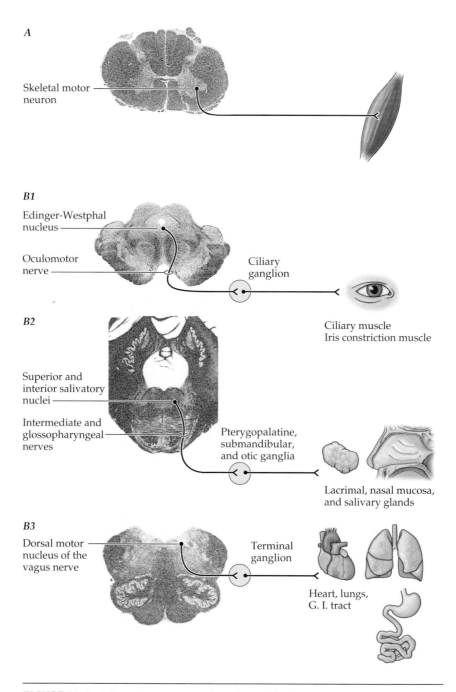

FIGURE 11–4 A. Somatic motor neurons have their cell body located in the central nervous system. Their axon projects directly to their peripheral targets, which are striated muscles. **B.** Parasympathetic preganglionic neurons are located in nuclei within the central nervous system, whereas postganglionic neurons are located in peripheral ganglia. **B1–B3** show examples of three parasympathetic functions: pupillary constriction (**B1**), secretions (**B2**), and visceral functions (**B3**).

separate neurons: preganglionic and postganglionic neurons (Figure 11–4B). Parasympathetic preganglionic neurons are located in the various nuclei that comprise the autonomic motor column; these neurons are also found in the sacral spinal cord (see Chapter 15). Parasympathetic postganglionic neurons are located in **peripheral autonomic ganglia.**

The autonomic motor column, which is lateral to the somatic skeletal motor column (Figure 11–2), contains four nuclei. The **Edinger-Westphal nucleus** is located in the midbrain and in the pretectal region, dorsal to the oculomotor nucleus (Figure 11–4B1). It participates in pupillary constriction and lens accommodation. The parasympathetic neurons in the nucleus send their axons into the **oculomotor (III) nerve** to synapse on postganglionic neurons in the **ciliary ganglion.** These neurons innervate the **ciliary muscle** and the **constrictor muscles of the iris.**

Parasympathetic preganglionic neurons are also located in nuclei of the caudal pons and medulla (Figure 11–4B2). Neurons of the **superior** and **inferior salivatory nuclei** are located in the pons and medulla. They are somewhat dispersed, not forming a discrete cell column. The axons of neurons of the superior salivatory nucleus course in the **intermediate nerve.** They synapse in two peripheral ganglia: (1) the **pterygopalatine** ganglion, where postganglionic neurons innervate the lacrimal glands and glands of the nasal mucosa, and (2) the **submandibular** ganglion, from which postganglionic parasympathetic neurons innervate the submandibular and sublingual salivary glands. The intermediate nerve is sometimes considered to be the sensory branch of the **facial nerve** because it contains afferent fibers, which are the axons of pseudounipolar neurons of the geniculate ganglion (see Chapters 6 and 9). The inferior salivatory nucleus contains parasympathetic preganglionic neurons whose axons course in the **glossopharyngeal nerve** and synapse on postganglionic neurons in the **otic ganglion** (Figure 11–4B2). Parasympathetic postganglionic neurons in the otic ganglion innervate the **parotid gland,** which secretes saliva.

The **dorsal motor nucleus of the vagus nerve** forms a column of parasympathetic preganglionic neurons beneath the floor of the **fourth ventricle** in the medulla (Figure 11–4B3). These neurons synapse in extracranial parasympathetic ganglia, called **terminal ganglia** (Figure 11–4B3). These ganglia are located in the viscera of the thoracic and abdominal cavities, including the gastrointestinal tract proximal to the splenic flexure of the colon. The functions of the vagal parasympathetic neurons include regulating heart rate (ie, slowing), gastric motility (ie, increasing), and bronchial muscle control (ie, contracting to constrict airway). (The colon distal to the splenic flexure is innervated by parasympathetic preganglionic neurons of the sacral spinal cord [see Chapter 15].)

The remaining sections of this chapter will focus on the cortical control of cranial motor nuclei and their regional anatomy in the pons and medulla.

The Functional Organization of the Corticobulbar Tract

The Cranial Motor Nuclei Are Controlled by the Cerebral Cortex and Diencephalon

Nuclei within the somatic skeletal and branchiomeric motor columns that innervate facial, tongue, jaw, laryngeal, and pharyngeal muscles are controlled by the cortical motor areas: the primary motor cortex, the supplementary motor area, the premotor cortex, and the cingulate motor area. These are the same cortical regions that control limb and trunk muscles (see Chapter 10). However, the cranial motor representations project to the various brain stem motor nuclei through the **corticobulbar tract,** one of the three components of the corticospinal system (Chapter 10). Nuclei that innervate extraocular muscles are controlled by different cortical areas and not by the corticobulbar tract and will be considered in Chapter 12. The nuclei comprising the autonomic motor column are influenced by projections from the cerebral cortex and **hypothalamus.** The autonomic nervous system and hypothalamus are considered in Chapter 15.

Of all the cortical motor areas, the **primary motor cortex** contributes the greatest number of axons to the corticobulbar tract. The cell bodies of these primary motor cortex axons are located within layer V of the cranial representation, which is the lateral precentral gyrus close to the **lateral sulcus** (see Figure 10–8). Their descending axons course within the internal capsule, along with but rostral to the corticospinal fibers. Corticobulbar neurons project to the pons and medulla. Their axons terminate either bilaterally or contralaterally, depending on the particular nucleus (see below). Muscles innervated by motor nuclei that receive a **bilateral projection** from the corticobulbar tract do not become weak after a unilateral lesion of the motor cortex, the internal capsule, or some other portion of its descending pathway. The projection from the intact side is sufficient for near-normal control of force production. This is not the case, however, for muscles receiving only a contralateral projection. In these instances, weakness reveals the unilateral damage. This relationship between the laterality of cortical control and the laterality of motor signs after unilateral damage is similar to that of the corticospinal system.

Bilateral Corticobulbar Tract Projections Innervate the Hypoglossal Nucleus, Trigeminal Nucleus, and Nucleus Ambiguus

The corticobulbar projection from the primary motor cortex to the hypoglossal nucleus is most commonly a bilateral one (Figure 11–5). Unilateral lesion of this projection, for example in the internal capsule, does not produce weakness of tongue muscles in the majority of people. In some individuals, however, contralateral tongue weakness does occur,

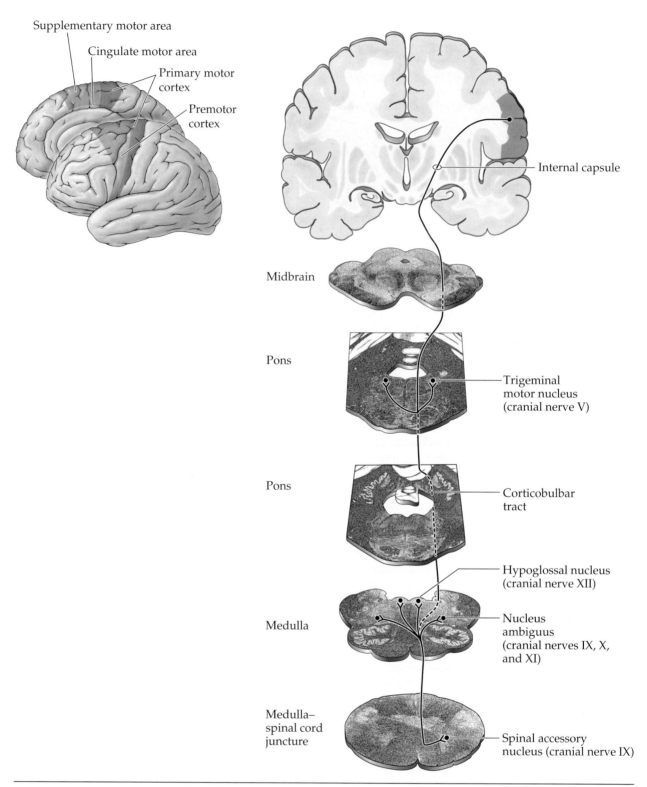

Supplementary motor area

Cingulate motor area

Primary motor cortex

Premotor cortex

Internal capsule

Midbrain

Pons — Trigeminal motor nucleus (cranial nerve V)

Pons — Corticobulbar tract

Hypoglossal nucleus (cranial nerve XII)

Medulla — Nucleus ambiguus (cranial nerves IX, X, and XI)

Medulla–spinal cord juncture — Spinal accessory nucleus (cranial nerve IX)

FIGURE 11–5 Cortical control of the branchiomeric motor cell column and hypoglossal nucleus. The top inset shows the locations of the primary motor cortex and three premotor areas: the supplementary motor area, the cingulate motor area, and the premotor cortex. Because most of these cranial motor nuclei receive a predominantly bilateral projection from the primary motor cortex, unilateral lesions have little or no effect. The spinal accessory nucleus is the exception. It receives a unilateral cortical projection. Lesion of this projection can produce unilateral weakness of the sternocleidomastoid muscle and part of the trapezius muscle.

suggesting a predominantly crossed (ie, unilateral) corticobulbar projection to the hypoglossal nucleus in these individuals. By contrast, a lesion of the hypoglossal nucleus or nerve consistently produces ipsilateral tongue paralysis. In the case of nucleus or nerve damage, when patients are asked to protrude their tongue, it deviates to the side of the lesion.

Because the primary motor cortex projects bilaterally to the trigeminal motor nuclei (Figure 11–5), unilateral cortical or descending pathway lesions do not produce weakness of the target muscles. Bilateral control by the primary motor cortex may reflect the fact that jaw muscles on both sides of the mouth are typically activated in tandem during most motor acts, for example, chewing or talking. This is similar to the bilateral control of axial muscles, for maintaining posture, by the medial descending spinal cord pathways (see Chapter 10).

The motor cortex also exerts bilateral control of motor neurons in the nucleus ambiguus (Figure 11–5), leading to the redundancy in their control, as discussed earlier. Whereas a unilateral lesion of the corticobulbar tract may not produce laryngeal and pharyngeal signs, brain stem lesions that damage the nucleus ambiguus and surrounding regions produce ipsilateral paralysis of pharyngeal and laryngeal muscles. Such damage results in hoarseness and swallowing impairments. Importantly, this also impairs the **airway protective reflex,** the automatic closure of the larynx during swallowing to prevent food and fluids from entering the trachea. When this reflex is impaired, small amounts of food or fluids can slip into the trachea, which can lead to aspiration pneumonia.

Unlike the nucleus ambiguus, which is under bilateral cortical control, the spinal accessory nucleus receives a predominantly ipsilateral cortical projection. This ipsilateral projection targets primarily the motor neurons of the sternocleidomastoid muscle, which turns the head to the opposite side. Interestingly, whereas the cortical projection is ipsilateral, the motor actions of the muscle produce a movement directed to the contralateral side.

Cortical Projections to the Facial Motor Nucleus Have a Complex Pattern

A facial nerve or nucleus lesion produces facial muscle paralysis over the entire **ipsilateral** face; this is a common occurrence in Bell's palsy, a viral infection of facial motor neurons. A unilateral lesion of the primary motor cortex, the internal capsule, or the descending cortical fibers produces differential effects on the voluntary control of upper and lower facial muscles. After the lesion, upper facial muscles retain voluntary control. A patient with such a lesion can furrow his or her brow symmetrically. In contrast, lower facial muscles contralateral to the side of the lesion become weak. A patient with such damage would smile asymmetrically when asked to smile by his or her physician. Surprisingly, if the patient were provoked to smile, for example by hearing a particularly

humorous joke, he or she could do so symmetrically, implying no facial weakness.

Knowledge of three features of the origin of corticobulbar neurons and the pattern of their connections helps to explain these peculiar effects. First, the primary motor cortex has dense contralateral projections to lower facial muscle motor neurons and sparse bilateral projections to upper facial motor neurons (Figure 11–6A). Thus, a lesion would be expected to weaken only the contralateral lower facial muscles. Second, motor neurons innervating upper facial muscles receive bilateral control by several premotor areas, especially the premotor cortex and cingulate motor region (Figure 11–6B). Third, the descending axons of these premotor regions are separated from those of the primary motor cortex; they are located farther rostrally in the corona radiata and internal capsule. They are typically spared with local cortical or internal capsule injury because they receive a different arterial supply (see Figure 3–6). As for the patient who is able to smile symmetrically after hearing a funny joke, that observation is also thought to be related to the intact premotor connections, especially those from the cingulate motor areas, which receive their major inputs from brain regions regulating emotions.

Regional Anatomy of Cranial Motor Nuclei and Corticobulbar Tract

The rest of this chapter focuses on the spatial relations between the cranial nerve motor nuclei innervating striated muscle, the corticobulbar tract, and key brain stem structures. In addition, this chapter further explains the three-dimensional organization of the brain stem.

Lesion of the Genu of the Internal Capsule Interrupts the Corticobulbar Tract

Similar to the corticospinal projection, neurons that form the corticobulbar tract originate from multiple cortical sites: the primary motor cortex, the supplementary motor area, the premotor cortex, and the cingulate motor area (see Figure 10–7). The corticobulbar projection descends in the genu and the posterior limb of the internal capsule, rostral to the corticospinal projection (Figure 11–7A, B). The various parts of the internal capsule are supplied by different cerebral artery branches (see Figure 3–6). The superficial portion is supplied by deep branches of the **middle cerebral artery.** The inferior part of the posterior limb is supplied by the **anterior choroidal artery,** and the inferior parts of the genu and anterior limbs are supplied primarily by deep branches of the **anterior cerebral artery.** In the midbrain, the descending cortical fibers, including the corticobulbar and corticospinal tracts, are together within the basis pedunculi (Figure 11–7C).

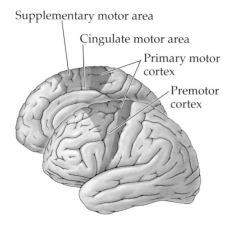

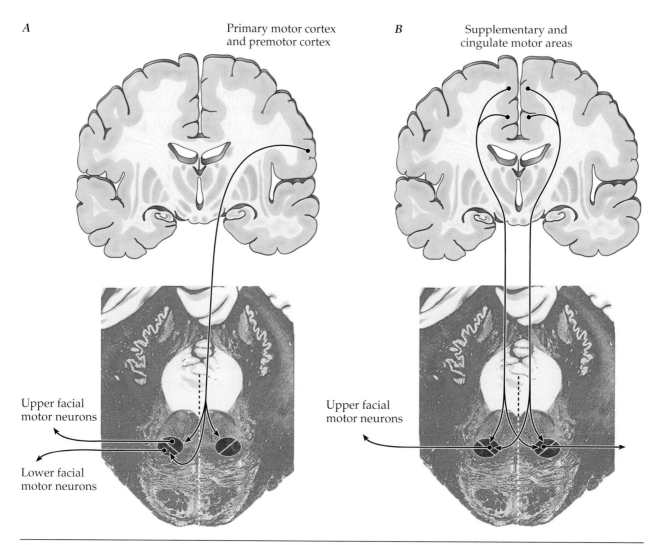

FIGURE 11–6 Pathways for the cortical control of facial motor neurons. **A.** Pathway from the primary motor and premotor cortical areas, which are both located on the lateral surface of the cortex. **B.** Pathway from the supplementary (*top*) and cingulate (*bottom*) motor areas, which are both located on the medial surface. The inset shows the locations of the primary motor cortex and the three premotor areas: the supplementary motor area, the cingulate motor area, and the premotor cortex.

A

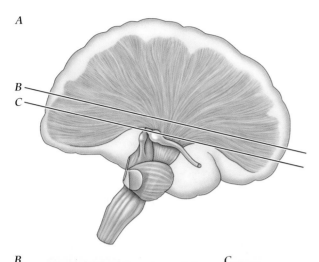

B   *C*

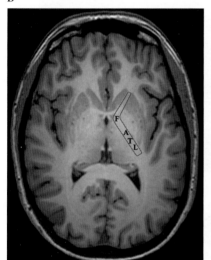   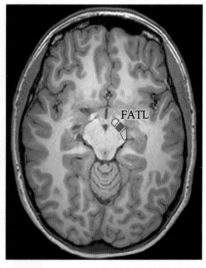

FIGURE 11–7 Internal capsule (**A**) and MRIs through internal capsule (**B**) and midbrain (**C**). The locations of the descending axons in the internal capsule and basis pedunculi are shown on the MRIs. The letters "FATL" abbreviate Face, Arm, Trunk, and Leg. In the midbrain, the descending cortical fibers (filled middle region in basis pedunculi) are flanked on either side by axons that originate in the cortex and synapse on neurons in the pontine nuclei (see Chapter 13). Within the filled regions, the order of descending axons are, from medial to lateral, face, arm, trunk, leg. Planes of section of MRIs in parts **B** and **C** are indicated in **A**. (**B, C**, Courtesy of Dr. Joy Hirsch, Columbia University.)

The Trigeminal Motor Nucleus Is Medial to the Main Trigeminal Sensory Nucleus

As the corticobulbar tract descends further, the projection becomes fragmented into innumerable small fascicles in the isthmus of the pons (Figure 11–8A). Farther caudally in the pons (Figure 11–8B), the fascicles coalesce to form a discrete bundle of descending cortical axons. This is at the level of the most rostral component of the branchiomeric motor column, the **trigeminal motor nucleus** (Figures 11–2 and 11–8B). The trigeminal motor nucleus is located lateral to the main trigeminal sensory nucleus (see Chapter 6). The trigeminal root fibers are located nearby (Figure 11–8B). The trigeminal motor nucleus is innervated bilaterally by the corticobulbar tract.

The Fibers of the Facial Nerve Have a Complex Trajectory Through the Pons

The pontine section shown in Figure 11–9A cuts through portions of the facial nerve. The axons leave the facial nucleus, where the motor neurons are located, and follow a path toward the floor of the fourth ventricle (Figure 11–9B). These fibers of the facial nerve are not seen in Figure 11–9A because they do not course in discrete and straight fascicles.

As the facial nerve fibers approach the ventricular floor, they first ascend close to the midline. Next, the fibers sweep around the medial, dorsal, and rostral aspects of the **abducens nucleus,** which contains motor neurons innervating the lateral rectus muscle, which abducts the eye (ie, looking away from the nose). This component is termed the **genu** of the facial nerve and, with the abducens nucleus, forms the **facial colliculus,** a surface landmark on the pontine floor of the fourth ventricle (Figure 11–9, inset). The facial nerve fibers then run ventrally and caudally to exit the pons at the **pontomedullary junction.** In addition to the axons of branchiomeric motor neurons, the facial nerve also contains visceral motor axons from the superior salivatory nucleus that innervate the **pterygopalatine** and **sub-mandibular** ganglia. The pterygopalatine ganglion innervates lacrimal glands and the nasal mucosa. The submandibular ganglion innervates submandibular and sublingual salivary glands.

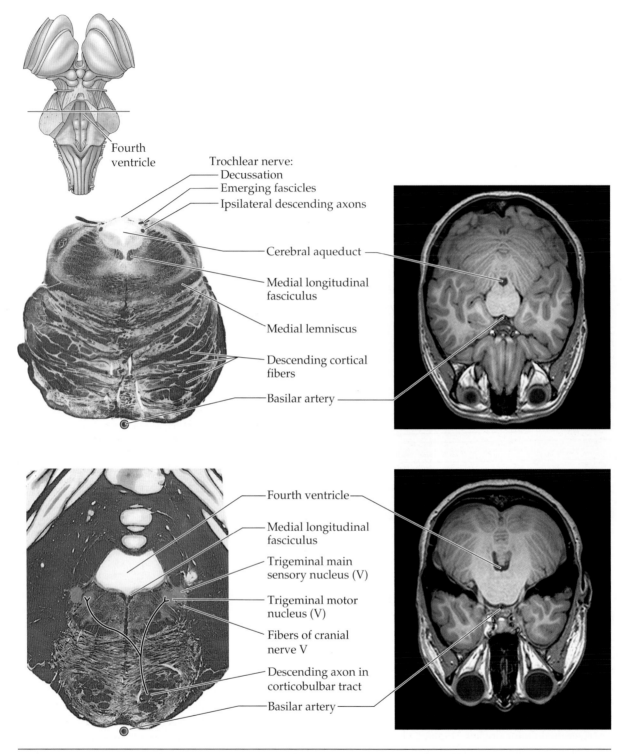

Fourth
ventricle

Trochlear nerve:
Decussation
Emerging fascicles
Ipsilateral descending axons

Cerebral aqueduct

Medial longitudinal
fasciculus

Medial lemniscus

Descending cortical
fibers

Basilar artery

Fourth ventricle

Medial longitudinal
fasciculus

Trigeminal main
sensory nucleus (V)

Trigeminal motor
nucleus (V)

Fibers of cranial
nerve V

Descending axon in
corticobulbar tract

Basilar artery

FIGURE 11–8 Myelin-stained transverse sections through the pons at the level of the isthmus (top, left) and trigeminal main sensory and motor nuclei (bottom, left). Corresponding MRIs are shown to the right. The inset shows the plane of section. (Courtesy of Dr. Joy Hirsch, Columbia University.)

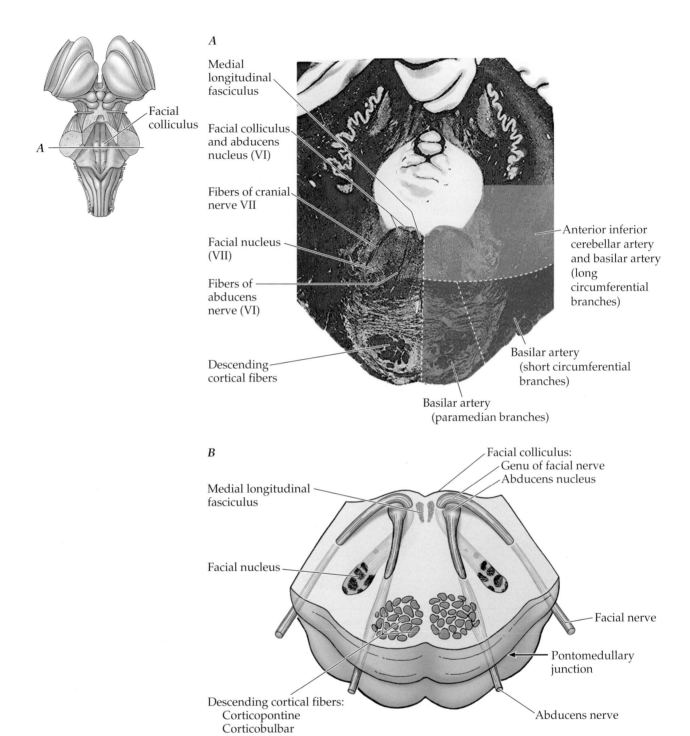

A.

Medial longitudinal fasciculus

Facial colliculus and abducens nucleus (VI)

Fibers of cranial nerve VII

Facial nucleus (VII)

Fibers of abducens nerve (VI)

Descending cortical fibers

Facial colliculus

A

Anterior inferior cerebellar artery and basilar artery (long circumferential branches)

Basilar artery (short circumferential branches)

Basilar artery (paramedian branches)

B

Facial colliculus:
Genu of facial nerve
Abducens nucleus

Medial longitudinal fasciculus

Facial nucleus

Facial nerve

Pontomedullary junction

Abducens nerve

Descending cortical fibers:
Corticopontine
Corticobulbar
Corticospinal

FIGURE 11–9 **A.** Myelin-stained transverse section through the pons at the level of the genu of cranial nerve VII. The arterial supply at this level is shown in **A. B.** The three-dimensional course of the facial nerve in the pons. The inset shows the plane of section in **A.** (**B,** Adapted from Williams PL, Warwick R. *Functional Neuroanatomy of Man.* New York, NY: W. B. Saunders; 1975.)

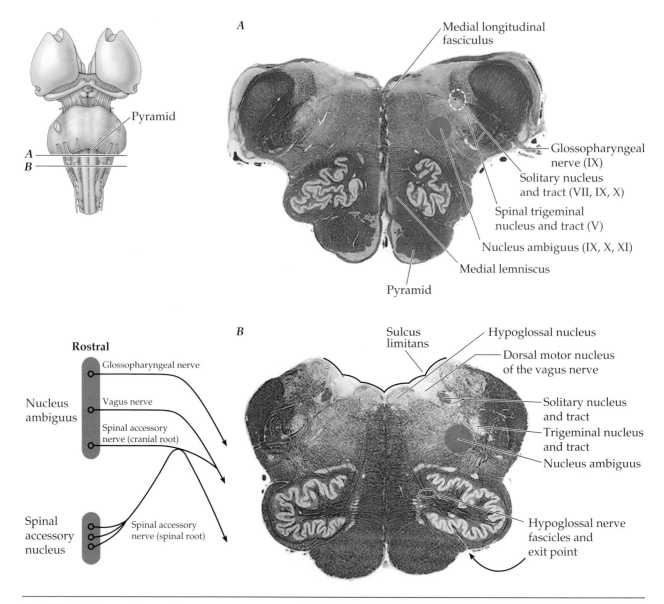

FIGURE 11–10   A. Myelin-stained transverse section at the level of exiting fibers of the glossopharyngeal (IX) nerve. **B.** Myelin-stained transverse section through the hypoglossal nucleus in the medulla. Top inset shows planes of section in **A** and **B.** Bottom inset shows the rostrocaudal organization of the nucleus ambiguus and spinal accessory nucleus.

The vascular supply to the pons is derived by separate paramedian, short circumferential, and long circumferential branches of the basilar artery (see Figure 3–3B2). At the level of the pons in Figure 11–9, the **anterior inferior cerebellar artery (AICA)** is the long circumferential branch. The more rostral pontine levels (Figure 11–8) also receive their blood supply from branches of the basilar artery.

The Glossopharyngeal Nerve Enters and Exits From the Rostral Medulla

The myelin-stained section through the rostral medulla is through the glossopharyngeal nerve root (Figure 11–10A). The motor axons of the glossopharyngeal nerve originate from neurons in two nuclei: Motor neurons innervating striated muscle (stylopharyngeus muscle) are located in the rostral portion of the **nucleus ambiguus;** autonomic motor neurons (parasympathetic preganglionic neurons) are located in the inferior salivatory nucleus. The parasympathetic preganglionic neurons innervate the otic ganglion, which, in turn, innervates the parotid gland for salivation.

From a clinical perspective, the glossopharyngeal nerve can be considered a sensory nerve because a unilateral lesion does not produce frank motor dysfunction (either somatic or visceral motor) on clinical examination. Recall that the glossopharyngeal nerve also contains gustatory and viscerosensory afferent fibers that terminate in the solitary nucleus as well as somatic sensory afferents that terminate in the trigeminal spinal nucleus (see Figure 11–10B).

A Level Through the Mid-medulla Reveals the Locations of Six Cranial Nerve Nuclei

The three cranial nerve motor nuclei in the mid-medulla—the hypoglossal nucleus, the dorsal motor nucleus of vagus, and the nucleus ambiguus—are medial to the three sensory nuclei at this level—the solitary, vestibular, and spinal trigeminal nuclei (Figure 11–10B). The cranial nerve sensory and motor nuclei are roughly separated by the sulcus limitans (Figure 11–10B). The hypoglossal and vagal nuclei are immediately beneath the floor of the fourth ventricle, whereas the nucleus ambiguus is deeper within the medulla (Figure 11–10B; see also Figure 11–13). The precise location of the nucleus ambiguus cannot be determined in myelin-stained sections; its approximate location is indicated in Figure 11–10B.

Infarction in the territory of different arterial branches interrupts the function of specific cranial nerve nuclei and brain stem pathways

In the medulla, different cranial nerve nuclei receive their arterial supply from specific branches of the vertebral-basilar system (Figure 11–12). The medial portion of the medulla is supplied by branches of the main portion of the vertebral artery. This region contains the hypoglossal nucleus, the medial lemniscus, and the pyramid. Infarction of this region of the medulla produces three deficits. First, tongue muscles are paralyzed on the side of the lesion because the **hypoglossal motor neurons** and **axons** are destroyed. Second, tactile sensation, vibration sense, and limb proprioception sense on the side opposite the lesion are impaired because the **medial lemniscus** is affected. Third, muscles of the limb on the side opposite the lesion are weak because corticospinal axons in the **pyramid** are affected.

The dorsolateral portion of the medulla is supplied by the **posterior inferior cerebellar artery (PICA)** (Figure 11–12). Six key sensory and motor signs—which comprise the **lateral medullary,** or **Wallenberg, syndrome**—can be produced when the territory of this artery becomes infarcted. We considered several sensory signs of this syndrome in Chapter 6, and

we will consider this syndrome further in Chapter 15. Among the sensory and motor signs, three are associated with damage to different cranial nerve nuclei:

- Difficulty in swallowing and hoarseness result from lesions of the **nucleus ambiguus.** An associated change, the loss of the gag reflex, is due either to lesions of the nucleus ambiguus (the efferent limb of the reflex) or to loss of pharyngeal sensation (cranial nerve IX) (the afferent limb).
- **Vertigo** (an illusion of a whirling movement; sometimes described as dizziness) and **nystagmus** (involuntary rhythmical oscillation of the eyes) are produced by **vestibular nuclear** lesions (see Chapter 12).
- Loss of pain and temperature senses on the ipsilateral face is due to lesions of the **spinal trigeminal nucleus** and **tract.**

The remaining signs result from damage to ascending or descending pathways that course through the dorsolateral medulla:

- Reduced pain and temperature senses on the contralateral limbs and trunk reflect lesion of the **anterolateral system.**
- Ipsilateral limb **ataxia** (jerky or uncoordinated movements) is due to lesions of the **inferior cerebellar peduncle,** which brings sensory information to the cerebellum (see Chapter 13).
- **Horner syndrome** results from damage to descending axons from the hypothalamus that regulate the functions of the sympathetic nervous system. (The precise location of these axons in the dorsolateral medulla is not known.) Horner syndrome consists of **pupillary constriction** due to unopposed actions of parasympathetic pupillary constrictors; **pseudoptosis** due to weakness of the tarsal muscle, a smooth muscle that assists the action of the levator palpebrae muscle (ptosis is drooping of the upper eyelid due to levator palpebrae muscle weakness); **reddening** of facial skin due to loss of sympathetic vasoconstrictor activity and resulting vasodilation; and **impaired sweating** due to loss of sympathetic control of the sweat glands (see Chapter 15).

Box 11–1

Cortical Control of Swallowing

Swallowing is a coordinated motor response that transports food and fluids from the mouth to the stomach. A swallow comprises multiple phases, beginning with the oral phase when the food is formed into a bolus and leading into the pharyngeal phase when the food bolus is transported into the esophagus. The final, or esophageal phase, carries the food into the stomach. The cerebral cortex plays an important role in initiating swallowing, especially during the oral phase. Brain stem centers organize the patterns of pharyngeal and esophageal muscle contraction for swallowing, much like spinal circuits organize limb muscle patterns for limb reflexes.

There are two key brain stem regions for swallowing. The first is the **solitary nucleus** (Figure 11–10B), which is important in

viscerosensory functions (see Chapter 6) and taste (see Chapter 9). It receives sensory information directly from the nerves innervating the mucous membranes of the pharynx and larynx, especially the superficial laryngeal nerve of the vagus nerve. The solitary nucleus projects to the second key region, comprising the **nucleus ambiguus** and the adjoining **reticular formation** (Figure 11–10B), which contain motor neurons and interneurons responsible for producing the muscle contractions for swallowing. These brain stem centers are also important for organizing the **airway protective reflex,** for closing the larynx during swallowing to prevent aspiration of food and fluids into the lungs.

(continued)

Box 11–1 (continued)

The frontal lobe motor areas are essential for initiating swallowing and for adapting the patterns of muscle contractions to different foods and fluids. The lateral precentral gyrus, containing the head representations of the primary motor and lateral premotor cortical areas, becomes active during swallowing (Figure 11–11A; transverse image). This activation occurs not only with voluntary swallowing but also during an autonomic and largely subconscious form of swallowing as saliva accumulates in the mouth. These cortical areas are activated bilaterally, reflecting the bilateral organization of the cortical projections to the nucleus ambiguus and the solitary nucleus.

Up to one third of patients who have strokes affecting cortical motor function experience **dysphagia,** a swallowing impairment, such as choking when starting to swallow. **Pulmonary aspiration** and malnutrition are two serious consequences of dysphagia. Why do some stroke victims have swallowing impairments if redundancy exists in the corticobulbar projection? Researchers have shown that the cortical representation of swallowing is asymmetrical, with dominant and nondominant hemispheres. In many people,

functional imaging shows an asymmetry in cortical activation during swallowing, suggesting that the side with the larger response is dominant for swallowing. Consistent with this idea, when the side with the larger response is stimulated noninvasively using transcranial magnetic stimulation, normal subjects show stronger contractions of pharyngeal and esophageal muscles from that side than the other. It is somewhat more common for the right hemisphere to be dominant (Figure 11–11B). (The side does not seem to depend on handedness.)

It has been suggested that stroke patients who develop dysphagia sustained a lesion to their dominant hemisphere and that they may recover effective swallowing because the nondominant intact hemisphere becomes dominant after the injury. The bilateral organization of the corticobulbar projections to the nucleus ambiguus might therefore provide an important anatomical substrate for recovery. Another mechanism for recovery of swallowing function is for other cortical regions on the same side, such as the cingulate motor area, to play a more important role after damage.

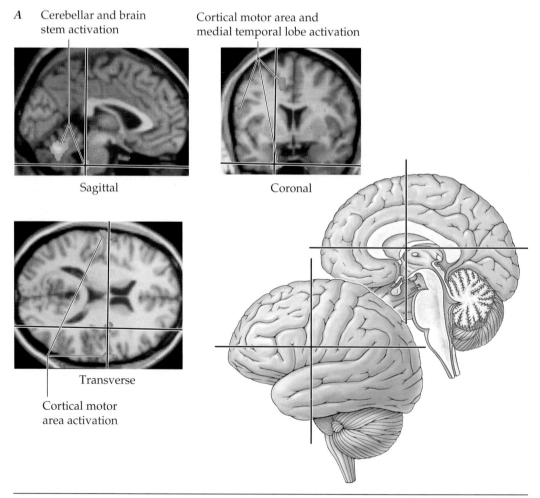

A   Cerebellar and brain stem activation

Cortical motor area and medial temporal lobe activation

Sagittal

Coronal

Transverse

Cortical motor area activation

FIGURE 11–11 Cortical control of swallowing. **A.** Functional magnetic resonance imaging scans. The inset in the center of the figure shows the planes of section on medial and lateral brain views. The transverse slice shows that there is bilateral motor cortical activation. There is also activation of subcortical structures, the cerebellum, and the brain stem.

B   Left   Right

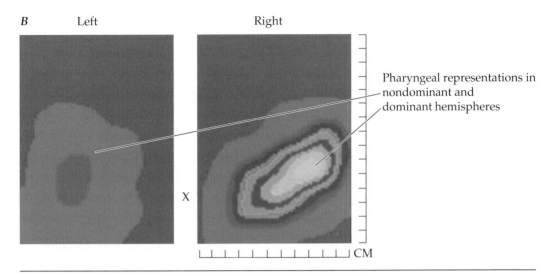

Pharyngeal representations in nondominant and dominant hemispheres

X

CM

FIGURE 11–11 *B.* Functional maps of the primary motor cortex areas where transcranial magnetic stimulation evokes contraction of pharyngeal and esophageal muscles. (Courtesy of Dr. Shaheen Hamdy, University of Manchester and the Medical Research Council; Hamdy S, Rothwell JC, Brooks DJ, Bailey D, Aziz Q, Thompson DG. Identification of the cerebral loci processing human swallowing with H215O PET activation. *J Neurophysiol.* 1999;81:1917-1926.)

The Spinal Accessory Nucleus Is Located at the Junction of the Spinal Cord and Medulla

The **pyramidal decussation** marks the boundary between the spinal cord and medulla (Figure 11–13B). The **spinal accessory nerve** contains axons of motor neurons whose cell bodies are located in the **spinal accessory nucleus** (Figure 11–13B). Recall that these motor neurons innervate the sternocleidomastoid muscle and the upper part of the trapezius muscle. Comparison of this section with the one through the cervical enlargement (eg, see Figure AII–5) reveals the similarity in location of the spinal accessory nucleus, on the one hand, and the ventral horn motor nuclei, on the other.

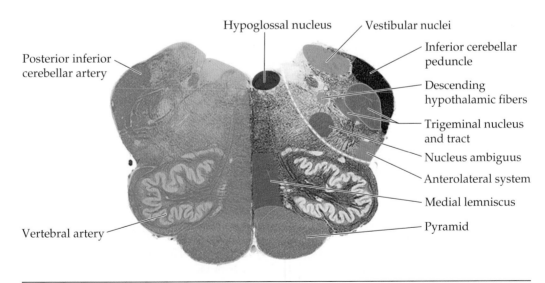

Hypoglossal nucleus — Vestibular nuclei

Posterior inferior cerebellar artery

Inferior cerebellar peduncle

Descending hypothalamic fibers

Trigeminal nucleus and tract

Nucleus ambiguus

Anterolateral system

Medial lemniscus

Vertebral artery

Pyramid

FIGURE 11–12 Arterial supply of the medulla. Occlusion of the posterior inferior cerebellar artery produces a complex set of neurological deficits, termed the lateral medullary, or Wallenberg, syndrome (see Chapter 6). Occlusion of the vertebral artery can produce a discrete set of limb sensory and motor signs.

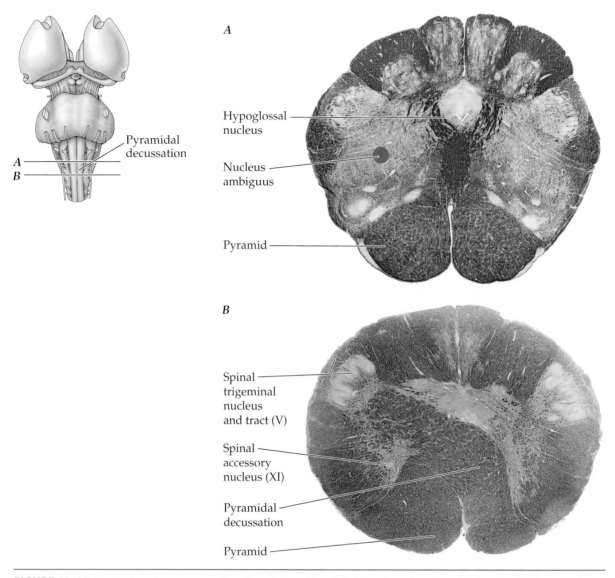

FIGURE 11–13 Myelin-stained transverse sections through the mid-medulla (**A**) and spinal cord–medulla junction (**B**). The inset shows planes of section in **A** and **B**.

Summary

There are three separate columns of cranial nerve motor nuclei (Figure 11–2), from medial to lateral: somatic skeletal motor, branchiomeric motor, and autonomic.

Somatic Skeletal Motor Nuclei

The somatic skeletal motor column is the most medial motor column. It comprises four nuclei, each of which contains motor neurons that innervate striated muscle derived from the *occipital somites.* The *oculomotor nucleus* (1) (Figure 11–2) contains motor neurons whose axons course in the *oculomotor (III) nerve* and innervate the following extraocular muscles: *medial rectus, superior rectus, inferior rectus,* and *inferior oblique.* The oculomotor nucleus also innervates the *levator palpebrae superioris muscle.*

The *trochlear nucleus* (2), via the *trochlear (IV) nerve,* innervates the *contralateral superior oblique muscle.* The *abducens nucleus* (3), via the *abducens (VI) nerve,* innervates the *lateral rectus muscle.* The *hypoglossal nucleus* (4) gives rise to axons that course in the *hypoglossal (XII) nerve* and innervate tongue muscles (Figures 11–2, 11–5, 11–10, and 11–12). The hypoglossal nucleus is the only nucleus of this column that receives a projection from the primary motor cortex.

Branchiomeric Motor Nuclei

The branchiomeric motor column is displaced ventrally from the floor of the fourth ventricle (Figures 11–2 and 11–3). It contains three nuclei, each of which innervates striated muscles derived from the branchial arches. The *trigeminal motor nucleus* (1) (Figures 11–5 and 11–8B) innervates the muscles of *mastication* via the *trigeminal (V) nerve*. This nucleus receives a bilateral projection from the motor cortex. The *facial nucleus* (2) (Figures 11–2 and 11–9) innervates the muscles of facial expression. The axons of facial motor neurons course in the *facial (VII) nerve*. Facial motor neurons that innervate lower face muscles receive a contralateral projection from the primary motor cortex. Motor neurons innervating upper facial muscles receive weak bilateral projections from the primary motor cortex but dense projections from premotor areas (Figure 11–6). The *nucleus ambiguus* (3) innervates the muscles of the *pharynx* and *larynx* predominantly via the *vagus (X) nerve* and to a lesser extent via the *glossopharyngeal (IX) nerve* and the cranial root of the *spinal accessory (XI) nerve* (Figure 11–5). The *spinal accessory nucleus* (spinal root) is in line with the nucleus ambiguus but is not part of the branchiomeric motor column. It innervates the sternocleidomastoid and trapezius muscles via the *spinal accessory (XI) nerve* (Figures 11–2 and 11–13B).

Autonomic Nuclei

The autonomic motor column contains four nuclei (Figure 11–2). Each nucleus contains *parasympathetic preganglionic neurons* (Figures 11–4 and 11–7). The *Edinger-Westphal nucleus* (1) is located in the midbrain. Its axons project via the *oculomotor nerve* to the *ciliary ganglion*, where postganglionic neurons innervate the constrictor muscles of the iris and the ciliary muscle (see Chapter 12). Axons from the *superior salivatory nucleus* (2) course in the *intermediate nerve* (a branch of the *facial nerve*). Via synapses in the pterygopalatine and submandibular ganglia, this nucleus influences the *lacrimal gland* and *glands of the nasal mucosa*. The *inferior salivatory nucleus* (3), via the *glossopharyngeal nerve*, synapses on postganglionic neurons in the *otic ganglion*. From there, postganglionic neurons innervate the *parotid gland*. Axons from the *dorsal motor nucleus of the vagus* (4) (Figures 11–10 and 11–13) course in the periphery in the *vagus nerve* and innervate *terminal ganglia* in most of the thoracic and abdominal viscera (proximal to the splenic flexure of the colon).

Selected Readings

Saper C, Lumsden A, Richerson GB, The sensory, motor, and reflex functions of the brain stem. In: Kandel ER, Schwartz JH, Jessell TM, Siegelbaum SA, Hudspeth AJ, eds. *Principles of Neural Science.* 5th ed. New York, NY: McGraw-Hill; in press.

Patten J. *Neurological Differential Diagnosis.* 2nd ed. London, UK: Springer-Verlag; 1996:448.

References

Akert K, Glickman MA, Lang W, et al. The Edinger-Westphal nucleus in the monkey: a retrograde tracer study. *Brain Res.* 1980;184:491-498.

Aviv J. The normal swallow. In: Carrau RL, ed. *Comprehensive Management of Swallowing Disorders.* San Diego, CA: Singular Publishing Group; 1999:23-29.

Broussard DL, Altschuler SM. Brainstem viscerotopic organization of afferents and efferents involved in the control of swallowing. *Am J Med.* 2000;108(Suppl 4a):79S-86S.

Chung CS, Caplan LR, Yamamoto Y, et al. Striatocapsular haemorrhage. *Brain.* 2000;123:1850-1862.

Geyer S, Matelli M, Luppino G, Zilles K. Functional neuroanatomy of the primate isocortical motor system. *Anat Embryol (Berl).* 2000;202(6):443-474.

Hamdy S, Rothwell JC. Gut feelings about recovery after stroke: the organization and reorganization of human swallowing motor cortex. *Trends Neurosci.* 1998;21:278-282.

Hamdy S, Rothwell JC, Brooks DJ, Bailey D, Aziz Q, Thompson DG. Identification of the cerebral loci processing human swallowing with H2^{15}O PET activation. *J Neurophysiol.* 1999;81:1917-1926.

Han BS, Hong JH, Hong C, et al. Location of the corticospinal tract at the corona radiata in human brain. *Brain Res.* 2010;1326:75-80.

Holodny AI, Watts R, Korneinko VN, et al. Diffusion tensor tractography of the motor white matter tracts in man: current controversies and future directions. *Ann N Y Acad Sci.* 2005;1064:88-97.

Hong JH, Son SM, Jang SH. Somatotopic location of corticospinal tract at pons in human brain: a diffusion tensor tractography study. *Neuroimage.* 2010;51(3):952-955.

Humbert IA, Robbins J. Normal swallowing and functional magnetic resonance imaging: a systematic review. *Dysphagia.* 2007;22(3):266-275.

Jang SH. A review of corticospinal tract location at corona radiata and posterior limb of the internal capsule in human brain. *NeuroRehabilitation.* 2009;24(3):279-283.

Jenny AB, Saper CB. Organization of the facial nucleus and corticofacial projection in the monkey: a reconsideration of the upper motor neuron facial palsy. *Neurology.* 1987;37:930-939.

Kidder TM. Esophago/pharyngo/laryngeal interrelationships: airway protection mechanisms. *Dysphagia.* 1995;10:228-231.

Kumar A, Juhasz C, Asano E, et al. Diffusion tensor imaging study of the cortical origin and course of the corticospinal tract in healthy children. *AJNR Am J Neuroradiol.* 2009;30(10):1963-1970.

Lowey AD, Saper CB, Yamondis ND. Re-evaluation of the efferent projections of the Edinger-Westphal nucleus in the cat. *Brain Res.* 1978;141:153-159.

Martin RE, Goodyear BG, Gati JS, Menon RS. Cerebral cortical representation of automatic and volitional swallowing in humans. *J Neurophysiol.* 2001;85:938-950.

Martin RE, Sessle BJ. The role of the cerebral cortex in swallowing. *Dysphagia.* 1993;8:195-202.

Matelli M, Luppino G, Geyer S, Zilles K. Motor cortex. In: Paxinos G, Mai JK, eds. *The Human Nervous System.* London: Elsevier; 2004:975-996.

Michou E, Hamdy S. Cortical input in control of swallowing. *Curr Opin Otolaryngol Head Neck Surg.* Jun 2009;17(3):166-171.

Miller AJ. Deglutition. *Physiol Rev.* 1982;62:129-184.

Miller AJ. The search for the central swallowing pathway: the quest for clarity. *Dysphagia.* 1993;8:185-194.

Morecraft RJ, Louie JL, Herrick JL, Stilwell-Morecraft KS. Cortical innervation of the facial nucleus in the non-human primate: a new interpretation of the effects of stroke and related subtotal brain trauma on the muscles of facial expression. *Brain.* 2001;124:176-208.

Morecraft RJ, McNeal DW, Stilwell-Morecraft KS, et al. Amygdala interconnections with the cingulate motor cortex in the rhesus monkey. *J Comp Neurol.* 2007;500(1):134-165.

Mosier KM, Liu WC, Maldjian JA, Shah R, Modi B. Lateralization of cortical function in swallowing: a functional MR imaging study. *AJNR Am J Neuroradiol.* 1999;20(8): 1520-1526.

Shaker R. Airway protective mechanisms: current concepts. *Dysphagia.* 1995;10:216-227.

Soros P, Inamoto Y, Martin RE. Functional brain imaging of swallowing: an activation likelihood estimation meta-analysis. *Hum Brain Mapp.* 2009;30(8):2426-2439.

Soros P, Lalone E, Smith R, et al. Functional MRI of oropharyngeal air-pulse stimulation. *Neuroscience.* 2008;153(4): 1300-1308.

Thompson ML, Thickbroom GW, Mastaglia FL. Corticomotor representation of the sternocleidomastoid muscle. *Brain.* 1997;120:245-255.

Törk I, McRitchie DA, Rikkard-Bell GC, Paxinos G. Autonomic regulatory centers in the medulla oblongata. In: Paxinos G, ed. *The Human Nervous System.* San Diego, CA: Academic Press; 1990:221-259.

Study Questions

1. Which statement below best describes the spatial relationship between cranial nerve motor and sensory nuclei in the medulla and pons?
    A. Motor nuclei are ventral to sensory nuclei
    B. Motor nuclei are dorsal to sensory nuclei
    C. Motor nuclei are medial to sensory nuclei
    D. Motor nuclei are lateral to sensory nuclei

2. Which of the following statements best describes the difference between innervation of skeletal muscle and smooth muscle by central nervous system neurons?
    A. Central nervous system neurons innervate skeletal muscle monosynaptically and innervate smooth muscle disynaptically via a synapse in peripheral ganglia.
    B. Central nervous system neurons innervate skeletal and smooth muscle monosynaptically.
    C. Central nervous system neurons innervate skeletal muscle disynaptically via a synapse in peripheral ganglia and innervate smooth muscle monosynaptically.
    D. Central nervous system neurons innervate skeletal and smooth muscle disynaptically via a synapse in peripheral ganglia.

3. After an internal capsule stroke, a person can loose some cranial nerve motor function. Typically, the lost function is expressed only on the contralateral side. Which statement below best explains this contralateral pattern?
    A. All corticobulbar projections are contralateral. Thus, a unilateral lesion will produce contralateral deficits.
    B. All corticobulbar projections are bilateral, but the contralateral projections are the strongest. When these strong connections are eliminated after a unilateral lesion, contralateral deficits occur.
    C. Some cranial motor nuclei receive contralateral corticobulbar projections, whereas others receive a bilateral projection. Nevertheless, the contralateral projections are the strongest, and when they are eliminated after a unilateral lesion, contralateral deficits occur.
    D. Cranial motor nuclei that receive bilateral corticobulbar projections are protected from gross impairment after unilateral corticobulbar lesions, whereas those receiving only a contralateral corticobulbar projection are not.

4. Which of the following best indicates the location of lost contralateral facial muscle control after a corticobulbar tract stroke?
   A. Upper facial muscles
   B. Lower facial muscles
   C. Upper and lower facial muscles
   D. Perioral and buccal muscles for assisting speech

5. A stroke affecting the corticobulbar tract will produce which of the following trigeminal motor impairments?
   A. Weakness or paralysis of contralateral muscles of mastication
   B. Weakness or paralysis of ipsilateral muscles of mastication
   C. Weakness or paralysis of muscles of mastication, bilaterally
   D. Minimal weakness because the trigeminal motor nucleus receives a bilateral corticobulbar tract innervation

6. Which of the following statements best describes the corticobulbar projection in the internal capsule?
   A. Corticobulbar axons receive an arterial supply from the posterior cerebral artery.
   B. Corticobulbar axons are located rostral to corticospinal axons.
   C. Corticobulbar axons descend in the anterior limb of the internal capsule.
   D. Corticobulbar axons intermingle with corticospinal axons in the posterior limb of the internal capsule.

7. A person has a developmental disorder in which some neurons fail to migrate from the ventricular surface during prenatal development. If this condition affects facial motor neurons, where would you expect to find facial motor neurons in this patient compared with a healthy person?

A. Dorsal
B. Ventral
C. Caudal
D. Lateral

8. A person has a stroke that damages the caudal part of the nucleus ambiguus. Which function is most impaired as a result of this lesion?
   A. Pharyngeal muscle control
   B. Laryngeal muscle control
   C. Tongue muscle control
   D. Blood pressure regulation

9. A person has a posterior inferior cerebellar artery (PICA) stroke. Which of the following indicates a likely motor impairment in this patient?
   A. Ipsilateral limb muscle weakness
   B. Ipsilateral tongue muscle weakness
   C. Ipsilateral laryngeal muscle weakness
   D. Ipsilateral facial muscle weakness

10. A person has a posterior inferior cerebellar artery (PICA) stroke. Which statement below best describes the pattern of sensory loss in this patient?
    A. Loss of pain and temperature on the contralateral limbs and trunk and the ipsilateral face
    B. Loss of pain and temperature on the contralateral limbs, trunk, and face
    C. Loss of pain and temperature on the contralateral limbs and trunk and the ipsilateral face, and loss of facial touch ipsilaterally
    D. Loss of pain and temperature on the contralateral limbs and trunk and the ipsilateral face, and loss of facial touch contralaterally

The Vestibular System and Eye Movements

CLINICAL CASE | One-and-One-Half Syndrome

A 30-year-old woman suddenly developed double vision that became worse upon looking to the right. She also indicated that she was unable to look to her left. On examination, when asked to look to the left, her eyes remained fixed forward, as she described. She was unable to abduct the left eye, and the right eye, which normally adducts on looking to the left, remained fixed forward (Figure 12–1A). When she was asked to look to the right, her left eye did not adduct (Figure 12–1B).

She had an MRI that revealed a mid-pontine lesion located close to the midline, just under the floor of the fourth ventricle (Figure 12–1B1). Normal MRI is shown in Figure 12–1B2, and a myelin-stained section through the pons is shown in Figure 12–1B3. In addition to this lesion, the patient had additional white matter lesions. Based on these neurological and radiological signs, as well as additional laboratory tests, the patient was diagnosed with multiple sclerosis.

Based on your reading of this chapter, you should be able to answer the following questions.

1. **Interruption of which components of the eye movement control circuit in this patient leads to the inability to look to the left?**

2. **Why does the left eye fail to adduct on looking to the right?**

Key neurological signs and corresponding damaged brain structures

Loss of ability to gaze to the left

The lesion included the left abducens nucleus. This damaged abducens muscle motor neurons, thereby paralyzing

—Continued next page

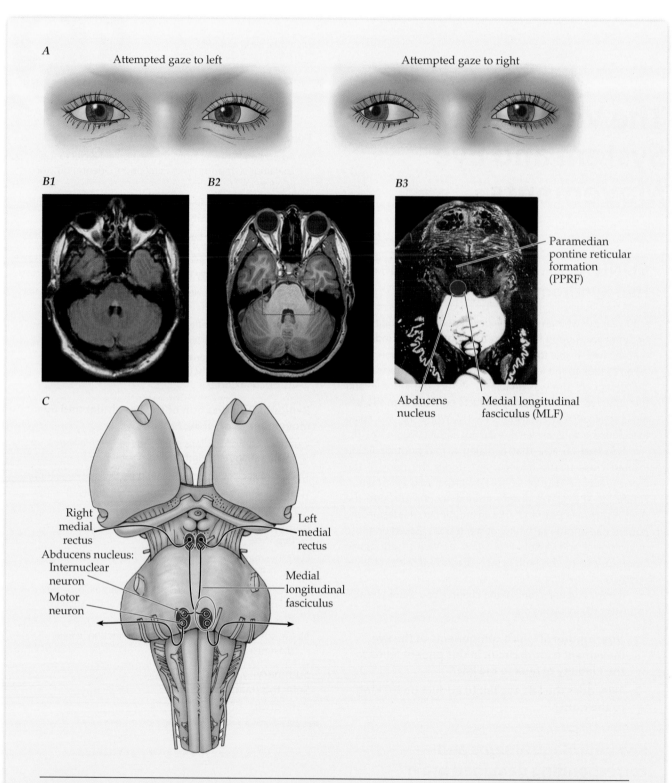

FIGURE 12–1 One-and-one-half syndrome. **A.** *Top.* Position of eyes when the patient is attempting to look to her left. Note that both eyes are fixed forward. *Bottom.* Position of eyes when patient is attempting to look to her right. The right eye abducts, but the left eye is fixed forward; there is no left eye adduction. **B.** Images of the pons. **B1.** MRI (**FLAIR**) of patient, showing lesion (bright region) (Reproduced with permission from Espinosa PS. Teaching NeuroImage: One-and-a-half-syndrome. *Neurology.* 2008;70[5]:e20.) **B2.** Normal MRI. **B3.** Myelin-stained section showing the locations of key structures and the approximate location of the lesion. **C.** Ventral brain stem view showing the circuit for horizontal gaze. The red ellipse indicates the extent of the lesion, which disrupts the left abducens nucleus and left MLF. (**B1,** Reproduced with permission from Espinosa PS. Teaching NeuroImage: One-and-a-half-syndrome. *Neurology.* 2008;70[5]:e20. **B2,** Courtesy of Dr. Joy Hirsch, Columbia University.)

that muscle. Adduction of the right eye was also absent. This is because the muscle control signals to look to the left originate in the left pons (Figures 12–1C and 12–7). When we want to look to the left, the paramedian pontine reticular formation, which receives commands from the cortex, sends signals to the left abducens nucleus. There are two neuron classes there: abducens motor neurons, which innervate the abducens muscle, and internuclear neurons, which project into the right MLF to command right medial rectus motor neurons to contract the medial rectus muscle to adduct the right eye. The lesion damages these neurons, as well as the motor neurons. Note that there is slight asymmetry to the left eye, showing a small amount of adduction, due to paralysis of the left lateral rectus muscle and the unopposed pulling of the intact right medial rectus muscle. Since multiple sclerosis is an inflammatory demyelinating condition, neurons are likely not degenerated but functionally impaired.

Inability to adduct the left eye on looking to the right

The lesion includes the MLF on the left side. Internuclear neurons from the opposite abducens nucleus project their axons into this MLF to reach left medial rectus motor neurons. Note that typically there is nystagmus, an abnormal oscillation or bobbing, of the abducting eye (see Figure 12–13).

References

Brust JCM. *The Practice of Neural Science*. New York, NY: McGraw-Hill; 2000.

Espinosa PS. Teaching NeuroImage: one-and-a-half-syndrome. *Neurology.* 2008;70:e20.

Shintani S, Tsuruoka S, Shiigai T. One-and-a-half syndrome associated with cheirooral syndrome. *Am J Neuroradiol.* 1996;17:1482-1484.

Uesaka Y, Nose H, Ida M. The pathway of gustatory fibers in the human ascends ipsilaterally. *Neurology.* 1998;50:827.

Wall M, Shirley HW. The one-and-a-half syndrome. A unilateral disorder of the pontine tegmentum: a study of 20 cases and review of the literature. *Neurology.* 1983;33:971-980.

During takeoff in a jet you experience a particularly salient function of the vestibular system: sensing body acceleration. Although perception of signals from the vestibular sensory organs occurs only under special circumstances, this system is operating continuously by controlling relatively automatic functions, such as maintaining balance when we are walking on uneven terrain or adjusting blood pressure when we stand up quickly. The vestibular system shares many brain stem circuits and functions with the neural systems for controlling the extraocular muscles that move the eyes. Eye movement must be precisely controlled to position the image of an object of interest over the fovea, where visual acuity is best (see Chapter 7). The vestibular and oculomotor systems coordinate the head and eyes during head movement. Consider your ability to maintain gaze on a friend's face in a crowded airport terminal as you run toward her. Your head bobs up and down, and from side to side, but you can maintain fixation effortlessly. The vestibular system detects your head motion, and the oculomotor system makes compensatory eye movements to stabilize the image of your friend on the retina. The actions of the two systems are coordinated automatically by the vestibuloocular reflex. In addition, the medial descending motor pathways (see Chapter 10) assist in this action by adjusting head position by controlling neck muscles. This happens without conscious awareness, apart from knowing where to fixate your gaze.

From a clinical perspective, the vestibular and eye movement control systems are also very tightly linked. An important part of testing the integrated functions of the brain stem involves careful assessment of a person's ability to coordinate eye movement during head motion. Assessment of vestibuloocular reflexes is an important part of examination of the comatose patient. This chapter also continues the examination of the cranial nerve nuclei, through which greater knowledge of brain stem regional anatomy will emerge, and the descending motor pathways. Such knowledge is essential for clinical problem solving, for example, in understanding behavioral deficits and identifying the locus of central nervous system damage after a stroke. Because each of the cranial nerve nuclei has a clearly identifiable sensory or motor function, the clinician can thoroughly test the integrity of such functions.

Functional Anatomy of the Vestibular System

Vestibular receptors sense head motion, both linear—such as that experienced during fast acceleration in an elevator or a jet—and angular—such as during turning. These receptors are located in five peripheral vestibular organs (Figure 12–2, inset): the three **semicircular canals,** which signal angular acceleration, and the **utricle and saccule,** which signal linear acceleration. Vestibular receptors are hair cells, which are innervated by bipolar neurons whose cell bodies are located in the **vestibular ganglion.** The axons of these bipolar neurons travel to the brain stem in the **vestibular division** of **cranial nerve VIII** and terminate in the **vestibular nuclei.** There are four separate vestibular nuclei: inferior, medial, lateral, and superior (Figure 12–2). The vestibular system comprises distinctive circuits that have the following major functions, each considered below: (1) perception, (2) blood pressure regulation, and (3) descending control of proximal and axial muscles. The vestibular system has a fourth major function in eye movement control; this is considered in the next section, on gaze control.

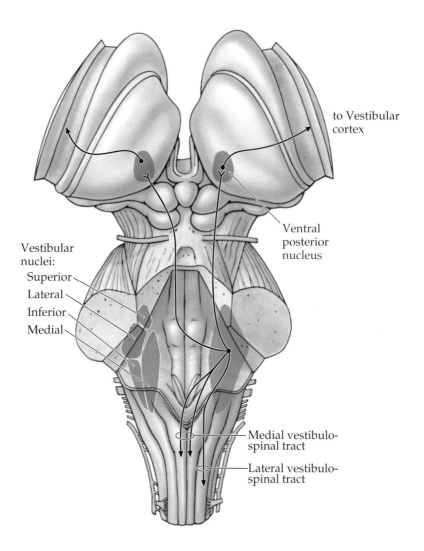

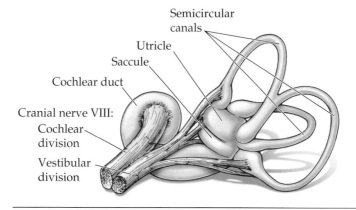

FIGURE 12–2 Dorsal view of brain stem showing overall organization of the vestibular system. Inset shows the peripheral vestibular and auditory organs.

An Ascending Pathway From the Vestibular Nuclei to the Thalamus Is Important for Perception, Orientation, and Posture

Originating primarily from the superior, medial, and inferior vestibular nuclei, the thalamic path ascends bilaterally to several sites within and around the **ventral posterior nucleus** (Figure 12–3B). Three major sites within the parietal lobe and insular cortex receive vestibular information (Figure 12–3A). The vestibular cortex in the (1) **retroinsular cortex** and (2) **posterior parietal lobe** play roles in conscious awareness of vestibular sensory activation and in sensing body orientation and the orientation of the world around us. A separate region, (3) **area 3a** (part of the primary somatic sensory cortex) is thought to participate in sensing head position in conjunction with proprioceptive afferents in neck muscles (see Chapter 4). Each of these cortical regions is also involved in controlling proximal muscles and posture, not directly like the corticospinal tract, but rather through their descending connections with vestibulospinal tract neurons, an indirect corticovestibulospinal tract.

The Vestibular System Regulates Blood Pressure in Response to Changes in Body Posture and Gravity

Blood pressure regulation is an integrated response involving primarily heart rate and vascular smooth muscle control. When we sit up quickly, blood must now flow against gravity. Maintenance of adequate blood flow to the brain is accomplished by a pressor reflex response, in which there are compensatory increases in heart rate and vascular smooth muscle tone. These responses are mediated by the autonomic nervous system (see Chapter 15). When this response is inadequate, such as when a person is taking certain medications for reducing blood pressure or diuretics, **orthostatic hypotension** can result. Vestibular regulation of blood pressure is accomplished through connections with the brain stem visceral integrative centers—the solitary, vagal, and parabrachial nuclei—that, in turn, regulate autonomic nervous system function (Figure 12–3A; see Chapters 6 and 15).

The Vestibular Nuclei Have Functionally Distinct Descending Spinal Projections for Axial Muscle Control

For axial muscle control, the vestibular nuclei receive information primarily from the cerebellum and cerebral cortex. The vestibular nuclei have two functionally distinct descending projections for balance and coordinating head and eye movements: the lateral and medial vestibulospinal tracts. These two descending motor pathways form a major portion of the **medial descending motor pathways.** The **lateral vestibulospinal tract,** which begins at the **lateral vestibular nucleus,** descends ipsilaterally in the white matter to all spinal levels (Figure 12–3C). This pathway is crucial for controlling posture and balance, which involves neck, back, hip, and leg muscles. Recall from Chapter 10 that even though a particular tract may have a unilateral projection, the medial descending pathways collectively exert a bilateral influence on proximal and axial muscle control because they synapse on commissural neurons (see Figure 10-16A). The **medial vestibulospinal tract,** which starts primarily at the **medial vestibular nucleus,** descends bilaterally in the white matter but only to the cervical and upper thoracic spinal cord (Figure 12–3B). The medial vestibulospinal tract plays a role in controlling head position in relation to eye position.

Functional Anatomy of Eye Movement Control

The position and movement of the eyes are controlled voluntarily and by vestibular reflexes. There are five types of eye movements:

1. **Vestibuloocular reflexes** use information from the semicircular canals to compensate for head motion by automatically adjusting eye position to maintain the direction of gaze.
2. **Saccades** are rapid movements that shift the fovea to an object of interest.
3. **Smooth pursuit movements** are slow and are used for tracking a moving object.
4. **Vergence movements** (either convergent or divergent) ensure that the image of an object of interest falls on the same place on the retina of each eye.
5. **Optokinetic reflexes** use visual information to supplement the effects of the vestibuloocular reflex.

With the exception of vergence, all eye movements are conjugate: The eyes move in tandem at the same speed and in the same direction. Vergence movements are disconjugate; the eyes move in opposite directions.

Each eye is controlled by six muscles, which operate as three functional pairs, with antagonistic mechanical actions (Figure 12–4A). The lateral and medial rectus muscles move the eye horizontally, abducting (looking away from the nose) and adducting (looking toward the nose), respectively. The superior and inferior rectus muscles elevate and depress the eye, particularly when the eye is abducted. Finally, the superior and inferior oblique muscles depress and elevate the eye, especially when the eye is adducted. Other actions of the extraocular muscles are indicated in Figure 12–4B.

The Extraocular Motor Neurons Are Located in Three Cranial Nerve Motor Nuclei

The **oculomotor nucleus** contributes most of the axons of the **oculomotor (III) nerve,** which exits the rostral midbrain. The

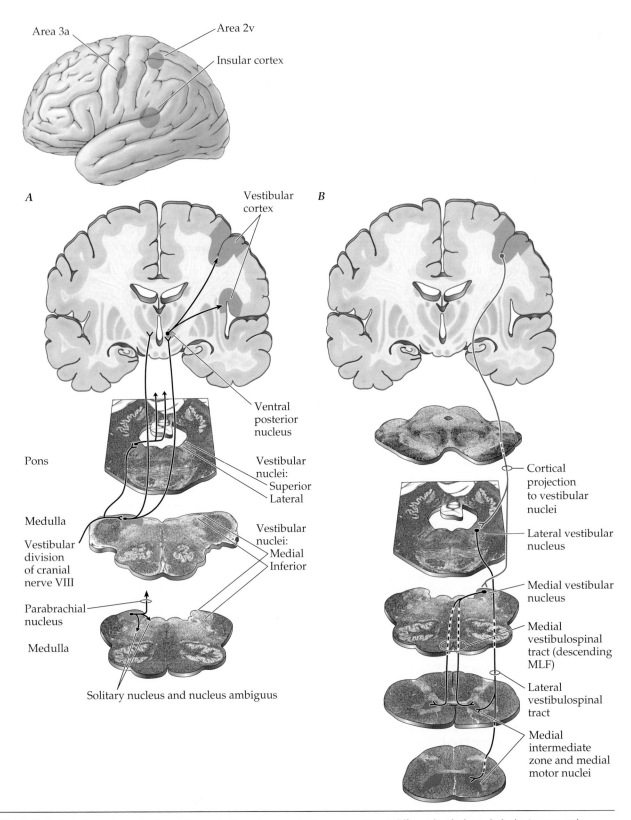

FIGURE 12–3 **A.** General organization of the vestibular system revealed in cross section at different levels through the brain stem and in coronal section through the diencephalon and cerebral hemispheres. **B.** The medial and lateral vestibulospinal tracts, together with the descending corticovestibular projection. The inset is a lateral view of the cerebral hemisphere, showing the locations of three key areas that receive vestibular inputs from the thalamus.

A

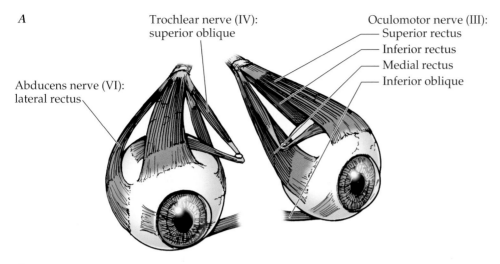

Trochlear nerve (IV):
superior oblique

Oculomotor nerve (III):
— Superior rectus
— Inferior rectus
— Medial rectus
— Inferior oblique

Abducens nerve (VI):
lateral rectus

B

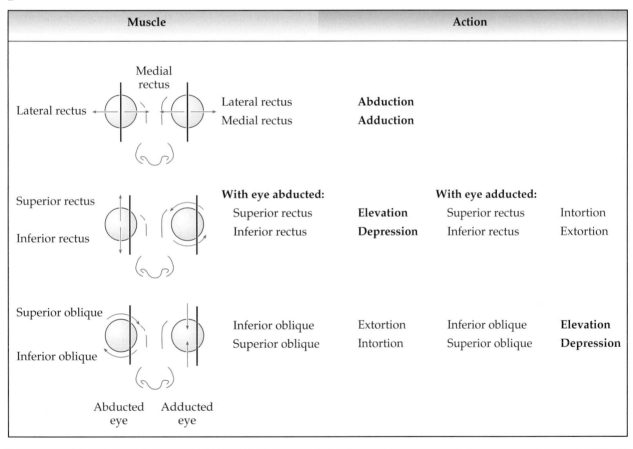

Muscle		Action		
Lateral rectus → ← Medial rectus	Lateral rectus	**Abduction**		
	Medial rectus	**Adduction**		
Superior rectus / Inferior rectus	**With eye abducted:**		**With eye adducted:**	
	Superior rectus	**Elevation**	Superior rectus	Intortion
	Inferior rectus	**Depression**	Inferior rectus	Extortion
Superior oblique / Inferior oblique	Inferior oblique	Extortion	Inferior oblique	**Elevation**
	Superior oblique	Intortion	Superior oblique	**Depression**
Abducted eye Adducted eye				

FIGURE 12–4 A. The two eyes with the various extraocular muscles and their innervation patterns. Not shown is the levator palpebrae, an eyelid elevator innervated by cranial nerve III. The extraocular muscles of both eyes operate as three functional pairs. The lateral and medial rectus muscles move the eye horizontally. The superior and inferior rectus muscles elevate and depress the eye, respectively (particularly when the eye is abducted). Finally, the inferior and superior oblique muscles elevate and depress the eye but to a greater extent when the eye is adducted. **B.** The mechanical actions of the extraocular muscles.

oculomotor nucleus (Figure 12–5) innervates four of the six extraocular muscles: **medial rectus, inferior rectus, superior rectus,** and **inferior oblique** (Figure 12–4). This nucleus also innervates the **levator palpebrae superioris muscle,** an eyelid elevator. (A contingent of autonomic nervous system axons travels in the oculomotor nerve to innervate smooth muscle; see Chapter 15.)

The other two extraocular motor nuclei are the trochlear and abducens nuclei (Figure 12–5). Motor neurons in the **trochlear nucleus** give rise to the fibers in the **trochlear (IV) nerve,** which innervate the **superior oblique muscle** (Figure 12–4). This cranial nerve is the only one that exits from the dorsal brain stem surface. The trochlear nerve is further

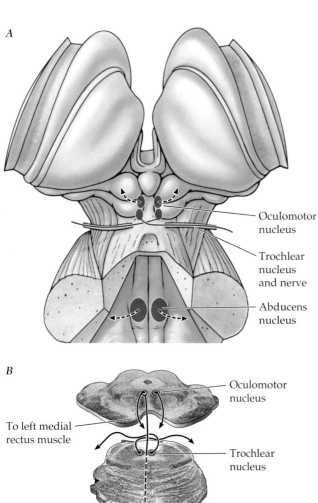

A

— Oculomotor
   nucleus

— Trochlear
   nucleus
   and nerve

— Abducens
   nucleus

B

— Oculomotor
   nucleus

To left medial
rectus muscle

— Trochlear
   nucleus

Medial
longitudinal
fasciculus

— Internuclear
   neuron

— Abducens
   motor
   neuron

To right lateral
rectus muscle

FIGURE 12–5 Extraocular muscle control. **A.** View of the dorsal brain stem, showing the locations of the oculomotor, trochlear, and abducens nuclei and depicting the course of the trochlear nerve within the brain stem. **B.** Transverse sections through the oculomotor, trochlear, and abducens nuclei. Axon of internuclear neuron travels in the contralateral medial longitudinal fasciculus.

distinguished because all of its axons **decussate** within the central nervous system. The **abducens nucleus** (Figure 12–5) contains the motor neurons that project their axons to the periphery through the **abducens (VI) nerve.** Abducens motor neurons innervate the **lateral rectus muscle** (Figure 12–4). Unlike spinal and other cranial nerve motor neurons, extra-ocular motor neurons are not controlled by the primary motor cortex.

The Vestibuloocular Reflex Maintains Direction of Gaze During Head Movement

Stable fixation can be maintained on an object during head movement because the vestibular system generates eye movement control signals that compensate for head movements. For example, horizontal rightward movement of the head generates leftward conjugate movement of the eyes (Figure 12–6A). This movement is produced by excitation of left lateral rectus motor neurons and right medial rectus motor neurons. The lateral and medial rectus motor neurons are directly activated by vestibular neurons (Figure 12–6B), demonstrating the importance of automatic control of eye movement by head movement. In addition, the medial rectus motor neurons are indirectly activated by the internuclear neurons in the left abducens nucleus (Figure 12–6B, thin line). Although not shown in Figure 12–6B, the circuit for vestibuloocular control also ensures that the mechanical action of the muscle that moves the eye, termed the agonist muscle, is not impeded by contraction of the antagonistic muscles (the muscles whose mechanical action is opposite that of the agonist muscle). This process occurs through inhibitory connections with the motor neurons of antagonistic muscles. For example, when the left lateral rectus motor neurons are excited, the left medial rectus motor neurons are inhibited.

Voluntary Eye Movements Are Controlled by Neurons in the Frontal Lobe and the Parietal-Temporal-Occipital Association Cortex

Saccades are triggered by neurons in the **frontal eye field,** a portion of cytoarchitectonic area 8 (see Figure 2–19). This cortical territory receives subcortical inputs from the basal ganglia and cerebellum, transmitted via thalamic neurons. The frontal eye field projects to the **superior colliculus** (Figure 12–7A). The axons of these frontal lobe projection neurons descend within the **anterior limb** and **genu of the internal capsule** to the brain stem. Superior colliculus neurons, in turn, project to distinct regions of the pontine and midbrain reticular formation that directly control saccades through their mono-synaptic connections to extraocular motor neurons. The frontal eye fields also project directly to these two reticular formation zones. For controlling horizontal saccades, the frontal eye fields project to neurons in the **paramedian pontine reticular formation** (Figure 12–7A, B). These neurons process control signals and, in turn, project to the abducens nucleus. The abducens nucleus is more than a motor nucleus because, in addition to containing lateral rectus motor neurons, it also contains **internuclear neurons** (Figure 12–7B). Signals from the paramedian pontine reticular formation trigger horizontal saccades by directly exciting lateral rectus motor neurons in the abducens nucleus and, via the internuclear neurons, indirectly exciting medial rectus motor neurons in the oculomotor

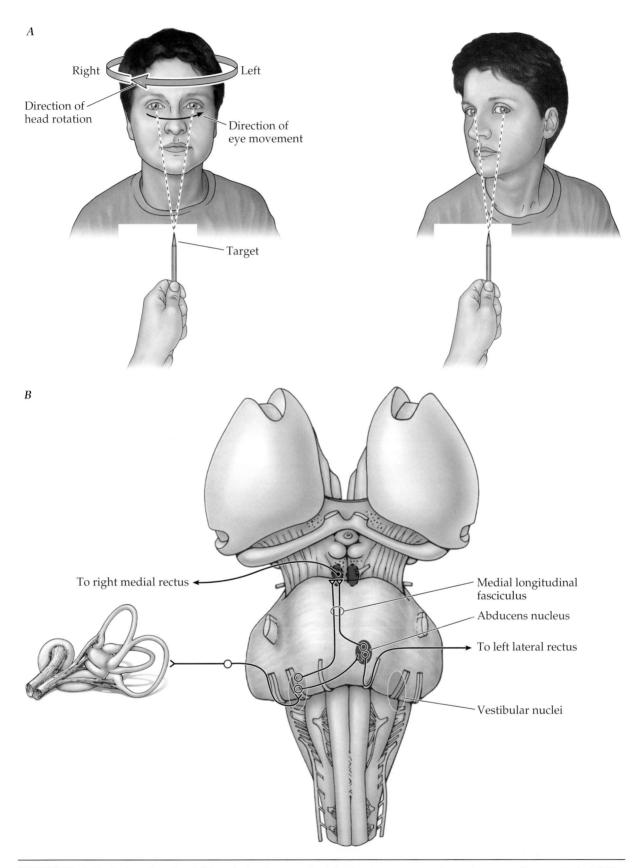

FIGURE 12–6 Vestibuloocular reflex. **A.** When the head turns to the right, the eyes compensate by turning an equal amount to the left. **B.** Ventral view of the brain stem, diencephalon, and basal ganglia, showing the circuit for the vestibuloocular reflex for the head turning to the right.

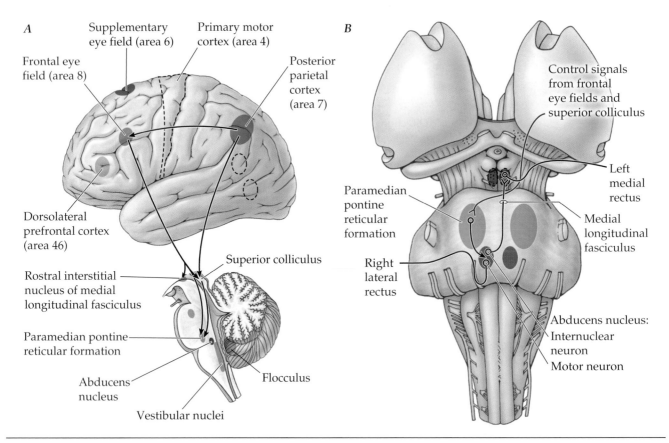

A.

Supplementary
eye field (area 6)

Primary motor
cortex (area 4)

Frontal eye
field (area 8)

Posterior
parietal
cortex
(area 7)

Dorsolateral
prefrontal cortex
(area 46)

Superior colliculus

Rostral interstitial
nucleus of medial
longitudinal fasciculus

Paramedian pontine
reticular formation

Abducens
nucleus

Flocculus

Vestibular nuclei

B.

Control signals
from frontal
eye fields and
superior colliculus

Left
medial
rectus

Paramedian
pontine
reticular
formation

Medial
longitudinal
fasciculus

Right
lateral
rectus

Abducens nucleus:
Internuclear
neuron
Motor neuron

FIGURE 12–7 *A.* Lateral view of the cerebral cortex and midsagittal view of the brain stem show the approximate location of structures involved in controlling saccadic eye movements. The middle temporal and middle superior temporal areas (dashed open ellipses) are part of the smooth pursuit system and described in Figure 12-8. The primary motor cortex is not involved in eye movement control. ***B.*** Ventral surface of the brain stem, diencephalon, and basal ganglia, showing the circuit for producing conjugate horizontal saccades to the right.

nucleus. For vertical saccades, the frontal eye fields project to the **rostral interstitial nucleus of the medial longitudinal fasciculus** in the midbrain reticular formation (Figure 12–7A). Neurons in this nucleus coordinate the muscles that produce vertical eye movements (Figure 12–5B). A portion of the **posterior parietal cortex** within area 7 participates in saccade generation through its role in visual attention: You must first attend to a stimulus before looking at it. This region projects through the **posterior limb of the internal capsule** to the superior colliculus.

Smooth pursuit movements have a remarkably different control circuit, one that involves higher-order **cortical visual areas,** for computing the speed of the moving target, and the **cerebellum** (Figure 12–8). The cortical control of smooth pursuit eye movements begins in the middle temporal (also termed V5) and middle superior temporal visual areas (see Figure 7–15). From the cortex, axons descend in the posterior limb of the internal capsule to engage a brain stem and cerebellar circuit comprising the **pontine nuclei,** the **flocculus** (a portion of the cerebellum; see Chapter 13), and the **vestibular nuclei** (Figure 12–8). All three extraocular nuclei receive input from the vestibular nuclei; the vestibular axons course in the **medial longitudinal fasciculus** (MLF). Axons in the MLF originating from the vestibular nuclei are also especially important in stabilizing eye position when the head is moved (see next section).

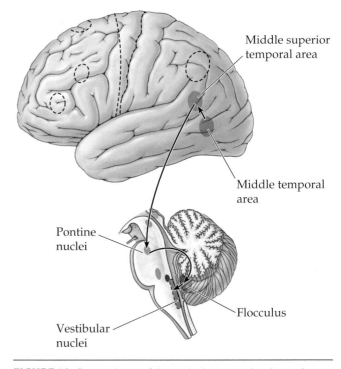

Middle superior
temporal area

Middle temporal
area

Pontine
nuclei

Flocculus

Vestibular
nuclei

FIGURE 12–8 Lateral view of the cerebral cortex and midsagittal view of the brain stem show the approximate location of structures involved in controlling smooth pursuit eye movements.

While the frontal eye field is essential for saccade generation, it also participates in smooth pursuit movements.

Regional Organization of the Vestibular and Eye Movement Control Systems

Vestibular Sensory Organs Are Contained Within the Membranous Labyrinth

The membranous labyrinth is filled with **endolymph,** an extracellular fluid resembling intracellular fluid in its ionic constituents: a high potassium concentration and a low sodium concentration (see Chapter 8). Vestibular receptor cells are hair cells, like auditory receptors, located in specialized regions of the semicircular canals (termed ampullae) (Figure 12–9, inset) and the saccule and utricle (termed maculae). The hair cells of the semicircular canals are covered by a gelatinous mass (termed the cupula) into which the stereocilia embed. Angular head movement induces the endolymph within the canals to flow, displacing the gelatinous mass, which in turn deflects the hair cell stereocilia. The utricle and saccule also have a gelatinous covering over hair cells in their maculae. Calcium carbonate crystals, embedded in the gelatin, rest on the stereocilia. Linear acceleration causes the crystals to deform the gelatinous mass, thereby deflecting the stereocilia. The saccule and utricle are sometimes called the **otolith organs** because otolith is the term for the calcium carbonate crystals. The semicircular canals, utricle, and saccule each have a different orientation with respect to the head, thereby conferring selective sensitivity to head movement in different directions. **Benign positional vertigo** is a condition in which calcium carbonate crystals move freely within the semicircular canals. Changing head position causes the crystals to stimulate the hair cells aberrantly, thereby causing vertigo.

Vestibular hair cells are innervated by the peripheral processes of vestibular bipolar neurons, the cell bodies of which are located in the **vestibular ganglion.** The central processes of these bipolar neurons, which form the **vestibular division** of **cranial nerve VIII,** course along with the cochlear division and enter the brain stem at the lateral pontomedullary junction (see Figure AI–6). Some vestibular axons project directly to the cerebellum (see Chapter 13). In fact, the vestibular sensory neurons are the only primary sensory neurons that have this privileged access to the cerebellum because of the special role of the vestibular system in controlling eye, limb, and trunk movements.

The Vestibular Nuclei Have Functionally Diverse Projections

The vestibular nuclei (Figure 12–10) occupy the floor of the fourth ventricle in the dorsolateral medulla and pons (Figure 12–2). This region is termed the **cerebellopontine angle.** The **posterior inferior cerebellar artery (PICA)** supplies blood to the vestibular nuclei (see Chapter 4). Occlusion of this artery can produce **vertigo,** an illusion of movement—typically whirling—of the patient or his or her surroundings. The vestibular nuclei have extensive intrinsic interconnections with components of the nuclear complex on the same and opposite sides that are important in the basic processing of vestibular signals. The **lateral vestibular nucleus** (also termed **Deiters' nucleus**) gives rise to the **lateral vestibulospinal tract,** important in maintaining balance. The **medial vestibular nucleus,** with a lesser contribution from the **superior** and **inferior vestibular nuclei,** gives rise to the **medial vestibulospinal tract,** for head and neck control. The inferior,

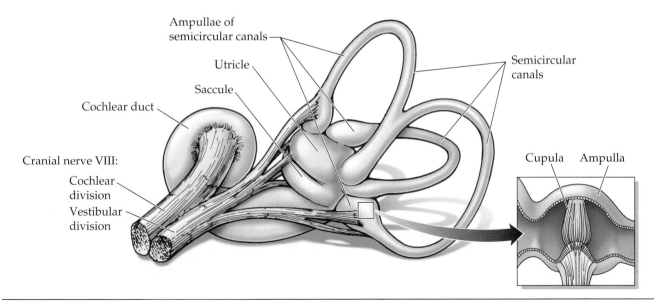

FIGURE 12–9 Organization of the peripheral vestibular system. Inset shows the ampulla of one semicircular canal.

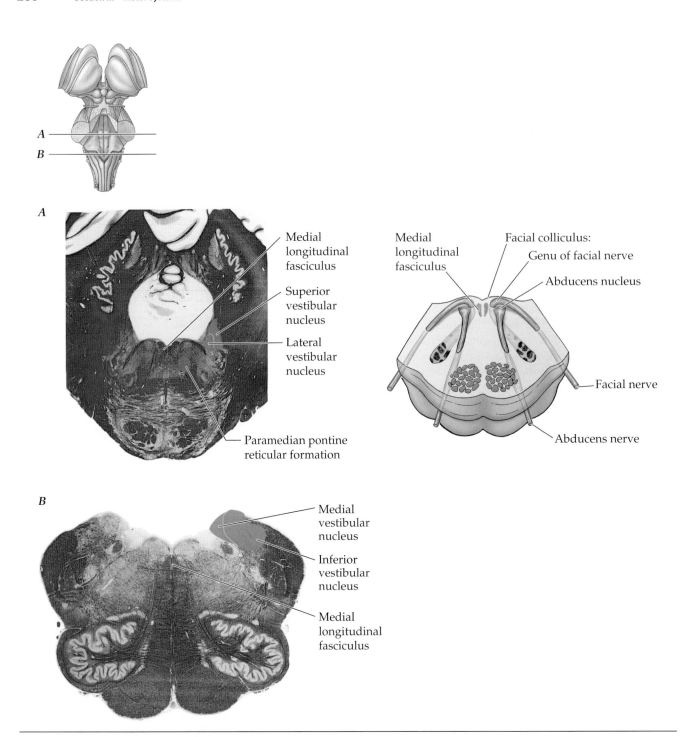

FIGURE 12–10 Myelin-stained transverse sections through the caudal pons (**A**) and medulla (**B**). The right inset shows the three-dimensional course of the facial and abducens nerves in the pons. The top inset shows the planes of section. (**Top inset,** Adapted from William PL, Warwick R. *Functional Neuroanatomy of Man.* Philadelphia, PA: W. B. Saunders, 1975.)

superior, and medial, but less so the lateral, vestibular nuclei also give rise to bilateral ascending projections to the thalamus. The **vestibular nuclei** also participate in the reflex stabilization of eye movements, the **vestibuloocular reflex** (Figure 12–6). Vestibular axons projecting to the extraocular motor nuclei travel in the MLF (Figures 12–10 and 12–11). Together with the cerebellum, the vestibular nuclei help to organize a blood pressor response to changes in gravity forces acting on the circulatory system.

The Extraocular Motor Nuclei Are Located Adjacent to the MLF in the Pons and Midbrain

The MLF is a myelinated pathway that runs close to the midline and beneath the fourth ventricle and cerebral aqueduct, throughout most of the brain stem. In the pons and medulla, it is closely associated with the extraocular motor nuclei: the abducens, trochlear, and oculomotor nuclei. The

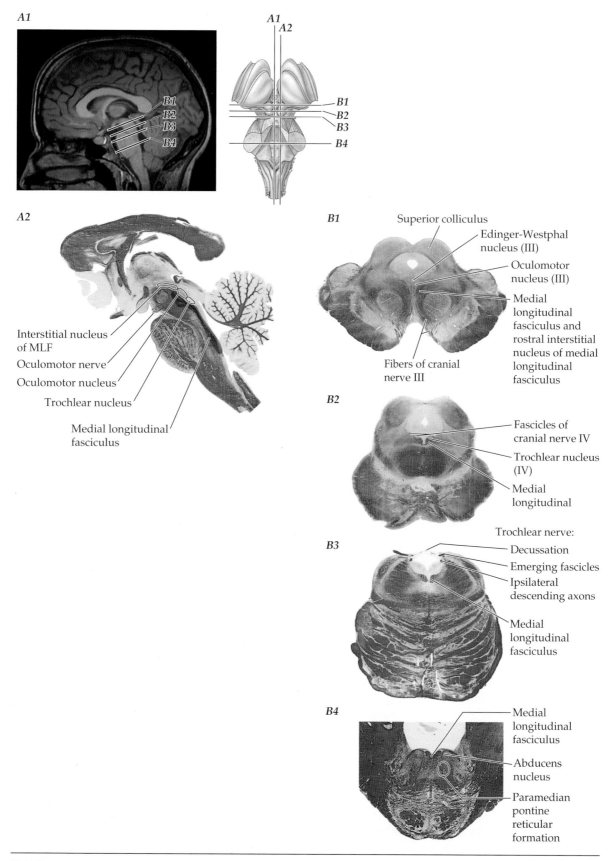

A1

A1
A2

B1
B2
B3
B4

A2

Interstitial nucleus
of MLF

Oculomotor nerve

Oculomotor nucleus

Trochlear nucleus

Medial longitudinal
fasciculus

B1
Superior colliculus
Edinger-Westphal
nucleus (III)
Oculomotor
nucleus (III)
Medial
longitudinal
fasciculus and
rostral interstitial
nucleus of medial
longitudinal
fasciculus
Fibers of cranial
nerve III

B2
Fascicles of
cranial nerve IV
Trochlear nucleus
(IV)
Medial
longitudinal

B3
Trochlear nerve:
Decussation
Emerging fascicles
Ipsilateral
descending axons
Medial
longitudinal
fasciculus

B4
Medial
longitudinal
fasciculus
Abducens
nucleus
Paramedian
pontine
reticular
formation

FIGURE 12–11 The MLF courses close to the midline in the brain stem. ***A1.*** MRI close to the midline showing the planes of transverse myelin-stained sections. ***A2.*** Midsagittal myelin-stained section closely matching the MRI. ***B.*** Sections through the rostral midbrain (***B1***), caudal midbrain (***B2***), midbrain-pons juncture (***B3***), and pons (***B4***).

rostrocaudal course of the MLF can be seen on a parasagittal myelin-stained section close to the midline (Figure 12–11A2).

Lesion of the oculomotor nucleus produces a down and out eye position

The oculomotor nucleus (Figure 12–11B1) innervates the medial, inferior, and superior rectus muscles; the inferior oblique muscle; and the levator palpebrae superioris muscle, an eyelid elevator. The motor axons run in the oculomotor nerve, coursing through the red nucleus and basis pedunculi en route to exiting into the interpeduncular fossa (Figure 12–12B). Oculomotor nerve damage produces a "down and out" resting eye position ipsilaterally, resulting from the unopposed actions of the lateral rectus muscle (producing the outward position) and the superior oblique muscle (producing the downward position).

There are three other important eye movement control centers in the midbrain. The first is the **superior colliculus,** essential for controlling saccadic eye movements (Figure 12–11B1). Receiving inputs directly from cortical eye movement control centers in the parietal and frontal lobes (Figure 12–7A), neurons in the deep layers of the superior colliculus project to the paramedian pontine reticular formation in the pons (for controlling horizontal saccades) and to the **interstitial nucleus of the MLF** (Figures 12–11B1 and 12–12A), the second midbrain control center. This nucleus organizes vertical eye movements through its connections with the oculomotor and trochlear nuclei. The third integrative center is the **interstitial nucleus of Cajal** (see Figure AII–15). This nucleus helps to coordinate eye and head movements, especially vertical and torsional movements. This nucleus contains neurons that project axons to the spinal cord (termed the interstitiospinal tract), for axial muscle control, and to the contralateral interstitial nucleus of Cajal (via the posterior commissure), for coordinating eye and axial muscle control bilaterally.

Knowledge of regional midbrain anatomy is clinically important because damage of the ventral midbrain produces a complex set of neurological deficits that disrupt eye movement control, facial muscle function, and limb movements. Branches of the **posterior cerebral artery** supply the ventral midbrain, and when these branches become occluded, the oculomotor nucleus, the third nerve, and the **basis pedunculi** are affected. In addition to producing the "down and out" eye position because of third nerve involvement, this damage results in limb and lower facial muscle weakness on the contralateral side because of involvement of the corticospinal and corticobulbar tracts in the basis pedunculi. Limb tremor can also occur due to damage of the red nucleus (see Figure 10–11) and nearby axons that connect the red nucleus and the cerebellum.

The trochlear nucleus is located in the caudal midbrain

Trochlear motor neurons, found in the **trochlear nucleus** (Figure 12–11B2), innervate the **superior oblique muscle** contralateral to its origin. The nucleus is located in the caudal midbrain at the level of the inferior colliculus, nested within the MLF. Trochlear motor axons course caudally along the lateral margin of the cerebral aqueduct and fourth ventricle, in the **periaqueductal gray matter.** The axons decussate in the rostral pons (Figure 12–5A), dorsal to the cerebral aqueduct, and emerge from the dorsal brain stem surface (Figure 12–5B). Lesion of the trochlear nerve paralyzes the superior oblique muscle, resulting in slight outward rotation of the eye (or extortion) because of the unopposed action of the inferior oblique muscle. The eye elevates slightly because of the unopposed action of the superior rectus muscle. A patient with this lesion compensates by tilting his or her head away from the side of the paralyzed muscle.

The abducens nucleus is located in the pons

The **abducens nucleus** (Figure 12–11B4) contains the motor neurons that innervate the **lateral rectus muscle.** The nucleus is located just beneath the floor of the fourth ventricle and is partially encircled by facial motor axons on their way to the periphery (Figure 12–10A, inset). The abducens nerve fibers course toward the ventral brain stem surface and exit the pons at the pontomedullary junction, medial to the facial nerve. Lesion of the abducens nerve paralyzes the ipsilateral lateral rectus muscle and results in the inability to abduct that eye.

Parasympathetic Neurons in the Midbrain Regulate Pupil Size

The Edinger-Westphal nucleus mediates two reflexes: pupil constriction in response to light and pupil constriction together with lens accommodation in response to near focusing. The **pupillary light reflex** is the constriction of the pupil that occurs when light hits the retina. Visual input from the retina passes, via the **brachium of superior colliculus,** directly to the **pretectal nuclei** (Figure 12–12). The pretectal nuclei project bilaterally to the **Edinger-Westphal nucleus,** which contains parasympathetic preganglionic neurons; pretectal axons cross to the contralateral side in the **posterior commissure.** Axons from the Edinger-Westphal nucleus travel with the oculomotor fibers in their path to synapse in the **ciliary ganglion** in the periphery. From there, postganglionic neurons innervate the constrictor muscles of the iris. The bilateral projection of pretectal neurons to the parasympathetic preganglionic neurons in the Edinger-Westphal nucleus ensures that illumination of one eye causes constriction of the pupil on the ipsilateral side (direct response in the lighted eye) as well as on the contralateral side (consensual response). Pupillary reflexes are an important component of assessing brain stem function during clinical examination, including examination of the comatose patient.

Pupillary dilation is mediated either by inhibition of the circuit for pupillary constriction or by the separate control of the iris by the sympathetic component of the autonomic nervous system (see Chapter 15). The pupillary dialator fibers

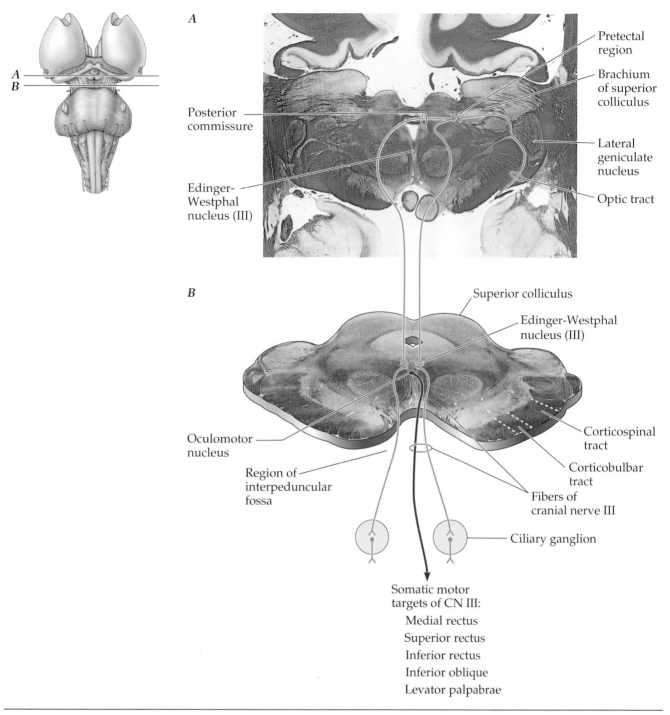

A

Posterior commissure

Edinger-Westphal nucleus (III)

Pretectal region

Brachium of superior colliculus

Lateral geniculate nucleus

Optic tract

B

Superior colliculus

Edinger-Westphal nucleus (III)

Oculomotor nucleus

Region of interpeduncular fossa

Corticospinal tract

Corticobulbar tract

Fibers of cranial nerve III

Ciliary ganglion

Somatic motor targets of CN III:
    Medial rectus
    Superior rectus
    Inferior rectus
    Inferior oblique
    Levator palpabrae

FIGURE 12–12 The circuit for the pupillary light reflex. Myelin-stained sections through the midbrain-diencephalic junction (**A**) and rostral midbrain (**B**). Signals from the optic nerve are transmitted to neurons in the pretectal nuclei at the level of the midbrain-diencephalon juncture. The pretectal nuclei project bilaterally to parasympathetic preganglionic neurons in the Edinger-Westphal nucleus. The next connection in the circuit is in the ciliary ganglia, where parasympathetic postganglionic neurons are located. These neurons innervate the smooth muscle in the eye. The dark green arrow is a reminder that somatic motor neurons are located in the oculomotor nucleus, which innervates the listed muscle. The inset shows planes of section in **A** and **B**.

join the third nerve close to the eye. As a consequence of this organization, damage to exiting fibers of the third nerve, such as by occlusion of a branch of the posterior cerebral artery, will spare the dilator fibers. Such a lesion produces pupillary dilation because of the unopposed action of the pupillary dilator fibers of the sympathetic nervous system, which are spared by the lesion.

Parasympathetic preganglionic neurons in the Edinger-Westphal nucleus of the midbrain participate in a second visual reflex, the **accommodation reflex,** which is the increase in lens curvature that occurs during near vision. This reflex is usually part of the **accommodation-convergence reaction,** a complex response that prepares the eyes for near vision by increasing lens curvature, constricting the pupils, and coordinating convergence of the eyes. These responses involve the integrated actions of the visual areas of the occipital lobe, along with motor neurons in the oculomotor nucleus that innervate the extraocular muscles and parasympathetic preganglionic neurons. Central nervous system pathology can distinguish different components of the visual reflexes. For example, in neurosyphilis the accommodation reaction is preserved but the light reflex is impaired. Patients with this condition have a classic neurological sign, the **Argyll Robertson pupils:** Their pupils are small and unreactive to light but get smaller when the patients accommodate. Distinct portions of the midbrain are supplied by paramedian, short circumferential, and long circumferential branches of the posterior cerebral artery (see Figure 4–4B1).

The action of levator palpebrae superioris muscle, an eyelid elevator, is assisted by the **tarsal muscle,** a smooth muscle under sympathetic nervous system control. Conditions that impair the functions of the sympathetic nervous system (see Chapter 15) can produce a mild drooping of the eyelid (pseudoptosis) resulting from weakness of the tarsal muscle. True ptosis is produced by weakness of the levator palpebrae muscle, the principal eyelid elevator. This effect can result from third nerve lesions or neuromuscular diseases, such as myasthenia gravis, an autoimmune disease that attacks the neuromuscular junction.

Eye Movement Control Involves the Integrated Functions of Many Brain Stem Structures

As discussed earlier, horizontal eye movements are controlled by signals from the frontal eye fields and superior colliculus to the paramedian pontine reticular formation that coordinate the actions of the lateral and medial rectus muscles. These circuits are well understood, so much so that lesions at different sites explain deficit horizontal eye movement control in humans (Figure 12–13). A lesion of the abducens nerve produces paralysis of the ipsilateral **lateral rectus muscle,** thereby preventing ocular abduction on the same side (Figure 12–13, lesion 1). The unopposed action of the medial rectus muscle can sometimes cause the affected eye to be adducted at rest (not shown in the figure).

Deficits after an abducens nerve lesion differ from those after a lesion of the abducens nucleus (Figure 12–13, lesion 2). As with the nerve lesion, the ipsilateral eye cannot be abducted because of destruction of the lateral rectus motor neurons. Here, too, the resting position of the eye may be adducted because of the unopposed action of the medial rectus muscle. The nuclear lesion has a second effect: The patient cannot contract the **contralateral medial rectus muscle** on horizontal gaze in the same direction as the side of the lesion. Hence, the patient cannot gaze to the lesion side. This is called **lateral gaze palsy,** and it occurs because the lesion also destroys the **internuclear neurons** that coordinate the lateral and medial rectus muscles (Figure 12–7B).

A more rostral lesion of the MLF, which spares the lateral rectus motor neurons but damages the axons of the internuclear neurons, produces **internuclear ophthalmoplegia** (Figure 12–13, lesion 3; at level of the pons in Figure 12–11B3). This lesion is characterized, on lateral gaze away from the side of the MLF lesion, by the lack of (or reduced) ability to contract the ipsilateral medial rectus muscle and thereby adduct that eye.

For lesions at sites 2 and 3 (Figure 12–13), a clever way to verify that the affected medial rectus muscle is not paralyzed is to demonstrate that the patient can converge both eyes to view an object at close distance. This eye movement requires activation of both medial rectus muscles. The neural mechanisms that coordinate convergence involve the **visual cortex** and **midbrain** integrative centers, not the internuclear cells of the abducens nucleus.

The Ventral Posterior Nucleus of the Thalamus Transmits Vestibular Information to the Parietal and Insular Cortical Areas

The vestibular nuclei project bilaterally to the thalamus. This ascending projection originates primarily from the medial, inferior, and superior vestibular nuclei. Unlike the auditory and somatic sensory systems, there is no single tract through which the ascending vestibular projection travels. Some fibers travel in the MLF, some in the lateral lemniscus, and others scattered in the brain stem gray matter. The principal thalamic target of the ascending vestibular projection is the **ventral posterior nucleus** (Figures 12–2, 12–3B, and 12–14). Although this nucleus is familiar as a somatic sensory relay, it serves other functions. The rostral region of the nucleus, adjacent to the ventral lateral nucleus (for motor control; see Chapter 10), receives vestibular input and projects to area 3a of the somatic sensory cortex, to integrate proprioceptive vestibular information. More dorsal and posterior parts of the nucleus, and adjoining nuclei, also receive vestibular information but project to the posterior parietal lobe and the retroinsular cortex, a region near the posterior end of the lateral fissure (Figure 12–14). There does not seem to be a single "primary" vestibular cortex, like some of the other sensory modalities. Rather,

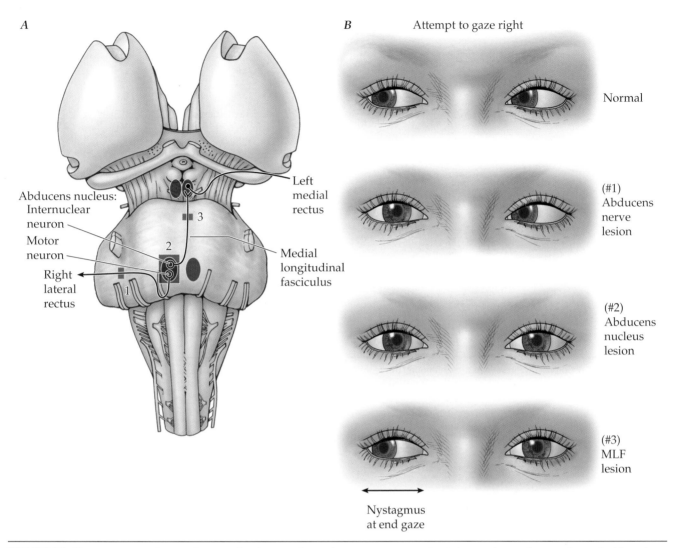

FIGURE 12–13 Brain stem mechanisms for controlling horizontal saccadic eye movements. **A.** Circuit for coordinating horizontal saccades. The red blocks indicate sites of lesion, producing the eye movement deficits shown in **B. B.** The four pairs of eyes illustrate eye position when an individual is asked to look to the right: (from top to bottom row) normal control of eyes, with a lesion of the right abducens nerve (lesion 1), with a lesion of the right abducens nucleus (lesion 2), and with a left medial longitudinal fasciculus lesion (lesion 3).

the vestibular cortical areas are interconnected to form a network that integrates vestibular inputs with joint proprioceptive information such as posture, orientation, and perception (eg, acceleration, vertigo). Many of these areas have descending projections to the vestibular nuclei, which, in turn, project to the spinal cord for controlling axial and proximal muscles. The organization of this system—corticovestibulospinal—is similar to the indirect corticospinal pathways from the frontal motor areas (see Figure 10–2).

Multiple Areas of the Cerebral Cortex Function in Eye Movement Control

Eye movements are not controlled by the primary motor cortex but rather by multiple regions in the frontal and parietal lobes. The **frontal eye fields,** corresponding to a portion of area 8, are the principal frontal lobe regions engaged in circuits for both saccadic and smooth pursuit movements (Figures 12–7 and 12–8). Two other frontal lobe areas contain neurons important for saccadic eye movements, the supplementary eye fields and the dorsolateral prefrontal cortex (Figure 12–14B). The frontal lobe eye movement control centers work together with neurons in the caudate nucleus (Figure 12–14A), a component of the basal ganglia (see Chapter 14). The parietal lobe site important for saccadic eye movements is located in area 7. This region receives visual information from the "where" pathway (see Figures 7–15 and 7–16). Two nearby areas, the middle temporal and middle superior temporal, which are also part of the where pathway, transmit visual information for guiding pursuit movements.

A

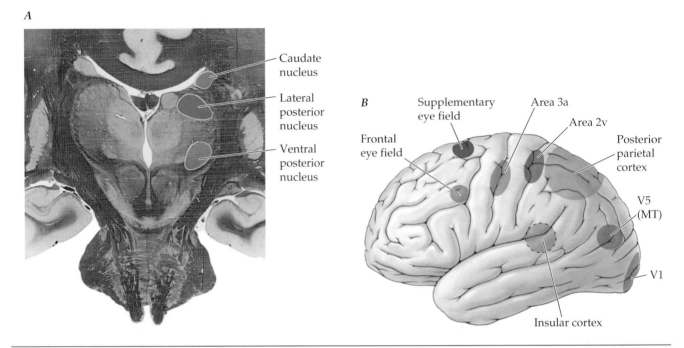

Caudate nucleus

Lateral posterior nucleus

Ventral posterior nucleus

B

Supplementary eye field

Area 3a

Area 2v

Frontal eye field

Posterior parietal cortex

V5 (MT)

V1

Insular cortex

FIGURE 12–14 *A.* Coronal myelin-stained section through the ventral posterior lateral nucleus, lateral posterior nucleus, and caudate nucleus. Each of these nuclei plays a role in eye movement control. ***B.*** Cortical vestibular and ocular motor centers in the cerebral cortex.

Summary

Vestibular System

Peripheral Vestibular Sensory Organs

There are five vestibular sensory organs: the three *semicircular canals,* the *utricle,* and the *saccule* (Figures 12–2 and 12–9). Receptor cells, located in specialized regions of the vestibular apparatus, are innervated by the distal processes of bipolar neurons located in the *vestibular ganglion.* The central processes of these bipolar neurons form the *vestibular division* of cranial nerve VIII (Figures 12–2 and 12–9). These fibers terminate in the vestibular nuclei, located beneath the floor of the fourth ventricle in the rostral medulla and caudal pons (Figure 12–2A).

Vestibular Nuclei and Their Projections

Four separate vestibular nuclei are located in the medulla and pons: the *inferior vestibular nucleus,* the *medial vestibular nucleus,* the *lateral vestibular nucleus,* and the *superior vestibular nucleus* (Figures 12–2A and 12–10). Neurons within the superior, lateral, and medial vestibular nuclei give rise to an ascending pathway to several sites within and around the *ventral posterior nucleus* of the thalamus (Figures 12–3 and 12–14). Three major sites within the parietal lobe and insular cortex receive and integrate

this information (Figures 12–3A and 12–14): (1) *area 3a,* which is thought to participate in head position and neck motor control, and (2) the *posterior parietal lobe* and (3) the *insular cortex,* which play roles in the sensing of body orientation and the orientation of the visual world.

There are two vestibulospinal tracts (Figure 12–3B). The *lateral vestibulospinal tract,* which descends to all spinal levels, originates from neurons within the *lateral vestibular nucleus* (Figure 12–10). This pathway is important for balance and posture. The *medial vestibulospinal tract,* which originates primarily from neurons within the *medial vestibular nucleus* (Figure 12–10), descends only to the cervical spinal cord. This pathway is important in controlling head position for gaze. Vestibulospinal tract neurons terminate on motor neurons that innervate *proximal limb* and *axial muscles* as well as on interneurons that synapse on these motor neurons.

Eye Movement Control

Extraocular Muscles

Each eye is controlled by six muscles, which operate as three functional pairs, with antagonistic actions (Figure 12–4). The *lateral* and *medial rectus muscles* move the eye horizontally, abducting (looking away from the nose) and adducting (looking toward the nose), respectively. The *superior* and *inferior rectus muscles* elevate and depress the eyes, respectively, but particularly when the eye is abducted. Finally, the *superior* and *inferior oblique muscles* depress and elevate the eye, especially when the eye is adducted.

Extraocular Motor Nuclei

The *oculomotor nucleus* innervates the *medial, inferior, and superior rectus muscles;* the *inferior oblique muscle;* and the *levator palpebrae superioris muscle.* The motor axons course in the oculomotor nerve (Figures 12–5, 12–11, and 12–12). Motor neurons in the *trochlear nucleus* give rise to the fibers in the *trochlear (IV) nerve,* which innervate the *superior oblique muscle* (see Figures 12–4, 12–10, and 12–11). This is the only cranial nerve that contains decussated axons and exits from the dorsal brain stem surface (Figure 12–5).

The *abducens nucleus* contains the motor neurons that project their axons to the periphery through the *abducens (VI) nerve* and innervate the *lateral rectus muscle* (Figures 12–4 and 12–9).

Brain Stem Centers and Cortical Areas for Eye Movement Control

Saccadic eye movements are controlled by neurons in the *frontal eye fields* (Figure 12–6A) that project to the *superior colliculus* (Figures 12–7B and 12–11B1) and to the pontine and midbrain reticular formation (Figure 12–7). The cortical axons descend in the *anterior limb of the internal capsule.* Neurons in the *paramedian pontine reticular formation* (Figures 12–7 and 12–10) coordinate horizontal saccades through their projections to lateral rectus motor neurons and *internuclear neurons* in the abducens nucleus (Figure 12–9), which project to medial rectus motor neurons in the oculomotor nucleus (Figures 12–6, 12–11, and 12–13B). Neurons in the *interstitial nucleus of the MLF* (Figures 12–11 and 12–13A) control vertical saccades. *Smooth pursuit eye movements* are also controlled by neurons in the frontal eye fields but through connections with the *pontine nuclei, cerebellum,* and *vestibular nuclei* (Figures 12–8 and 12–14).

Selected Readings

Goldberg M. The control of gaze. In: Kandel ER, Schwartz JH, Jessell TM, Siegelbaum SA, Hudspeth AJ, eds. *Principles of Neural Science.* 5th ed. New York, NY: McGraw-Hill; in press.

Goldberg M, Hudspeth J. The vestibular system. In: Kandel ER, Schwartz JH, Jessell TM, Siegelbaum SA, Hudspeth AJ, eds. *Principles of Neural Science.* 5th ed. New York, NY: McGraw-Hill; in press.

Patten J. *Neurological Differential Diagnosis.* 2nd ed. London: Springer-Verlag; 1996:446.

References

Akbarian S, Grusser OJ, Guldin WO. Thalamic connections of the vestibular cortical fields in the squirrel monkey (Saimiri sciureus). *J Comp Neurol.* 1992;326(3):423-441.

Bankoul S, Neuhuber WL. A direct projection from the medial vestibular nucleus to the cervical spinal dorsal horn of the rat, as demonstrated by anterograde and retrograde tracing. *Anat Embryol (Berl).* 1992;185(1):77-85.

Bronstein AM, Lempert T. Management of the patient with chronic dizziness. *Restor Neurol Neurosci.* 2010;28(1):83-90.

Büttner U, Büttner-Ennever JA. Present concepts of oculomotor organization. In: Büttner-Ennever JA, ed. *Neuroanatomy of the Oculomotor System.* Amsterdam: Elsevier Science Publishers; 1988:3-164.

Büttner-Ennever JA, Henn V. An autoradiographic study of the pathways from the pontine reticular formation involved in horizontal eye movements. *Brain Res.* 1976;108:155-164.

Buttner-Ennever JA, Horn AKE. Reticular formation: eye movements, gaze, and blinks. In: Paxinos G, Mai JK, eds. *The Human Nervous System.* London: Elsevier; 2004:480-510.

Cohen B, Yakushin SB, Holstein GR, et al. Vestibular experiments in space. *Adv Space Biol Med.* 2005;10:105-164.

Dieterich M. Functional brain imaging: a window into the visuo-vestibular systems. *Curr Opin Neurol.* 2007;20(1):12-18.

Dieterich M, Bense S, Stephan T, Brandt T, Schwaiger M, Bartenstein P. Medial vestibular nucleus lesions in Wallenberg's syndrome cause decreased activity of the contralateral vestibular cortex. *Ann N Y Acad Sci.* 2005;1039:368-383.

Dieterich M, Brandt T. Functional brain imaging of peripheral and central vestibular disorders. *Brain.* 2008;131(Pt 10): 2538-2552.

Dieterich M, Brandt T. Imaging cortical activity after vestibular lesions. *Restor Neurol Neurosci.* 2010;28(1):47-56.

Eberhorn AC, Horn AK, Fischer P, Buttner-Ennever JA. Proprioception and palisade endings in extraocular eye muscles. *Ann N Y Acad Sci.* 2005;1039:1-8.

Fukushima K. Corticovestibular interactions: anatomy, electrophysiology, and functional considerations. *Exp Brain Res.* 1997;117(1):1-16.

Guldin WO, Grusser OJ. Is there a vestibular cortex? *Trends Neurosci.* 1998;21:254-259.

Gunny R, Yousry TA. Imaging anatomy of the vestibular and visual systems. *Curr Opin Neurol.* 2007;20(1):3-11.

Highstein SM, Holstein GR. The anatomy of the vestibular nuclei. *Prog Brain Res.* 2006;151:157-203.

Huisman AM, Ververs B, Cavada C, Kuypers HG. Collateralization of brainstem pathways in the spinal ventral horn in rat as demonstrated with the retrograde fluorescent double-labeling technique. *Brain Res.* 1984;300(2):362-367.

Karnath HO, Ferber S, Dichgans J. The neural representation of postural control in humans. *Proc Natl Acad Sci USA.* 2000;97:13931-13936.

Kokkoroyannis T, Scudder CA, Balaban CD, Highstein SM, Moschovakis AK. Anatomy and physiology of the primate interstitial nucleus of Cajal I: efferent projections. *J Neurophysiol.* 1996;75:725–739.

Krauzlis RJ. The control of voluntary eye movements: new perspectives. *Neuroscientist.* 2005;11(2):124-137.

Lackner JR, DiZio P. Vestibular, proprioceptive, and haptic contributions to spatial orientation. *Annu Rev Psychol.* 2005;56:115-147.

Lang W, Kubik S. Primary vestibular afferent projections to the ipsilateral abducens nucleus in cats. An autoradiographic study. *Exp Brain Res.* 1979;37(1):177-181.

Leigh RJ, Zee DS. *The Neurology of Eye Movements.* 4th ed. New York, NY: Oxford University Press; 2006.

Lobel E, Kleine JF, Bihan DL, Leroy-Willig A, Berthoz A. Functional MRI of galvanic vestibular stimulation. *J Neurophysiol.* 1998;80:2699-2709.

Miyamoto T, Fukushima K, Takada T, De Waele C, Vidal PP. Saccular projections in the human cerebral cortex. *Ann N Y Acad Sci.* 2005;1039:124-131.

Pierrot-Deseilligny C, Gaymard B. Eye movements. In: Kennard C, ed. *Clinical Neurology.* New York, NY: Churchill Livingstone; 1992:27-56.

Pierrot-Deseilligny C, Muri RM, Nyffeler T, Milea D. The role of the human dorsolateral prefrontal cortex in ocular motor behavior. *Ann N Y Acad Sci.* 2005;1039:239-251.

Rub U, Jen JC, Braak H, Deller T. Functional neuroanatomy of the human premotor oculomotor brainstem nuclei: insights from postmortem and advanced in vivo imaging studies. *Exp Brain Res.* 2008;187(2):167-180.

Shiroyama T, Kayahara T, Yasui Y, Nomura J, Nakano K. Projections of the vestibular nuclei to the thalamus in the rat: a Phaseolus vulgaris leucoagglutinin study. *J Comp Neurol.* 1999;407(3):318-332.

Simpson JI. The accessory optic system. *Annu Rev Neurosci.* 1984;7:13-41.

Sparks DL. The brainstem control of saccadic eye movements. *Nat Rev Neurosci.* Dec 2002;3(12):952-964.

Sugiuchi Y, Izawa Y, Ebata S, Shinoda Y. Vestibular cortical area in the periarcuate cortex: its afferent and efferent projections. *Ann N Y Acad Sci.* 2005;1039:111-123.

Wolfson L. Gait and balance dysfunction: a model of the interaction of age and disease. *Neuroscientist.* 2001;7(2):178-183.

Study Questions

1. After a brain stem stroke, a person experiences vertigo. Which of the listed arteries likely produced this neurological sign?
   A. Superior cerebellar
   B. Posterior inferior cerebellar
   C. Vertebral
   D. Posterior spinal

2. The ascending vestibular pathway projects to the _____ nucleus of the thalamus, where _____ information is integrated with vestibular sensory messages for perception.
   A. ventral posterior; proprioceptive
   B. medial geniculate; auditory
   C. medial dorsal; cognitive
   D. ventral posterior; visceral sensory

3. The vestibulospinal tracts are part of which of the following descending systems?
   A. Lateral
   B. Medial
   C. Ventral
   D. Lateral and medial

4. Ocular depression is produced by contraction of which of the following extraocular muscles?

   A. Inferior rectus
   B. Inferior rectus and medial rectus
   C. Inferior rectus and inferior oblique
   D. Inferior rectus and superior oblique

5. A person has a lesion that damaged the oculomotor nerve. Which of the following best describes the position of the affected eye in this person?
   A. Elevated and adducted
   B. Elevated and abducted
   C. Depressed and abducted
   D. Depressed and adducted

6. Palsy of the fourth nerve does not produce _____.
   A. horizontal diplopia
   B. tortional diplopia
   C. a head tilt away from the affected eye to compensate for weakened ocular intortion
   D. vertical diplopia that becomes worse when looking toward the tip of the nose

7. Horizontal saccadic eye movements are driven by which of the following brain stem regions?
   A. The cerebellum
   B. The interstitial nucleus of the MLF and the oculomotor nucleus

C. The paramedial pontine reticular formation and the abducens nucleus

D. The superior colliculus and oculomotor nuclei

8. What pathway is important for transmitting vestibular information from the vestibular nuclei to the oculomotor nucleus?

A. Medial lemniscus

B. Dorsal longitudinal fasciculus

C. Medial longitudinal fasciculus

D. Solitary tract

9. Horizontal saccades are to smooth pursuit eye movements as

A. the paramedial pontine reticular formation is to the cerebellum.

B. interstitial nucleus of the MLF is to the superior colliculus.

C. vestibular nuclei are to the cerebellum.

D. prepositus nucleus is to the superior colliculus.

10. On looking to the right, a person experiences diplopia. The right eye is normally abducted, but the left eye does not adduct. Vergence is normal. Lesion of which of the following structures likely produces this sign?

A. Right abducens nucleus

B. Left abducens nucleus

C. Right MLF

D. Left MLF

The Cerebellum

CLINICAL CASE | Friedreich Ataxia

A 10-year-old boy first presented to his pediatrician with difficulty walking. He was an only child, of French-Canadian parents. His parents reported that recently he has difficulty standing still, is constantly shifting his position, and difficulty running. They reported normal motor development initially, but that now he seems clumsy. On examination, he was observed to have a wide-based gait with occasional shifting of position to maintain balance. Sitting and standing were noted to be associated with titubation. He was referred to a child neurologist. After further workup and genetic testing, he was diagnosed with Friedreich ataxia, a progressive spinocerebellar ataxia. Friedreich ataxia is an autosomal recessive disorder, due to a chromosome 9 mutation that, in virtually all cases, is an expansion of a GAA trinucleotide repeat within the gene that codes for the mitochondrial protein frataxin.

He was seen regularly by his neurologist who noted progression in motor signs to include upper extremity ataxia, dysdiadochokinesia, and intention tremor. When asked to maintain a standing posture with his eyes closed, he began to sway and loose his balance (positive Romberg sign). He had no tendon reflexes, such as the knee-jerk or biceps reflexes. Friedreich ataxia patients often have cardiomyopathy, and most patients die as a result of cardiac arrhythmia or congestive heart failure.

Figure 13–1A is an MRI from a young Friedreich ataxia patient. Compared with the MRI from a healthy person (Figure 13–1B), the most notable feature is narrowing of the cervical spinal cord.

Answer the following questions based on your reading of the case and the chapter.

1. **Why does the patient have a positive Romberg sign, and how is this related to the loss of tendon reflexes?**

2. **What could account for the wide-based gait and ataxia?**

—Continued next page

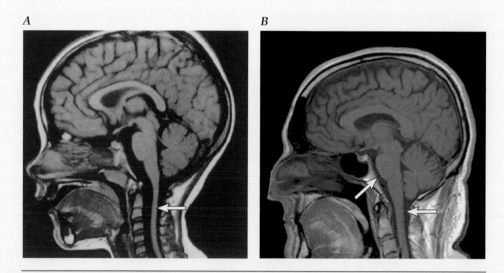

FIGURE 13–1 Friedreich ataxia. **A.** MRI from a person with Friedreich ataxia. Note thinning of the cervical spinal cord (arrow). **B.** MRI from a healthy person. Note normal cervical spinal cord (lower arrow). Other arrow points to the base of the pons, which contains pontine nuclei that project axons to the cerebellum. (**A,** Reproduced with permission from Fauci AS, Kasper DL, Braunwald E, et al., eds. *Harrison's Principles of Internal Medicine*. 18th ed. New York, NY: McGraw-Hill, Inc; 2012. **B,** Courtesy of Dr. Joy Hirsch, Columbia University.)

Key neurological signs and corresponding damaged brain structures

Proprioceptive and reflex signs

The cervical spinal cord in the patient is thin compared with a healthy person. Thinning is produced by degeneration of large-diameter somatic sensory afferents; unmyelinated fibers are spared. The degeneration is in the dorsal columns. Whereas the degeneration is accompanied by gliosis, it is insufficient to maintain the normal size of the cord. The dorsal roots show thinning as well. With this large-diameter fiber loss, there is associated loss of tendon reflexes and limb proprioception. Patients with this sensory loss rely on vision to help maintain balance. Often patients have impairment in tactile sensation.

Ataxia

The loss of limb proprioceptive information leads to incoordination. Further, there is loss of neurons in Clarke's column, which transmit proprioceptive and other mechanosensory information to the cerebellum; these neurons give rise to the dorsal spinocerebellar tract (Figure 13–6B). Together these factors contribute to ataxia. To compensate for both the balance impairment and impaired lower extremity coordination, patients adopt a broad-based, slowed gait. Interestingly, Friedreich ataxia patients may not show extensive cerebellar degeneration for most of the course of the disease. Thus, the ataxia may be more related to the somatic sensory loss. In this way, it is similar to motor disturbances in neurosyphilis (see Clinical Case in Chapter 4). Absence of early cerebellar degeneration contrasts with cerebellar degenerative conditions, such as olivopontocerebellar atrophy, which does show extensive degeneration.

The cerebellum is a fascinating brain structure; more so than many because several of its properties and organizational principles are unexpected. It is a little brain unto itself; roughly half of the neurons in the central nervous system are located in the cerebellum, and when stretched out, it is more than several square meters. That so much of the central nervous system is devoted to the cerebellum means that its functions are particularly important or complex, requiring so much neural power; indeed, it is likely both. It is no surprise that early anatomists termed this structure the cerebellum, which means little brain in Latin. Its microscopic structure is nearly crystalline in its organization, providing insight into a similarity in the way it processes information across this large brain region.

We know that the cerebellum plays a key role in movement, and it does so by regulating the functions of the motor pathways (see Figure 10–2). When this major brain structure is damaged, movements that were smooth and steered accurately become uncoordinated and erratic. Important insights into the general role of the cerebellum in motor control can be gained by considering that the cerebellum receives information from most of the sensory systems and from virtually all other components of the limb and eye movement systems. With these connections, the cerebellum is poised to compare information about the intention of an upcoming movement, by receiving information from the motor pathways, with what actually occurs, by retrieving information from the sensory systems. Research has shown that the cerebellum may compute control signals to correct for differences between intent and action, or errors. The cerebellum, in turn, provides a major input to the brain stem and cortical pathways for limb, trunk, and eye movement control.

The cerebellum also receives information from areas of the central nervous system that do not play a direct role in movement control, such as the parietal association cortex and the limbic association cortex. How is this finding reconciled with its important role in movement control? Many areas of association cortex, as well as higher-order sensory areas, help in the planning of movements—for example, by allowing an individual's motivation state of being thirsty to influence when to reach for a glass of water or by allowing the determination of the location of the glass to ensure reaching accuracy. However, the cerebellum serves nonmotor functions, too. Indeed, cerebellar damage can produce impairments in language, decision making, and affect that cannot be attributed to motor defects. Contributing to the surprise of the cerebellum, it is involved in many diverse functions, like the central nervous system itself.

Gross Anatomy of the Cerebellum

Because the three-dimensional organization of the cerebellum is so complex (Figure 13–2), rivaling that of the cerebral hemispheres and diencephalon, its gross anatomy is considered before its functional organization. Located dorsal to the pons and medulla (Figure 13–2A, B), the cerebellum is separated from the overlying cerebral cortex by a tough flap in the dura, the **cerebellar tentorium** (Figure 13–3B; see Figure 3–15). The inferior surface of the cerebellum is incompletely divided by the posterior cerebellar incisure (Figure 13–2C). The cerebellum comprises an outer cortex containing neuronal cell bodies overlying a region that contains predominantly myelinated axons. The cerebellar cortex contains an extraordinary number of neurons and a rich array of neuron types (see below).

Two shallow grooves running from rostral to caudal divide the cerebellar cortex into the **vermis,** located along the midline, and **two hemispheres** (Figure 13–2). This anatomical distinction marks the specific functional divisions of the cerebellar cortex (see below). Like the cerebral cortex, the cerebellar cortex is highly convoluted. These characteristic folds, termed **folia,** are equivalent to the gyri of the cerebral cortex. They vastly increase the amount of cerebellar cortex that can be packed into the posterior cranial fossa (see Figure 3–15).

The cerebellar cortex is organized into groups of folia, termed **lobules,** that are separated from one another by fissures. In a sagittal section through the vermis, the lobules appear to radiate from the apex of the roof of the fourth ventricle (Figure 13–3A, inset). Anatomists recognize 10 lobules, whose nomenclature is used largely by specialists studying the cerebellum. Two fissures are particularly deep and divide the various lobules into **three lobes** (Figures 13–2 and 13–3A). The **primary fissure** separates the **anterior lobe** from the **posterior lobe.** The **flocculonodular lobe** is separated from the posterior lobe by the **posterolateral fissure.** This lobe consists of the **nodulus,** located on the midline (equivalent to the vermis of the flocculonodular lobe), and the two **flocculi,** on either side. The anterior lobe is important in the control of limb and trunk movements, whereas the posterior lobe may be somewhat more important in movement planning and in the nonmotor functions of the cerebellum. The flocculonodular lobe plays a key role in maintaining balance and controlling eye movement.

Beneath the cerebellar cortex is the **white matter,** which contains axons coursing to and from the cortex (Figure 13–3). The branching pattern of the white matter of the cerebellum inspired early anatomists to refer to it as the **arbor vitae** (Latin for "tree of life"); hence, the name *folia* (Latin for "leaves") rather than *gyri,* used to describe cerebral cortex convolutions. Embedded within the cerebellar white matter are four bilaterally paired nuclei, the **deep cerebellar nuclei: the fastigial nucleus,** the **globose nucleus,** the **emboliform nucleus,** and the **dentate nucleus.** The globose and emboliform nuclei are collectively termed the **interposed nuclei.** These nuclei are shown on the cerebellar cortex surface (Figure 13–2A), as if it were transparent; they are also shown in the schematic transverse section through the pons and cerebellum (Figure 13–4). It is tempting to think that the functional relation between the deep nuclei and cortex of the cerebellum is similar to that of the thalamus and cerebral cortex. But that is wrong; we will see that neurons in the cerebellar cortex send connections to the deep nuclei, not the reverse as with the thalamus and cerebral cortex.

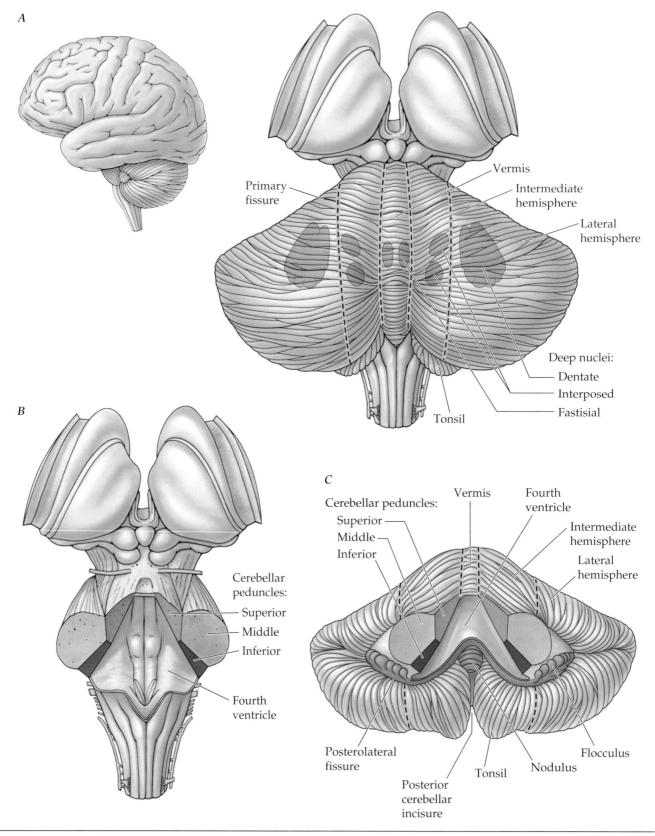

A

B

Primary
fissure

Vermis

Intermediate
hemisphere

Lateral
hemisphere

Deep nuclei:

Dentate

Interposed

Fastisial

Tonsil

Cerebellar
peduncles:

Superior

Middle

Inferior

Fourth
ventricle

C

Cerebellar peduncles:

Superior

Middle

Inferior

Vermis

Fourth
ventricle

Intermediate
hemisphere

Lateral
hemisphere

Posterolateral
fissure

Posterior
cerebellar
incisure

Tonsil

Nodulus

Flocculus

FIGURE 13–2 *A.* Dorsal view of the brain stem and cerebellum. The borders between the vermis and intermediate and lateral parts of the cerebellar hemisphere are shown. These three parts of the cerebellar cortex also correspond to functional subdivisions. *B.* The three cerebellar peduncles are revealed when the cerebellum is removed. *C.* The cerebellum, viewed from the ventral surface. Inset (*A*) shows lateral view of brain.

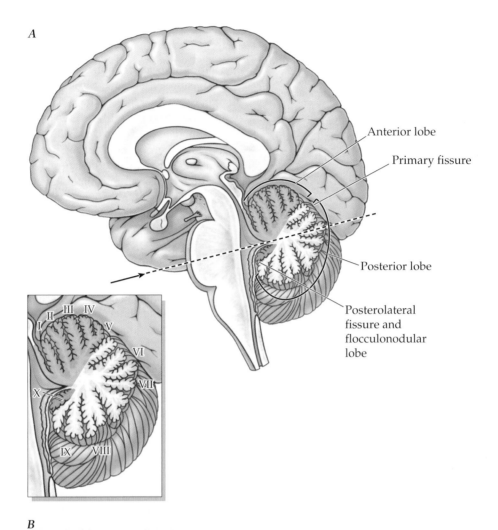

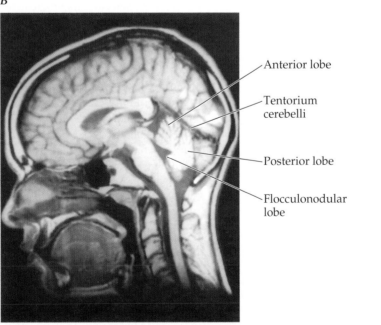

FIGURE 13-3   A. Midsagittal cut through the brain, revealing the cerebellar vermis. The inset shows the 10 cerebellar lobules. Lobules I through V comprise the anterior lobe, VI through IX comprise the posterior lobe, and X comprises the flocculonodular lobe. **B.** Midsagittal MRI, showing the three cerebellar lobes.

Axons projecting to and from the cerebellum course through the **peduncles** (Figure 13–2B, C): The **superior cerebellar peduncle** contains mostly efferent axons, the **middle cerebellar peduncle** contains only afferent axons, and the **inferior cerebellar peduncle** contains both afferent and efferent axons. An alternate nomenclature is often used for the cerebellar peduncles in the clinical and scientific literature. The superior cerebellar peduncle is also called the brachium conjunctivum; the middle cerebellar peduncle, the brachium pontis; and the inferior cerebellar peduncle, the restiform body. The various peduncles are distinguished in Figure 13–2B, C because each one has been given a different cut surface in the drawing. Three distinct peduncles would not be apparent had a single cut been drawn.

Functional Anatomy of the Cerebellum

The Cerebellum Has a Basic Circuit

Figure 13–4 shows the circuits of the cerebellum. There are two major sets of inputs to the cerebellum—termed **climbing** and **mossy fibers**—and, with some exceptions, both sets of inputs are directed to neurons in the deep nuclei and cortex. Climbing fibers originate from a single nucleus, the **inferior olivary nucleus** (see Figure 13–11B); mossy fibers originate from many different brain stem and spinal cord nuclei. In the cortex, climbing fibers synapse on Purkinje neurons, which generate a cerebellar cortex output signal by projecting to neurons in the deep nuclei. Interestingly, many neurons of the vestibular nuclei have similar connections as the deep cerebellar nuclei, receiving inputs from climbing fibers and Purkinje neurons (see below). This points to common developmental origins of the two sets of nuclei.

Mossy fibers engage a network of cerebellar excitatory and inhibitory interneurons (Figure 13–4A). The excitatory interneurons, in turn, synapse on Purkinje neurons, also leading to a cerebellar cortex output signal. The inhibitory interneurons help to regulate Purkinje neurons activity, making it easier—with less inhibition—or harder with more, for the climbing and mossy fibers to generate a cortical output signal. Surprisingly, the Purkinje neuron is an inhibitory projection neuron.

All Three Functional Divisions of the Cerebellum Display a Similar Input-Output Organization

The cerebellum has three functional divisions, each consisting of a portion of the cerebellar cortex and one or more deep nuclei (Figures 13–2 and 13–5). Each functional division of the cerebellum uses the same basic circuit to carry out its own tasks, the circuit shown in Figure 13–4A. However, each functional division differs from the others with respect to the specific input sources and the specific structures to which it

projects. The divisions are named for their major sources of information:

- The **spinocerebellum,** which receives highly organized somatic sensory inputs from the spinal cord, is important in controlling the posture and movements of the trunk and limbs (Figure 13–5A). The spinocerebellum comprises the **vermis;** the adjoining **intermediate hemisphere,** of both the anterior and posterior lobes; and the **fastigial and interposed nuclei.** This division also receives information from structures other than the spinal cord; a portion receives trigeminal and other sensory cranial nerve information. A portion of the vermis of the posterior lobe may play a role in nonmotor functions.

- The **cerebrocerebellum,** which receives input indirectly from the cerebral cortex, participates in the planning of movement and nonmotor functions. This division consists of the **lateral hemisphere,** in both the anterior and posterior lobes, and the **dentate nucleus.**

- The **vestibulocerebellum,** which receives input directly from the **vestibular labyrinth** as well as the **vestibular nuclei,** helps in maintaining balance and controlling head and eye movements. This cerebellar division corresponds to the **flocculonodular lobe.** There is no deep cerebellar nucleus for the vestibulocerebellum. Instead, the **vestibular nuclei** serve a similar role.

The spinocerebellum projects to the lateral and medial motor systems

The **spinocerebellum** is important in the control of body musculature. It is somatotopically organized: The vermis controls axial and proximal muscles and the intermediate hemisphere, limb muscles (Figure 13–5A). This mediolateral somatotopic arrangement recalls the somatotopic organization of the ventral horn, where medial motor neurons innervate **axial** and **proximal limb muscles,** and those located laterally innervate more **distal muscles** (see Figure 10–3). As with the descending motor pathways, the components of the spinocerebellum that control the distal limb are predominantly crossed, whereas the components controlling proximal and axial muscles have a more bilateral organization.

The organization of the spinocerebellum that captures both its salient and clinical features (see later section on the motor effects of cerebellar damage) is shown in Figure 13–6. It receives somatic sensory information primarily from mechanoreceptors, especially those that innervate muscle (see Table 4–1), from the limbs and trunk, via ipsilateral spinocerebellar tracts. The **dorsal spinocerebellar tract** originates from **Clarke's nucleus** and transmits sensory information from the leg and lower trunk to the cerebellar nuclei and cortex. By contrast, the **cuneocerebellar tract** originates from the **accessory cuneate nucleus.** It transmits sensory information from the arm and upper trunk. Several cerebellar conditions, including **Fredrich ataxia,** produce limb and trunk control

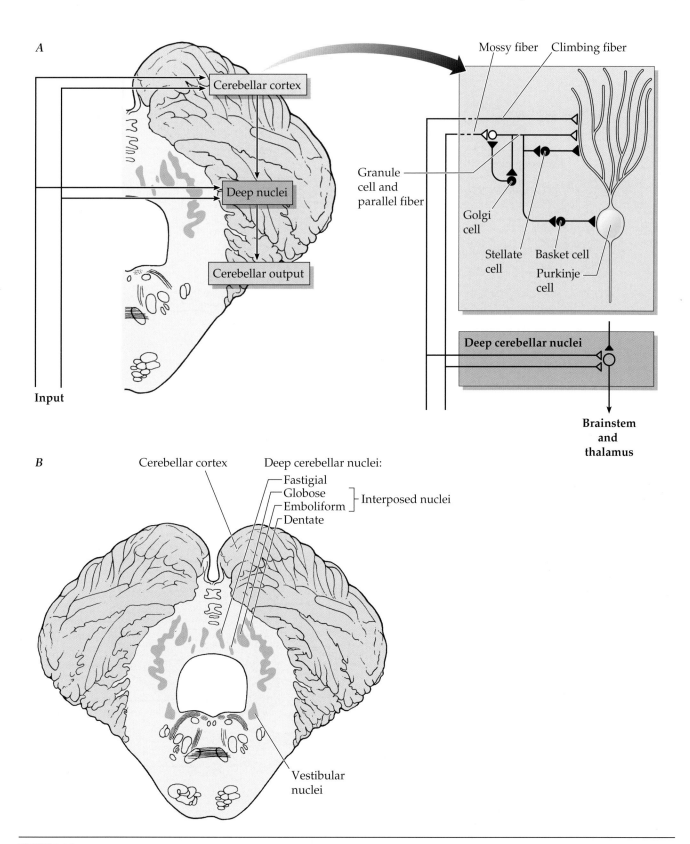

FIGURE 13–4 Schematic transverse section through the pons and cerebellum, illustrating the salient features of cerebellar circuitry (**A**). The breakout image to the right shows the basic cerebellar circuit, which is present in all parts of the cerebellar cortex. Open cell bodies and synapses are excitatory and filled cell bodies and synapses are inhibitory. Part **B** shows the location of the deep cerebellar nuclei. The vestibular nuclei are also shown because they are anatomically equivalent to the deep cerebellar nuclei for the flocculonodular lobe. They receive inputs from Purkinje cells and the inferior olivary nucleus.

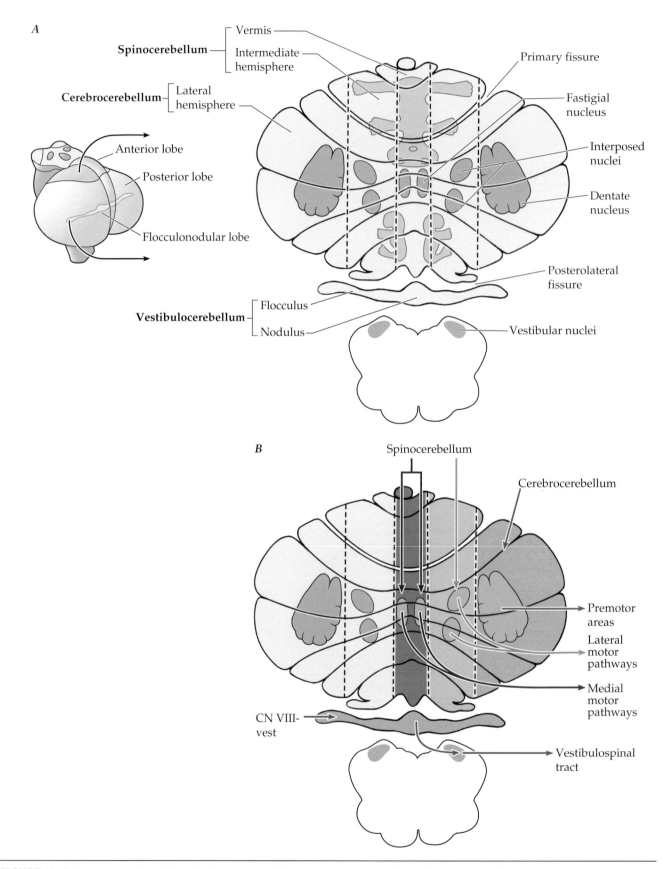

FIGURE 13–5 The anatomy (**A**) and three functional divisions (**B**) are shown in schematic views of the cerebellum. The topographic organization of somatic sensory inputs to the spinocerebellum is also shown in **A**. These inputs are somatotopically organized. Visual, auditory, and vestibular inputs are directed predominantly to the "head" areas. The deep cerebellar nuclei are shaded dark brown. The nuclei are labeled in Figure 13-2. Inset shows how the schematic "flattened out" view is constructed. (**Inset in A** modified from Kandel E, Schwartz JH, Jessell T, eds. *Principles of Neural Science*. 4th ed. New York, NY: McGraw-Hill.)

impairments by causing degeneration in these ascending cerebellar pathways (see clinical case in this chapter). Ataxia is a kind of incoordination that occurs following many different kinds of cerebellar disease.

The axons of both of these tracts travel through the **inferior cerebellar peduncle** (Figure 13–6); they are examples of mossy fibers, forming connections with diverse cerebellar neurons. For limb control, the spinocerebellar axons synapse on neurons in the interposed nuclei. Information also projects to neurons of the **intermediate hemisphere** of the cerebellar cortex, where Purkinje neurons project to the interposed nuclei (Figure 13–5B). The interposed nuclei project from the cerebellum, through the **superior cerebellar peduncle,** to the magnocellular component of the red nucleus and, predominantly, via the ventrolateral nucleus of the thalamus, to motor areas of the frontal lobe (Figures 13–3B). These components of the motor systems give rise to the **lateral descending pathways:** the rubrospinal and lateral corticospinal tracts. The logic of the laterality of these connections ensures that somatic sensory information from one limb is projected to the side of the spinocerebellum that, in turns, projects to the parts of the lateral motor pathways that control the same limb.

For proximal muscle control, including the trunk and upper back, the circuitry is more bilaterally organized (Figures 13–5B and 13–7). Here the dorsal spinocerebellar and cuneocerebellar tracts project both to the fastigial nuclei and the **vermis** of the cerebellar cortex, which, in turn, also projects to the fastigial nuclei (Figure 13–7). This deep nucleus influences motor neurons primarily through their projections onto the **medial descending pathways,** the reticulospinal (Figure 13–7) and vestibulospinal tracts (Figure 12–3B). The fastigial nucleus has also a small ascending projection, via a thalamic relay, to cells of origin of the ventral corticospinal tract in primary and premotor cortical areas. This efferent projection exits through the superior cerebellar peduncle. Some Purkinje neurons of the vermis send their axons to the vestibular nuclei (see following section on vestibulocerebellum).

Two other spinocerebellar pathways (Figure 13–6B,)—the ventral and rostral spinocerebellar tracts, for the lower and upper halves of the body—are thought to transmit internal feedback signals for correcting inaccurate movements rather than somatic sensory information. Many of the axons that decussate in the spinal cord cross again in the superior cerebellar peduncle to terminate in the ipsilateral cerebellum; these axons are "doubly crossed." There are also **trigeminocerebellar pathways** that originate from the **spinal trigeminal nuclei,** principally from parts of the interpolar and oral nuclei (see Chapter 6).

The cerebrocerebellum projects to premotor and association cortical areas

The **cerebrocerebellum** (Figures 13–5B and 13–8) is primarily involved in the planning of movement and is interconnected with diverse regions of the **cerebral cortex.** The major input to the cerebrocerebellum is from the **contralateral cerebral cortex,** not only from the motor areas but also from the sensory and association areas (Figure 13–8). This projection is relayed by neurons in the ipsilateral **pontine nuclei** (Figure 13–8A, and inset). The pontine nuclei, in turn, project to the contralateral cerebellar cortex through the **middle cerebellar peduncle.** Purkinje neurons of the cerebrocerebellum project to the **dentate nucleus,** the largest and most lateral of the deep nuclei. Neurons in the dentate nucleus project their axons to two main motor control centers. The first is the motor relay nucleus of the thalamus, the ventrolateral nucleus, and from here, to the primary motor cortex and premotor areas. The logic of the laterality of these connections is that the cerebral cortex controlling one limb also projects to the cerebrocerebellum controlling the same limb.

The second motor control center to which the dentate nucleus projects is the **red nucleus;** however, it projects to the **parvocellular division,** not to the magnocellular division. Whereas the magnocellular portion of the red nucleus gives rise to the rubrospinal tract (see Chapter 10), the parvocellular division projects to the ipsilateral **inferior olivary nucleus,** the source of climbing fiber input to the cerebellum (see below). The parvocellular red nucleus forms a loop: first connecting to the ipsilateral olive, from there to the contralateral dentate, and then back to the same parvocellular red nucleus via a decussation in the superior cerebellar peduncle. Whereas the function of this loop is not known, damage along the loop can produce tremor.

Recent functional imaging and clinical studies in humans suggest that the most ventrolateral and posterior portion of the dentate nucleus participates in nonmotor functions, including cognition and language. There may be a distinctive anatomical correlate for the role of the dentate nucleus in higher brain functions. In the monkey, where anatomical tracer studies can be conducted, a portion of the dentate nucleus is analogous to the ventrolateral dentate in the human. Different sets of neurons in this portion of the monkey's dentate nucleus project—via integrative thalamic nuclei, including the medial dorsal nucleus—to the association cortex: to **prefrontal association cortex,** involved in **working memory,** where information that is used to plan and shape upcoming behaviors is temporarily stored; and to **posterior parietal association cortex,** the interface of visual perception, attention, and motor action. Thus, the cerebrocerebellum has the connections to mediate several higher brain functions.

The vestibulocerebellum projects to brain stem centers for controlling eye and head movements

The **vestibulocerebellum** is crucial for controlling gaze, through the combined control of eye and head movements (Figures 13–5B and 13–9). This cerebellar division receives information from **primary vestibular afferents** and secondary vestibular neurons in the **vestibular nuclei.** In fact, the vestibular afferents are the only primary sensory neurons that project directly to the cerebellum. The cortical component of the vestibulocerebellum projects to the vestibular nuclei: the lateral, medial, inferior, and superior vestibular nuclei

A

B

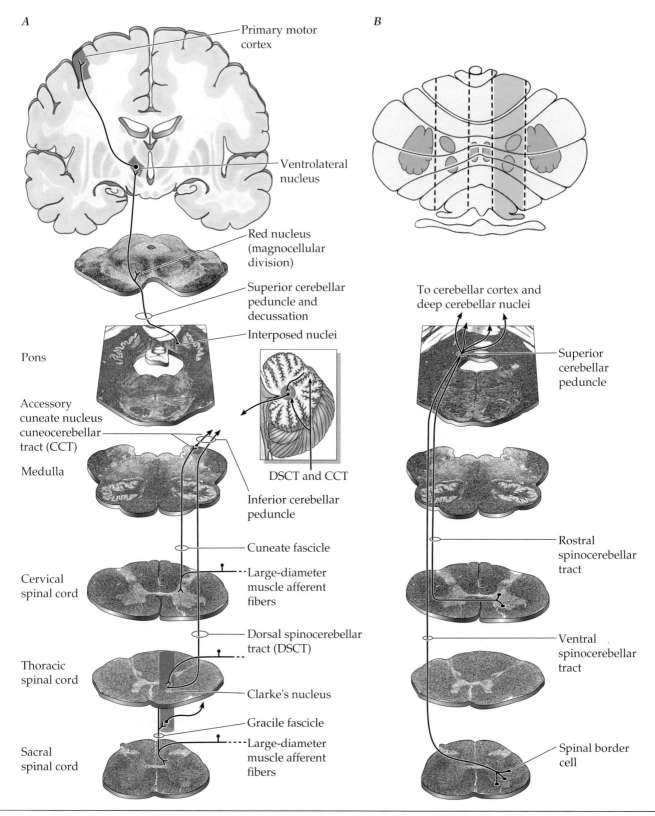

Primary motor cortex

Ventrolateral nucleus

Red nucleus (magnocellular division)

Superior cerebellar peduncle and decussation

Interposed nuclei

Pons

Accessory cuneate nucleus cuneocerebellar tract (CCT)

Medulla

DSCT and CCT

Inferior cerebellar peduncle

Cuneate fascicle

Cervical spinal cord

Large-diameter muscle afferent fibers

Dorsal spinocerebellar tract (DSCT)

Thoracic spinal cord

Clarke's nucleus

Gracile fascicle

Sacral spinal cord

Large-diameter muscle afferent fibers

To cerebellar cortex and deep cerebellar nuclei

Superior cerebellar peduncle

Rostral spinocerebellar tract

Ventral spinocerebellar tract

Spinal border cell

FIGURE 13–6 Key features of the input-output organization of the lateral spinocerebellum, which is important for controlling the limbs. Part **A** shows the dorsal and cuneocerebellar tracts projecting to the cerebellum (lower four sections). The upper sections show the cerebellar output path. Part **B** shows the ventral and rostral spinocerebellar tracts. The output of the lateral spinocerebellum is shown in **A**. The inset shows the cerebellar cortex and deep nuclei; the lateral spinocerebellum is highlighted.

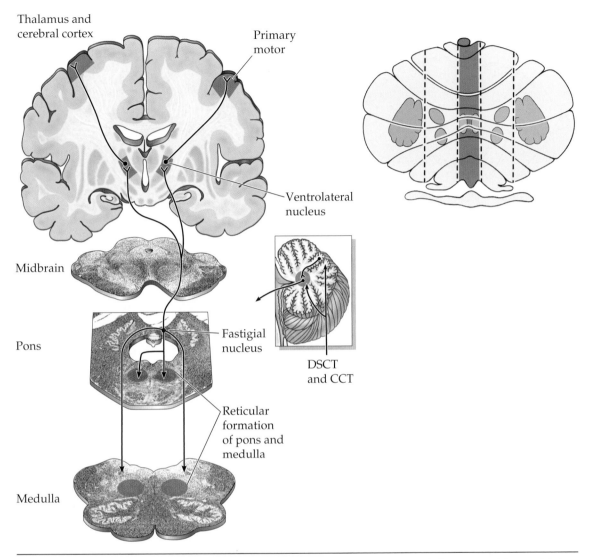

FIGURE 13–7 Salient features of the vermis of the spinocerebellum. The inset shows the cerebellar cortex and deep nuclei; the vermis of the spinocerebellum is highlighted.

(Figure 13–9). As we saw in Chapter 12, the vestibular nuclei are important for smooth pursuit eye movements as well as the vestibuloocular reflexes. The vestubulocerebellum participates in coordinating neck muscle function with eye control, via the **medial vestibulospinal tract;** maintaining balance, via the **lateral vestibulospinal tract;** and maintaining eye movement control, via fibers in the **medial longitudinal fasciculus** to extraocular motor nuclei.

Damage to the Cerebellum Produces Limb Motor Signs on the Same Side as the Lesion

There are three classic signs of cerebellar damage: ataxia, tremor, and nystagmus. **Ataxia** is inaccuracy in the speed, force, and distance of movement. In reaching for an object, a patient with cerebellar damage overshoots (hypermetria) or undershoots (hypometria) the target. Ataxia of gait produces staggering and lurching. Ataxia is due to impairments in interjoint coordination. **Tremor** is involuntary oscillation of the limbs or trunk. Cerebellar tremor is characteristically present when the patient is trying to perform a movement requiring skill, such as touching the examiner's finger or bringing a forkful of food to the mouth. **Nystagmus** is a rhythmic involuntary oscillation of the eyes. Ataxia and nystagmus typically occur after damage to cerebellar inputs, such as the spinocerebellar tracts or the inferior cerebellar peduncle. In contrast, tremor is more often a consequence of damage to the cerebellar output pathways, such as the superior cerebellar peduncle. However, combinations of signs typically occur with damage to the cerebellum depending on the site and size of the lesion.

Knowledge of the anatomy of the descending projection pathways is crucial for understanding why unilateral cerebellar damage typically produces **ipsilateral limb motor signs.** Ipsilateral signs occur because both the cerebellar efferent projections and the descending pathways (ie, the targets of cerebellar action) are crossed. The combined decussations

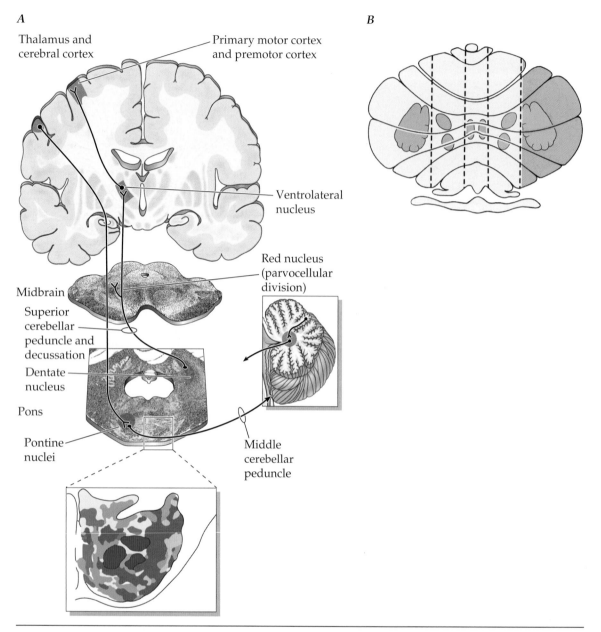

FIGURE 13–8 Afferent and efferent connections of the cerebrocerebellum (*A*) and the portion of the cerebellar cortex that corresponds to this cerebellar division (*B*). Note that the major input to the pontine nuclei is from large areas of the cerebral cortex, although input from only a single site is shown. Most cortical regions project to the cerebellum, via the pontine nuclei (see inset). Different cortical areas project to distinct sets of pontine nuclei, represented as different shades in the schematic inset of ventral pons. The darkest gray areas correspond to descending cortical axons. (Adapted from Schmahmann JD, Pandya DN. The cerebrocerebellar system. *Int Rev Neurobiol.* 1997;41:31-60.)

result in a system of connections that is "doubly crossed" (Figure 13–10). Damage to cerebellar input from the spinal cord also produces ipsilateral signs because the principal spinocerebellar pathways, the dorsal spinocerebellar and cuneocerebellar tracts, ascend ipsilaterally. Thus, whether damage occurs to cerebellar inputs or outputs, or to the cerebellum itself, neurological signs are present on the ipsilateral side.

Occlusion of the **posterior inferior cerebellar artery (PICA)** infarcts the **inferior cerebellar peduncle** as well as most of the **deep cerebellar nuclei.** Two key signs related to this infarction are nystagmus (also a consequence of damage to the

vestibular nuclei) and ipsilateral limb ataxia. These are the key cerebellar signs associated with the **lateral medullary, or Wallenberg, syndrome** (see Clinical Cases for Chapters 6 and 15). Somatic sensory deficits are also present with PICA occlusion because infarction of the dorsolateral medulla interrupts ascending fibers of the anterolateral system (see Chapter 5) as well as the trigeminal spinal tract and nucleus (see Chapter 6). Importantly, even though the cerebellum receives sensory information, especially somatic sensory information, patients do not have loss of sensation; for example, they do not report sensory threshold changes, numbness, or visual blind spots.

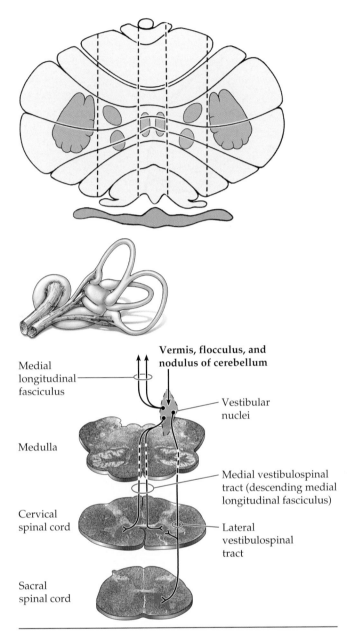

Medial longitudinal fasciculus

Vermis, flocculus, and nodulus of cerebellum

Vestibular nuclei

Medulla

Medial vestibulospinal tract (descending medial longitudinal fasciculus)

Cervical spinal cord

Lateral vestibulospinal tract

Sacral spinal cord

FIGURE 13–9 Afferent and efferent connections of the vestibulocerebellum. The inset shows the structure of the inner ear. The otolith organs provide the major input to the vestibulocerebellum (see Figure 12–2).

Although the principal signs of cerebellar damage are motor, patients with cerebellar damage may also have behavioral impairments that cannot be attributed to a primary motor impairment. This phenomenon has been described as the cerebellar "cognitive affective syndrome." The syndrome is characterized by impairments in executive functions (eg, planning behaviors), abstract reasoning, visuospatial reasoning, and working memory. Some patients have personality changes, with a blunting of affect. This syndrome is more prominent in patients with lesions of posterior lobe hemisphere (cognitive and language impairments) and posterior lobe vermis (defective affect). These changes could be due to impairments in processing information from diverse cortical regions—such as association areas, including limbic association cortex—carried

by the corticopontine projection. It could also be related to damaging cerebellar regions that project to the dorsolateral prefrontal and other association areas. Interestingly, there are cerebellar structural changes in patients with **autism spectrum disorder,** a condition presenting with deficits in social interaction, impaired verbal and nonverbal communication, and expression of stereotyped patterns of behavior. This is a common neuropsychiatric disorder affecting about 1 in 150 individuals. Further, many of the genes associated with autism spectrum disorder are expressed in the cerebellum. While controversial, there is a growing body of basic and clinical evidence asserting the cerebellum's role in nonmotor functions and neuropsychiatric disorders.

Regional Anatomy of the Cerebellum

The rest of this chapter examines the regional anatomy of the connections and cellular organization of the cerebellum. Sections through key levels, from caudal to rostral, are used to illustrate the locations of spinocerebellar tracts, the histology of the cerebellar cortex, the deep nuclei, and the efferent projections to the brain stem and thalamus.

Spinal Cord and Medullary Sections Reveal Nuclei and Paths Transmitting Somatic Sensory Information to the Cerebellum

Clarke's nucleus and the accessory cuneate nucleus are the principal nuclei that relay somatic sensory information to the spinocerebellum. **Clarke's nucleus** is found in the medial portion of the intermediate zone of the spinal cord gray matter (lamina VII) (Figure 13–11). This nucleus forms a column with a limited rostrocaudal distribution (Figure 13–6). In the human, Clarke's nucleus spans the **eighth cervical segment** (C8) to approximately the **second lumbar segment** (L2) and relays somatic sensory information from the lower limb and lower trunk. Because the caudal boundary of the nucleus is rostral to the lumbosacral enlargement, afferent fibers from most of the lower extremity first enter and ascend in the gracile fascicle (Figure 13–6). Then they leave the white matter to terminate in Clarke's nucleus. The **dorsal spinocerebellar tract** originates from Clarke's nucleus. The tract ascends in the outermost portion of the ipsilateral lateral column (Figure 13–11C) and enters the cerebellum via the **inferior cerebellar peduncle** (Figure 13–11A, B). The other pathway from the lower limb, the **ventral spinocerebellar tract,** is lateral to the ascending fibers of the anterolateral system (Figure 13–11C). The ventral spinocerebellar tract originates from diverse neurons in the ventral horn. The ventral spinocerebellar tract is a crossed spinal pathway, entering the cerebellum via the **superior cerebellar peduncle,** where some of the axons re-cross (Figure 13–12).

The caudal medulla contains the **accessory cuneate nucleus** (Figure 13–11A, B), which is rostral to the cuneate nucleus, important for perception (see Chapter 4). (The

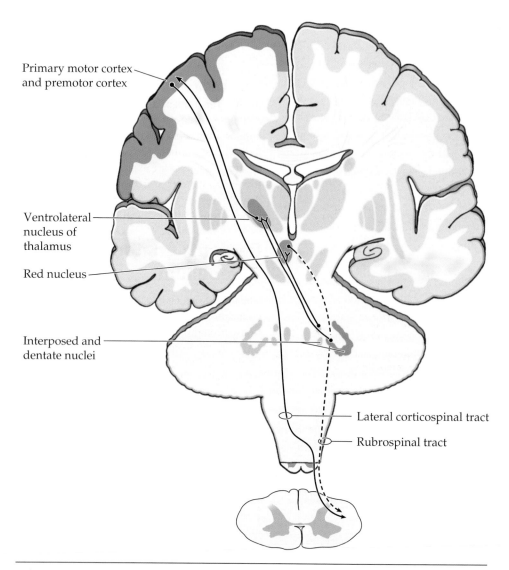

Primary motor cortex
and premotor cortex

Ventrolateral
nucleus of
thalamus

Red nucleus

Interposed and
dentate nuclei

Lateral corticospinal tract

Rubrospinal tract

FIGURE 13–10 The "doubly crossed" arrangement of the efferent projections of the cerebellum. Note that the cerebellar projection to the magnocellular division of the red nucleus is from the interposed nuclei (globose and emboliform nuclei), and the projection to the parvocellular division (not shown) originates in the dentate nucleus.(Adapted with permission from Parent A. *Carpenter's Human Neuroanatomy.* 9th ed. Williams & Wilkins; 1996.)

accessory cuneate nucleus is also termed the external cuneate nucleus.) The accessory cuneate nucleus relays somatic sensory information from the upper trunk and upper limb to the cerebellum, not for perception but for controlling movements. To reach the accessory cuneate nucleus, afferent fibers from the upper trunk, arm, and back of the head first course rostrally within the cervical spinal cord in the **cuneate fascicle** of the dorsal column (Figure 13–11A). The entire course of the cuneocerebellar tract is within the **inferior cerebellar peduncle.**

The Inferior Olivary Nucleus Is the Only Source of Climbing Fibers

The inferior olivary nucleus (Figure 13–11B), from which all **climbing fibers** originate, is a collection of three subnuclei (see Figure AII–8) that have somewhat different connections. It forms an elevation on the ventral surface of the medulla

termed the **olive** (Figure AI–6). The inferior olivary nucleus consists of a convoluted sheet of neurons surrounded by the axons of the central tegmental tract, which originated from the ipsilateral parvocellular division of the red nucleus (see below). Neurons in the inferior olivary nucleus are electrically coupled, resulting in a synchrony of action among local groups of olivary neurons. The principal division of the nucleus (Figure 13–11B) is the largest in humans. Interestingly, in animals this division is associated with the cerebrocerebellum.

Dorsal to the inferior olivary nucleus is the **lateral reticular nucleus** (Figure 13–11B), which gives rise to a mossy fiber projection to the cerebellum. The lateral reticular nucleus receives sensory information from mechanoreceptors of the limbs and trunk as well as information from the motor cortex, by branches of corticospinal tract axons. Like neurons of the ventral spinocerebellar tract, the lateral reticular nucleus is thought to participate in correcting for movement errors.

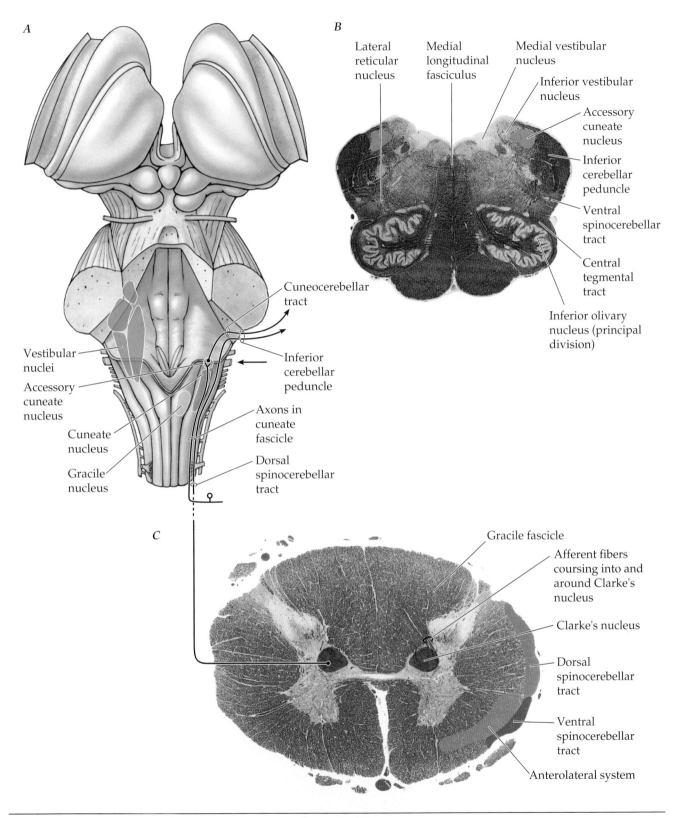

A

B

Lateral reticular nucleus

Medial longitudinal fasciculus

Medial vestibular nucleus

Inferior vestibular nucleus

Accessory cuneate nucleus

Inferior cerebellar peduncle

Ventral spinocerebellar tract

Central tegmental tract

Inferior olivary nucleus (principal division)

Cuneocerebellar tract

Inferior cerebellar peduncle

Axons in cuneate fascicle

Dorsal spinocerebellar tract

Vestibular nuclei

Accessory cuneate nucleus

Cuneate nucleus

Gracile nucleus

C

Gracile fascicle

Afferent fibers coursing into and around Clarke's nucleus

Clarke's nucleus

Dorsal spinocerebellar tract

Ventral spinocerebellar tract

Anterolateral system

FIGURE 13–11   Brain stem (*A, B*) and spinal cord (*C*) nuclei transmitting somatic sensory information to the cerebellum. *A.* Key pathways for information from the dorsal spinocerebellar and cuneocerebellar tracts. *B.* Myelin-stained transverse section through the medulla, at the level of the accessory cuneate nucleus and inferior olivary nucleus. The arrow in *A* indicates the plane of section in *B.* Myelin-stained section through the upper lumbar cord (*C*). Note, the anterolateral system axons are located immediately medial to those of the ventral spinocerebellar tract.

The Vestibulocerebellum Receives Input From Primary and Secondary Vestibular Neurons

Purkinje neurons of the flocculonodular lobe send their axons primarily to the **vestibular nuclei** (Figure 13–11A, B), rather than to the deep cerebellar nuclei, as do Purkinje neurons in other regions of the cerebellum. (Exceptions exist; some Purkinje neurons of the flocculonodular lobe synapse in the fastigial nucleus, and some within the anterior and posterior lobe vermis synapse in the vestibular nuclei.) The vestibular nuclei are the anatomical equivalent of the deep cerebellar nuclei of the vestibulocerebellum because they share two similarities in the sources of afferent input, both: receive a projection from the inferior olivary nucleus and are monosynaptically inhibited by Purkinje neurons.

The flocculonodular lobe projects to the medial, inferior, and superior vestibular nuclei. These nuclei—especially the medial vestibular nucleus—give rise to the medial vestibulospinal tract, for coordinating head and eye movements (Chapter 12). The fastigial nucleus projects primarily to the lateral vestibular nucleus, which gives rise to the lateral vestibulospinal tract, for controlling axial muscles to maintain balance and posture. The vestibular nuclei also contribute to the **medial longitudinal fasciculus** (Figures 13–11A, 13–12, and 13–15B), which plays a key role in eye muscle control through projections to the extraocular motor nuclei (see Chapter 12). Thus,

the vestibulocerebellum has direct control of head and eye position via its influence on the vestibular nuclei.

The Pontine Nuclei Provide the Major Input to the Cerebrocerebellum

The pontine nuclei (Figure 13–12; also Figures 13–8 and 13–15B3, 4) relay information from the cerebral cortex to the cerebrocerebellum. Virtually the entire cerebral cortex projects to the pontine nuclei (see below). Corticopontine neurons originate in layer V of the cerebral cortex, the same layer that gives rise to the corticospinal and corticobulbar neurons. The descending axons course within the internal capsule and basis pedunculi to synapse in the ipsilateral pontine nuclei. The axons of neurons of the pontine nuclei decussate in the pons and enter the cerebellum via the **middle cerebellar peduncle** (Figure 13–12).

The Intrinsic Circuitry of the Cerebellar Cortex Is the Same for the Different Functional Divisions

The cellular constituents and synaptic connections of the cerebellar cortex are among the best understood of the central nervous system (see Box 13–1). The cerebellar cortex consists of three cell layers, progressing from its external surface inward

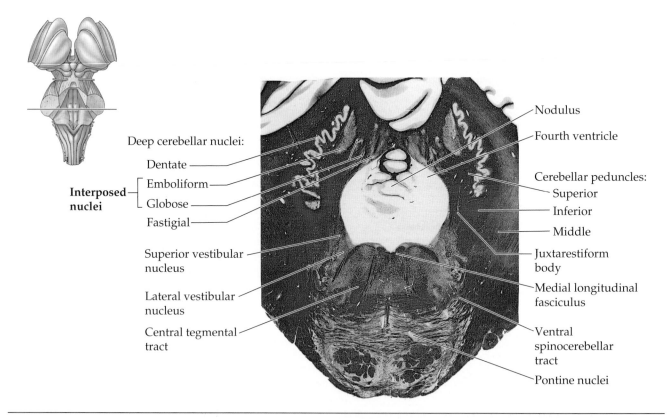

FIGURE 13-12 Myelin-stained transverse section through the caudal pons and deep cerebellar nuclei. The inset shows the plane of section.

Box 13–1

Inhibitory Circuitry of the Cerebellum

The Purkinje neuron is an inhibitory projection neuron: When it discharges, it hyperpolarizes the neurons in the deep cerebellar nuclei or vestibular nuclei with which it synapses. How then can neurons in the deep cerebellar nuclei and vestibular nuclei transmit control signals to the motor pathways when they are only inhibited by Purkinje neuron? The climbing fibers as well as many mossy fibers (from the spinal cord and reticular formation) make direct excitatory synaptic connection onto neurons in the deep nuclei (Figure 13–14A). (Anatomical data suggest that most mossy fibers from the pontine nuclei bypass the deep nuclei, synapsing only in the cortex.) It is thought that these direct inputs to the deep nuclear neurons increase their excitability and help to maintain their background neuronal activity at a high level. Also, intrinsic cell membrane properties, such as high resting inward ionic currents, help to maintain high levels of activity in these neurons. This continuously high level of neural activity is then reduced, or "sculpted," by the inhibitory actions of the Purkinje neurons. Similarly, for the vestibular nuclei, direct excitatory inputs from vestibular afferents and membrane properties help to maintain a high background level of activity.

The activity of Purkinje neurons is inhibited by two groups of interneurons (Figures 13–13B and 13–14A): **stellate neurons,** located in the outer portion of the molecular layer, and **basket neurons,** located close to the border between the molecular and Purkinje layers. Because its synapse is located on the cell body, the basket neuron is very effective in inhibiting the Purkinje neuron. These neurons receive their predominant input from parallel fibers. The action of these inhibitory interneurons "disinhibits" Purkinje neurons; they will exert less inhibition on neurons in the deep nuclei and vestibular nuclei.

The third cerebellar cortical inhibitory interneuron is the **Golgi neuron,** which inhibits the granule neuron. This inhibitory synapse is made in the granular layer, in a complex structure termed the **cerebellar glomerulus** (Figure 13–13C; clear zones seen under high magnification). Synaptic glomeruli ensure specificity of connections because this entire synaptic complex is contained within a **glial capsule.** An inventory of the synaptic action of the interneurons of the cerebellar cortex demonstrates that all but the granule neuron are inhibitory (Table 13–1).

(Figure 13–13): the **molecular layer,** the **Purkinje layer,** and the **granular layer,** which is adjacent to the white matter. The cerebellar cortex contains five types of neurons, and they each have a different laminar distribution and are excitatory or inhibitory (Figure 13–13B; Table 13–1): (1) Purkinje neuron, (2) granule neuron, (3) basket neuron, (4) stellate neuron, and (5) Golgi neuron. The Purkinje neuron is the projection neuron of the cerebellar cortex; it is located in the Purkinje layer. All others are interneurons.

The same two basic circuits are present throughout the cortex of the spinocerebellum, cerebrocerebellum, and vestibulocerebellum; one receiving excitatory input from the climbing and the other, from the mossy fibers. **Climbing fibers** originate entirely from the **inferior olivary nuclear complex** (Figure 13–11B) and synapse on Purkinje neurons (Figure 13–14). Climbing fibers make multiple synapses with one Purkinje neuron. Remarkably, each Purkinje neuron receives input from only a single climbing fiber. Individual climbing fibers branch to make contact with no more than about 10 Purkinje neurons.

The other circuit begins with the **mossy fibers;** the **Purkinje neuron** is also the target, but not directly (Figure 13–14). Mossy fibers first synapse on **granule neurons**—the only excitatory interneurons in the cerebellum. Located in the granular layer (Figure 13–13), granule neurons have an axon that ascends through the Purkinje layer into the molecular layer. Here the axon bifurcates to form the **parallel fibers,** which synapse on Purkinje neurons (Figure 13–14) and other cerebellar interneurons (Table 13–1). Note that the micrograph of the Purkinje neuron (Figure 13–14) is in the plane of the dendritic tree; the right side of the drawing is at right angles to the dendritic tree. Owing to the planar dendritic tree of Purkinje neurons, one parallel fiber will synapse only a few

times with a Purkinje neuron, as the axon passes through its dendrites. That axon may synapse on hundreds of Purkinje neurons that are stacked along the folium. Each Purkinje neuron receives synapses from thousands of parallel fibers. The efficacy of parallel fiber input onto a given Purkinje neuron is increased immediately after Purkinje neuron activation by a climbing fiber. Purkinje neurons of the spinocerebellum and cerebrocerebellum project their axons through the cerebellar white matter to synapse on neurons in the deep cerebellar nuclei (Figure 13–12). To reach the vestibular nuclei, Purkinje neuron axons of the vestibulocerebellum travel through the inferior cerebellar peduncle.

The cerebellum is thought to have a modular functional organization organized, in part, by the projections of climbing fibers. Within the different sagittal functional zones (eg, Figure 13–5), there are **microzones** in which small clusters of Purkinje neurons receive climbing fiber inputs that have similar physiological characteristics, such as processing somatic sensory information from the same body part. The Purkinje neurons in the microzone, in turn, project to a group of neurons in a deep nucleus or vestibular nucleus that receive similar inputs from the olive. Within each functional division there are many microzones. It is thought that each microzone subserves a different aspect of the overall functions of the broader zone, such as regulating the coordination and strength of contraction of different hand muscles within arm representation of the spinocerebellum.

The Deep Cerebellar Nuclei Are Located Within the White Matter

The deep cerebellar nuclei can be identified in the transverse section through the pons and cerebellum shown in

A

B

Basket neuron

Stellate neuron

Purkinje neuron

Parallel fiber

Molecular layer
Purkinje layer
Granular layer
White matter

Golgi neuron

Granule neuron

C

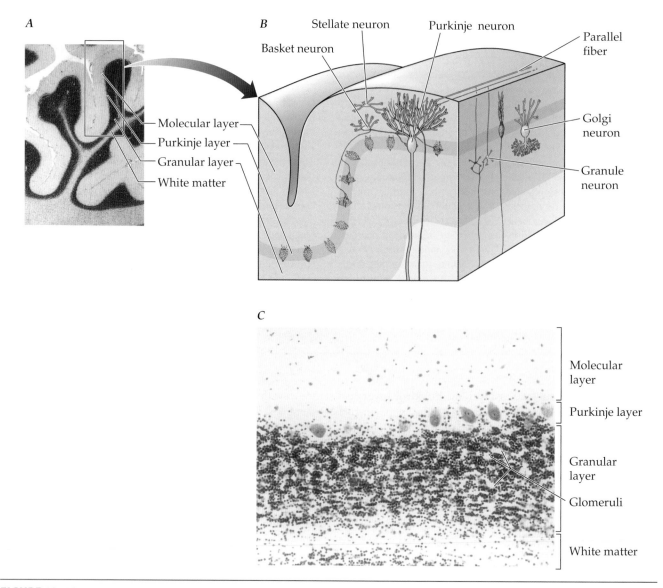

Molecular layer

Purkinje layer

Granular layer

Glomeruli

White matter

FIGURE 13–13 Nissl-stained section (low-magnification) through the cerebellar cortex (*A*); schematic drawing of a cerebellar folium (*B*). High-magnification view of the cerebellar cortex (*C*).

Figure 13–12, from medial to lateral: fastigial, globose, emboliform, and dentate nuclei. Recall that the globose and emboliform nuclei collectively are termed the interposed nuclei. The efferent projections of the deep nuclei course through the inferior and superior cerebellar peduncles.

The fastigial, interposed, and dentate nuclei have differential projections that reflect their functions in maintaining balance, controlling limb movement, and planning movement, respectively. The major targets of the output of the fastigial nucleus are the vestibular nuclei and the reticular formation, two components of the medial descending pathways that control balance and posture. The major targets of the interposed nuclei are the **magnocellular division** of the red nucleus, where the rubrospinal tract originates and, via the thalamus, the **motor cortex.** The major targets of the dentate nucleus are the **parvocellular division** of the red

nucleus, which sends its axons to the ipsilateral inferior olivary nucleus via the **central tegmental tract** (shown at its termination in Figure 13–11A), and, via the thalamus, areas of cortex involved in motor planning. Note that the two divisions of the red nucleus cannot be clearly distinguished. The parvocellular division is much larger than the magnocellular division.

The ascending projections from the deep nuclei course in the **superior cerebellar peduncle** (Figures 13–12 and, 13–15B4). The superior cerebellar peduncle decussates in the caudal midbrain, at the level of the inferior colliculus (Figure 13–15A, B2). The axons continue rostrally, either synapsing with the two divisions of the red nucleus or passing through the nucleus en route to the motor thalamic nuclei. Collectively, the projections from the deep cerebellar nuclei to the thalamus are termed the **cerebellothalamic tract.**

Table **13-1** Neurons and circuits of the cerebellar cortex

Neuron type	Laminar distribution	Synaptic action	Input	Postsynaptic target
Projection neuron				
Purkinje	Purkinje	Inhibitory	Climbing fiber	Deep nuclei; vestibular nuclei
			Mossy fibers→granule neuron-parallel fibers	Deep nuclei; vestibular nuclei
Interneurons				
Granule	Granular	Excitatory	Mossy fibers	Purkinje, stellate, basket, and Golgi neurons
Basket	Molecular	Inhibitory	Parallel fibers	Purkinje neurons
Stellate	Molecular	Inhibitory	Parallel fibers	Purkinje neurons
Golgi	Granular	Inhibitory	Parallel fibers	Granule neurons
Principal circuits				
Climbing fiber (+)→Purkinje neuron (–)→Deep cerebellar nuclei or vestibular nuclei				
Mossy fiber (+)→Granule neuron (+)→ Purkinje neuron (–)→Deep cerebellar nuclei or vestibular nuclei				
Interneuronal circuits				
Granule neuron (+)→Basket cell (–)→Purkinje neuron				
Granule neuron (+)→Stellate cell (–)→Purkinje neuron				
Granule neuron (+)→Golgi cell (–)→Granule neuron				

The Ventrolateral Nucleus Relays Cerebellar Output to the Premotor and Primary Motor Cortical Areas

The portion of the thalamus that receives mostly cerebellar input and transmits this information to the motor areas of the frontal lobe, **ventrolateral nucleus,** is separate from the thalamic sensory nuclei. The ventrolateral nucleus (Figure 13–16) is difficult to identify. One clue that makes identification a bit easier is the presence of the **thalamic fasciculus.** This band of myelinated fibers contains axons of the cerebellothalamic tract as well as axons of the basal ganglia projection to the thalamus (see Chapter 14).

The ventrolateral nucleus is large and has many component divisions that have distinctive connections, primarily with the frontal lobe but also to the parietal lobe. The interposed and dentate nuclei project to the part of the ventrolateral nucleus that relays information mostly to the **primary motor cortex (area 4)** and the **premotor cortex (lateral area 6).** In addition, the dentate nucleus projects to other parts of the ventrolateral nucleus that project to posterior parietal cortex and the medial dorsal thalamus, which transmits information to the prefrontal cortex. The projections from the dentate nucleus interdigitate with but do not overlay the terminations from the interposed nuclei.

The Cerebellum Is Important for Many Nonmotor Functions

Transneuronal viral tracing studies in the monkey have revealed extensive connections between the dentate nucleus and diverse regions of the prefrontal and posterior parietal cortex, basically, nonmotor areas. These projections originate from the dentate nucleus. Routing through the thalamus, the projections target several regions within the prefrontal cortex and posterior parietal cortex. Whereas cerebellar damage in humans produces characteristic motor signs, as described earlier, damage of the posterior lobe can result in cognitive and affective changes. The projections of the cerebellum to prefrontal and posterior parietal cortex in monkey help to explain these nonmotor functions in the human. Also important for the nonmotor cerebellar functions are the descending corticopontine projections from cerebral cortical regions for cognition and affect (eg, Figure 13–7; discussed further below). In the monkey, only about 40% of the dentate nucleus is devoted to motor system connections. This leaves an intriguingly large portion of the nucleus for nonmotor connections and functions. Considering the increased complexity of the human brain, the nonmotor functions of the cerebellum—and the interplay between these functions and movement control—will very likely be an important direction for clinical and basic studies in the future.

The Corticopontine Projection Brings Information From Diverse Cortical Areas to the Cerebellum for Motor Control and Higher Brain Functions

Cerebral cortical regions to which the deep cerebellar nuclei project, via the thalamus, in turn project back to the cerebellum via the corticopontine projection (Figure 13–7). This forms a "closed loop," in which a particular functional region of the

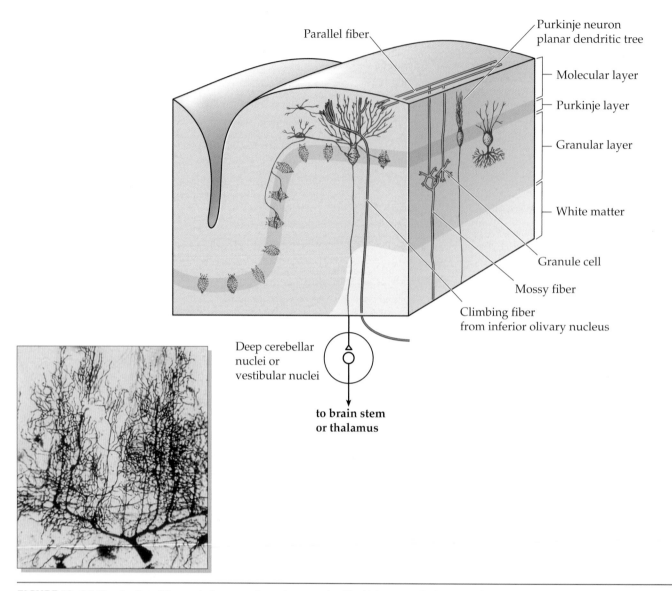

FIGURE 13–14 The circuitry of the cerebellar cortex. Inset shows a stained Purkinje neuron (Golgi stain). There are two major excitatory inputs to the cerebellum: climbing fibers and mossy fibers. Whereas the climbing fibers synapse directly on Purkinje neurons, the mossy fibers first synapse on granule neurons, which in turn give rise to the parallel fibers, which synapse on Purkinje neurons.

cerebellum, for example the hand control zone of the spino-cerebellum, projects to an area of the cerebral cortex involved in the same function. We will see a similar predominantly closed loop organization for the basal ganglia (Chapter 14). There is little evidence for the alternative "open loop" organization, in which a cerebellar functional region communicates with cortical areas serving a different function.

In the human, diffusion tensor imaging (DTI; see Figure 2–7) has revealed that the densest of the corticopontine projections arise from the frontal lobe (Figure 13–17), which includes the primary motor cortex (area 4), the premotor areas (area 6) (see Figure 10–8), and the prefrontal association cortex. Additional projections also arise from association cortex in the parietal, occipital, and temporal lobes and from parts of the limbic cortical areas (which play important roles in emotions; see Chapter 16). Also using DTI, the topographic organization of the axons in the human basis pedunculi can be elucidated. Surprisingly, the largest region of the basis pedunculi contains descending axons from nonmotor areas (Figure 13–17). This amplifies what was discussed earlier, that the nonmotor functions of the cerebellum are likely to be very important.

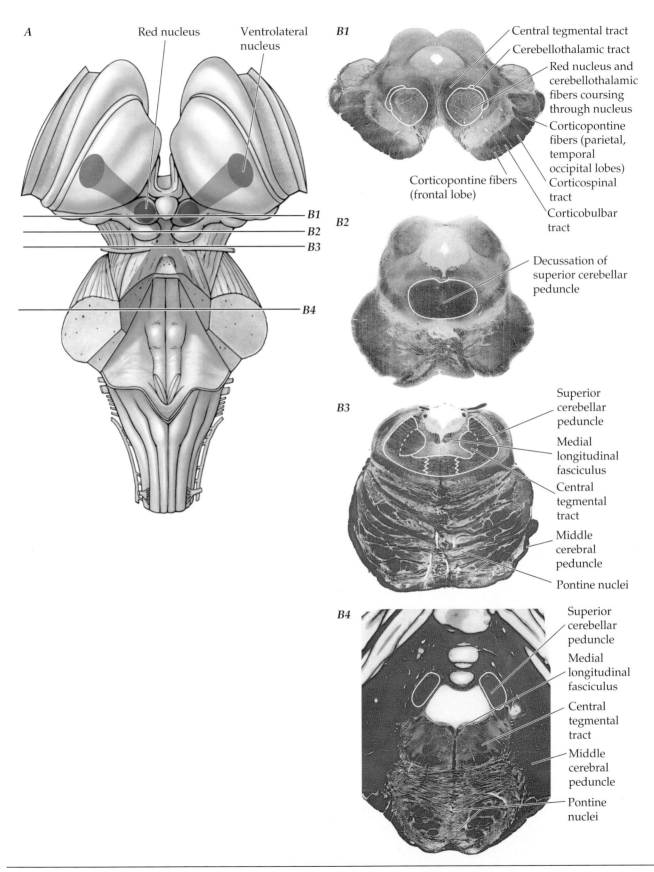

FIGURE 13–15 The superior cerebellar peduncle is the principal output path of the cerebellum. **A.** Location of the superior cerebellar peduncle and associated axons from the cerebellum to the thalamus (pale red shading) in relation to the red nucleus and ventrolateral nucleus of the thalamus. **B.** Transverse myelin-stained sections through the rostral midbrain (**B1**), caudal midbrain (**B2**), pons-midbrain junction (isthmus, **B3**), and rostral pons (**B4**).

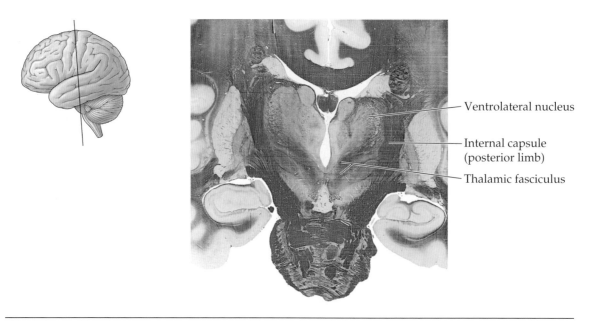

FIGURE 13–16 Myelin-stained coronal section through the ventrolateral nucleus. The inset shows the plane of section.

Ventrolateral nucleus

Internal capsule (posterior limb)

Thalamic fasciculus

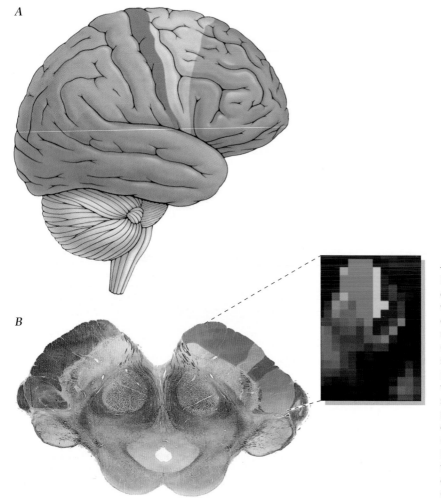

A

B

FIGURE 13–17 The corticopontine projection originates from most areas of the cerebral cortex, whereas the corticospinal projection originates only from the premotor (yellow), primary motor (dark gray-blue), and somatic sensory (light gray-blue) cortical areas (*A*). Part *B* shows schematically the locations of the descending projections in the basis pedunculi from the various cortical areas. The inset in *B* shows the somatotopic organization of the corticopontine projection in the basis pedunclui based on diffusion tensor imaging (DTI) data in humans. (From Ramnani N, Behrens TE, Johansen-Berg H, et al. The evolution of prefrontal inputs to the cortico-pontine system: diffusion imaging evidence from Macaque monkeys and humans. *Cereb Cortex.* 2006;16[6]:811-818.)

Cerebellar Anatomy

The cerebellar cortex overlies the white matter (Figures 13–2 and 13–13). The cerebellar cortex contains numerous *folia,* which are grouped into three *lobes* (Figures 13–2 and 13–3): the *anterior lobe,* the *posterior lobe,* and the *flocculonodular lobe.* Embedded within the white matter of the cerebellum are four bilaterally paired deep nuclei, from medial to lateral (Figures 13–2 and 13–3): the *fastigial nucleus,* the *globose nucleus,* the *emboliform nucleus,* and the *dentate nucleus.* The globose and emboliform nuclei are collectively termed the *interposed nuclei.* The cerebellar cortex consists of three cell layers, from the cerebellar surface to the white matter (Figure 13–13): *molecular, Purkinje,* and *granular layers.* Five neuron classes are found in the cerebellar cortex (Figures 13–4 and 13–14; Table 13–1): (1) *Purkinje neurons* (Figures 13–4, 13–13, and 13–14), the *projection neurons* of the cerebellum—which are *inhibitory;* (2) *granule neurons,* the only *excitatory interneurons* in the cerebellum; and the (3) *basket,* (4) *stellate,* and (5) *Golgi neurons*—the three *inhibitory interneurons.*

Cerebellar Circuits

Two principal classes of afferent fibers reach the cerebellum to give rise to the two main circuits: *climbing fibers* (Figures 13–4 and 13–14), which are the axons of neurons of the *inferior olivary nuclei* (Figure 13–11B), and *mossy fibers,* which originate from numerous sources, including the *pontine nuclei* (Figure 13–15B4), *reticular formation nuclei, vestibular nuclei* (Figure 13–11), and *spinal cord* (Figure 13–11C). Most climbing and mossy fiber inputs are directed to both the deep cerebellar nuclei and the cerebellar cortex (Figure 13–4). The climbing fibers make monosynaptic connections with the Purkinje neurons; the mossy fibers synapse on granule neurons, which in turn synapse on Purkinje neurons via their *parallel fibers.* The Purkinje neurons project from the cerebellar cortex to the deep nuclei (Figure 13–12) and the vestibular nuclei (Figure 13–11).

Cerebellar Functional Divisions

The cerebellum is divided into three functional regions (Figures 13–2 and 13–5): the spinocerebellum, the cerebrocerebellum, and the vestibulocerebellum. Unilateral cerebellar damage produces ipsilateral limb motor signs due to decussation of cerebellar output pathways and decussation of the lateral motor pathways (Figure 13–10).

The *spinocerebellum* (Figures 13–6 and 13–7), which is important in posture and limb movement, is subdivided into two cortical regions that also have functional counterparts: The medial *vermis* subserves control of *axial and girdle muscles,* and the *intermediate hemisphere* controls *limb muscles.* The principal inputs to the spinocerebellum originate from the spinal cord. Somatic sensory information from the leg and lower trunk is transmitted to the cerebellum by the *dorsal spinocerebellar tract* (Figure 13–6A), via *Clarke's nucleus,* and from the upper trunk, arm, and neck, by the *cuneocerebellar tract,* via the *accessory cuneate nucleus* (Figure 13–11B). Other pathways convey internal feedback signals. Purkinje neurons of the vermis project to the *fastigial nucleus* (Figures 13–7 and 13–12), which influences *medial descending pathways:* the reticulospinal, vestibulospinal, and ventral corticospinal tracts. The projection to the lower brain stem is via the *inferior cerebellar peduncle* (Figure 13–11B), and the thalamic projection is via the *superior cerebellar peduncle* (Figure 13–15). The *intermediate hemisphere* projects to the interposed nuclei (Figure 13–12), which in turn influence *lateral descending pathways:* the rubrospinal and lateral corticospinal tracts. All projections from the spinocerebellum course through the superior cerebellar peduncle.

The *cerebrocerebellum* (Figure 13–8) plays a role in planning movements; its cortical component is the *lateral hemisphere.* The cerebral cortex projects to the *pontine nuclei* (Figure 13–12), which provide the main input to the cerebrocerebellum. Purkinje neurons of this functional division project to the *dentate nucleus* (Figure 13–12). From there, dentate neurons project to the contralateral *parvocellular red nucleus* (Figure 13–15B1) and the *ventrolateral nucleus* of the thalamus (Figures 13–10 and 13–16), both via the *superior cerebellar peduncle.* The principal projections of the ventrolateral nucleus are to the *primary motor cortex (area 4)* and the *premotor cortex (lateral area 6)* (see Figure 10–7). The dentate nucleus also projects, via the thalamus, to the prefrontal and parietal association cortex to mediate nonmotor functions.

The *vestibulocerebellum* (Figures 13–5 and 13–9) is important in eye and head movement control; the cortical component corresponds anatomically to the *flocculonodular lobe.* It receives input from the *vestibular nuclei* and *primary vestibular afferents* and projects back to the vestibular nuclei via the *inferior cerebellar peduncle* (Figure 13–11B).

Selected Readings

Lisberger S, Thach T. The cerebellum. In: Kandel ER, Schwartz JH, Jessell TM, Siegelbaum SA, Hudspeth AJ, eds. *Principles of Neural Science*. 5th ed. New York, NY: McGraw-Hill; in press.

Patten J. *Neurological Differential Diagnosis*. 2nd ed. London: Springer-Verlag; 1996:448.

References

Angevine JB Jr., Mancall EL, Yakovlev PI. *The Human Cerebellum: An Atlas of Gross Topography in Serial Sections*. Boston, MA: Little Brown; 1961.

Apps R, Garwicz M. Anatomical and physiological foundations of cerebellar information processing. *Nat Rev Neurosci*. 2005;6(4):297-311.

Apps R, Hawkes R. Cerebellar cortical organization: a one-map hypothesis. *Nat Rev Neurosci*. 2009;10(9):670-681.

Bostan AC, Dum RP, Strick PL. The basal ganglia communicate with the cerebellum. *Proc Natl Acad Sci USA*. 2010;107(18):8452-8456.

Dean P, Porrill J, Ekerot CF, Jorntell H. The cerebellar microcircuit as an adaptive filter: experimental and computational evidence. *Nat Rev Neurosci*. 2010;11(1):30-43.

Dietrichs E, Walberg F. Cerebellar nuclear afferents: where do they originate? *Anat Embryol*. 1987;177:165-172.

Eccles JC, Ito M, Szentágothai J. *The Cerebellum as a Neuronal Machine*. Berlin, Germany: Springer-Verlag; 1967.

Gibson AR, Robinson FR, Alam J, Houk JC. Somatotopic alignment between climbing fiber input and nuclear output of the cat intermediate cerebellum. *J Comp Neurol*. 1987;260:362-377.

Glower DM, West RA, Lynch JC, Strick PL. The inferior parietal lobule is the target of output from the superior colliculus, hippocampus, and cerebellum. *J Neurosci*. 2001;21:6283-6291.

Gowen E, Miall RC. The cerebellum and motor dysfunction in neuropsychiatric disorders. *Cerebellum*. 2007;6(3):268-279.

Habas C, Cabanis EA. Cortical projections to the human red nucleus: a diffusion tensor tractography study with a 1.5-T MRI machine. *Neuroradiology*. 2006;48(10):755-762.

Habas C, Kamdar N, Nguyen D, et al. Distinct cerebellar contributions to intrinsic connectivity networks. *J Neurosci*. 2009;29(26):8586-8594.

Holmes GP. The cerebellum of man. *Brain*. 1939;62(1):1-30.

Hoover JE, Strick PL. The organization of cerebellar and basal ganglia outputs to primary motor cortex as revealed by retrograde transneuronal transport of herpes simplex virus type 1. *J Neurosci*. 1999;19:1446-1463.

Horn KM, Pong M, Gibson AR. Functional relations of cerebellar modules of the cat. *J Neurosci*. 2010;30(28):9411-9423.

Hoshi E, Tremblay L, Feger J, Carras PL, Strick PL. The cerebellum communicates with the basal ganglia. *Nat Neurosci*. 2005;8(11):1491-1493.

Jueptner M, Weiller C. A review of differences between basal ganglia and cerebellar control of movements as revealed by functional imaging studies. *Brain*. 1998;121:1437-1449.

Kim SS-G, Ugurbil K, Strick PL. Activation of cerebellar output nucleus during cognitive processing. *Science*. 1994;265:949-951.

Leiner HC, Leiner AL, Dow RS. Cognitive and language functions of the human cerebellum. *Trends Neurosci*. 1993;16:444-447.

Levisohn L, Cronin-Golomb A, Schmahmann JD. Neuropsychological consequences of cerebellar tumour resection in children: cerebellar cognitive affective syndrome in a paediatric population. *Brain*. 2000;123:1041-1050.

Massion J. Red nucleus: past and future. *Behav Brain Res*. 1988;28:l-8.

Matsushita M, Hosoya Y, Ikeda M. Anatomical organization of the spinocerebellar system in the cat, as studied by retrograde transport of horseradish peroxidase. *J Comp Neurol*. 1979;184:81-106.

Middleton FA, Strick PL. Anatomical evidence for cerebellar and basal ganglia involvement in higher cognitive function. *Science*. 1994;266:458-461.

Middleton FA, Strick PL. Dentate output channels: motor and cognitive components. *Prog Brain Res*. 1997;114:553-566.

Nakano K, Takimoto T, Kayahara T, Takeuchi Y, Kobayashi Y. Distribution of cerebellothalamic neurons projecting to the ventral nuclei of the thalamus: an HRP study in the cat. *J Comp Neurol*. 1980;194:427-439.

Ramnani N, Behrens TE, Johansen-Berg H, et al. The evolution of prefrontal inputs to the cortico-pontine system: diffusion imaging evidence from Macaque monkeys and humans. *Cereb Cortex*. 2006;16(6):811-818.

Schell GR, Strick PL. The origin of thalamic inputs to the arcuate premotor and supplementary motor areas. *J Neurosci*. 1984;4:539-560.

Schmahmann JD. An emerging concept: the cerebellar contribution to higher function. *Arch Neurol*. 1991;48:1178-1187.

Schmahmann JD. From movement to thought: anatomic substrates of the cerebellar contribution to cognitive processing. *Human Brain Mapping*. 1996;4:174-198.

Schmahmann JD, Doyon J, McDonald D, et al. Three-dimensional MRI atlas of the human cerebellum in proportional stereotaxic space. *Neuroimage*. 1999;10(3 Pt 1):233-260.

Schmahmann JD, Pandya DN. Course of the fiber pathways to pons from parasensory association areas in the rhesus monkey. *J Comp Neurol*. 1992;326:159-179.

Schmahmann JD, Pandya DN. The cerebrocerebellar system. *Int Rev Neurobiol.* 1997;41:31-60.

Schmahmann JD, Sherman JC. The cerebellar cognitive affective syndrome. *Brain.* 1998;121:561-579.

Schmahmann JD, Weilburg JB, Sherman JC. The neuropsychiatry of the cerebellum: insights from the clinic. *Cerebellum.* 2007;6(3):254-267.

Stoodley CJ, Schmahmann JD. Evidence for topographic organization in the cerebellum of motor control versus cognitive and affective processing. *Cortex.* 2010;46(7): 831-844.

Strick PL, Dum RP, Fiez JA. Cerebellum and nonmotor function. *Annu Rev Neurosci.* 2009;32:413-434.

Tan J, Simpson JI, Voogd J. Anatomical compartments in the white matter of the rabbit flocculus. *J Comp Neurol.* 1995;356(1):1-22.

Taroni F, DiDonato S. Pathways to motor incoordination: the inherited ataxias. *Nat Rev Neurosci.* 2004;5(8):641-655.

Thach WT, Goodkin HP, Keating JG. The cerebellum and the adaptive coordination of movement. *Annu Rev Neurosci.* 1992;15:403-442.

Turner BM, Paradiso S, Marvel CL, et al. The cerebellum and emotional experience. *Neuropsychologia.* 2007;45(6): 1331-1341.

Voogd J. Cerebellum and precerebellar nuclei. In: Paxinos G, Mai JK, eds. *The Human Nervous System.* London: Elsevier; 2004:322-392.

Voogd J, Gerrits NM, Ruigrok TJ. Organization of the vestibulocerebellum. *Ann N Y Acad Sci.* 1996;781:553-579.

Voogd J, Glickstein M. The anatomy of the cerebellum. *TINS.* 1998;21(9):370-375.

Wylie DR, De Zeeuw CI, DiGiorgi PL, Simpson JI. Projections of individual Purkinje cells of identified zones in the ventral nodulus to the vestibular and cerebellar nuclei in the rabbit. *J Comp Neurol.* 1994;349(3):448-463.

Study Questions

1. A person has a tumor in the posterior fossa, on the dorsal surface of the cerebellum. Which of the following statements best describes the location of the tumor?
   A. Between the cerebellum and the occipital lobe
   B. Between the cerebellum and medulla
   C. Between the cerebellum and temporal lobe
   D. Between the cerebellum and tentorium

2. From lateral to medial, the anterior and posterior lobes of the cerebellar cortex connect with the deep nuclei in the following order:
   A. dentate, interposed, fastigial
   B. fastigial, interposed, dentate
   C. dentate, fastigial, vestibular
   D. fastigial, interposed, dentate, vestibular

3. Which of the following is the principal synaptic target of Purkinje cells of the nodulus?
   A. Dentate nuclei
   B. Interposed nuclei
   C. Fastigial nuclei
   D. Vestibular nuclei

4. A person had a unilateral cerebellar stroke. Which of the following best explains the laterality (ie, side of body on which ataxia presents) of ataxia during reaching?
   A. Contralateral, because cerebellar output is not decussated and the descending motor pathways are crossed
   B. Ipsilateral, because cerebellar output decussates and the descending pathways cross
   C. Bilateral, because the cerebellar output decussates and the descending pathways cross
   D. Bilateral, because the descending pathways are bilateral

5. Which of the following circuits traces the connection, via the cerebellum, from the right posterior parietal cortex to the spinal cord?
   A. Triple crossed: right posterior parietal cortex→right pons→left cerebellum→right thalamus→right motor cortex→left spinal cord
   B. Double crossed: right posterior parietal cortex→right pons→right cerebellum→left thalamus→left motor cortex→right spinal cord
   C. Triple crossed: right posterior parietal cortex→left pons→right cerebellum→right thalamus→right motor cortex→left spinal cord
   D. Double crossed: right posterior parietal cortex→left pons→left cerebellum→left thalamus→left motor cortex→right spinal cord

6. The principal output nuclei of the vestibulocerebellum are
   A. dentate nuclei
   B. interposed nuclei
   C. fastigial nuclei
   D. vestibular nuclei

7. It is discovered at autopsy that a person with Friedreich ataxia, a progressive spinocerebellar ataxia, had extensive degeneration of Clarke's nucleus. This produced denegation of which of the following pathways?
   A. Cuneocerebellar tract
   B. Dorsal spinocerebellar tract
   C. Ventral spinocerebellar tract
   D. Spinothalamic tract

8. A person has olivopontocerebellar atrophy, with extensive degeneration of the inferior olivary nucleus and the pontine nuclei, as well as parts of the cerebellum. Which of the following connections is likely to be lost in this person?
   A. Between mossy fibers and Purkinje cells
   B. Between mossy fibers and basket cells
   C. Between climbing fibers and Purkinje cells
   D. Between climbing fibers and granule cells

9. A person has a rare (fictitious, for the purpose of questioning) cerebellar degenerative disorder producing loss of connections from the dentate nucleus to the red nucleus. Which of the following would best describe the impact that this condition has on motor control?
   A. Loss of the principal input to rubrospinal neurons in the magnocellular red nucleus
   B. Loss of the principal input to rubro-olivary neurons in the parvocellular red nucleus
   C. Loss of mossy fibers from the red nucleus to the cerebellum
   D. Loss of climbing fibers from the red nucleus to the cerebellum

10. The cerebellum is thought to be a site of dysfunction in several neuropsychiatric diseases, such as schizophrenia and autism. Which of the following statements best describes how information from frontal and temporal lobe areas involved in cognition and emotion can be influenced by cerebellar processing?
    A. Frontotemporal association areas must transmit information first to premotor and motor areas, which project to the pontine nuclei and then the cerebellum.
    B. Frontotemporal association areas must transmit information first to the posterior parietal association cortex, which projects to the pontine nuclei and then the cerebellum.
    C. Frontotemporal association areas transmit information directly to the pontine nuclei and then the cerebellum.
    D. Frontotemporal association areas project directly to the cerebellar cortex as mossy fibers.

Chapter 14

The Basal Ganglia

CLINICAL CASE | Hemiballism

A 65-year-old man with a history of hypertension suddenly developed involuntary, violent, ballistic movements of his right arm and leg. The movements primarily involved flexion and rotation of the proximal parts of the limbs. MRI showed a small hemorrhagic lesion in the subthalamic nucleus on the left side (Figure 14–1A).

Answer the following questions based on your reading of this chapter and relevant sections from other chapters.

1. **Explain why the aberrant ballistic movements are on the contralateral side.**

2. **Occlusion of which cerebral artery and branch could produce a lesion such as the one shown in Figure 14–1?**

Key neurological signs and corresponding damaged brain structures

Subthalamic nucleus circuitry

The subthalamic nucleus is part of the indirect pathway. It receives GABA-ergic inputs from the external segment of the globus pallidus and projects to the internal segment of the globus pallidus. From there, information is directed to the motor thalamus, and then the motor cortex, which controls movements contralaterally, via the corticospinal tract. Additionally, the subthalamic nucleus receives dense glutamatergic inputs from the motor cortex, primarily on the ipsilateral side. Whereas the cortical-basal ganglia circuitry is ipsilateral, it exerts its movement control influence on the contralateral side because the corticospinal tract is predominantly crossed. The nucleus is somatotopically organized; the lesion shown in Figure 14–1A is sufficiently large to affect both its arm and leg areas of the small nucleus.

Because the subthalamic nucleus normally activates an inhibitory structure—the internal segment of the globus pallidus—when it is lesioned it is reasoned that this inhibition is less. Hemiballism is thus thought to be produced by disinhibition; it is a release phenomenon. It

—Continued next page

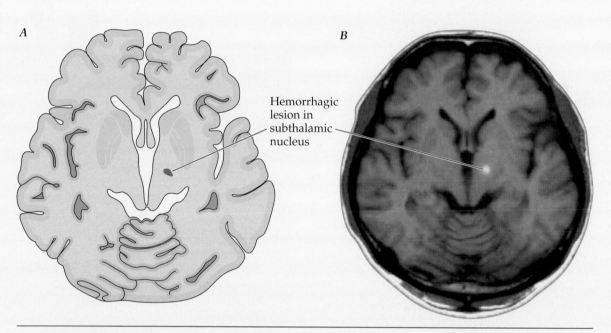

A

B

Hemorrhagic
lesion in
subthalamic
nucleus

FIGURE 14–1 Hemiballism. *A.* Schematic drawing in the plane of the MRI showing the location of the subthalamic nucleus and lesion. *B.* MRI from a person with a small hemorrhagic lesion of the left subthalamic nucleus. (Reproduced with permission from Nishioka H, Taguchi T, Nanri K, Ikeda Y. Transient hemiballism caused by a small lesion of the subthalamic nucleus. *J Clin Neurosci.* 2008;15:1416-1418.)

is not known why this is reflected in the violent proximal movements, so much a signature of subthalamic nucleus damage.

The largest portion of the subthalamic nucleus is devoted to limb and trunk motor functions. In addition, smaller regions of the nucleus are more important for eye movement control, emotional, and cognitive functions. These regions are parts of the ocular motor, limbic, and cognitive loops of the basal ganglia.

References

Brust JCM. *The Practice of Neural Science.* New York, NY: McGraw-Hill; 2000.

Kitajima M, Korogi Y, Kakeda S, et al. Human subthalamic nucleus: evaluation with high-resolution MR imaging at 3.0 T. *Neuroradiology.* 2008;50(8):675-681.

Nishioka H, Taguchi T, Nanri K, Ikeda Y. Transient hemiballism caused by a small lesion of the subthalamic nucleus. *J Clin Neurosci.* 2008;15(12):1416-1418.

Hamani C, Saint-Cry JA, Fraser J, Kaplitt M, Lozano A. The subthalamic nucleus in the context of movement disorders. *Brain.* 2004;127:4-20.

The basal ganglia are a collection of subcortical nuclei that have captured the fascination of clinicians and scientists for well over a century because of the remarkable range of behavioral dysfunction associated with basal ganglia disease. Movement control deficits are among the key signs, ranging from the paucity and slowing of movement in Parkinson disease and the writhing movements of Huntington disease to the bizarre tics of Tourette syndrome and distorted postures of dystonia. Unmistakingly, these clinical findings indicate that one important set of basal ganglia functions is regulating our motor actions. How do the basal ganglia fit into an overall view of the organization of the motor systems? Unlike the motor cortex and several brain stem nuclei, which have direct connections with the spinal cord and motor neurons, the basal ganglia influence movements by acting on the descending pathways; this is similar to the cerebellum.

In addition to producing movement control deficits, basal ganglia disease can also impair intellectual capacity and affect, pointing to important roles in cognition and emotion. Dementia is an early disabling consequence of Huntington disease and can be present in patients with advanced stages of Parkinson disease. The basal ganglia play important roles in aspects of drug addiction and psychiatric disease.

Although the basal ganglia continue to be among the least understood of all brain structures, their mysteries are now yielding to modern neurobiological techniques for elucidating neurochemistry and connections. For example, the basal ganglia contain virtually all of the major neuroactive agents that have been discovered in the central nervous system. Although the reason for this biochemical diversity remains elusive, such knowledge can be used to treat some forms of basal ganglia disease. Indeed, the discovery that the brains of patients with

Parkinson disease are deficient in dopamine quickly led to the development of drug replacement therapy. Knowledge about connections of the basal ganglia with the rest of the brain has led to a major revision of the traditional views of basal ganglia organization and function. Discoveries about basal ganglia circuitry and pathways have even led to therapeutic neurosurgical and neurophysiological procedures.

This chapter first considers the constituents of the basal ganglia and their three-dimensional shapes, partly from a developmental context. Next, their functional organization is surveyed, emphasizing the distinctive roles of the basal ganglia in movement control, cognition, and emotions. (Chapter 16 revisits the basal ganglia in relation to emotions and psychiatric disease.) Finally, this chapter examines the regional anatomy of the basal ganglia using a series of myelin-stained sections and MRI slices through the cerebral hemispheres and brain stem.

Organization and Development of the Basal Ganglia

Separate Components of the Basal Ganglia Process Incoming Information and Mediate the Output

The many components of the basal ganglia are best learned, in a general way, from the outset; then their functional and clinical anatomy can be mastered. As we will focus on later in the context of their connections, the components of the basal ganglia can be divided into three categories: input, output, and intrinsic nuclei (Table 14–1). The **input nuclei** receive afferent connections from brain regions other than the basal ganglia, in particular the cerebral cortex, and in turn project to the intrinsic and output nuclei. There are three input nuclei, merged into a single structure termed the **striatum** (Figure 14–2): (1) the caudate nucleus, (2) the putamen, and (3) the nucleus accumbens. The functions of the striatum do not correspond precisely to its component anatomical parts. Most of the **caudate nucleus** participates in eye movement control and cognition, whereas the **putamen** participates mostly in control of limb and trunk movements. Emotions are mediated by the **nucleus accumbens**, together with adjoining parts of the caudate nucleus and putamen; the emotional striatum is commonly termed the ventral striatum. Given that the striatum is really a composite of three nuclei, it is not surprising that it has a complex shape.

The **output nuclei** project to regions of the diencephalon and brain stem that are not part of the basal ganglia. There are three nuclei on the output side of the basal ganglia (Table 14–1; Figure 14–2B1, B2): the **internal segment of the globus pallidus,** associated mostly with the putamen and limb and trunk control; the **substantia nigra pars reticulata,** primarily involved in cognition and eye movements along with the caudate nucleus, and a portion of the **ventral pallidum,** important for emotions with the ventral striatum. These nuclei are located deep within the base of the brain; they are shown schematically in Figure 14–2 in relation to a transparent view of the striatum.

The **intrinsic nuclei** are also located deep within the base of the brain; their connections are largely restricted to the basal ganglia (Table 14–1; Figure 14–2). The basal ganglia have five intrinsic nuclei: the **external segment of the globus pallidus,** a portion of the **ventral pallidum** (separate from the output part), the **subthalamic nucleus,** the **substantia nigra pars compacta,** and the **ventral tegmental area** (Figure 14–2). Their connections are closely related to the input and output nuclei.

The Complex Shapes and Fractionation of Basal Ganglia Components Are Understood by How the Basal Ganglia Develop

Learning the numerous components and subdivisions of the basal ganglia is a challenge. Taking a developmental perspective helps to understand two key features of the anatomy of the basal ganglia: the complex three-dimensional shape and fractionation of the components of the basal ganglia into subdivisions. The caudate nucleus develops a **C-shape,** largely as a consequence of cerebral cortex development. As the cortex expands caudally and inferiorly, forming the occipital and temporal lobes (Figure 14–3A), underlying structures—including the caudate nucleus and lateral ventricle—follow. This expansion and change in shape are produced by the birth and migration of cells along predetermined axes. This imparts a distinctive shape of the caudate nucleus in relation to the shapes of the other two striatal components. The C-shape of the caudate nucleus results in three components: head, body, and tail (Figure 14–3C).

A second developmental process contributes to formation of some of the basal ganglia subdivisions. Development of

Table **14–1** **Components of the Basal Ganglia**

Input nuclei (striatum)[1]	1. Caudate nucleus
	2. Putamen
	3. Nucleus accumbens
Output nuclei	1. Globus pallidus—internal segment[2]
	2. Ventral pallidum—output part
	3. Substantia nigra pars reticulata
Intrinsic nuclei	1. Globus pallidus—external segment
	2. Ventral pallidum—intrinsic part
	3. Subthalamic nucleus
	4. Substantia nigra pars compacta
	5. Ventral tegmental area

[1]The striatum is also termed the neostriatum.

[2]The putamen and internal and external segments of the globus pallidus together are also termed the lenticular nucleus because their form is similar to that of a lens.

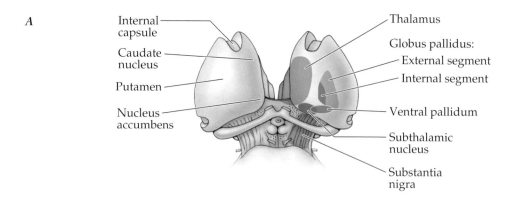

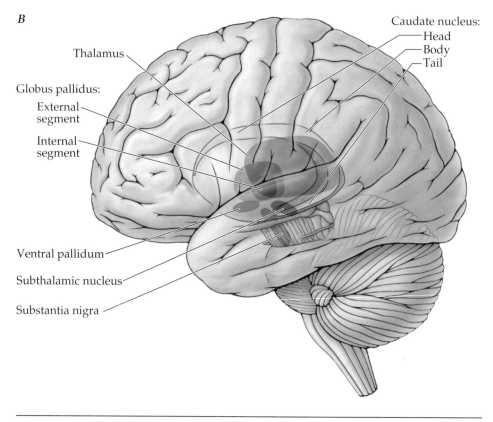

FIGURE 14–2 Nuclei of the basal ganglia are shown in relation to the thalamus and internal capsule. **A.** Frontal view. **B.** Lateral view.

axon projection to and from the cerebral cortex in the **internal capsule** divides many basal ganglia components into separate nuclei, thereby increasing the complexity of the nomenclature. Figure 14–3B, schematic coronal sections through the developing forebrain, shows a single developing striatum (Figure 14–3B1) and separation of the caudate nucleus (head and body) and the putamen by the internal capsule. Three developing axon projections within the internal capsule are key, those from (1) the thalamus to the cortex (ie, to layer 4); (2) the cortex (layer 6) back to the thalamus; and (3) the cortex (layer 5) to the striatum, brain stem, and spinal cord. For the striatum, these internal capsule axons incompletely divide

the striatum into the three components, leaving behind **cell bridges** (Figure 14–3C). Throughout its entire course, the caudate nucleus is medial to the internal capsule, and the putamen, lateral. Figure 14–4A shows the course of the corticospinal tract in the internal capsule; its path can be followed between the head of the caudate and the putamen. The nucleus accumbens is largely that portion of the striatum rostral and inferior to the anterior limb of the internal capsule. The tail of the caudate nucleus is separated from the putamen by additional projection fibers.

The internal capsule also separates the internal segment of the globus pallidus and the substantia nigra pars reticulata,

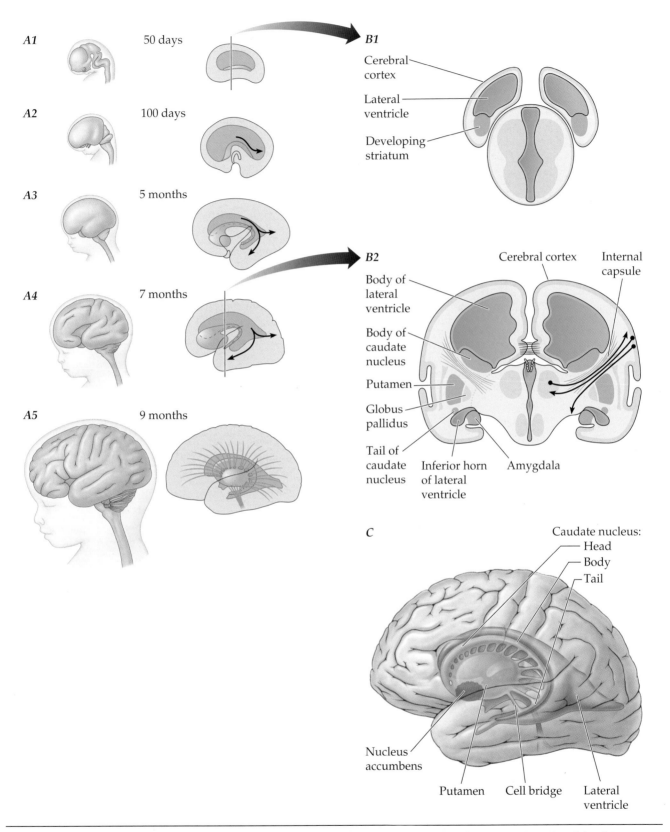

FIGURE 14–3 Development of the basal ganglia. **A.** Lateral views of the developing brain and head at different prenatal ages (**A1–A4**) and term. Schematic diagrams of the cerebral hemisphere, lateral ventricle, and striatum accompany each age. The fibers in **A5** (right) are of the internal capsule. **B.** Brain sections through 50-day embryo (**B1**) and 7-month embryo (**B2**). Schematic ascending and descending axons in the internal capsule are shown in **B2**. **C.** The striatum in relation to the ventricular system in the mature brain. The striatum consists of the caudate nucleus, putamen, and nucleus accumbens. Only the caudate nucleus has a C-shape, which is similar to that of the lateral ventricle. The nucleus accumbens is located ventromedially primarily on the medial striatal surface.

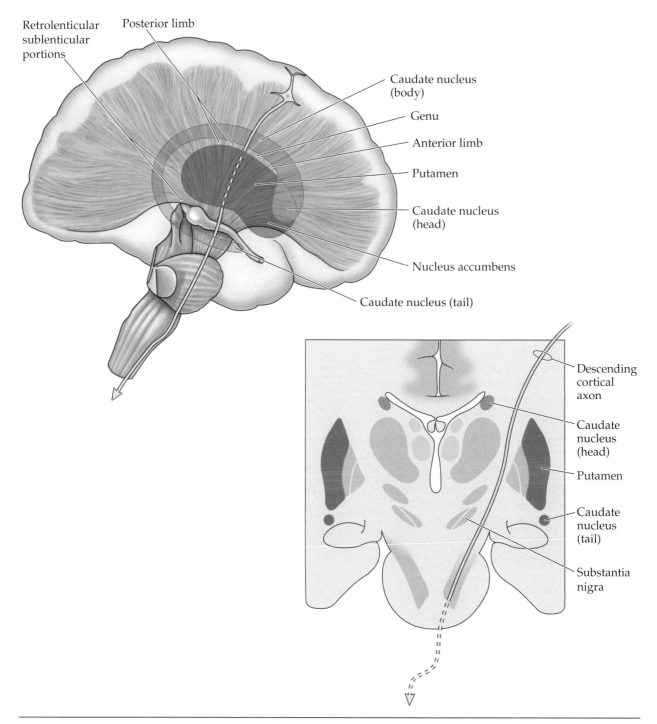

FIGURE 14–4 Internal capsule. **A.** Lateral view showing striatum and corticospinal tract axon. **B.** Drawing of coronal slice through the posterior limb of the internal capsule showing path of a descending cortical axon.

similar to the striatal cell bridges, shown in maturity in Figure 14–3. In humans, cells of the substantia nigra pars reticulata and internal segment of the globus pallidus are scattered between each other within the internal capsule (see Figure 14–15). In addition to being part of the same structure but separated by the internal capsule, the morphology, neurotransmitter content, and connections of neurons in the internal segment of the globus pallidus and the substantia nigra pars reticulata are similar.

Although not understood from a simple developmental perspective, the anterior commissure separates the external segment of the globus pallidus from the ventral pallidum. However, many neurons in the ventral pallidum have connections and a neurochemistry similar to the globus pallidus external segment—like that of an intrinsic nucleus—and others, especially in the more caudal ventral pallidum, have properties like the internal segment of the globus pallidus, an output nucleus.

Functional Anatomy of the Basal Ganglia

Direct and Indirect Pathways Form Common Circuits Throughout All Functional Divisions of the Basal Ganglia

The general organization of the basal ganglia from input to output is shown in Figure 14–5. Like the cerebellum, a basic circuit describes the basal ganglia, irrespective of motor, cognitive, or emotional function. As described, the basal ganglia are divided into input, output, and intrinsic nuclei (Figure 14–5A). Beginning with all areas of the cerebral cortex, information passes through the input nuclei and then the output nuclei. Connections with the thalamus target several nuclei that, in turn, project to different areas of the frontal lobe. These differential projections confer the distinctive functions of the basal ganglia (discussed below). Connections with the brain stem motor control centers target the **pedunculopontine nucleus,** important in gait control, and the **superior colliculus,** for saccadic eye movements. As an example of the flow of information through the basal ganglia, follow the path in Figure 14–5B, from the frontal lobe, to the putamen, globus pallidus internal segment, thalamus, and back to the cerebral cortex (to primary motor cortex).

There are functionally and clinically important connections with the intrinsic nuclei. The external segment of the globus pallidus and the subthalamic nucleus are part of a basal ganglia circuit that receives input from other basal ganglia nuclei and in turn projects back (Figure 14–5A). The **substantia nigra pars compacta** and the **ventral tegmental area** contain dopaminergic neurons that project to the striatum, as well as to portions of the cortex (Figure 14–5A). Dopamine has a neuromodulatory action on striatal neurons. There are many different dopamine receptor subtypes and, depending on the particular subtype present on the postsynaptic neuron, dopamine either depolarizes or hyperpolarizes striatal neurons.

The output of the basal ganglia depends on two complementary pathways

Whereas the basal ganglia have a daunting complexity, there is a logic to the connections that helps explain their overall actions. A pair of complementary circuits—termed the direct and indirect pathways—have opposing actions on their downstream structures. The connections from the striatum to the output nuclei and then to the thalamus and brain stem, described above, comprise the **direct path** (Figure 14–5A, B),

which promotes the actions of the basal ganglia. By contrast, connections from the striatum to three intrinsic nuclei—the external segment of the globus pallidus, part of the ventral pallidum, and the subthalamic nucleus—comprise the **indirect path** (Figure 14–5A, B inset), which inhibits the actions of the basal ganglia. In Figure 14–5B (inset) follow the path from the striatum, globus pallidus external segment, subthalamic nucleus, and then globus pallidus internal segment. For the components of the basal ganglia that control limb and trunk movements, eye movements, and facial muscles, the direct path enables these actions and the indirect path puts the brakes on. Box 14–1 shows schematically how neuronal activity changes in the direct and indirect paths as information from the cortex is processed from one structure to the next. Aberrant direct path functions in many movement disorders appear to drive excessive muscle tone, tics, and habitual behaviors, and aberrant indirect path functions produce debilitating akinesia, bradykinesia, and rigidity in Parkinson disease. It is thought that similar facilitatory and suppressive actions influence the nonmotor functions of the basal ganglia as well. We consider below how the complementary actions of the direct and indirect paths occur, in the context of the diversity of neurotransmitter actions in the basal ganglia.

Knowledge of Basal Ganglia Connections and Neurotransmitters Provides Insight Into Their Function in Health and Disease

Many neurotransmitters and **neuromodulatory** substances are present in the various basal ganglia nuclei (Figure 14–6). The excitatory neurotransmitter **glutamate** is used by corticostriatal neurons (the major input to the basal ganglia), thalamic neurons that project to the striatum, and the projection neurons of the subthalamic nucleus. Surprisingly, the major neurotransmitter of the basal ganglia is γ-aminobutyric acid, or **GABA,** which is **inhibitory.** In the striatum, the projection neurons, termed **medium spiny neurons** because they have abundant dendritic spines (see Figure 1–2), use GABA as their neurotransmitter. The axons of these neurons project to the two segments of the globus pallidus, the ventral pallidum, and the substantia nigra pars reticulata. Medium spiny neurons also contain neuropeptides, with two distinct neuron classes containing either **enkephalin** or **substance P** (and **dynorphin**). Enkephalin thus marks indirect path striatal neurons and substance P, direct path. When one understands that direct and indirect path neurons have a different neurochemistry, it is easier to appreciate that they can be differentially vulnerable to pathological processes. Projection neurons of the internal and external segments of the globus pallidus and the substantia nigra pars reticulata also contain GABA. Thus, the output of the basal ganglia, similar to that of the cerebellar cortex, is inhibitory. The significance of this common synaptic organization is not yet apparent.

Neurons in the substantia nigra pars compacta and the ventral tegmental area contain **dopamine.** The activity and

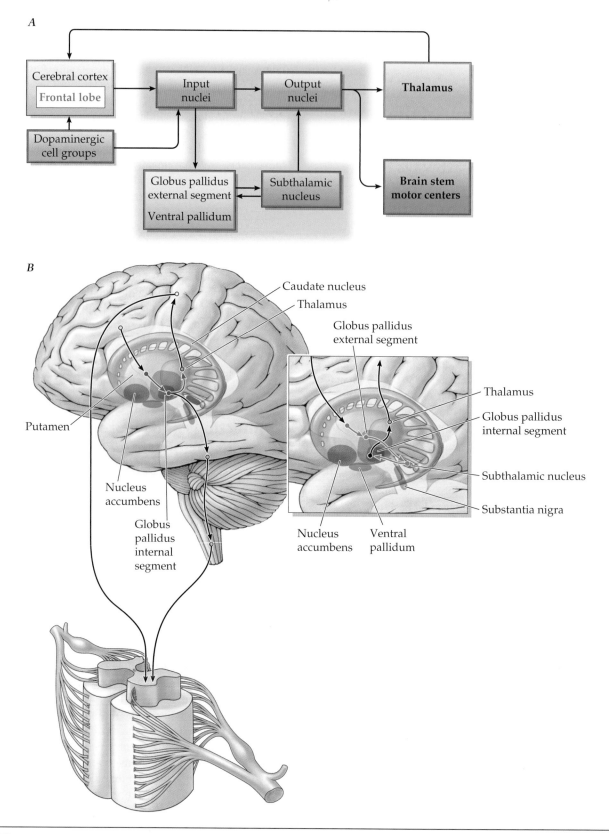

FIGURE 14–5 Direct and indirect paths of the basal ganglia. **A.** Block diagram. The input nuclei are the components of the striatum; they receive input from all cortical areas. The output nuclei are the globus pallidus internal segment, the substantia nigra pars reticulata, and part of the ventral pallidum. Blue shading is the direct path. Green shading shows the indirect path. Whereas the basal ganglia receive input from all cortical areas, the return path from the thalamus is directed only to the frontal lobe. Note, dopaminergic cell groups innervate both the cerebral cortex and the striatum. Connections to the brain stem are directed to the superior colliculus, for eye movement control, and the pedunculopontine nucleus, for gait control. **B.** Circuitry of the direct path. Follow the path from cortex: (1) back to cortex; and (2) to brain stem. Note how both paths eventually end in the spinal cord. Inset shows the indirect path that terminates in the internal globus pallidus. Motor pathways to the spinal cord are also shown.

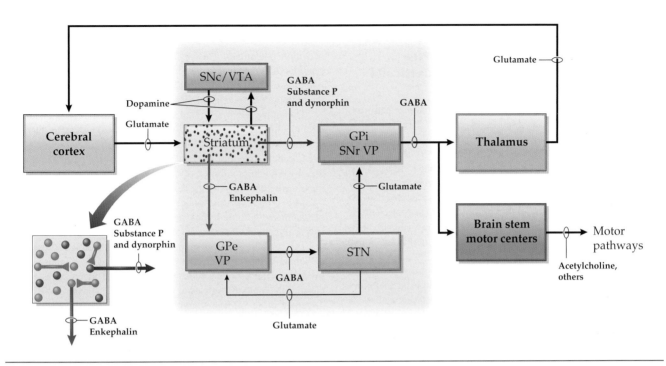

FIGURE 14–6 The neurotransmitters of the basal ganglia are shown in relation to the organization of basal ganglia circuits. Neurons in the striatum that contain GABA, substance P, and dynorphin (purple) give rise to the direct path, projecting to the internal segment of the globus pallidus. Neurons that contain GABA and enkephalin (green) give rise to the indirect path and project to the external segment of the globus pallidus. GABA, γ-aminobutyric acid; GPe, external segment of the globus pallidus; GPi, internal segment of the globus pallidus; SNc, substantia nigra pars compacta; SNr, substantia nigra pars reticulata; STN, subthalamic nucleus; VP, ventral pallidum; VTA, ventral tegmental area.

function of the postsynaptic targets of these nuclei, the striatum and portions of the frontal lobe, are under important regulation by dopamine. Dopamine can be excitatory or inhibitory depending on the balance of dopamine receptor subtypes present on the postsynaptic neuron's membrane. **Acetylcholine** is another common neurotransmitter in the basal ganglia; it is present in striatal interneurons. Striatal cholinergic interneurons play an important role in regulating diverse basal ganglia functions, including plasticity.

Parkinson disease is a hypokinetic movement disorder

In Parkinson disease, there is a major impairment in initiating movements, termed **akinesia,** and a reduction in the extent and speed of movements, called **bradykinesia** (see Figure 14–7C1). These are called **hypokinetic signs** because movements become impoverished. In addition, patients exhibit a resting **tremor,** and when an examiner moves their limbs, a characteristic stiffness or **rigidity** can be noted. The dopaminergic neurons in the substantia nigra pars compacta and the ventral tegmental area degenerate in Parkinson disease, and striatal dopamine is profoundly reduced. The term *substantia nigra* means black substance. This name derives from the presence of the black pigment **neuromelanin,** a polymer of the catecholamine precursor dihydroxy-phenylalanine (or dopa), which is contained in the neurons of the pars compacta. Not surprisingly, neuromelanin is not present in the substantia

nigra pars compacta of Parkinson patients. Dopaminergic neurons in other parts of the central nervous system are also destroyed in Parkinson disease. Dopamine loss in the basal ganglia, however, apparently produces the most debilitating neurological signs. Dopamine replacement therapy using a precursor to dopamine, **L-dopa,** leads to a dramatic improvement in the neurological signs of Parkinson disease.

Researchers have an important tool in the study of Parkinson disease. They discovered that a certain kind of synthetic heroin produces a permanent clinical syndrome in humans that is remarkably similar to Parkinson disease. This substance contains the neurotoxin MPTP (l-methyl-4-phenyl-1,2,3,6-tetrahydropyridine), which is a meperidine derivative that kills the dopaminergic neurons of the substantia nigra pars compacta (as well as other dopaminergic neurons in the central nervous system). When monkeys are given MPTP, they too develop parkinsonian signs, including akinesia, bradykinesia, rigidity, and tremor.

There are several hyperkinetic movement disorders

Huntington disease is a hyperkinetic disorder (see Figure 14–7C2). One **hyperkinetic sign** of this disorder is **chorea,** which is characterized by involuntary rapid and random movements of the limbs and trunk. Involuntary distal limb movements, such as writhing of the hand, or **athetosis,** may also occur. Patients with Huntington disease also develop

Box 14–1

Knowledge of the Intrinsic Circuitry of the Basal Ganglia Helps to Explain Hypokinetic and Hyperkinetic Signs

Knowledge of dysfunction in the direct and indirect pathways in the skeletomotor loop (Figures 14–5 to 14–7) is helping to explain the mechanisms of disordered movement control in basal ganglia disease and to develop more effective therapies. As discussed earlier, the direct path promotes movements, and the indirect path inhibits movements. Projection neurons of the putamen in the direct path synapse on neurons in the **internal segment of the globus pallidus,** which project to the ventrolateral and ventral anterior nuclei of the thalamus. This circuit contains two inhibitory neurons, in the putamen and globus pallidus. Thus, a brief period of cortical excitation of the putamen (see neural responses in boxes marked cerebral cortex and striatum; Figure 14–7A) is transformed into an inhibitory message (pause in neural activity) in the internal segment of the globus pallidus because striatal neurons are inhibitory. However, because the output of the internal segment of the globus pallidus is also inhibitory, the amount of inhibition of the thalamus from the internal segment of the globus pallidus is reduced. Inhibition of an inhibitory signal is termed **disinhibition;** functionally, this double negative is equivalent to excitation. The thalamic response shown is transiently released from inhibition and fires a burst of action potentials. In a motor behavior such as reaching for a glass of water, neurons in premotor areas, as well as corticospinal tract neurons in primary motor cortex, are thought to be excited by the actions of the direct path.

The indirect path has the opposite effect on the thalamus and cerebral cortex as the direct path. Putamen neurons of the indirect path, which are inhibitory because they contain GABA, project to the **external segment of the globus pallidus.** Excitation of the striatal neurons inhibits the external segment of the globus pallidus (pause in action potentials). Because the output of the external segment of the globus pallidus is inhibitory, indirect path neurons of the putamen disinhibit the subthalamic nucleus (burst

of action potentials). This disinhibition will excite the internal segment of the globus pallidus and substantia nigra pars reticulata (which are both inhibitory) and thereby increase the strength of the inhibitory output signal directed to the thalamus.

Dopamine excites striatal neurons of the direct path and inhibits striatal neurons of the indirect path. Despite these different actions on striatal neurons, the effect of dopamine on either path is to reduce the inhibitory output of the basal ganglia, thereby reducing inhibition of the thalamus. This effect promotes movement generation by the thalamocortical circuits.

The power of this model is that it helps to explain the mechanisms of some **hypokinetic** and **hyperkinetic signs** seen in basal ganglia disease. Dopamine is deficient in Parkinson disease, which produces hypokinetic signs. Reduced striatal dopamine in Parkinson disease would be expected to diminish the excitatory effects of the direct path on cortical motor areas and enhance the inhibitory effects of the indirect path (Figure 14–7C1). Together these effects would drastically reduce the thalamic signals to the cortex. For the premotor and motor cortical areas, this would reduce cortical outflow along the corticospinal and corticobulbar tracts and reduce production of motor behaviors (ie, hypokinesia).

In hyperkinetic disorders, the opposite changes take place (Figure 14–7C2): There are enhanced excitatory effects of the indirect path on the cortex. (Note that the output of the substantia nigra pars compactor may be normal.) In Huntington disease, recent studies suggest that striatal neurons of the indirect path, which contain both GABA and enkephalin, are lost (low neural response). This cell loss would result in greater thalamic outflow to the cortex by decreasing striatal inhibition of the external segment of the globus pallidus. Hemiballism, another hyperkinetic disorder, is produced by a subthalamic nucleus lesion. This nucleus normally exerts an excitatory action on the internal segment of the globus pallidus. When the subthalamic nucleus becomes lesioned, the internal segment of the globus pallidus would be expected to inhibit the thalamus less (thin dashed line), thereby increasing outflow to the cerebral cortex.

---

dementia. Huntington disease is inherited as an autosomal dominant disorder. In most patients, Huntington disease presents during midlife. The Huntington gene is located on the short arm of chromosome 4 and codes for a protein, huntingtin, whose function is not yet known. The gene mutation that causes Huntington disease is an expansion of the nucleotide sequence of CAG (>35 repeats) at the 5′ end. This is translated into huntingtin having an excessively long polyglutamine repeat that makes medium spiny neurons particularly vulnerable to cell death. This mutation, which is present in all cells of the body but apparently affecting primarily medium spiny neuron function, also leads to the dysfunction and death of neurons in other brain regions, including the cortex. Although neurodegeneration is widespread in Huntington disease, pathological changes occur earliest in striatal neurons that contain enkephalin, which are part of the indirect path (Figure 14–6). Interestingly, several neurodegenerative diseases are associated with a polyglutamine repeat mutation.

Another hyperkinetic disorder is **hemiballism** (see the clinical case in this chapter). This remarkable clinical disturbance occurs after damage to the **subthalamic nucleus,** an intrinsic basal ganglia nucleus. Hemiballism causes patients to make uncontrollable, rapid **ballistic** (or flinging) **movements** of the contralateral limbs. These movements are produced by motion at proximal limb joints, such as the shoulder and elbow.

Parallel Circuits Course Through the Basal Ganglia

One important aspect of basal ganglia circuitry is that they comprise parallel anatomical loops. Three important points relate to the general organization of these parallel circuits:

1. Each loop originates from multiple cortical regions that have similar general functions.

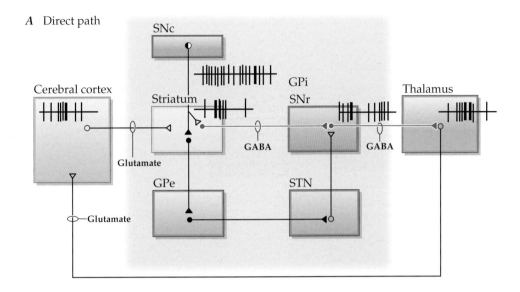

A Direct path

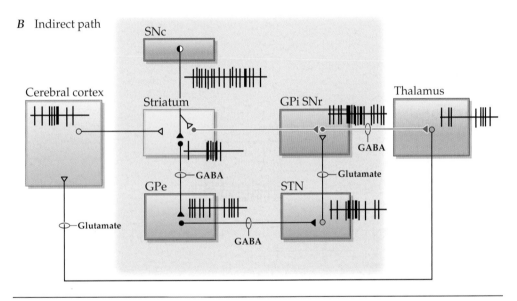

B Indirect path

FIGURE 14–7 Functional basal ganglia circuits in health and disease. Summary of the direct (*A*) and indirect (*B*) paths of the healthy basal ganglia. Filled neuronal cell bodies and terminals indicate inhibitory actions, and open cell bodies indicate excitatory actions. Schematic action potential records are shown by each structure. The vertical line is an action potential; the horizontal line is the baseline. Neural activity for each circuit can be followed, beginning with a phasic excitatory input from the cortex and the resulting phasic change in the thalamus. Changes in activity in the diseased circuits are shown for hypokinetic (*C1*) and hyperkinetic (*C2*) neurological signs. The thickness of the lines indicates relative changes in the number of neurons and strength of connections. Thicker means stronger connections and more activity; thinner means fewer and weaker connections. Schematic neural responses are also shown. Unlike *A* and *B,* which are the neural responses to discrete cortical input signals, the responses in *C1* and *C2* reflect changes in continuous activation patterns produced by disease. These paths follow only tonic changes in neural activation, because phasic changes are not well characterized. GPe, external segment of the globus pallidus; GPi, internal segment of the globus pallidus; SNc, substantia nigra pars compacta; SNr, substantia nigra pars reticulata; STN, subthala-mic nucleus.

C1   Hypokinetic

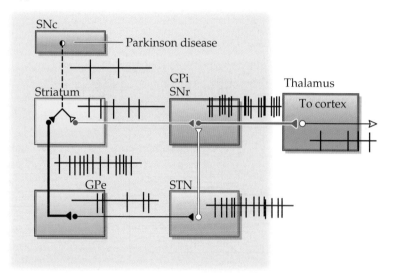

C2   Hyperkinetic

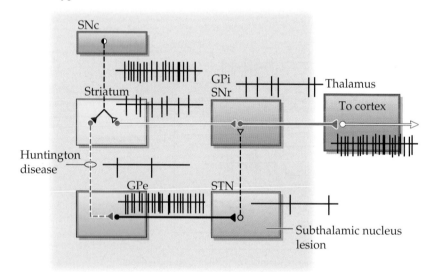

(Continued)—**FIGURE 14–7**

2. Each loop passes through different basal ganglia and thalamic nuclei, or separate portions of the same nucleus. These include the motor thalamic nuclei—the **ventrolateral nucleus** (a part distinct from the one receiving cerebellar input), and the **ventral anterior nucleus**—and the **medial dorsal nucleus,** which serves cognition, emotions, and eye movements.

3. Each loop targets separate portions of the **frontal lobe.**

Through their diverse connections, each loop mediates a different set of functions. Although many parallel loops originate from various cortical areas, anatomical and physiological studies have focused on four major loops (Figure 14–8): the skeletomotor, oculomotor, prefrontal cortex (or cognitive), and limbic loops. Each of these loops comprises many subcircuits. The **skeletomotor loop** plays important roles in the control of facial, limb, and trunk musculature (Figure 14–8A1). Inputs originate from the primary somatic sensory and frontal motor areas and project back to the frontal motor areas (Figure 14–8B). Animal experiments show separate circuits within the skeletomotor loop, originating from the different motor, premotor, and somatic sensory areas, passing through different parts of the globus pallidus, and ultimately terminating in different premotor and motor areas. The **oculomotor loop** plays a role in the control of saccadic eye movements. Key inputs derive from the frontal eye field, which is important in the production of rapid conjugate eye movements through brain stem projections, and the posterior parietal association cortex, which processes visual information for controlling the speed and direction of eye movements

(Figure 14–8A2). The output of this loop is to the frontal eye movement control centers (Figure 14–8; see Chapter 12). More is known about the organization of these two movement control loops than about the other two loops.

The **associative loop** plays a role in cognition and executive behavioral functions, such as strategic planning of behavior. Receiving inputs from diverse association areas, this loop projects primarily to the dorsolateral prefrontal cortex, and some premotor regions as well (Figure 14–8A3, B). Though principally involved in thought and reasoning and in the highest level of organizing goal-directed behaviors, the prefrontal cortex has relatively direct connections with premotor areas involved in movement planning.

The **limbic loop** participates in the motivational regulation of behavior and in emotions. The term *limbic* derives from the limbic system, the brain system that comprises the principal structures for emotions. The limbic association cortex and the hippocampal formation provide the major input to the limbic loop. The limbic loop engages the most distinct set of basal ganglia circuits: the **ventral striatum**—which includes the nucleus accumbens and ventromedial portions of the caudate nucleus and putamen—and the **ventral pallidum** (Figure 14–8A4). The limbic association cortex in the anterior cingulate gyrus is the major frontal lobe recipient of the output of the limbic loop (Figure 14–8B).

Integration of Information Between the Basal Ganglia Loops

Behaviors result from integration of complex sensory, cognitive, and motivational information. It is therefore not surprising that, in addition to the parallel loops (Figures 14–8 and 14–9A), the basal ganglia have also many different ways to integrate information between loops. Three kinds of basal ganglia integrative circuits are highlighted (Figure 14–9B). First, there is overlap in the input connections—those between the cortex and the striatum—as well as within intrinsic circuitry. Second, there appears to be integrative subregions, or "nodal points of convergence" within the basal ganglia loops. For example, while most connections of the dorsolateral prefrontal cortex are to the parts of the striatum in the associative loop, there are smaller focal projections to parts of the ventral striatum for integrating cognition with emotions and reward and to dorsal regions for linking basic eye and limb muscle control with more complex behaviors. Third, the descending corticothalamic projection, which we first examined in detail in the sensory systems (see Figure 4–11and Figure 2–18), is more widespread than the ascending thalamocortical projection.

In organizing behavior, the various parallel circuits of the basal ganglia appear to have distinct functions. This is how we think the loops function for initiating and controlling when you reach for a glass of water. The limbic loop participates in the initial decision to move, motivated by thirst. The prefrontal cortex loop participates in formulating the goal plan, for example, how, where, and when to reach for the water. The oculomotor

and skeletomotor loops assist in the programming and execution of the particular behaviors to achieve the goal. For example, these loops are important in coordinating eye and limb movements to accurately direct your hand to the glass. When we are very thirsty, our movements are faster and more reactive. We think that the integrative connection from the limbic loop to the motor loop is one way for this to happen.

Regional Anatomy of the Basal Ganglia

The rest of this chapter examines the regional anatomy of the parts of the brain that contain the components and associated nuclei of the basal ganglia. This examination begins with a horizontal slice through the cerebral hemispheres and diencephalon because it permits visualization of the various components of the internal capsule, which form major subcortical landmarks. From there, the chapter moves on to coronal slices through the basal ganglia and thalamus. Finally, we consider the brain stem targets of the basal ganglia. In addition to explaining the regional anatomy of the basal ganglia, this discussion also provides an overall view of the deep structures of the cerebral hemispheres.

The Anterior Limb of the Internal Capsule Separates the Head of the Caudate Nucleus From the Putamen

In horizontal section, the **internal capsule** is shaped like an arrowhead pointed toward the midline (Figure 14–4A). The internal capsule contains ascending thalamocortical fibers and descending cortical fibers. The three main segments of the internal capsule are the **anterior limb,** the **posterior limb,** and the **genu,** which connects the two limbs (Figure 14–4). Complementing the three main segments of the internal capsule are the retrolenticular and sublenticular portions. They are named for their locations with respect to the **lenticular nucleus,** which comprises the putamen and globus pallidus.

The anterior limb separates the **head of the caudate nucleus** from the **putamen.** This limb contains axons projecting to and from the prefrontal association cortex and the various premotor cortical areas. The posterior limb separates the **putamen** and the **globus pallidus** (lenticular nucleus) laterally, from the **thalamus** and **caudate nucleus,** medially. The posterior limb contains the corticospinal tract, probably most of the corticobulbar tract, as well as the projections to and from the somatic sensory areas in the parietal lobe. Only coronal sections through the posterior limb cut through the thalamus. The key structures can be seen in the MRI (Figure 14–10B), which is the same plane as the myelin-stained section (see inset in Figure 14–10).

An important feature of the complex three-dimensional structure of the caudate nucleus can be identified in Figure 14–10A. Because the caudate nucleus has a C-shape, it can

A

1. Skeletomotor loop

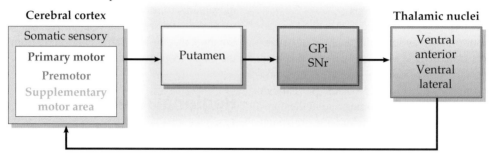

2. Oculomotor loop

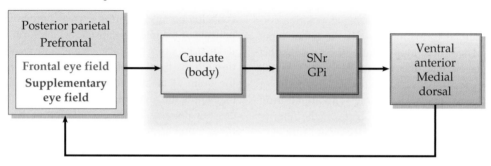

3. Associative loop

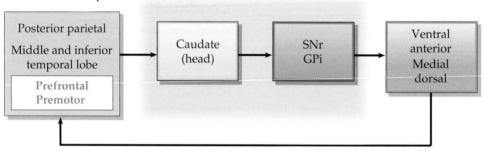

4. Limbic loop

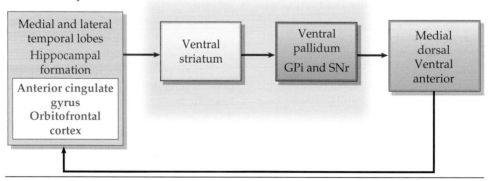

FIGURE 14–8 There are four principal input-output loops through the basal ganglia. **A.** Block diagrams illustrating the general organization of the loops. (1) Skeletomotor loop, (2) oculomotor loop, (3) associative loop, and (4) limbic loop. GPi, internal segment of the globus pallidus; SNr, substantia nigra pars reticulata.

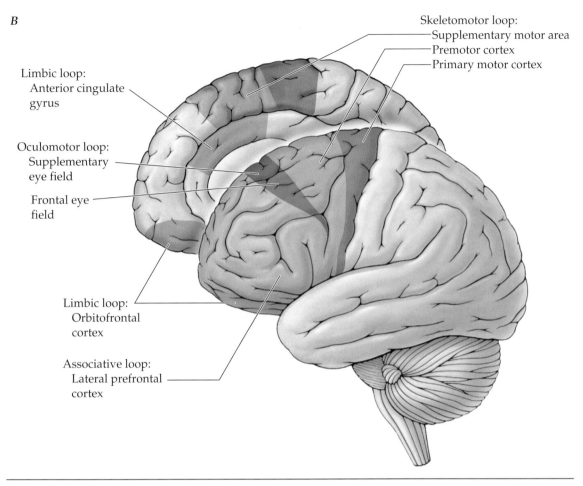

B

Limbic loop:
Anterior cingulate
gyrus

Oculomotor loop:
Supplementary
eye field

Frontal eye
field

Limbic loop:
Orbitofrontal
cortex

Associative loop:
Lateral prefrontal
cortex

Skeletomotor loop:
Supplementary motor area
Premotor cortex
Primary motor cortex

Continued—**FIGURE 14–8 B.** Lateral and medial views of the cerebral cortex, illustrating the approximate location of the target regions in the frontal lobe. The medial orbitofrontal cortex is ventral to the lateral prefrontal cortex.

be seen in two locations in this section. The head of the caudate nucleus is located rostromedially, and the tail of the caudate nucleus is located caudolaterally. (The body of the caudate nucleus is dorsal to the plane of section.) In certain coronal sections, the caudate nucleus is also seen in two locations (dorsomedially and ventrolaterally) (see below). Whereas it is too small to identify, the approximate location of the tail of the caudate is shown in the MRI (Figure 14-10B).

The Three Components of the Striatum Are Located at the Level of the Anterior Horn of the Lateral Ventricle

A coronal slice through the anterior limb of the internal capsule reveals the three components of the striatum (Figure 14–11): the **caudate nucleus** (at this level, the head of the caudate nucleus), the **putamen,** and the **nucleus accumbens.** Although the internal capsule courses between the caudate nucleus and the putamen, **striatal cell bridges** link the two structures. As a further reminder that the three striatal components are not separate structures, the nucleus

accumbens together with the ventromedial portions of the caudate nucleus and putamen (Figure 14–11A) comprise the **ventral striatum,** the striatal component of the limbic loop (Figure 14–8A4). (The olfactory tubercle is sometimes included within the ventral striatum; it is located on the basal surface of the forebrain. A portion of the tubercle receives olfactory inputs.) The **septum pellucidum** is a pair of thin connective tissue membranes that form the medial walls of the anterior horn and body of the lateral ventricles on the two sides (Figure 14–11A). Between the two septa is a cavity in which fluid may accumulate.

The head of the caudate nucleus bulges into the anterior horn of the lateral ventricle (Figure 14–11A, B). Gross changes in the structure of the caudate nucleus in a patient with Huntington disease also can be seen (Figure 14–11C). Patients with Huntington disease exhibit a loss of **medium spiny neurons.** This cell loss is most noticeable in the progression of the disease as a reduction in the size of the head of the caudate nucleus. Note the loss of the characteristic bulge of the head of the caudate nucleus into the lateral ventricle in the Huntington disease patient (Figure 14–11C).

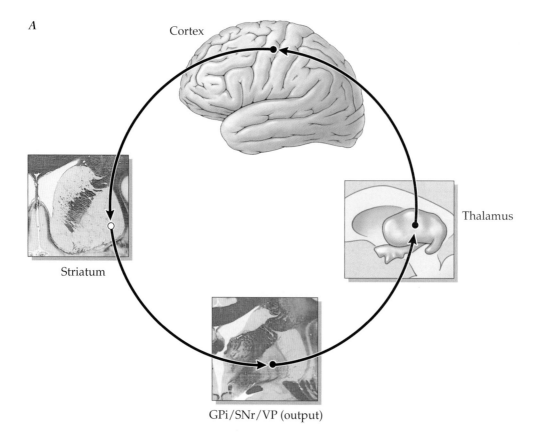

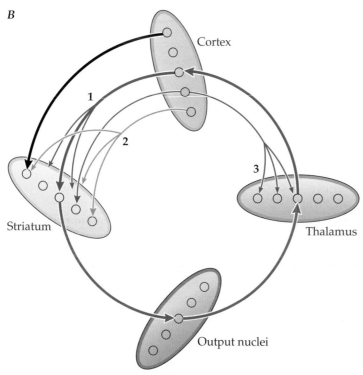

FIGURE 14–9 Integration of information in the basal ganglia. **A.** General organization of single parallel loop. The corticostriatal projection (top) targets the striatum (left). From the striatum, the direct path targets the output nuclei (bottom), which, in turn, project to the thalamus (right) and then back to the cortex. **B.** Schematic showing three circuit features where integration across loops takes place. (1) At the borders between the specific loops. (2) Special interloop connections. (3) At the level of corticothalamic terminations. GPi, internal segment of the globus pallidus; SNr, substantia nigra pars reticulata; VP, ventral pallidum.

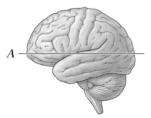

A

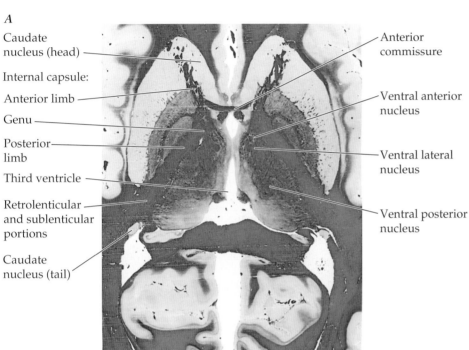

Caudate
nucleus (head)

Internal capsule:

Anterior limb

Genu

Posterior
limb

Third ventricle

Retrolenticular
and sublenticular
portions

Caudate
nucleus (tail)

Anterior
commissure

Ventral anterior
nucleus

Ventral lateral
nucleus

Ventral posterior
nucleus

B

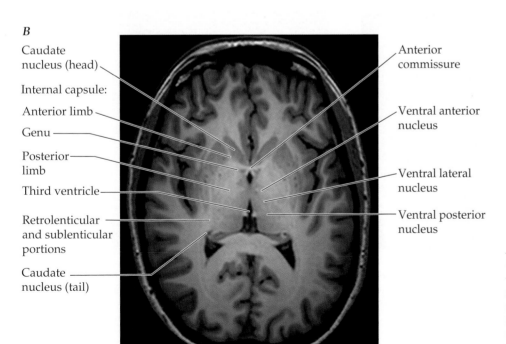

Caudate
nucleus (head)

Internal capsule:

Anterior limb

Genu

Posterior
limb

Third ventricle

Retrolenticular
and sublenticular
portions

Caudate
nucleus (tail)

Anterior
commissure

Ventral anterior
nucleus

Ventral lateral
nucleus

Ventral posterior
nucleus

FIGURE 14–10 Horizontal section
through basal ganglia. **A.** Myelin-stained
section. **B.** T1-weighted MRI In the same
plane as the myelin-stained section in
part **A.** Inset in **A** shows the approximate
plane of the myelin-stained section in **A**
and the MRI in **B.** (**B,** Courtesy of Dr. Joy
Hirsch, Columbia University.)

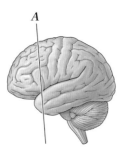

A

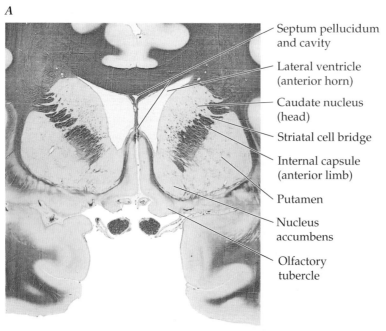

Septum pellucidum and cavity

Lateral ventricle (anterior horn)

Caudate nucleus (head)

Striatal cell bridge

Internal capsule (anterior limb)

Putamen

Nucleus accumbens

Olfactory tubercle

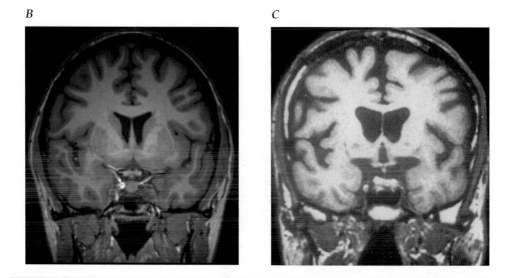

B   *C*

FIGURE 14–11 Coronal sections through head of caudate nucleus. *A.* Myelin-stained section. *B.* MRI from healthy person. *C.* MRI from patient with Huntington disease. (MRI in part **B** courtesy of Dr. Joy Hirsch, Columbia University; MRI in part **C** courtesy of Dr. Susan Folstein.)

The striatum has a compartmental organization

Whereas in myelin-stained sections the three striatal components appear identical and homogeneous, staining for neurotransmitters and neuromodulators or specific afferent connections reveals heterogeneity. Cholinergic markers, for example, stain a **matrix** of tissue that contains a higher concentration surrounding patches, also called **striosomes,** of low marker concentration (Figure 14–12A). The axon terminations of cortical and dopaminergic neurons also have a nonuniform distribution of their striatal terminations. For example, projections from the prefrontal association cortex to the head of the caudate nucleus, comprising part of the associative loop, form patches of dense terminations (Figure 14–12B; inset shows corticostriatal neurons, red). Complementary projections from the posterior parietal cortex also form termination patches, but they interdigitate with those from the prefrontal cortex (Figure 14–12B inset; blue). Callosal neurons are also shown in the schematic (green) because they are labeled by the technique shown in Figure 14–12B. Importantly, compartments related to particular connections and neurochemical distributions appear to be independent, overlapping in some areas and separate in others. The functional significance of fractionating the striatum into compartments related to the different markers and inputs has remained elusive and is among the most important of the many unresolved questions concerning basal ganglia organization.

The External Segment of the Globus Pallidus and the Ventral Pallidum Are Separated by the Anterior Commissure

The external segment of the globus pallidus and part of the ventral pallidum, as discussed earlier, are intrinsic basal ganglia nuclei that send their axons to the subthalamic nucleus. These two structures are likely one and the same, but separated by the anterior commissure (Figure 14–13A). This commissure interconnects specific structures of the temporal lobe. Another portion of the ventral pallidum contains the output neurons that project to the thalamus. Circuits routing through the external segment of the globus pallidus are part of the skeletomotor, cognitive, and oculomotor loops; the circuits through the ventral pallidum are part of the limbic loop.

The Ansa Lenticularis and the Lenticular Fasciculus Are Output Tracts of the Internal Segment of the Globus Pallidus

The putamen, external segment of the globus pallidus, and internal segment of the globus pallidus are separated from one another by thin white matter laminae (Figure 14–14; see AII–20 for their nomenclature). The internal segment of the globus pallidus is a major output of the basal ganglia (Figure 14–14A). Neurons of this nucleus project their axons to

the thalamus (and brain stem, see below), through two anatomically separate pathways: the **lenticular fasciculus** and the **ansa lenticularis.** The axons of the lenticular fasciculus course directly through the internal capsule, but these axons are not clearly visualized until they collect medial to the internal capsule (Figure 14–14B). The internal capsule appears to be a barrier for fibers of the ansa lenticularis; these fibers course around it to reach the thalamus (Figure 14–14A, B). The ansa lenticularis and lenticular fasciculus converge beneath the thalamus and join fibers of the cerebellothalamic tract to form the **thalamic fasciculus** (Figure 14–14B). Deep brain stimulation (DBS) of the internal segment of the globus pallidus is a common treatment of Parkinson disease and dystonia, a rare genetic movement disorder (see later section on basal ganglia circuitry and DBS).

The three major thalamic targets of the output nuclei of the basal ganglia (Figure 14–8A) can be identified in Figures 14–14 and 14–15: the **medial dorsal nucleus,** the **ventral lateral nucleus,** and the **ventral anterior nucleus.** Most of the fibers of the deep cerebellar nuclei also terminate in the ventral lateral nucleus but in a separate portion than axons from the basal ganglia. Two intralaminar thalamic nuclei (see Chapter 2), the **centromedian** and **parafascicular nuclei,** are anatomically closely related to the basal ganglia because they provide a major direct input to the striatum (like that of cortex). These thalamic nuclei also project to the frontal lobe, which is the cortical target of the basal ganglia. Because the intralaminar nuclei have widespread cortical projections, they are considered diffuse-projecting thalamic nuclei and not relay nuclei (see Chapter 2).

Lesion of the Subthalamic Nucleus Produces Hemiballism

Ventral to the thalamus is the subthalamic region, which consists of a disparate collection of nuclei. The major nucleus in this brain region is the **subthalamic nucleus** (Figure 14–15A). A lesion of the subthalamic nucleus produces **hemiballism,** a hyperkinetic disorder, characterized by ballistic movements of the contralateral limbs (see clinical case and Box 14–1; Figure 14–7C2). The connections of the subthalamic nucleus are complex. Receiving input from the external segment of the globus pallidus as well as from the motor cortex, the subthalamic nucleus projects back to both the **external** and **internal segments of the globus pallidus** (Figure 14–15). The subthalamic nucleus is also reciprocally connected with the ventral pallidum (Figure 14–13). The subthalamic nucleus, along with the internal segment of the globus pallidus, is a key target of DBS for treatment of Parkinson disease (see later section on DBS).

Very little is known of the function of the **zona incerta** (Figure 14–15), a nuclear region interposed between the subthalamic nucleus and the thalamus. The zona incerta receives projections from a variety of sources, including the spinal cord and cerebellum. Many of the neurons in the zona incerta contain GABA and have diffuse cortical projections.

A

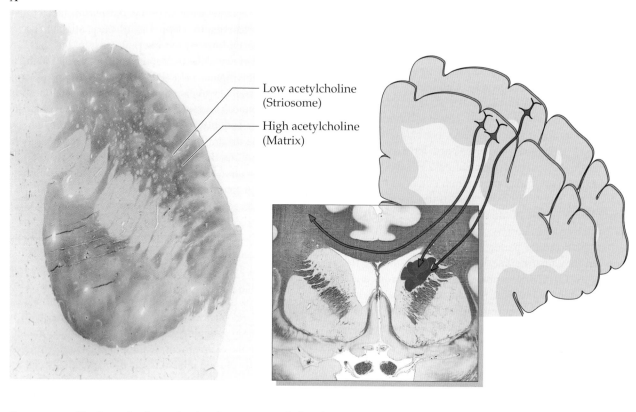

Low acetylcholine
(Striosome)

High acetylcholine
(Matrix)

B

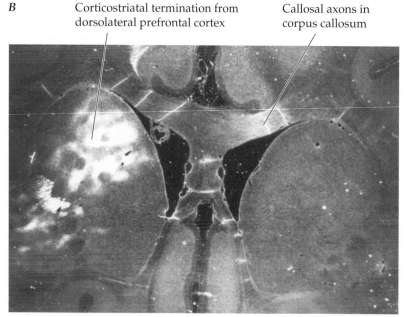

Corticostriatal termination from
dorsolateral prefrontal cortex

Callosal axons in
corpus callosum

FIGURE 14–12 Striosome-matrix organization of the striatum. **A.** Histochemical localization of acetylcholinesterase in the striatum. Regions of high acetylcholinesterase concentration are within the striosomes, and low concentration, in the matrix. **B.** Patchy distribution of labeled corticostriatal axon terminals in the head of the caudate nucleus of the rhesus monkey. Labeling in part **B** was achieved by injection of a radioactive tracer, consisting of a mixture of 3H-proline and 3H-leucine, into the cortex. Tracer was incorporated into cortical neurons and transported anterogradely to their axons and terminals. This process resulted in an intricate pattern of labeling in the caudate nucleus. Axons were labeled in the white matter, including in the corpus callosum, because the tracer labels callosal neurons as well as a variety of descending projection neurons. The inset shows how labeled callosal neurons send their axon into the corpus callosum. Ipsilateral corticocortical projections from different parts of cortex are shown terminating within different parts of the striatum. (**A,** Courtesy of Dr. Suzanne Haber, University of Rochester School of Medicine. **B,** Courtesy of Dr. Patricia Goldman-Rakic; Goldman-Rakic PS. Neuronal plasticity in primate telencephalon: anomalous projections induced by prenatal removal of frontal cortex. *Science.* 1978;202[4369]:768-770.)

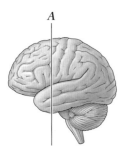

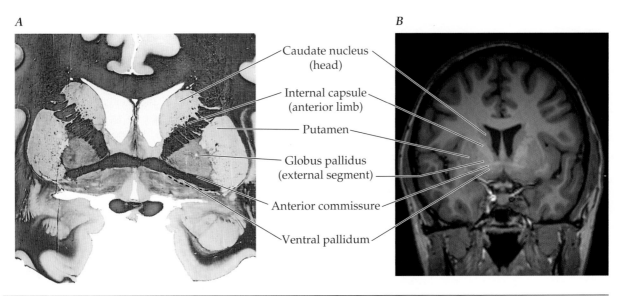

Caudate nucleus (head)

Internal capsule (anterior limb)

Putamen

Globus pallidus (external segment)

Anterior commissure

Ventral pallidum

A

B

FIGURE 14–13 Myelin-stained coronal section through the external segment of the globus pallidus and ventral pallidum. The inset shows the plane of section (**A**) and corresponding MRI (**B**). (**B,** Courtesy of Dr. Joy Hirsch, Columbia University.)

The Substantia Nigra Contains Two Anatomical Divisions

The posterior limb of the internal capsule separates the internal segment of the globus pallidus from the substantia nigra, a separation that can be seen in coronal section (Figure 14–15). Like separation of the components of the striatum, cell bridges can be seen within the internal capsule, between the **substantia nigra pars reticulata** and internal segment of the globus pallidus. The substantia nigra pars reticulata and internal segment of the globus pallidus appear to be part of the same basal ganglia output nucleus that becomes largely separated by axons of the internal capsule. They are not identical, however. The substantia nigra pars reticulata is part of the oculomotor and cognitive/associative loops; it also projects to the superior colliculus (Figure 14–16A), which is important in controlling **saccadic eye movements** (see Chapter 12). The substantia nigra pars reticulata, which is adjacent to the basis pedunculi (Figures 14–15 and 14–16), contains GABA (Figure 14–6) and, like the internal segment of the globus pallidus, projects to the thalamus and pedunculopontine nucleus (see below).

The other division of the substantia nigra is the **substantia nigra pars compacta;** it consists of neurons containing dopamine. The projection of these neurons to the striatum forms the **nigrostriatal tract.** Dopaminergic neurons that project

to the different striatal regions are topographically organized. The activity of many of the substantia nigra pars compacta neurons, shown in animal studies, is related to salient stimuli, such as a tone that predicts receiving a food reward, rather than particular features of the movement the animals perform. This salience reflects key inputs from the **amygdala,** which is involved in motivation and emotions, the **reticular formation,** which is involved in arousal, and serotonergic connections from the **raphe nuclei.**

The substantia nigra pars compacta is not the only midbrain region that contains dopamine. The **ventral tegmental area** is dorsomedial to the substantia nigra, beneath the floor of the interpeduncular fossa (Figure 14–16A). Dopaminergic neurons in the ventral tegmental area send their axons to the striatum via the **medial forebrain bundle** (see Chapters 15 and 16) as well as to the frontal lobe (see Figure 2–3B1).

The Pedunculopontine Nucleus Is Part of a Parallel Path From the Basal Ganglia to Brain Stem Locomotor Control Centers

Whereas much of the output of the basal ganglia is directed to the thalamus, and then back to the cerebral cortex, a

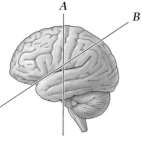

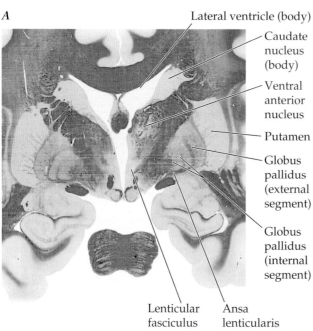

A

Lateral ventricle (body)

Caudate nucleus (body)

Ventral anterior nucleus

Putamen

Globus pallidus (external segment)

Globus pallidus (internal segment)

Lenticular fasciculus

Ansa lenticularis

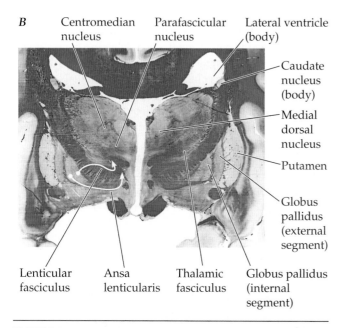

B

Centromedian nucleus

Parafascicular nucleus

Lateral ventricle (body)

Caudate nucleus (body)

Medial dorsal nucleus

Putamen

Globus pallidus (external segment)

Lenticular fasciculus

Ansa lenticularis

Thalamic fasciculus

Globus pallidus (internal segment)

FIGURE 14–14 Myelin-stained coronal (**A**) and oblique (**B**) sections through the internal and external segments of the globus pallidus. The inset shows the planes of section.

second output circuit involves the **pedunculopontine nucleus** (Figure 14–16B). This is the descending projection of the basal ganglia, and it is thought to play an important role in locomotor function. The pedunculopontine nucleus has diverse functions, including regulating arousal, through diffuse ascending projections to the thalamus and cortex, and movement control, through descending projections. In animals, activation of the pedunculopontine nucleus promotes locomotor behaviors, whereas inhibition retards locomotor behaviors. It projects to brain stem locomotor centers and also has a small direct spinal projection. As discussed below, the pedunculopontine nucleus is a target of deep brain stimulation to alleviate the locomotor disturbances in Parkinson disease. Many of the neurons in this nucleus are **cholinergic,** including those projecting to the thalamus. The dorsal raphe nucleus, also located in the caudal midbrain-rostral pons (Figure 14–16B), gives rise to an ascending **serotonergic** projection to the striatum. In addition to projecting to the striatum, the dorsal raphe nucleus has extensive projections to most of the cerebral cortex and to other forebrain nuclei.

Stimulation-based Treatments for Movement and Nonmovement Disorders Rely on Knowledge of the Regional Anatomy and Circuitry of the Basal Ganglia

There is a long history of neurosurgical procedures to alleviate motor signs of severe basal ganglia disease, with the most effective being lesion of the internal segment of the globus pallidus produced by a technique termed *electrocoagulation*. This surgical procedure, termed **pallidotomy,** eliminated the abnormal output of the basal ganglia, thereby helping the remaining portions of the motor systems to function better. More recently, pallidotomy is a procedure of last resort in patients, only when L-dopa becomes less effective.

Deep brain stimulation, or **DBS,** has largely superseded pallidotomy, especially in developed countries. DBS is a neurophysiological approach to treating basal ganglia and other diseases, often with remarkably positive outcomes. The DBS electrode is implanted within the internal segment of the globus pallidus or the subthalamic nucleus, often bilaterally. By selection of the proper stimulation frequency and amplitude, neural activity of the aberrant output circuitry is altered and many of the parkinsonian signs are ameliorated. DBS of the internal segment of the globus pallidus is now routinely used for treatment of dystonia.

Knowledge that different portions of the internal globus pallidus and subthalamic nucleus are parts of the different functional basal ganglia loops has allowed neurosurgeons to position DBS electrodes for treatment of nonmotor disorders, as well, such as obsessive-compulsive disorders and Tourette syndrome. Because of their important interconnections with the cerebral cortex, DBS is also being explored for affective disorders (see Chapter 16).

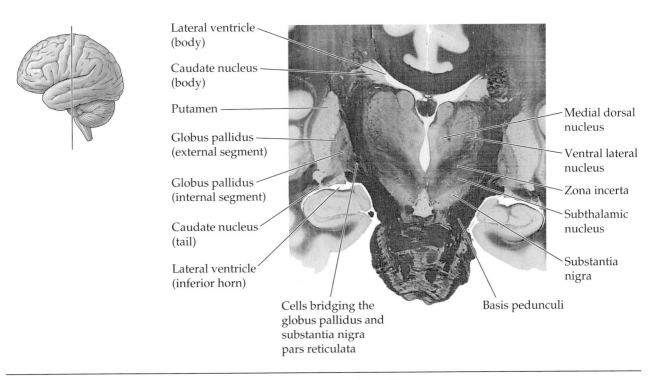

Lateral ventricle (body)

Caudate nucleus (body)

Putamen

Globus pallidus (external segment)

Globus pallidus (internal segment)

Caudate nucleus (tail)

Lateral ventricle (inferior horn)

Medial dorsal nucleus

Ventral lateral nucleus

Zona incerta

Subthalamic nucleus

Substantia nigra

Cells bridging the globus pallidus and substantia nigra pars reticulata

Basis pedunculi

FIGURE 14–15 Myelin-stained section through the internal segment of the globus pallidus.

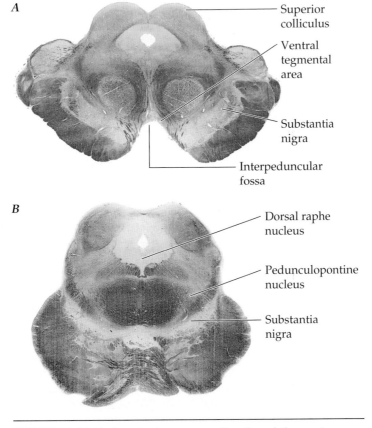

A

Superior colliculus

Ventral tegmental area

Substantia nigra

Interpeduncular fossa

B

Dorsal raphe nucleus

Pedunculopontine nucleus

Substantia nigra

FIGURE 14–16 Myelin-stained transverse sections through the superior colliculus (*A*) and the inferior colliculus (*B*).

Surprisingly, despite extensive use of DBS, we do not yet know the mechanism of its therapeutic action, for either movement or nonmovement disorders. DBS probably does not simply activate neurons. Rather, it modulates the activity of local neurons in the neighborhood of the electrode—both facilitation and suppression depending on a neuron's location—and these local effects are passed on to wider brain regions via monosynaptic and polysynaptic circuits. DBS may even function like a pacemaker, to change an abnormally slow and highly synchronized level of neuronal activity in the diseased brain—signatures of a resting functional state—to faster levels of activity, characteristic of a more active state.

The Vascular Supply of the Basal Ganglia Is Provided by the Middle Cerebral Artery

As described in Chapter 3, the vascular supply to the deep structures of the cerebral hemispheres—the **thalamus, basal ganglia,** and **internal capsule**—is provided by branches of the internal carotid artery and the three cerebral arteries. Most of the striatum is supplied by perforating branches of the middle cerebral artery; however, rostromedial regions are supplied by deep branches of the anterior cerebral artery (see Figure 3–7). Collectively, these branches of the anterior and middle cerebral arteries are termed the **lenticulostriate arteries.** Most of the globus pallidus is supplied by the **anterior choroidal artery,** which is a branch of the internal carotid artery.

Summary

Basal Ganglia Nuclei

The basal ganglia contain numerous component nuclei that can be divided into three groups based on their connections (Table 14–1; Figure 14–5): input nuclei, output nuclei, and intrinsic nuclei. The *input nuclei* consist of the *caudate nucleus,* the *putamen,* and the *nucleus accumbens* (Figures 14–2 and 14–11) and collectively are termed the *striatum.* The ventromedial portions of the caudate nucleus and putamen, together with the nucleus accumbens, comprise the *ventral striatum.* The *output nuclei* include the *internal segment of the globus pallidus* (Table 14–1; Figures 14–5, 14–13, and 14–14), a portion of the *ventral pallidum* (Figure 14–13), and the *substantia nigra pars reticulata* (Figures 14–15 and 14–16). The *intrinsic nuclei* comprise the *external segment of the globus pallidus* (Figure 14–13), a portion of the *ventral pallidum,* the *subthalamic nucleus* (Figure 14–15), the *substantia nigra pars compacta* (Figures 14–15 and 14–16), and the *ventral tegmental area* (Figure 14–16A).

Basal Ganglia Functional Loops

The basic input-output pathway through the basal ganglia links wide regions of the cerebral cortex with, in sequence, the input nuclei of the basal ganglia (striatum), the output nuclei, the thalamus, and a portion of the frontal lobe (Figure 14–5B). There are four key functional loops through the basal ganglia (Figure 14–8): the skeletomotor, oculomotor, associative, and limbic loops. The *skeletomotor* and *oculomotor loops* play important roles in the control of facial, limb, and trunk musculature and extraocular muscles; the *associative loop* may subserve tasks such as cognition and executive behavioral functions; and the *limbic loop* may function in the regulation of behavior and in emotions. The skeletomotor, oculomotor, and prefrontal cortex loops begin in the *somatic sensory, motor,* and *association areas* of the cerebral cortex and pass through the *caudate nucleus* and *putamen* (Figure 14–8). The output nuclei of these loops are the *internal segment of the globus pallidus* (Figure 14–14) and the *substantia nigra pars reticulata* (Figures 14–15 and 14–16). They, in turn, synapse in the *ventrolateral, ventral anterior,* and *medial dorsal nuclei* of the thalamus (Figures 14–15 and 14–16). The internal segment of the globus pallidus projects to the thalamus via two pathways: the *ansa lenticularis* and the *lenticular fasciculus* (Figure 14–15B). However, components of the various loops synapse on neurons located in different nuclei or in different portions of the same nuclei. The internal segment of the globus pallidus also projects to the pedunculopontine nucleus, which plays a role in arousal and movement control.

The *limbic loop* (Figure 14–8) begins in the *limbic association cortex.* The *ventral striatum,* which comprises the nucleus accumbens and the ventromedial parts of the caudate nucleus and putamen (Figure 14–11), is the principal input nucleus of the limbic loop; the output and thalamic nuclei of the limbic loop are the *ventral pallidum* (Figure 14–13) and the *medial dorsal nucleus* (Figure 14–15).

The cortical targets of the four loops are (Figure 14–8B) *supplementary motor areas, premotor cortex,* and *primary motor cortex* for the skeletomotor loop; *frontal* and *supplementary eye fields* for the oculomotor loop; *prefrontal association cortex* for the association loop; and *anterior cingulate gyrus* (and *orbitofrontal gyri*) for the limbic loop.

Selected Readings

Wichmann T, DeLong MR. The basal ganglia. In: Kandel ER, Schwartz JH, Jessell TM, Siegelbaum SA, Hudspeth AJ, eds. *Principles of Neural Science.* 5th ed. New York, NY: McGraw-Hill; in press.

References

Albin RL, Mink JW. Recent advances in Tourette syndrome research. *TINS.* 2006;29(3):175-182.

Alexander GE, Crutcher MD. Functional architecture of basal ganglia circuits: neural substrates of parallel processing. *Trends Neurosci.* 1990;13:266-271.

Bergman H, Feingold A, Nini A, et al. Physiological aspects of information processing in the basal ganglia of normal and parkinsonian primates. *Trends Neurosci.* 1998;21:32-38.

Bjorklund A, Dunnett SB. Dopamine neuron systems in the brain: an update. *TINS.* 2007;30(5):194-202.

Bolam JP, Hanley JJ, Booth PA, Bevan MD. Synaptic organisation of the basal ganglia. *J Anat.* 2000;196:527-542.

Bostan AC, Dum RP, Strick PL. The basal ganglia communicate with the cerebellum. *Proc Natl Acad Sci USA.* 2010;107(18):8452-8456.

Bostan AC, Strick PL. The cerebellum and basal ganglia are interconnected. *Neuropsychol Rev.* 2010;20(3):261-270.

Breakefield XO, Blood AJ, Li Y, Hallett M, Hanson PI, Standaert DG. The pathophysiological basis of dystonias. *Nat Rev Neurosci.* 2008;9(3):222-234.

Brundin P, Li JY, Holton JL, Lindvall O, Revesz T. Research in motion: the enigma of Parkinson's disease pathology spread. *Nat Rev Neurosci.* 2008;9(10):741-745.

Cattaneo E, Zuccato C, Tartari M. Normal huntingtin function: an alternative approach to Huntington's disease. *Nat Rev Neurosci.* 2005;6(12):919-930.

Charara A, Smith Y, Parent A. Glutamatergic inputs from the pedunculopontine nucleus to midbrain dopaminergic neurons in primates: phaseolus vulgaris-leucoagglutinin anterograde labeling combined with postembedding glutamate and GABA immunohistochemistry. *J Comp Neurol.* 1996;364:254-266.

Conn PJ, Battaglia G, Marino MJ, Nicoletti F. Metabotropic glutamate receptors in the basal ganglia motor circuit. *Nat Rev Neurosci.* 2005;6(10):787-798.

DeLong MR. Primate modes of movement disorders of basal ganglia origin. *Trends Neurosci.* 1990;13:281-285.

Duzel E, Bunzeck N, Guitart-Masip M, Wittmann B, Schott BH, Tobler PN. Functional imaging of the human dopaminergic midbrain. *TINS.* 2009;32(6):321-328.

Gerfen CR. The neostriatal matrix: multiple levels of compartmental organization. *Trends Neurosci.* 1992;15:133-139.

Guridi J, Lozano AM. A brief history of pallidotomy. *Neurosurgery.* 1997;41(5):1169-1180; discussion 1180-1183.

Gusella JF, Wexler NS, Conneally PM, et al. A polymorphic DNA marker genetically linked to Huntington's disease. *Nature.* 1983;306:234-238.

Haber SN. Neurotransmitters in the human and nonhuman primate basal ganglia. *Hum Neurobiol.* 1986;5:159-168.

Haber SN. Integrative networks across basal ganglia circuits. In: Steiner H, Kuei T, eds. *Handbook of Basal Ganglia Structure and Function.* San Diego, CA: Elsevier; 2010:409-427.

Haber SN, Fudge JL, McFarland N. Striatonigrostriatal pathways in primates form an ascending spiral from the shell to the dorsolateral striatum. *J Neurosci.* 2000;20:2369-2382.

Haber SN, Groenewegen HJ, Grove EA, et al. Efferent connections of the ventral pallidum: evidence of a dual striato-pallidofugal pathway. *J Comp Neurol.* 1985;235:322-335.

Haber SN, Johnson Gdowski M. The basal ganglia. In: Paxinos G, Mai JK, eds. *The Human Nervous System.* London: Elsevier; 2004.

Haber SN, Knutson B. The reward circuit: linking primate anatomy and human imaging. *Neuropsychopharmacology.* 2010;35(1):4-26.

Haber SN, McFarland NR. The concept of the ventral striatum in nonhuman primates. *Ann NY Acad Sci.* 1999;877:33-48.

Haber SN, Watson SJ. The comparative distribution of enkephalin, dynorphin and substance P in the human globus pallidus and basal forebrain. *Neuroscience.* 1985;4:1011-1024.

Hammond C, Bergman H, Brown P. Pathological synchronization in Parkinson's disease: networks, models and treatments. *TINS.* 2007;30(7):357-364.

Hoover JE, Strick PL. Multiple output channels in basal ganglia. *Science.* 1993;259:819-821.

Hoover JE, Strick PL. The organization of cerebellar and basal ganglia outputs to primary motor cortex as revealed by retrograde transneuronal transport of herpes simplex virus type 1. *J Neurosci.* 1999;19:1446-1463.

Hoshi E, Tremblay L, Feger J, Carras PL, Strick PL. The cerebellum communicates with the basal ganglia. *Nat Neurosci.* 2005;8(11):1491-1493.

Karachi C, Yelnik J, Tande D, Tremblay L, Hirsch EC, Francois C. The pallidosubthalamic projection: an anatomical substrate for nonmotor functions of the subthalamic nucleus in primates. *Mov Disord.* 2005;20(2):172-180.

Kowianski P, Dziewiatkowski J, Kowianska J, Morys J. Comparative anatomy of the claustrum in selected species: a morphometric analysis. *Brain Behav Evol.* 1999;53:44-54.

Krack P, Hariz MI, Baunez C, Guridi J, Obeso JA. Deep brain stimulation: from neurology to psychiatry? *TINS.* 2010;33(10):474-484.

Kringelbach ML, Jenkinson N, Owen SL, Aziz TZ. Translational principles of deep brain stimulation. *Nat Rev Neurosci.* 2007;8(8):623-635.

Macchi G, Jones EG. Toward an agreement on terminology of nuclear and subnuclear divisions of the motor thalamus. *J Neurosurg.* 1997;86:670-685.

Mata IF, Wedemeyer WJ, Farrer MJ, Taylor JP, Gallo KA. LRRK2 in Parkinson's disease: protein domains and functional insights. *TINS.* 2006;29(5):286-293.

McFarland N, Haber SN. Organization of thalamostriatal terminals from the ventral motor nuclei in the macaque. *J Comp Neurol.* 2001;429:321-336.

McHaffie JG, Stanford TR, Stein BE, Coizet V, Redgrave P. Subcortical loops through the basal ganglia. *TINS.* 2005;28(8):401-407.

Mena-Segovia J, Bolam JP, Magill PJ. Pedunculopontine nucleus and basal ganglia: distant relatives or part of the same family? *TINS.* 2004;27(10):585-588.

Middleton FA, Strick PL. Anatomical evidence for cerebellar and basal ganglia involvement in higher cognitive function. *Science.* 1994;266:458-461.

Middleton FA, Strick PL. The temporal lobe is a target of output from the basal ganglia. *Proc Natl Acad Sci USA.* 1996;93:8683-8687.

Middleton FA, Strick PL. Basal ganglia and cerebellar loops: motor and cognitive circuits. *Brain Res Brain Res Rev.* 2000;31:236-250.

Nandi D, Aziz TZ, Giladi N, Winter J, Stein JF. Reversal of akinesia in experimental parkinsonism by GABA antagonist microinjections in the pedunculopontine nucleus. *Brain.* 2002;125(Pt 11):2418-2430.

Pahapill PA, Lozano AM. The pedunculopontine nucleus and Parkinson's disease. *Brain.* 2000;123:1767-1783.

Paus T. Primate anterior cingulate cortex: where motor control, drive and cognition interface. *Nat Rev Neurosci.* 2001;2:417-424.

Percheron G. Thalamus. In: Paxinos G, Mai JK, eds. *The Human Nervous System.* London: Elsevier; 2004:592-676.

Pisani A, Bernardi G, Ding J, Surmeier DJ. Re-emergence of striatal cholinergic interneurons in movement disorders. *TINS.* 2007;30(10):545-553.

Poirier LJ, Giguère M, Marchand R. Comparative morphology of the substantia nigra and ventral tegmental area in the monkey, cat and rat. *Brain Res Bull.* 1983;11:371-397.

Reiner A, Albin RL, Anderson KD, D'Amato CJ, Penney JB, Young AB. Differential loss of striatal projection neurons in Huntington disease. *Proc Natl Acad Sci USA.* 1988;85:5733-5737.

Romanski LM, Giguere M, Bates JF, Goldman-Rakic PS. Topographic organization of medial pulvinar connections with the prefrontal cortex in the rhesus monkey. *J Comp Neurol.* 1997;379:313-332.

Schell GR, Strick PL. The origin of thalamic inputs to the arcuate premotor and supplementary motor areas. *J Neurosci.* 1984;4:539-560.

Schutz W, Romo R. Dopamine neurons of the monkey midbrain: contingencies of response to stimuli eliciting immediate behavioral reactions. *J Neurophysiol.* 1990;63:607-624.

Selemon LD, Goldman-Rakic PS. Longitudinal topography and interdigitation of corticostriatal projections in the rhesus monkey. *J Neurosci.* 1985;5:776-794.

Stern CE, Passingham RE. The nucleus accumbens in monkeys (Macaca fascicularis): I. The organization of behaviour. *Behav Brain Res.* 1994;61:9-21.

Weinberger M, Hamani C, Hutchison WD, Moro E, Lozano AM, Dostrovsky JO. Pedunculopontine nucleus microelectrode recordings in movement disorder patients. *Exp Brain Res.* 2008;188(2):165-174.

Yeterian EH, Van Hoesen GW. Cortico-striate projections in the rhesus monkey: the organization of certain cortico-caudate connections. *Brain Res.* 1978;139:43-63.

Yin HH, Knowlton BJ. The role of the basal ganglia in habit formation. *Nat Rev Neurosci.* 2006;7(6):464-476.

1. A person received a gunshot to the side of the head. Identify the structures on one side of the brain, marked by the line of dots on the myelin-stained section below, that the bullet would have damaged. Also, note the salient function or connection of the structure.

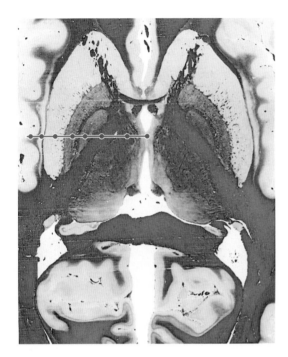

2. The output nuclei of the basal ganglia send projections to the diencephalon and brain stem. Which of the following lists two output nuclei of the basal ganglia?
   A. Globus pallidus internal, globus pallidus external
   B. Caudate nucleus, nucleus accumbens
   C. Substantia nigra par reticulata, substantia nigra pars compacta
   D. Globus pallidus internal, substantia nigra par reticulata

3. Which of the following lists components of the same functional loop of the basal ganglia?
   A. Frontal eye fields, body of caudate nucleus, ventral pallidum, ventral lateral nucleus of the thalamus
   B. Orbitofrontal cortex, nucleus accumbens, ventral pallidum, medial dorsal nucleus of the thalamus
   C. Primary motor cortex, putamen, globus pallidus internal segment, medial dorsal nucleus of the thalamus
   D. Hippocampus, ventral striatum, globus pallidus internal segment, ventral lateral nucleus

4. Which of the following describes the action of dopamine on striatal neurons of the direct and indirect paths?
   A. Facilitates activity, suppresses activity
   B. Facilitates activity, no effect on activity
   C. Suppresses activity, facilitates activity
   D. No effect on activity, facilitates activity

5. A person has a small stroke that interrupts axons of the ansa lenticularis. This stroke would produce retrograde degeneration of neurons in which of the following structures?
   A. Substantia nigra pars compacta
   B. Globus pallidus external segment
   C. Globus pallidus internal segment
   D. Subthalamic nucleus

6. Midbrain dopaminergic neurons have major actions on neurons in which of the following structures?
   A. Striatal neurons only
   B. Striatal neurons and cortical neurons
   C. Striatal neurons, globus pallidus internal segment neurons, and cortical neurons
   D. Striatal neurons, globus pallidus internal segment neurons, globus pallidus external segment neurons, and cortical neurons

7. Which of the following statements best matches the structure and neurons with the correct neurotransmitter?
   A. Substantia nigra pars compacta and GABA
   B. Globus pallidus external segment and glutamate
   C. Subthalamic nucleus and glutamate
   D. Caudate nucleus and dopamine

8. A man developed significant personality changes and clumsiness late in his fourth decade of life. His father had dementia and bilateral choreoform movements at the time of his death, which was in his early 60s. The man's mother is currently healthy. Which of the following neuropsychiatric conditions is most likely affecting the son?
   A. Huntington disease
   B. Parkinson disease
   C. Hemiballism
   D. Schizophrenia

9. Which of the following is a target of deep brain stimulation for treatment of basal ganglia movement disorders?
   A. Globus pallidus external segment
   B. Globus pallidus internal segment
   C. Caudate nucleus
   D. Putamen

10. The internal segment of the globus pallidus has projections to which of the following brain stem structures?
   A. Pedunculopontine nucleus
   B. Superior colliculus
   C. Dorsal raphe nucleus
   D. Red nucleus

INTEGRATIVE SYSTEMS

IV

Chapter 15

The Hypothalamus and Regulation of Bodily Functions

CLINICAL CASE | Lateral Medullary Syndrome and Horner Syndrome

A 69-year-old hypertensive man suddenly developed vertigo and left facial numbness. He is unable to stand unassisted.

His sensory and motor functions were tested at the emergency room. Pain and temperature sensations are markedly decreased on the left side of his face, including the left side of his oral cavity. Tactile sensation is preserved bilaterally on his face. Pain and temperature sensations are diminished on the right side of the scalp, neck, limbs, and trunk. Touch and limb propriosensation were normal bilaterally. There is a loss of the gag reflex on the left.

On finger-nose-finger testing of the left arm and heel-to-shin testing of the left leg, his movements are ataxic. He has difficulty making rapidly alternating movements (dysdiadochokinesia) with the left arm. Corresponding right limb functions are normal. He has difficulty standing, and the limited walking he is able to accomplish is associated with a broad-based gait. His voice sounds hoarse. He is able to extend his tongue along the midline.

On further examination, the patient also is noted to have mild ptosis on the left. His pupils were reactive to light, but his left pupil was smaller than the right. Finally, the left side of his face feels dry and warm to touch.

Figure 15–1A is an MRI of the medulla, and Figure 15–1B, a nearby myelin-stained section. The bright dorsolateral region in part A is the site of an infarction.

Answer the following questions on the basis of your reading of this chapter and prior chapters on sensory and motor functions of the dorsolateral medulla.

1. **Occlusion of which artery would infarct the medullary region shown on the MRI?**

—Continued next page

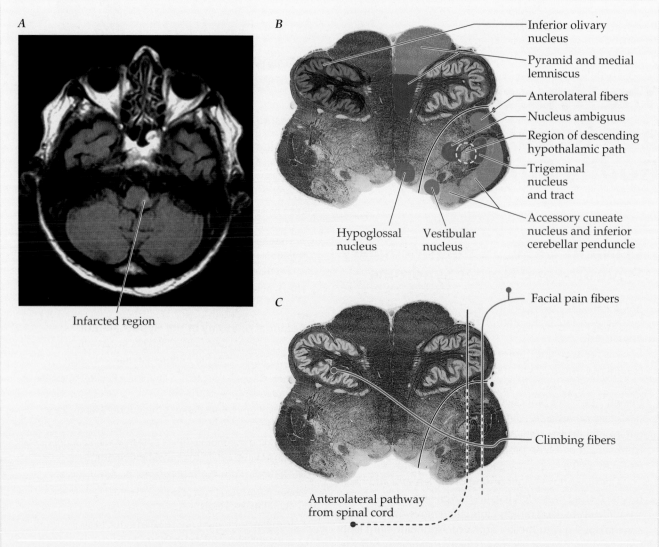

FIGURE 15–1 Lateral medullary syndrome. **A.** MRI from a person with an infarction of the posterior inferior cerebellar artery. **B.** Myelin-stained section. **C.** Myelin-stained section with schematic showing the pathways affected by the infarction. Note, all images show the ventral side up.

2. **Indicate the particular nucleus or tract that, after damage by infarction, produces: (1) ipsilateral facial pain loss, (2) contralateral loss of limb and trunk pain, (3) ataxia, (4) hoarse voice, and (5) ipsilateral ptosis.**

Key neurological signs and corresponding damaged brain structures

Distribution of the posterior inferior cerebellar artery

The site of lesion corresponds to the distribution of the posterior inferior cerebellar artery. The territory supplied by this artery receives little collateral circulation (see Chapter 3). This means that blood flow from a functioning neighboring artery does not take over, as in many regions of the brain. Remaining areas of the medulla at this level are supplied by small, direct branches from the vertebral artery.

Alternating loss of pain and temperature on the left side of the face and right limbs and trunk with preservation of touch

The lesion produced a classical sign. Ipsilateral loss of facial pain and temperature sensation is due to interruption of the spinal trigeminal tract, as well as part of the spinal trigeminal nucleus (caudal nucleus). Contralateral loss of pain and temperature sensation on the neck, limbs, and trunk is due to interruption of the anterolateral system, which decussates in the spinal cord (Figure 15–1C). This pattern was considered in the Chapter 6 clinical case in which tactile and limb position senses are preserved because the dorsal column-medial lemniscal system is located outside of the distribution of the posterior inferior cerebellar artery.

Hoarse voice

Several cranial nerve motor nuclei are located within the territory of the posterior inferior cerebellar artery; especially nucleus ambiguus, which contains pharyngeal and laryngeal motor neurons. The hoarse voice is produced by unilateral paralysis of laryngeal muscles. The patient is unable to close off the trachea and build pressure within the lungs, for his voice to project. This lesion often disrupts the laryngeal closure reflex, in which the vocal cords close when the surrounding region is stimulated by solid food or liquid. Normally, this reflex prevents aspiration of materials into the lungs (see Chapter 11). The loss of the gag reflex is likely due to lesion of the nucleus ambiguus, although the solitary nucleus and trigeminal nuclei are affected, which can impede the function of the afferent limb of the reflex, which is carried by the glossopharyngeal nerve. There may also be swallowing impairments, but this was not tested.

Ataxia and dysdiadochokinesia

Three major inputs to the cerebellum travel through the inferior cerebellar peduncle, which is supplied by the posterior inferior cerebellar artery: climbing fibers from the inferior olivary nucleus and the cuneocerebellar and dorsal spinocerebellar tracts. The cuneocerebellar tract originates from within the infarcted zone. Loss of these key cerebellar paths leads to the observed motor signs. Moreover, the posterior inferior cerebellar artery also supplies parts of the cerebellar cortex and deep nuclei. Thus, these signs can be due to direct involvement of the cerebellum, in addition to its input pathways. Strength is usually preserved after infarction

of the posterior inferior cerebellar artery. This is because the corticospinal tract travels in the pyramids, which are not supplied by the posterior inferior cerebellar artery.

Vertigo

Vertigo is a classic sign of vestibular nerve and nuclei damage. This results because of an imbalance in vestibular signaling. However, cerebellar involvement can produce vertigo. Damage to the dorsolateral medulla and cerebellum can often produce nystagmus.

Pupillary signs, ptosis, and facial dryness and warmth

Pupils and eyelid control are functions of the midbrain. How can they be affected with a medullary lesion? This is because the descending pathway from the hypothalamus to the spinal cord that controls aspects of sympathetic nervous system function travels in the dorsolateral medulla (see Figure 15–1B; dashed circle). The sympathetic nervous system produces pupillary dilatation. Pupillary constriction occurs in the patient because of the loss of sympathetic drive to the ciliary muscle, and now, unopposed actions of the parasympathetic nervous system. Mild ptosis (termed pseudoptosis) is due to the loss of sympathetic control of smooth muscle that assists the mechanical action of the levator palpebrae muscle. Sweating is also a sympathetic nervous system function; its loss produces dryness. Loss of sympathetic vasoconstriction results in arterial vasodilation.

Reference

Brust JCM. *The Practice of Neural Science.* New York, NY: McGraw-Hill; 2000.

Choi K-D, Oh S-Y, Park S-H, Kim J-H, Koo J-W, Kim JS. Head-shaking nystagmus in lateral medullary infarction. *Neurology.* 2007;68:1337-1344.

Kim JS, Moon SY, Park S-H. Ocular lateropulsion in Wallenberg syndrome. *Neurology.* 2004;62:2287.

The hypothalamus is crucial for maintaining normal organ function and for producing many of the behaviors necessary to meet basic needs such as feeding, drinking, mating, and sleeping. The hypothalamus thus ensures survival of both the individual and its species. Virtually every body organ depends on the hypothalamus for some aspect of control, including the heart, lungs, gastrointestinal tract, and genitourinary organs. The hypothalamus helps organize the body's reactions to disease, such as fever production in response to infection. Skeletal muscle depends on the hypothalamus for regulating its blood supply; even bone mass seems to depend on hypothalamic regulation. In animals, the hypothalamus controls complex behaviors, like sexual responsiveness, maternal care (eg, nursing), and aggression. Whereas it can only be speculated how much of similar human behaviors depend on

the hypothalamus, it is now becoming clear that the hypothalamus is important in regulating aspects of human social behavior. The list goes on and on! Compared with just about every other region of the nervous system, each of which serves a small set of functions, the hypothalamus accomplishes a bewilderingly wide range of tasks. We will see that it does this largely by using information about the body's internal state, about emotions, and about critical environmental stimuli, to control hormone production and the autonomic nervous system, and to regulate the moment-to-moment functions of neural circuits for arousal.

This chapter first considers hypothalamic gross anatomy. Next, the chapter surveys its functional organization, highlighting several key aspects. Additional important functions of the hypothalamus are examined when we learn about its regional anatomy, later in the chapter. Chapter 16 revisits the hypothalamus and its role in motivational and appetitive behavior, along with other brain structures that comprise the limbic system for emotions.

Gross Anatomy of the Hypothalamus

The hypothalamus is a tiny diencephalic structure, about 1-cm square, that is located ventral and anterior to the thalamus (Figure 15–2). The third ventricle separates the two halves of the hypothalamus. On its medial, or ventricular, surface the hypothalamus is distinguished from the thalamus by a shallow groove, the **hypothalamic sulcus.** Anteriorly, part of the hypothalamus extends a bit beyond the anterior wall of the third ventricle. (The anterior wall of the third ventricle is the location of the most anterior portion of the developing central nervous system, or the lamina terminalis; Figure 15–2.) The hypothalamus reaches caudally, just beyond the mammillary bodies, paired hypothalamic nuclei on its ventral surface (Figure 15–3).

We will learn that the functions of the hypothalamus are organized by projection neurons in discrete nuclei, or small groups of nuclei, that interface with different effector systems and circuits in other parts of the central nervous system. These hypothalamic nuclei are arranged into three mediolateral zones, each with distinctive functions (Figures 15–3 and 15–4; Table 15–1):

1. The **periventricular zone** is the most medial and comprises thin nuclei that border the third ventricle. This zone is important in regulating the release of **endocrine hormones** from the anterior pituitary gland.

2. The **middle zone,** which is interposed between the periventricular and lateral zones, serves diverse functions. It contains nuclei that regulate the release of **vasopressin** and **oxytocin** from the posterior pituitary gland. It is also a major site for neurons that regulate the **autonomic nervous system.** The body's biological clock is set by neurons in this zone, as are aspects of the control of wakefulness.

3. The **lateral zone** is separated from the medial zone by the **fornix,** a C-shaped tract that interconnects limbic system structures (see Figure 1–11A). This zone contains neurons that integrate information from other hypothalamic nuclei and telencephalic structures engaged in emotions. This is also a region important for regulating sleep and wakefulness and feeding.

The nuclei of the hypothalamus are located at discrete anterior-posterior positions (Table 15–1). This describes an orthogonal regional organization that will be the basis for examining sections through the hypothalamus later in the chapter. Historically, this organization was stressed because scientists recognized distinctive differences between the functions of the anterior and posterior hypothalamus. Now, we recognize these differences in the context of discrete hypothalamic nuclei rather than its gross anatomy. Whereas the boundaries between the anterior-posterior regions are not precise, a general knowledge of their locations is essential for an understanding of the three-dimensional organization of the hypothalamus.

- The **anterior** part of the hypothalamus, located dorsal and rostral to the optic chiasm (see Figure 15–3, inset), includes the preoptic area, with its numerous preoptic nuclei. The preoptic area is sometimes considered separate from the hypothalamus. But because its functions are intimately related to other, more caudal, hypothalamic functions, it is best to consider them together. The principal nucleus for circadian rhythms is also located in the anterior hypothalamus.

- The **middle** hypothalamus is between the optic chiasm and the mammillary bodies. This portion contains the infundibular stalk, from which the pituitary gland arises. The nuclei for anterior and posterior pituitary hormone release are mostly located here.

- The **posterior** portion includes the mammillary bodies and nuclei dorsal to them.

Functional Anatomy of the Hypothalamus

Separate Parvocellular and Magnocellular Neurosecretory Systems Regulate Hormone Release From the Anterior and Posterior Lobes of the Pituitary

The pituitary gland is connected to the ventral surface of the hypothalamus by the **infundibular stalk** (Figure 15–4A). In humans, two major anatomical divisions of the pituitary gland mediate the release of distinct sets of hormones (Figure 15–5): the **anterior lobe** (also called the adenohypophysis; see Table 15–2) and the **posterior lobe** (or neurohypophysis). A third lobe, the intermediate lobe, although prominent in many simpler mammals, is vestigial in humans.

The anterior and posterior lobes are parts of two distinct neurosecretory systems, and hormone release from these lobes is regulated by different populations of hypothalamic neurons. The anterior lobe is part of the **parvocellular neurosecretory system** (Figure 15–5A). This system contains small-diameter hypothalamic neurons (hence the term parvocellular) that are located in numerous nuclei. They regulate hormone release by epithelial secretory cells of the anterior pituitary. Parvocellular neurosecretory neurons are located predominantly in nuclei of the **periventricular zone.** By contrast, the posterior lobe is part of the **magnocellular neurosecretory system** (Figure 15–5B). Here, axons of large-diameter hypothalamic neurons in two nuclei project to and release peptide hormones

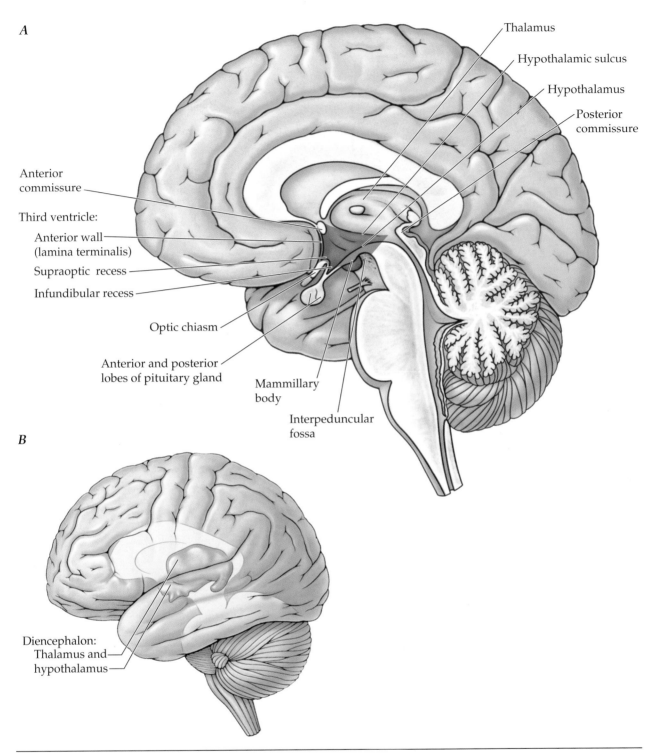

FIGURE 15–2 A. Midsagittal view of the brain, showing key structures in and around the hypothalamus. **B.** Semitransparent lateral surface of the cerebral hemisphere and brain stem, illustrating the location of the hypothalamus and thalamus.

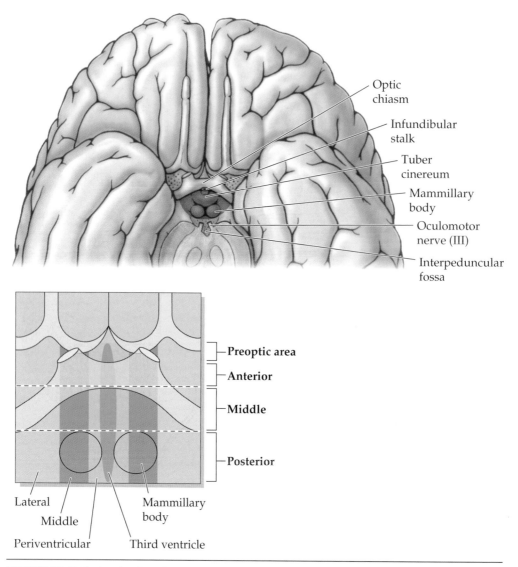

Optic
chiasm

Infundibular
stalk

Tuber
cinereum

Mammillary
body

Oculomotor
nerve (III)

Interpeduncular
fossa

Preoptic area

Anterior

Middle

Posterior

Lateral

Middle

Periventricular

Mammillary
body

Third ventricle

FIGURE 15–3 The basal surface of the brain showing the hypothalamus and nearby structures. The inset shows schematically the divisions of the hypothalamus in relation to the ventricle and anatomical landmarks.

into the posterior lobe. Rostrocaudally, parvocellular neurosecretory neurons are located in all the three hypothalamic regions, whereas the magnocellular neurosecretory neurons are mostly located in the middle zone.

Regulatory peptides released into the portal circulation by hypothalamic neurons control secretion of anterior lobe hormones

The process by which the hypothalamus stimulates anterior lobe secretory cells to release their hormones (or to inhibit release) is quite unlike mechanisms of neural action considered in earlier chapters. Rather than synapse on anterior lobe secretory cells, the hypothalamic parvocellular neurosecretory neurons terminate on capillaries of the **pituitary portal circulation** in the floor of the third ventricle (Figure 15–5A).

A portal circulatory system is distinguished by the presence of separate **portal veins** interposed between two sets of capillaries. The first set is located in a region termed the **median eminence,** which is part of the proximal infundibular stalk. The portal veins are located in the distal part of the infundibular stalk. The second set of capillaries is found in the anterior pituitary. (In the systemic circulation, such as the vascular supply of the rest of the brain, capillary beds are interposed between arterial and venous systems.)

Parvocellular neurons release chemicals, most of which are peptides, that either promote (**releasing hormones**) or inhibit (**release-inhibiting hormones**) the release of hormones from anterior lobe secretory cells (Table 15–2). Release or release-inhibiting hormones are carried to the anterior lobe in the portal veins (Figure 15–5A), where they act directly on epithelial secretory cells.

A

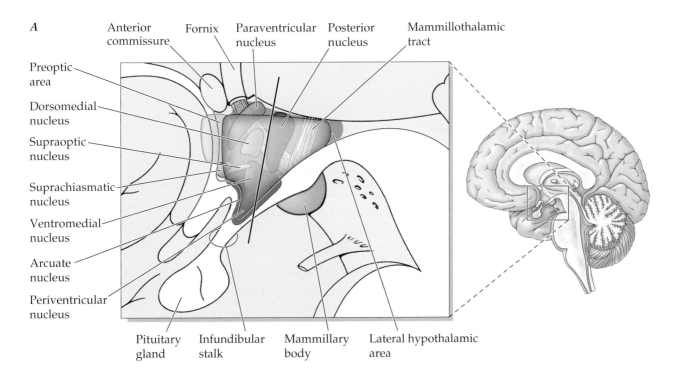

B

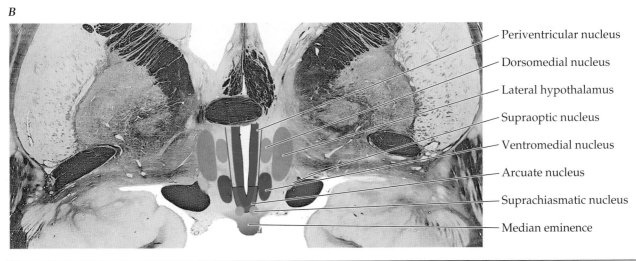

FIGURE 15–4   *A.* The major nuclei are illustrated in a cutaway view of the hypothalamus. The inset shows the region illustrated in the cross-sectional view (***B***). The arcuate and periventricular nuclei comprise the periventricular zone; they form a thin veil beneath the walls and floor of the third ventricle. The middle and lateral zones are the two other hypothalamic zones. The line shows the approximate plane of section in ***B***. ***B.*** Myelin-stained coronal section through the hypothalamus. The approximate locations of the key hypothalamic nuclei are shown. The periventricular and arcuate nuclei comprise the periventricular zone. The other nuclei form the middle and lateral hypothalamic zones.

An analogy can be drawn between the capillaries in the median eminence and the integrative function of spinal motor neurons (see Chapter 10). Separate descending pathways and spinal interneuronal systems synapse on the motor neuron. Thus, the motor neuron is the final common pathway for the integration of neuronal information controlling skeletal muscle. The final common pathway for control of anterior lobe hormone release comprises the capillaries of the median eminence. This is because different hypothalamic neurons secrete

releasing or release-inhibiting hormones into the capillaries of the median eminence (Figure 15–5A), and summation of neurohormones occurs at this vascular site.

The distribution of neurons that project to the median eminence has been examined extensively in rodents. Although these neurons are widespread, the major sources are located in nuclei within the **periventricular zone** (Figures 15–4 and 15–5A). Among the major sources, and some of the hormones they release, are the following:

Table **15–1**   The functions of major hypothalamic nuclei

Nucleus	Mediolateral zone	Key functions
Anterior Hypothalamus		
Preoptic nuclei:		
Ventrolateral	Lateral	Sleep-wakefulness
Medial	Periventricular	Parvocellular hormone control
	Middle	Thermoregulation
Middle Hypothalamus		
Paraventricular	Periventricular and middle	Magnocellular hormones (oxytocin, vasopressin); parvocellular; direct autonomic control, including urination
Supraoptic	Middle	Magnocellular hormones (oxytocin, vasopressin)
Arcuate	Periventricular	Parvocellular hormones; visceral functions
Suprachiasmatic	Middle	Circadian rhythm
Ventromedial	Middle	Appetitive/consummatory behaviors
Dorsomedial	Middle	Feeding, drinking, and body weight regulation
Periventricular	Periventricular	Parvocellular hormones
Posterior Hypothalamus		
Mammillary[a]		Memory
Tuberomammillary	Lateral	Sleep-wakefulness (histamine)
Lateral Hypothalamus[b]		
Lateral hypothalamic and perifornical areas	Lateral	Various, including arousal, food intake; contain orexin

[a]The mammillary bodies, while anatomically part of the hypothalamus, neither interconnect nor function with other hypothalamic nuclei. They are therefore not considered to be part of the medioloateral functional zones.

[b]The lateral hypothalamus is present throughout the rostrocaudal extent of the hypothalamus.

- The **arcuate nucleus** contains neurons that release gonadotropin-releasing hormone, luteinizing hormone–releasing hormone, somatostatin, and adrenocorticotropic hormone.

- Neurons in the **periventricular portion** of the **parvocellular nucleus** (the part that lies along the third ventricle) contain corticotropin-releasing hormone (CRH).

- The **periventricular nucleus** provides gonadotropin-releasing hormone, luteinizing hormone–releasing hormone, and dopamine (which inhibits prolactin release).

- The **medial preoptic area** contains parvocellular neurons that secrete luteinizing hormone–releasing hormone.

In addition, there are extrahypothalamic sources of releasing and release-inhibiting neurohormones. For example, the septal nuclei (see Chapter 16) are a source of gonadotropin-releasing hormone. Interestingly, many of these neurohormones are also found in hypothalamic neurons that do not project to the median eminence and in neurons in other regions of the central nervous system. This widespread distribution of neurohormones indicates that they are **neuroactive compounds** at these other sites and not just chemicals that regulate anterior pituitary hormone release. Individual neurons of the parvocellular system, as in the magnocellular system (see below), may synthesize and release more than one peptide. This peptide synthesis and release may be regulated by circulating hormones in the blood. This is one way in which environmental factors, such as prolonged exposure to stressful situations, may alter the neurohormonal composition in the portal circulation and thereby influence anterior pituitary hormone release. Note that the blood-brain barrier is less of an obstacle in the hypothalamus than in most other brain regions (see Figure 3–16B).

Hypothalamic neurons project to the posterior lobe and release vasopressin and oxytocin

Posterior pituitary hormones, **vasopressin** and **oxytocin,** are the neurosecretory products of hypothalamic neurons; they have diverse functions on body organs. The peptide vasopressin elevates blood pressure, for example, through its action on vascular smooth muscle. Vasopressin also promotes water reabsorption from the distal tubules of the kidney to reduce urine volume. Another name for vasopressin is **antidiuretic hormone** (sometimes called ADH). Oxytocin is a peptide

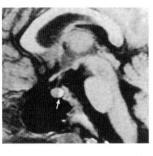

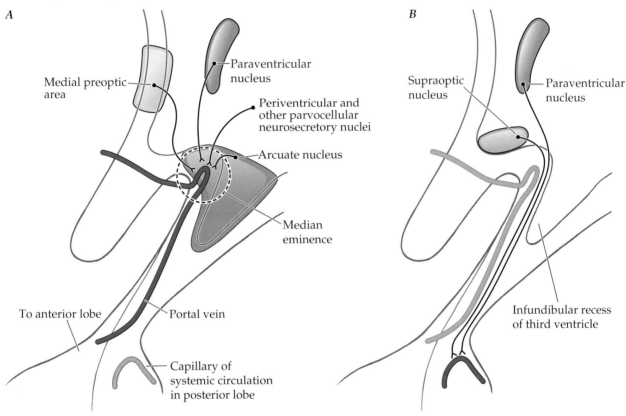

FIGURE 15–5   A. Parvocellular neurosecretory system. **B.** Magnocellular neurosecretory system. Inset shows an MRI that distinguishes the anterior and posterior pituitary lobes of the pituitary gland. (**A,** reproduced from Sartor K. *MR Imaging of the Skull and Brain.* New York, NY: Springer; 1992.)

Table **15–2** **Anterior pituitary hormones and substances that control their release**

Anterior pituitary hormones	Releasing hormones (RH)	Release-inhibiting hormones (RIH)
Growth hormone	Growth hormone RH	Somatostatin (growth hormone RIH)
Lutenizing hormone	Gonadotrophin RH	
Follicle-stimulating hormone	Gonadotrophin RH	
Thryotropin	Thryotropin RH (or TRH)	Somatostatin (growth hormone RIH)
Prolactin	Prolactin RH	Prolactin RIH; dopamine
Adrenocorticotropic hormone (ACTH)	Corticotropin RH (CRH)	
Melanocyte-stimulating hormone (MSH)	Melanocyte-stimulating hormone RH	Melanocyte-stimulating hormone RIH

with a chemical structure nearly identical to that of vasopressin, differing by amino acids at only two sites. Oxytocin is best known for its actions on female organs, where it functions to stimulate uterine contractions and to promote ejection of milk from the mammary glands. There are other important behavioral actions of vasopressin and oxytocin. Both are important for pair bonding in monogamous animals of both sexes, although most studies focus on oxytocin in females and vasopressin in males. Both peptides also are important in other aspects of social behavior, such as vasopressin in social recognition and oxytocin in formation of interpersonal trust.

In the hypothalamus, both vasopressin and oxytocin are synthesized primarily in two nuclei, the **paraventricular nucleus** and the **supraoptic nucleus** (Figure 15–5B). Experiments in animals have shown that the paraventricular nucleus comprises at least three distinct cell groups. As described earlier, there are parvocellular neurosecretory neurons in the portion of the nucleus that apposes the third ventricle. Lateral to these neurons are the **magnocellular neurosecretory neurons** that synthesize and release the two posterior lobe neurohormones. A third neuron group, typically considered magnocellular because of their morphology not hormonal function, gives rise to a descending brain stem and spinal projection for regulating autonomic nervous system functions (see next section). The supraoptic nucleus consists only of magnocellular neurosecretory neurons. However, a small number of oxytocin-containing neurons of both the paraventricular and supraoptic nuclei project to several other brain regions, where they are thought to regulate aspects of social behavior.

Both vasopressin and oxytocin are synthesized from larger prohormone molecules. The prohormone molecules from which vasopressin and oxytocin derive contain additional proteins, called **neurophysins.** It was once thought that vasopressin was synthesized in one nucleus and oxytocin in the other. With the use of immunocytochemical techniques, however, it has been established that different cells in each nucleus produce one or the other hormone.

The axons of the paraventricular and the supraoptic magnocellular neurons in the **infundibular stalk** (Figures 15–4A and 15–5B) do not make synaptic contacts with other neurons. Rather, they terminate on **fenestrated capillaries** in the **posterior lobe** of the pituitary. (Fenestrations, or pores, make capillaries leaky. Recall that the posterior lobe of the pituitary [see also Figure 3–16] is one of the brain regions lacking a blood-brain barrier. Thus, neurohormones can pass freely into the capillaries through the fenestrations.)

Immunocytochemical studies also have shown that magnocellular neurons, like their parvocellular counterparts, contain other peptides that act on neurons in the central nervous system and on peripheral organs. These other peptides also may be released into the circulation along with oxytocin or vasopressin and have coordinated actions on diverse structures. Vasopressin itself is an example of a brain peptide that has a diversity of coordinated functions at different sites. For example, it is a blood-borne hormone that influences the function of specific peripheral target organs, such as the kidney,

and it is a neuroactive peptide involved in control of the autonomic nervous system (see below).

An understanding of the projections from other brain regions to magnocellular hypothalamic neurons provides insight into how the brain controls neurohormone release. For example, magnocellular neurons that contain vasopressin are important for regulating blood volume. These neurons receive inputs from three key sources that each serve a related function.

- First, magnocellular neurons receive an indirect projection from the **solitary nucleus.** This pathway conveys **baroreceptor** input from the glossopharyngeal and vagus nerves (see Chapter 6) to the hypothalamus, providing important afferent signals for controlling blood pressure and blood volume.

- The second major input source is from two **circumventricular organs,** the **subfornical organ** and the **organum vasculosum of the lamina terminalis** (see Figure 3–16). The circumventricular organs do not have a blood-brain barrier. As discussed in Chapter 3, the blood-brain barrier is a specific permeability barrier between capillaries in the central nervous system and the extracellular space. This barrier protects the brain from the influence of many neuroactive chemicals circulating in the blood. Without a blood-brain barrier, neurons in subfornical organ and the organum vasculosum of the lamina terminalis are capable of sensing plasma osmolality and circulating chemicals and thereby can regulate blood pressure and blood volume through their hypothalamic projections.

- The **preoptic area** provides the third input to the magnocellular neurons. This region is implicated in the central neural mechanisms for regulating the composition and volume of body fluids and thus indirectly affects the control of blood pressure.

The Parasympathetic and Sympathetic Divisions of the Autonomic Nervous System Originate From Different Central Nervous System Locations

The hypothalamus regulates the **autonomic nervous system.** The autonomic nervous system controls several organ systems of the body: cardiovascular and respiratory, gastrointestinal, exocrine, and urogenital. Two divisions of the autonomic nervous system—the **parasympathetic** and **sympathetic nervous systems**—originate from different parts of the central nervous system. Similar to the control of skeletal muscle, visceral control by the sympathetic and parasympathetic systems relies on both relatively simple reflexes, involving the spinal cord and brain stem, and more complex control by higher levels of the central nervous system, especially the hypothalamus.

The **enteric nervous system** is sometimes considered a third division of the autonomic nervous system. It is located entirely in the periphery. This system provides the intrinsic innervation of the gastrointestinal tract and mediates the complex coordinated reflexes for peristalsis. It is thought that the enteric nervous system functions independent of the hypothalamus and the rest of the central nervous system.

The next section reviews the anatomical organization of the sympathetic and parasympathetic divisions. An understanding of how these autonomic divisions connect to their target organs is essential before considering their higher-order regulation by the hypothalamus.

Sympathetic and parasympathetic system innervation of body organs differs from the way the somatic nervous system innervates skeletal muscle

The innervation of skeletal muscle is mediated directly by motor neurons located in spinal and cranial nerve motor nuclei (Figure 15–6, left side of spinal cord). Further, skeletal muscle is controlled primarily by the contralateral cerebral cortex (Figure 15–6, red line) and various brain stem motor control nuclei (see Chapter 10). For the autonomic innervation of the viscera, two neurons link the central nervous system with organs in the periphery: the **preganglionic neuron** and the **postganglionic neuron**. Visceral control is mediated by the ipsilateral hypothalamus (Figure 15–6, black line) and brain stem nuclei. This is shown for the sympathetic nervous system in Figure 15–6 (right side of spinal cord; see Figure 11–4); more is known about the central control of the sympathetic than parasympathetic nervous system. The cell body of the sympathetic preganglionic neuron is located in the central nervous system, and its axon follows a tortuous course to the periphery. From the ventral root and through various peripheral neural conduits, the axon of the preganglionic neuron finally synapses on postganglionic neurons in **peripheral ganglia** (Figure 15–6). A notable exception is the adrenal medulla, which receives direct innervation by preganglionic sympathetic neurons. This exception is related to the fact that adrenal medullary cells, like postganglionic neurons, develop from the neural crest (see Chapter 6).

Two major differences exist in the neuroanatomical organization of the sympathetic and parasympathetic divisions (Figure 15–7). First is the location of the preganglionic neurons in the central nervous system; second is the location of the peripheral ganglia. **Sympathetic preganglionic neurons** are found in the intermediate zone of the spinal cord, between the first thoracic and third lumbar spinal cord segments. Most of the neurons are located in the **intermediolateral nucleus** (Figure 15–6) (also called the **intermediolateral cell column** because, like Clarke's column, this nucleus has an extensive rostrocaudal organization; Figure 15–7, left).

In contrast, **parasympathetic preganglionic neurons** are found in the brain stem and the second through fourth sacral spinal cord segments (Figure 15–7, right). The general organization of the parasympathetic brain stem nuclei was described in Chapter 11 in the discussion of cranial nerve nuclei. Most brain stem preganglionic neurons are located in four nuclei:

(1) Edinger-Westphal nucleus, (2) superior salivatory nucleus, (3) inferior salivatory nucleus, and (4) dorsal motor nucleus of the vagus. Others are scattered in the reticular formation. The parasympathetic preganglionic neurons in the sacral spinal cord are found in the intermediate zone, at sites analogous to those of sympathetic preganglionic neurons.

The second major difference in the neuroanatomy of the sympathetic and parasympathetic divisions is the location of the peripheral ganglia in which the postganglionic neurons are located. Parasympathetic ganglia, often called **terminal ganglia,** are located on or near their target organs. In contrast, sympathetic ganglia are found closer to the spinal cord. Postganglionic sympathetic neurons are located in **paravertebral ganglia,** which are part of the sympathetic trunk, and in **prevertebral ganglia** (Figure 15–7).

Hypothalamic nuclei regulate the functions of the autonomic nervous system through descending visceromotor pathways

The autonomic nervous system implements important aspects of hypothalamic control of body functions. How does the hypothalamus regulate the functions of the autonomic nervous system? The answer, perhaps surprising, is related to how the brain controls voluntary movement. As discussed in Chapter 10, distinct areas of the cerebral cortex and brain stem nuclei give rise to the descending motor pathways that regulate the excitability of motor neurons and interneurons (Figure 15–6). These spinal projections transmit control signals to steer voluntary movements and regulate spinal reflexes. Visceral motor functions—mediated by the autonomic nervous system—are subjected to a similar control by the brain (Figure 15–6). The descending autonomic pathways originate from the hypothalamus and various brain stem nuclei. The major hypothalamic nucleus for controlling sympathetic and parasympathetic functions is the **paraventricular nucleus** (Figure 15–8). The neurotransmitters used by this pathway include glutamate and the peptides **vasopressin and oxytocin,** the same peptides released by the magnocellular neurosecretory system. The neurons giving rise to the descending pathway, however, are distinct from those projecting to the posterior pituitary. Other hypothalamic sites contribute axons to the descending visceromotor pathways. These areas include neurons in the lateral hypothalamic zone, the dorsomedial hypothalamic nucleus, and the posterior hypothalamus. The visceromotor pathway descends laterally—and primarily ipsilaterally—through the hypothalamus in the **medial forebrain bundle,** which is located in the lateral zone. The descending axons leave the bundle and then run in the **dorsolateral tegmentum** in the midbrain, pons, and medulla (Figure 15–8). As is discussed below, lesions of the dorsolateral brain stem tegmentum can produce characteristic autonomic changes because of damage to these descending hypothalamic axons. The descending autonomic pathway synapses on brain stem parasympathetic nuclei, such as the dorsal motor nucleus of the vagus, spinal sympathetic neurons in the intermediolateral nucleus of the

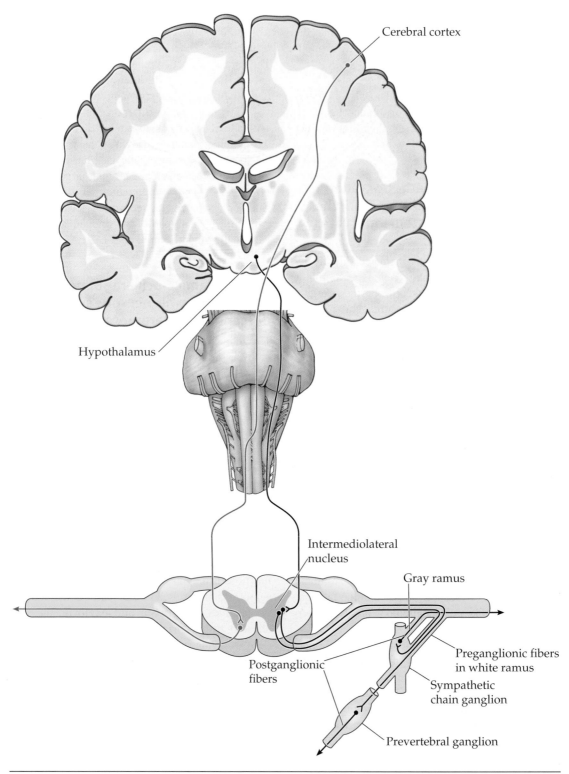

Cerebral cortex

Hypothalamus

Intermediolateral nucleus

Gray ramus

Postganglionic fibers

Preganglionic fibers in white ramus

Sympathetic chain ganglion

Prevertebral ganglion

FIGURE 15–6 The circuits for skeletal muscle control and visceral organ innervation by the sympathetic nervous system. For the viscera, control is exerted primarily from the hypothalamus. Preganglionic sympathetic autonomic neurons are located in the intermediate zone of the spinal cord. Their axons exit the spinal cord through the ventral roots and project to ganglia in the sympathetic trunk (paravertebral ganglia) through the spinal nerves and white rami. The axons of postganglionic neurons in the sympathetic ganglia course to the periphery through the rami and spinal nerves. The white and gray rami contain, respectively, the myelinated and unmyelinated axons of preganglionic and postganglionic autonomic neurons. A postganglionic neuron in a prevertebral ganglion is also shown with input from a preganglionic neuron. For somatic muscle control, control derives from the descending motor paths; the corticospinal tract is shown. Muscle is innervated directly by motor neurons in the ventral horn. Note that for skeletal muscle control, only the direct path from the cerebral cortex to motor neurons is shown. In addition, there are indirect paths that relay in the brain stem and via spinal cord interneurons.

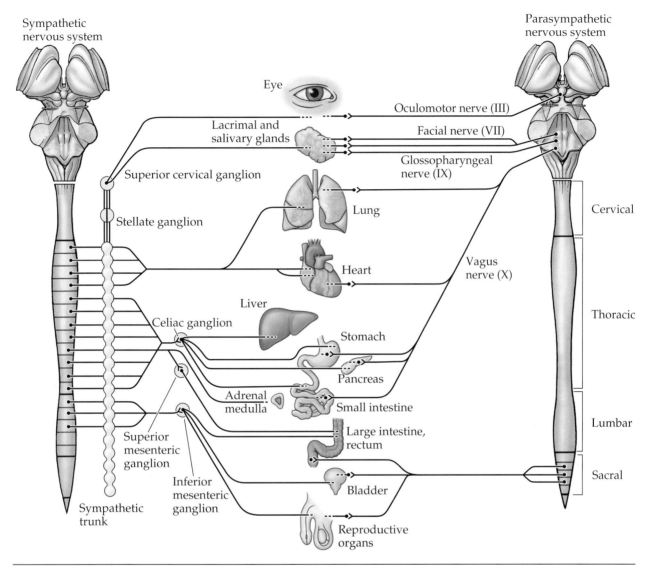

FIGURE 15–7 Organization of the autonomic nervous system. The sympathetic nervous system is shown at left, and the parasympathetic nervous system is shown at right. Note that the postganglionic neurons for the sympathetic nervous system are located in sympathetic trunk ganglia and prevertebral ganglia (eg, celiac ganglion). The postganglionic neurons for the parasympathetic nervous system are located in terminal ganglia close to the target organ. (Adapted from Schmidt RF, Thews G, eds. *Human Physiology*. 2nd ed. Berlin, Heidelberg: Springer-Verlag; 1989.)

thoracic and lumbar segments, and spinal parasympathetic neurons in the sacral cord (Figure 15–8).

The visceral and somatic motor systems communicate with one another to mediate coordinated responses. When we are preparing to increase muscular exertion, there are anticipatory increases in blood pressure and heart rate. There is evidence that some somatic motor control centers, in addition to projecting to spinal somatic muscle control regions, also project to the intermediolateral nucleus to help coordinate visceral and vascular responses with skeletal muscle contraction. Many of the brain stem nuclei described earlier, including the solitary and parabrachial, receive convergent connections from centers controlling somatic muscle and visceral structures, such as the kidney. This is a way to make sure that metabolic byproducts of muscular action are properly excreted.

Hypothalamic Nuclei Coordinate Integrated Visceral Responses to Body and Environmental Stimuli

Most bodily functions necessary for survival have important hypothalamic control. So far, this chapter has considered the substrates for basic hypothalamic control of endocrine hormone release (both anterior and posterior pituitary) and visceromotor control by the autonomic nervous system. The hypothalamus also plays a key role in coordinating endocrine and autonomic control, together with somatic motor functions, to produce highly integrated and purposeful responses. The hypothalamus engages in five major integrative functions, each with clear neuroanatomical substrates: (1) regulation of blood pressure and body fluid electrolyte composition, (2)

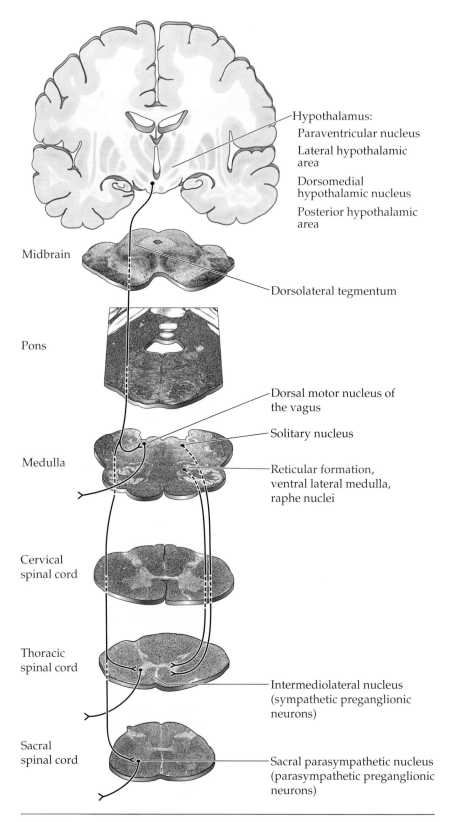

FIGURE 15–8 Regions of origin, course, and termination sites of descending hypothalamic pathways.

temperature regulation, (3) regulation of energy metabolism, (4) reproductive functions, and (5) organization of a rapid response to emergency situations. For each of these regulatory functions, the hypothalamus senses environmental or body signals and uses this information, first, to organize an appropriate response and, then, to command other brain regions to implement the response. Complex environmental stimuli, such as recognizing a threatening situation or assessing the social context, require extensive processing by telencephalic structures, including the amygdala and the cerebral cortex. This information, which is transmitted to the hypothalamus, can trigger organized and stereotypic behavioral and visceral responses.

Five major brain stem structures work together with the hypothalamus to help regulate the autonomic nervous system and coordinate responses. They do so by projecting to other brain stem viscerosensory and visceromotor nuclei, as well as by projecting directly to brain stem and spinal cord sympathetic and parasympathetic nuclei.

- The **solitary nucleus** (see Figure 15–13C) relays viscerosensory information from the glossopharyngeal and vagus nerves to the hypothalamus, as well as to the parabrachial nucleus (see Figure 15–13B), the thalamus, and other forebrain structures (see Chapter 6). It also has a component that projects directly to the intermediolateral nucleus.

- The **parabrachial nucleus** receives viscerosensory information from the solitary nucleus and, in turn, projects to diverse forebrain centers involved in various homeostatic functions, such as food and water intake. The parabrachial nucleus connects with the paraventricular and other hypothalamic nuclei.

- Neurons in the **ventrolateral medulla** (see Figure 15–13C) give rise to an **adrenergic projection** to brain stem and spinal autonomic nuclei. These neurons play an important role in regulating blood pressure.

- Neurons of the **pontomedullary reticular formation** have dense projections to autonomic preganglionic neurons in the brain stem and spinal cord. Because many of these neurons also project to spinal motor and premotor neurons, they may coordinate complex behavioral responses such as defense reactions that involve both visceral and somatic changes. For example, when you are startled by an unexpected, loud noise, many of your skeletal muscles respond and your blood pressure rises.

- The serotonergic **dorsal raphe nucleus** receives strong inputs from the hypothalamus and provides serotonin throughout the forebrain. Other, more caudally located raphe nuclei project to spinal and brain stem autonomic nuclei. One function of the raphespinal system is to suppress dorsal horn pain transmission (see Chapter 5) in relation to the individual's emotional state.

The Hypothalamus Coordinates Circadian Responses, Sleep, and Wakefulness

Sleep is a recurring change in the functional state of the brain, a state in which responsiveness is reduced. A decreased ability to react to stimuli distinguishes sleep from quiet wakefulness. Sleep impacts many bodily functions, such as respiration and metabolism; also, we are usually immobile during sleep, indicating an important influence over somatic muscle control. Sleep is essential. No species is known not to sleep. Without sleep, people and animals suffer dearly; ultimately sleep deprivation is fatal. Given the importance of sleep to the individual, it is not surprising that the hypothalamus plays a central role in its regulation. As sleep impacts so many bodily functions, the integrated capacity for the hypothalamus to regulate neuroendocrine, autonomic, and somatic functions makes it well suited for regulating wakefulness.

Circadian signals from the suprachiasmatic nucleus regulate sleep and wakefulness through connections with other hypothalamic nuclei

The hypothalamus is the brain region essential for establishing the circadian functions of the body, including sleep and wakefulness. It does so through connections within the hypothalamus as well as descending projections to brain stem structures that regulate arousal and motor control, on the one hand, and ascending projections to telencephalic structures for cognition and emotion, on the other. The brain's clock is in the **suprachiasmatic nucleus** of the hypothalamus (Figure 15–9A), located directly above the optic chiasm. The actions of neurons in this nucleus are governed by a genetically-controlled molecular circadian clock. All neurons in this nucleus keep the same time, a time that is set by daylight signals arising directly by connections from a unique class of retinal ganglion neuron that contain the photopigment melanopsin. Recall, light sensitivity of most retinal ganglion neurons is conferred by the input from photoreceptors, relayed by bipolar neurons (see Figure 7–7). The suprachiasmatic nucleus, in turn, connects with other hypothalamic neurons, so that their functions are entrained to the circadian rhythm. For example, diurnal regulation of melatonin from the pineal gland occurs through a projection to the paraventricular nucleus to regulate the sympathetic nervous system, which projects to the pineal gland (Figure 15–9A).

The preoptic area helps switch from wakefulness to sleep

The key hypothalamic region for switching from wakefulness to sleep is the preoptic area sleep center (Figure 15–9B), in particular the ventral lateral preoptic nucleus. Many preoptic neurons that regulate sleep are GABAergic. Through their connections, they are thought to inhibit brain stem neurons

A. Circadian rhythms

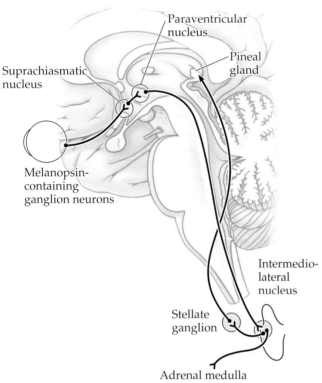

B. Sleep and wakefulness

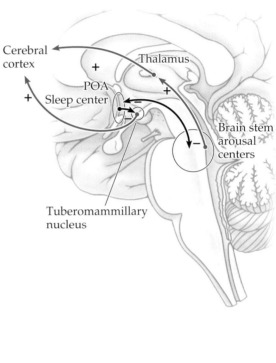

C. REM sleep

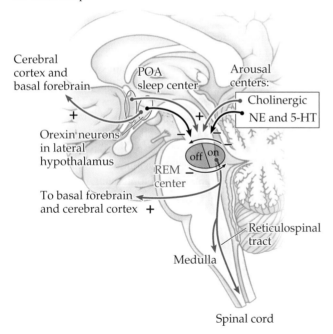

FIGURE 15–9 Sleep circuits of the brain. **A.** Circadian rhythms and the suprachiasmatic nucleus. The suprachiasmatic nucleus receives visual information that sets the clock. This nucleus projects to other hypothalamic nuclei to implement circadian functions. This example is for circadian control of melatonin release from the pineal gland. **B.** Preoptic area (POA) sleep center and sleep and wakefulness. The principal component of the preoptic sleep center is the ventrolateral preoptic nucleus. This nucleus is key to the switch from wakefulness to sleep. The preoptic nucleus acts on the brain stem arousal center, which includes the cholinergic pedunculopontine nucleus, the serotonergic dorsal raphe nucleus, and the noradrenergic locus ceruleus. This is shown as the negative sign by the brain stem-directed arrow in the arousal center. **C.** Rapid eye movement (REM) sleep control is extraordinarily complex, regulated by orexin neurons in the lateral hypothalamus, the preoptic sleep center, and several brain stem nuclei comprising the brain stem arousal center. The plus signs indicate structures that promote entry into REM sleep, whereas the negative signs indicate structures that retard entry.

that maintain arousal. The preoptic sleep center also has dense connections with the **tuberomammillary nucleus** of the hypothalamus, which uses **histamine** as its neurotransmitter to activate neurons in wide areas of the forebrain. Recall that a common side effect of antihistamines for allergic reactions is drowsiness. The preoptic sleep center also connects with brain stem nuclei important for arousal, including the locus ceruleus and the dorsal raphe nucleus (see Chapter 2, Figure 2–3), which use noradrenaline and 5-HT, respectively. Another component of the brain stem arousal center is the **pedunculopontine nucleus,** which uses acetylcholine as its neurotransmitter. Through projections especially to the thalamus, cholinergic neurons of the pedunculopontine nucleus help to activate thalamocortical circuits. Recall that the pedunculopontine nucleus is a target for deep brain stimulation in Parkinson disease, where it is used predominantly in ameliorating bradykinesia. When these various brain stem arousal nuclei are inhibited by the preoptic sleep center (brain stem-directed arrow, Figure 15–9), the arousal level of the brain decreases, and this helps to bring on sleep. Many of its brain stem targets, in turn, inhibit the preoptic sleep center (hypothalamus-directed arrow, Figure 15–9); this inhibition is thought to enable the brain to switch back into wakefulness.

Orexin neurons in the lateral hypothalamus help switch from non-REM to REM sleep

While we sleep, we cycle through different stages, or depths. One sleep stage is called rapid eye movement or **REM sleep.** Most of our dreams are during REM sleep. In addition to the occurrence of rapid eye movements during dreaming, REM sleep is also characterized by muscle atonia and a paradoxically high level of forebrain arousal (ie, the electroencephalogram, or EEG, is desynchronized). Muscle atonia prevents us from acting out our dreams. REM sleep is orchestrated by antagonistic sets of REM-on and REM-off neurons in the REM sleep center in the rostral pontine tegmentum (Figure 15–9C). REM-on neurons drive forebrain activity up—likely contributing to dreaming—and trigger muscle atonia, through direct and indirect reticulospinal projections that inhibit motor neurons. Importantly, motor neurons for respiratory muscles are not inhibited. REM-off neurons have the opposite functions.

The switch from non-REM to REM sleep is under important hypothalamic and brain stem regulation. Cholinergic neurons in the brain stem arousal center promote entry into REM sleep, while serotonergic and noradrenergic brain stem arousal neurons inhibit entry (Figure 15–9C). The hypothalamus also has antagonistic control. The preoptic sleep center helps turn on REM sleep (Figure 15–9C). Another set of hypothalamic neurons in the lateral hypothalamus that contain the peptide **orexin** inhibits entry into REM sleep. Not surprisingly, orexin neurons also have diverse forebrain projections that are important in maintaining arousal, just like their hypothalamic and brain stem counterparts that use histamine, acetylcholine, 5-HT, and noradrenaline.

Orexin may be central to the sleep disorder **narcolepsy.** Narcolepsy is a condition in which the person suddenly experiences excessive daytime sleepiness. One of the signs of narcolepsy is sudden switch from waking to sleep atonia, termed **cataplexy.** Often, the switch is triggered by a strong emotion, such as laughing. Mutation in an orexin receptor produces narcolepsy in animals. Some people with narcolepsy have reduced numbers of orexin-containing neurons in the brain, suggesting that orexin is associated with this sleep disorder. It has been suggested that narcolepsy could be an autoimmune disease in which the immune system mistakes orexin receptors for a foreign protein.

Regional Anatomy of the Hypothalamus

We now consider the regional anatomy of the hypothalamus from rostral to caudal. Three levels are considered, through the anterior, middle, and posterior parts of the hypothalamus. Then we will follow the descending visceromotor projection into the brain stem and spinal cord.

The Preoptic Area Influences Release of Reproductive Hormones From the Anterior Pituitary

The preoptic area is the most anterior part of the hypothalamus (Figures 15–4 and 15–10). It contains many small nuclei that serve five key functions. First, neurons in the medial preoptic area contain gonadotropin-releasing hormone. These neurons are believed to regulate pituitary reproductive hormone release because they project to the **median eminence.** Second, nuclei in the medial preoptic area and anterior hypothalamus of animals show sexual dimorphism (ie, morphological differences in males and females). In rats, gender affects the size of a sexually dimorphic nucleus as well as the architecture of neurons within the nucleus. Moreover, the size of this nucleus is dependent on perinatal exposure to gonadal steroids. This is an interesting example of how sexual differentiation alters brain morphology. In humans, identification of sexual dimorphism in the hypothalamus and other forebrain regions is controversial, with evidence existing for and against sex differences in the preoptic area and anterior hypothalamus. Part of the problem in identifying sex differences is that the human preoptic area has a complex organization, with numerous small and sometimes poorly differentiated nuclei. One of the nuclei reported to show sexual dimorphism in the human is part of the interstitial nuclei of the anterior hypothalamus, a small nucleus located at the level of the section shown in Figure 15–10. A third function of the preoptic area, discussed earlier, is in regulating sleep and wakefulness (Figure 15–9). Fourth, the preoptic area is important for regulating urination (discussed in a later section). Finally, the preoptic area, along with the posterior hypothalamus, is involved in thermoregulation. Neural circuits in the preoptic area dissipate heat, through coordinated actions on the autonomic nervous system, to produce vasodilation and increased sweating, and,

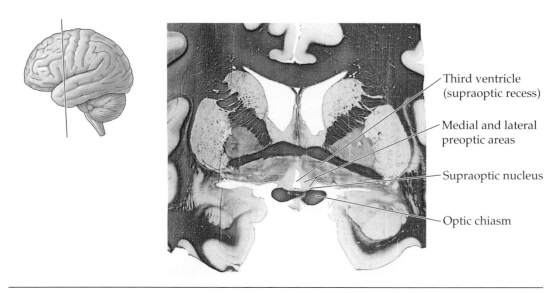

Third ventricle (supraoptic recess)

Medial and lateral preoptic areas

Supraoptic nucleus

Optic chiasm

FIGURE 15–10 Myelin-stained coronal section through the anterior hypothalamus, showing the preoptic area. The inset shows the plane of section.

in animals, on the somatic motor system, to promote panting. By contrast, the posterior hypothalamus is involved in heat conservation (see section on posterior hypothalamus).

The **suprachiasmatic nucleus** is located dorsal to the optic chiasm. As discussed earlier, neurons in the suprachiasmatic nucleus act as circadian clocks. They receive a direct projection from the **retina—the retinohypothalamic tract—** thereby allowing visual stimuli to synchronize (or reset) the internal clock (or circadian rhythm) of the body. The clinical significance of normal circadian rhythms and the function of the suprachiasmatic nucleus are just beginning to be appreciated. For example, defects in circadian rhythms are believed to underlie some sleep disorders and certain forms of depression, notably **seasonal affective disorder.**

Section Through the Median Eminence Reveals Parvocellular and Magnocellular Nuclei

The three mediolateral zones are shown schematically in Figure 15–11B, which is a coronal section through the proximal portion of the infundibular stalk. The infundibular stalk connects the basal hypothalamic surface with the pituitary gland. The **median eminence,** which contains the primary capillaries of the hypophyseal portal system, is located in the proximal portion of the infundibular stalk (Figure 15–4). Recall that the blood-brain barrier is absent in the median eminence (see Figure 3–16). As discussed, parvocellular neurosecretory neurons project to the median eminence. Releasing and release-inhibiting hormones secreted by the parvocellular neurosecretory neurons pass directly into the portal circulation through fenestrations, or pores, in the capillaries of the median eminence. Portal veins carry releasing and release-inhibiting

hormones to the anterior lobe of the pituitary. Note that the lobes of the pituitary gland have different developmental histories. The anterior lobe is of nonneural **ectodermal** origin, developing from a diverticulum in the roof of the developing oral cavity, called **Rathke's pouch.** In contrast, the posterior lobe develops from the **neuroectoderm.** Early in development, the ectodermal and neuroectodermal portions fuse to form a single structure.

The **arcuate nucleus** is located in the periventricular hypothalamic region (Figure 15–4). Parvocellular neurons in the arcuate nucleus contain various releasing and release-inhibiting hormones. In addition, many neurons in the arcuate nucleus contain β-**endorphin,** an endogenous opiate cleaved from the large peptide **proopiomelanocortin.** Some of these neurons may play a role in opiate analgesia because they project to the periaqueductal gray matter, where electrical stimulation produces analgesia (see Chapter 5). Neurons in the arcuate nucleus are sensitive to three circulating hormones that play important roles in the control of feeding: insulin, leptin, and ghrelin. Because the blood-brain barrier in the arcuate nucleus is weak compared to most other brain regions, circulating peptides have access to arcuate neurons. **Insulin,** produced by the pancreas, circulates in relation to body energy balance (ie, the difference between energy consumed and energy expended). **Leptin** is produced by adipocytes in proportion to the amount of body fat. Both leptin and insulin are signals that act to inhibit food intake and increase energy expenditure. Both are normally available during times of plenty. Reductions in leptin and insulin, usually signaling anorexia, are stimuli to increase food intake and inhibit energy expenditure. **Ghrelin,** which is produced by **enteroendocrine cells** of the stomach, promotes feeding. Fasting stimulates its release; therefore, it has the opposite effects of insulin and

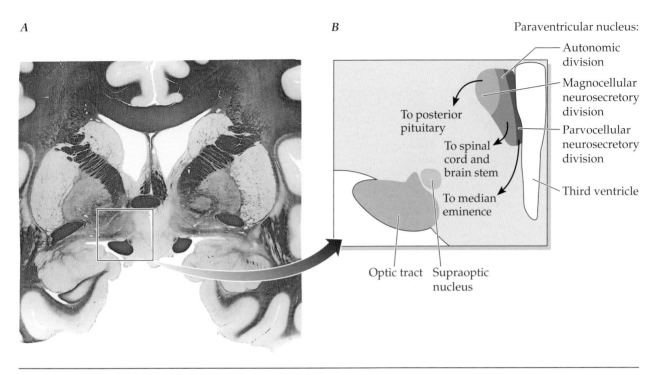

FIGURE 15–11 **A.** Myelin-stained coronal section through the infundibular stalk. **B.** Paraventricular nucleus organization.

leptin. In addition, neurons in the **arcuate nucleus** contain peptide neurotransmitters that have strong effects on feeding. For example, neuropeptide Y is contained in arcuate neurons and promotes feeding when injected intracerebrally into laboratory animals. Another major nucleus important in feeding is located in the rostrocaudal middle of the hypothalamus, the **ventromedial hypothalamic nucleus** (Figure 15–4). This nucleus receives input from a major limbic system structure, the **amygdala** (see Chapter 16). The ventral medial hypothalamus is also involved in regulating other appetite and consummatory behaviors.

Magnocellular neurosecretory cells of the paraventricular and supraoptic nuclei (Figure 15–11) project to the posterior lobe of the pituitary gland to release vasopressin and oxytocin onto systemic capillaries in the posterior lobe of the pituitary (Figure 15–5B). The axons travel down the infundibular stalk to contact capillaries that are part of the systemic circulation in the posterior lobe. Damage to the infundibular stalk, such as after traumatic head injury, may cut the axons of magnocellular neurosecretory cells as they pass to the posterior pituitary. This damage results in **diabetes insipidus,** in which excessive amounts of urine are produced. Fortunately the condition can be temporary because the cells are capable of forming a new, functional posterior lobe with nearby capillaries.

In addition to projecting to the posterior pituitary lobe, the paraventricular and supraoptic nuclei project to other brain regions. Importantly, both of these nuclei also use vasopressin and oxytocin at these other synapses. Recall that the paraventricular nucleus has a complex organization. In addition to the

magnocellular division, it contains a **parvocellular** division that projects to the median eminence and an **autonomic division** that projects to brain stem and spinal cord nuclei containing autonomic preganglionic neurons (Figure 15–11B). Many neurons in each subdivision contain vasopressin or oxytocin. Release of vasopressin or oxytocin at the various target sites of neurons in the paraventricular nucleus may serve similar sets of functions. For example, vasopressin can be used by the projections of the paraventricular nucleus to the medulla, for regulating blood pressure, and the projections to the interme-diolateral nucleus, for regulating blood volume by the kidney. The supraoptic nucleus also comprises vasopressin- and oxytocin-containing neurons and, like the paraventricular nucleus, also has projections to sites other than the posterior lobe. For example, some oxytocin-containing neurons of the supraoptic nucleus project to the nucleus accumbens; this projection is part of a reward circuit. Oxytocin-containing neurons are not just located in the paraventricular and supraoptic nuclei; they are also located in the lateral hypothalamus and the bed nucleus of the stria terminalis, a component of the limbic system (see Chapter 16). Note that while there are magnocellular neurons with diverse projections, only neurons that project to the posterior pituitary lobe are considered magnocellular **neurosecretory** cells.

Many hypothalamic neurons in the lateral zone (see Figure 15–12B) also have widespread projections to the cerebral cortex. One population of lateral hypothalamic neurons is particularly intriguing because the neurons contain peptides, termed **orexins** (or termed hypocretins), that, as discussed

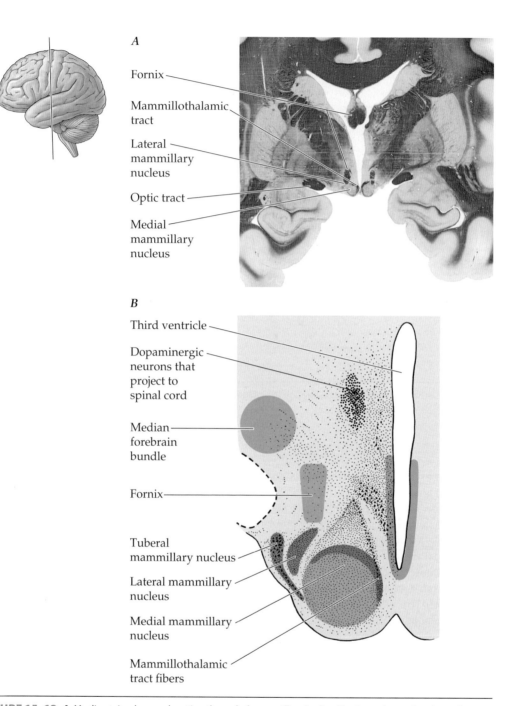

A

Fornix

Mammillothalamic tract

Lateral mammillary nucleus

Optic tract

Medial mammillary nucleus

B

Third ventricle

Dopaminergic neurons that project to spinal cord

Median forebrain bundle

Fornix

Tuberal mammillary nucleus

Lateral mammillary nucleus

Medial mammillary nucleus

Mammillothalamic tract fibers

FIGURE 15–12 **A.** Myelin-stained coronal section through the mamillary bodies. The inset shows the plane of section. **B.** Schematic drawing of Nissl-stained section through the posterior hypothalamus and mammillary bodies. Green shading indicates the periventricular zone.

earlier, are essential for regulating sleep and arousal. The lateral hypothalamus is also important in feeding and food-seeking behavior. Lesions of the lateral hypothalamus in laboratory animals can cause reduced food intake and weight loss. This role in food intake also involves the orexin neurons. In addition to being the only brain area that contains orexin, the lateral hypothalamus is the only site containing neurons with **melanin-concentrating hormone,** another factor important in feeding behavior.

The Posterior Hypothalamus Contains the Mammillary Bodies

A section through the posterior hypothalamus reveals the mammillary nuclei (or bodies) (Figure 15–12). Each mammillary body contains two nuclei: the prominent **medial mammillary nucleus** and the smaller lateral mammillary nucleus. Remarkably, the mammillary bodies establish virtually no intrahypothalamic connections. By contrast, most other hypothalamic nuclei have extensive intrahypothalamic connections. This shows that the function of the mammillary bodies is unlike that of the other hypothalamic nuclei. They receive their major input from a portion of the hippocampal formation, via the **fornix** (Figures 15–4 and 15–12A; see Chapter 16). The efferent projections of the mammillary bodies are carried primarily in the **mammillothalamic tract,** which projects to the anterior nuclei of the thalamus (see Figure AII–19). The mammillary bodies also have a descending projection to the midbrain and pons, the **mammillotegmental tract.** Whereas the mammillothalamic tract originates from the medial and lateral mammillary nuclei, the mammillotegmental tract originates only from the lateral nucleus. The outputs of the mammillary bodies are considered part of the limbic system and are discussed further in Chapter 16.

Another nucleus in the posterior hypothalamus, the **tuberomammillary nucleus** (Figure 15–12B), contains histamine. Like the brain stem monoamine systems, noradrenalin, dopamine, and serotonin, histaminergic neurons in the tuberomammillary nucleus have widespread projections. This system is important in maintaining arousal. Blockade of histamine reduces cortical neuronal responsiveness, and antihistamine therapy in humans can produce drowsiness if the drug crosses the blood-brain barrier. The tuberomammillary nucleus is important in regulating sleep and wakefulness (Figure 15–9).

Other nuclei within the posterior hypothalamus do not contribute in a major way to neuroendocrine function. Rather, this region plays a role in regulating autonomic functions and mediating integrated behavioral responses to environmental stimuli. For example, the posterior hypothalamus is important in conserving body heat, which includes promoting vasoconstriction and shivering in response to low temperatures. This is also the only region to contain dopaminergic neurons that project directly to the spinal cord. Whereas the normal functions of these neurons are not yet known, loss of this dopaminergic projection has been implicated in **restless legs syndrome,** a disorder in which patients experience abnormal sensations in their legs that prompt the urge to move their legs to quell the sensation. The abnormal sensations and movements are more common during rest and sleep.

Descending Autonomic Fibers Course in the Periaqueductal Gray Matter and in the Lateral Tegmentum

Hypothalamic regulation of the autonomic nervous system is mediated, in large part, by descending projections to four sets of neurons: (1) brain stem parasympathetic nuclei, (2) brain stem visceral integrative nuclei (solitary nuclei, ventrolateral medulla, and parabrachial nucleus; Figure 15–13C), (3) sympathetic neurons in the intermediolateral nucleus in thoracic and lumbar spinal segments (see Figure 15–15A), and (4) parasympathetic neurons in the intermediate zone of the sacral spinal cord (see Figure 15–15B). The major path from the hypothalamus taken by the descending autonomic pathway

is through the **medial forebrain bundle** (MFB), which is in the lateral zone (Figure 15–12B). This path is a conduit for axons from diverse sources, including ascending and descending connections between the brain stem, the hypothalamus, and the cerebral hemisphere. Neurons in the lateral zone tend not to be organized into distinct nuclei but rather are interspersed along the MFB. The MFB becomes dispersed in the brain stem, where the descending autonomic pathway courses in the lateral tegmentum (Figure 15–13A). (The term *medial forebrain bundle* is reserved for the portion in the hypothalamus only.) The Edinger-Westphal nucleus, which contains parasympathetic preganglionic neurons innervating the ciliary ganglion, is located at this level.

Another hypothalamic pathway, the **dorsal longitudinal fasciculus,** contains ascending viscerosensory and descending fibers. This pathway courses within the gray matter along the wall of the third ventricle, in the midbrain periaqueductal gray matter and the gray matter in the floor of the fourth ventricle. Although diffuse in the diencephalon and midbrain, fibers constituting this pathway can be identified in the pons and in the medulla (in the dorsal portion of the hypoglossal nucleus; Figure 15–13C).

Nuclei in the Pons Are Important for Bladder Control

The pons is an important site for bladder control, receiving control signals from the preoptic area: Neurons in the **medial preoptic area** project to a cluster of neurons in the dorsolateral pons that trigger **urination.** These neurons project to the parasympathetic bladder motor neurons and interneurons that inhibit urethral sphincter motor neurons. Separate pontine neurons, located laterally and ventrally, that excite urethral sphincter motor neurons are implicated in circuitry to prevent urination (ie, sphincter contraction). A positron emission tomography (PET) scan obtained while a human subject urinated is shown in Figure 15–14A, whereas a scan from a subject who was unable to voluntarily urinate during the scan—presumably because sphincter tone was too high—is shown in Figure 15–14B. These two scans reveal two distinct regions of the pons that control urination. Surprisingly, only the right pons became activated, suggesting cerebral lateralization of this function.

Dorsolateral Brain Stem Lesions Interrupt Descending Sympathetic Fibers

Several key structures for controlling the autonomic nervous system are located in the medulla (Figure 15–13C). The **dorsal motor nucleus of the vagus** contains parasympathetic preganglionic neurons that innervate the various terminal ganglia. This nucleus was considered in Chapter 11. The **solitary nucleus,** considered in Chapter 6, is the major brain stem relay for visceral afferent fibers. Different populations of projection neurons in the solitary nucleus ascend to the

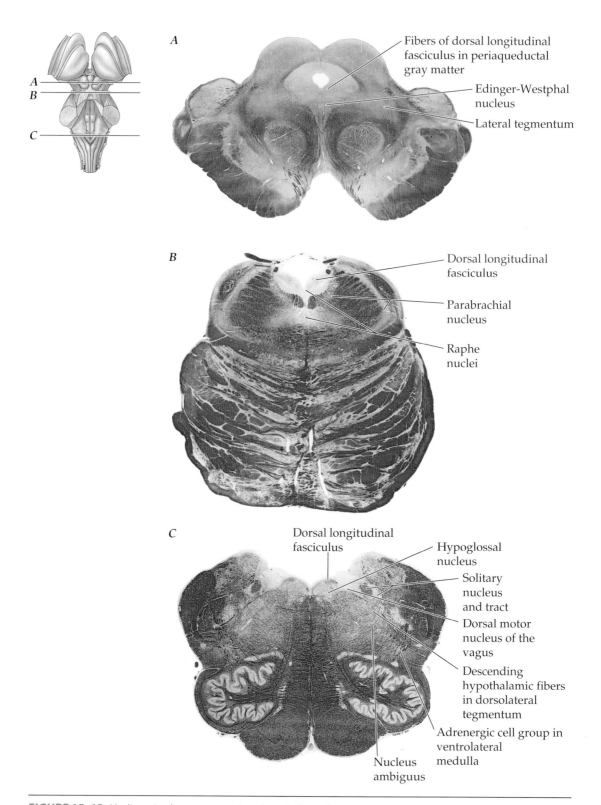

A

Fibers of dorsal longitudinal fasciculus in periaqueductal gray matter

Edinger-Westphal nucleus

Lateral tegmentum

B

Dorsal longitudinal fasciculus

Parabrachial nucleus

Raphe nuclei

C

Dorsal longitudinal fasciculus

Hypoglossal nucleus

Solitary nucleus and tract

Dorsal motor nucleus of the vagus

Descending hypothalamic fibers in dorsolateral tegmentum

Adrenergic cell group in ventrolateral medulla

Nucleus ambiguus

FIGURE 15–13 Myelin-stained transverse sections through the midbrain (*A*), pons (*B*), and medulla (*C*). In contrast to the dorsal longitudinal fasciculus, which is a discrete tract, the medial forebrain bundle is located only in the hypothalmus. Axons in the bundle extend and descend within the lateral brain stem, but they do not form a discrete tract.

A   *B*

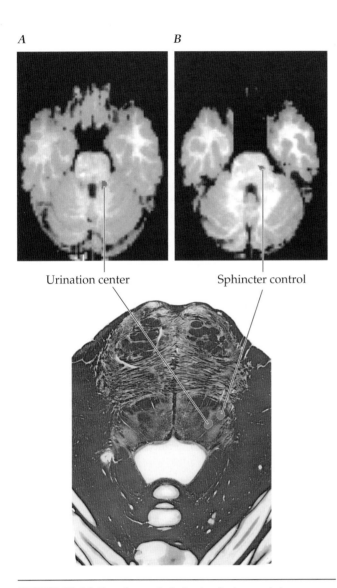

Urination center   Sphincter control

FIGURE 15–14 Neural control of urination. Positron emission tomography (PET) scans through the rostral pons show activation of two zones that play distinct roles in urination. **A.** The area that excites parasympathetic motor neurons that control muscles of the bladder wall and inhibit the sphincter motor neurons. This scan was obtained while the subject urinated. **B.** The area thought to prevent urination by exciting sphincter motor neurons, which are somatic motor neurons of the ventral horn. This scan was obtained while the subject was asked to urinate but was unable do to so on command. This was presumably because the sphincter muscles were contracting. Pontine control of urination is exerted via axons that travel in the reticulospinal tract. The inset shows the approximate locations of these zones on a transverse myelin-stained section through the pons. The section is inverted to match the orientation of the pons in the PET scans. (Adapted from Blok BF, Willemsen AT, Holstege G. A PET study on brain control of micturition in humans. *Brain.* 1997;120 [1]:111-121.)

parabrachial nucleus (Figure 15–13B) and the hypothalamus and descend to the spinal cord. Adrenergic neurons in the ventrolateral medulla project to the intermediolateral cell column for blood pressure control.

Damage to the dorsolateral pons or medulla can produce **Horner syndrome,** a disturbance in which the functions of

the sympathetic nervous system become impaired (see clinical case in this chapter; see also Box 15–1). Surprisingly, parasympathetic functions are spared (see below). Such damage typically occurs as a consequence of occlusion of the **posterior inferior cerebellar artery (PICA)** (see Figure 3–3B3). The most common signs of Horner syndrome and their causes are as follows:

- **Ipsilateral pupillary constriction** (miosis), resulting from the unopposed action of the pupillary constrictor innervation by the parasympathetic Edinger-Westphal nucleus (see Chapter 12).
- **Partial dropping of the eyelid, or pseudoptosis,** produced by removal of the sympathetic control of the smooth muscle (tarsal muscle) assisting the action of the levator palpebrae muscle.
- **Decreased sweating** and **increased warmth and redness of the ipsilateral face,** related to reduced sympathetic control of facial blood flow.

It is not understood why damage to the dorsal motor nucleus of the vagus following PICA occlusion does not produce parasympathetic signs. Perhaps the parasympathetic functions of the nucleus are not well lateralized and the intact side can take over the functions of the damaged side.

Preganglionic Neurons Are Located in the Lateral Intermediate Zone of the Spinal Cord

The descending autonomic fibers from the hypothalamus course in the lateral column of the spinal cord, within the region of the lateral corticospinal tract (Figure 15–15), and terminate in the intermediolateral nucleus (or cell column) of the thoracic and lumbar cord (Figure 15–15A) to regulate sympathetic functions. This is where sympathetic preganglionic motor neurons are located. Projections to the intermediate zone of the second through fourth sacral segments regulate parasympathetic functions (Figure 15–15B). This is where parasympathetic preganglionic motor neurons are located. Additional sympathetic and parasympathetic preganglionic neurons are scattered medially in the intermediate zone. At certain thoracic levels, the intermediolateral nucleus extends into the lateral column (Figure 15–15A), which explains why this region is sometimes called the **intermediate horn** of the spinal cord gray matter. The inset in Figure 15–15 shows the columnar shape of the intermediolateral nucleus. This organization is similar to that of Clarke's nucleus (see Figure 13–6) and the cranial nerve nuclei (see Figure 6–6). Because important control of the sympathetic nervous system is present in divisions of the central nervous system, it is not surprising that damage at different levels can produce Horner syndrome (Box 15–1). Somatic motor neurons that innervate the urinary sphincter are located in **Onuf's nucleus,** in the ventral horn of the sacral spinal cord.

Box 15–1

Lesions in Diverse Locations Can Produce Horner Syndrome

Unfortunately, Horner syndrome alone provides little information to the clinician for localizing the site of a lesion. The syndrome can be produced by a lesion anywhere along the descending autonomic pathway (Figure 15–16A), from the hypothalamus, the dorsolateral brain stem, the dorsolateral white matter of the spinal cord, and the intermediolateral nucleus. Horner syndrome can also be produced by a lesion in the periphery, where axons of the sympathetic postganglionic neurons course to reach the head, beginning with the route to the superior cervical ganglion and ending with the target organs of the head (Figure 15–16). How can the clinician distinguish between damage to one or another

level? The answer lies in identifying other neurological signs that may accompany Horner syndrome. A medullary lesion—for example, produced by PICA occlusion—that produces Horner syndrome also will produce other signs associated with the **lateral medullary syndrome** (see clinical case in this chapter; also Figure 6–12); these include loss of pain and temperature on the contralateral limbs and trunk and ipsilateral face, as well as ipsilateral limb ataxia, vertigo, and ipsilateral loss of taste. A spinal cord lesion producing Horner syndrome will also cause ipsilateral paralysis because the descending autonomic pathway is near the axons of the lateral corticospinal tract (Figures 15–15A and 15–16). The ascending postganglionic sympathetic fibers ascend, in part, along the carotid artery. Peripheral tumors in this region may lead to Horner syndrome.

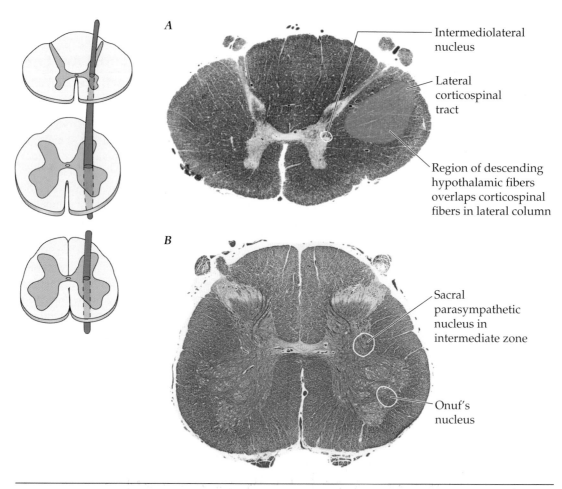

A

Intermediolateral nucleus

Lateral corticospinal tract

Region of descending hypothalamic fibers overlaps corticospinal fibers in lateral column

B

Sacral parasympathetic nucleus in intermediate zone

Onuf's nucleus

FIGURE 15–15 Myelin-stained transverse sections through the thoracic (*A*) and sacral (*B*) spinal cord. The inset shows the columnar configuration of the intermediolateral cell column.

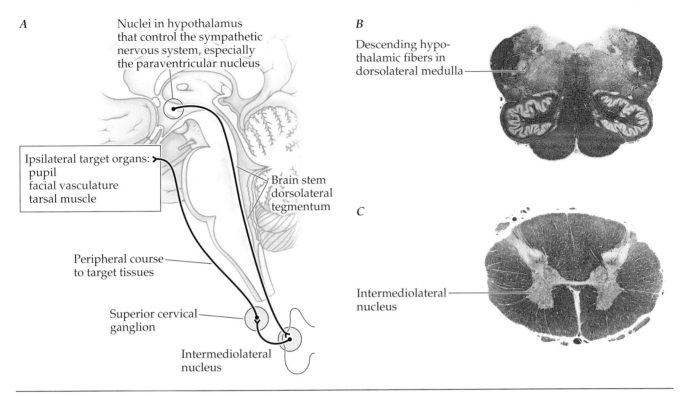

A

Nuclei in hypothalamus that control the sympathetic nervous system, especially the paraventricular nucleus

Ipsilateral target organs:
pupil
facial vasculature
tarsal muscle

Brain stem dorsolateral tegmentum

Peripheral course to target tissues

Superior cervical ganglion

Intermediolateral nucleus

B

Descending hypothalamic fibers in dorsolateral medulla

C

Intermediolateral nucleus

FIGURE 15–16 Horner syndrome. **A.** Circuit for Horner syndrome begins in the hypothalamus, where nuclei control the autonomic nervous system. There is loss of certain cranial sympathetic functions in Horner syndrome. An important nucleus for controlling sympathetic functions is the paraventricular nucleus. Lesion along the descending pathway in the brain stem and spinal cord can produce Horner syndrome. Also, damage in the periphery—often produced by tumors or enlarged lymph nodes—can disrupt the axons of the sympathetic postganglion neurons en route to target organs in the head. **B.** Myelin-stained section through the medulla. **C.** Myelin-stained section through the thoracic spinal cord.

Summary

General Hypothalamic Anatomy

The hypothalamus is a part of the diencephalon. On the midline it is bounded by the *rostral wall of the third ventricle* rostrally and the *hypothalamic sulcus* dorsally. The preoptic area extends farther anteriorly (Figure 15–4). The lateral boundary is the *internal capsule*. The hypothalamus has a mediolateral anatomical and functional organization, with separate *periventricular, medial,* and *lateral zones* (Figure 15–4).

Neuroendocrine Control

Neuroendocrine control by the hypothalamus is mediated by separate *parvocellular and magnocellular neurosecretory systems,* which control hormone release from the anterior and posterior pituitary, respectively (Figure 15–5).

Parvocellular neurosecretory neurons (Figure 15–5A) regulate anterior lobe hormone release by secreting *releasing or release-inhibiting hormones* (Table 15–2) into the

portal circulation in the *median eminence* (Figure 15–5). The major parvocellular nuclei, which are largely located in the periventricular zone, are the *periventricular nuclei,* the *arcuate nucleus,* the *paraventricular nucleus* (medial, or periventricular, part, only), and the *medial preoptic area.* Additional hypothalamic and extrahypothalamic sites project to the median eminence and release gonadotropin-releasing hormones.

Two nuclei form the magnocellular system: the magnocellular division of the *paraventricular nucleus* and the *supraoptic nucleus* (Figures 15–4, 15–5B, and 15–11). Axons from the magnocellular neurons in these nuclei project into the *infundibular stalk,* which connects the pituitary gland with the brain (Figure 15–5). Their termination site is the posterior lobe, where they release *vasopressin and oxytocin* directly into the systemic circulation. Separate neurons in the paraventricular and supraoptic nuclei synthesize either vasopressin or oxytocin (Figure 15–11). Both parvocellular and magnocellular neurons colocalize additional neuroactive peptides.

Autonomic Nervous System and Visceromotor Functions

The autonomic nervous system has two anatomical components: the *sympathetic division and the parasympathetic* division. The *enteric nervous system* is the intrinsic innervation of the gut. For the sympathetic and parasympathetic divisions, two neurons link the central nervous system with their target organs (Figures 15–6, 15–7, and 15–8): a *preganglionic neuron,* located in the central nervous system, and a *postganglionic neuron,* located in peripheral ganglia. The sympathetic division originates from the spinal cord, between the first thoracic and third lumbar segments (Figure 15–7). Preganglionic neurons of this division are located in the *intermediolateral nucleus* (Figure 15–15A). The parasympathetic division originates from the brain stem and the sacral spinal cord. Four parasympathetic nuclei in the brain stem contain preganglionic neurons (see Chapters 11 and 12): the Edinger-Westphal nucleus, the superior salivatory nucleus, the inferior salivatory nucleus, and the dorsal motor nucleus of the vagus. The lateral intermediate zone of the second through fourth sacral segments contains parasympathetic preganglionic neurons (Figure 15–15B).

Hypothalamic control of the autonomic nervous system is through descending pathways whose axons synapse on preganglionic neurons (Figures 15–6 and 15–8). The major source of this projection is the autonomic division of the *paraventricular nucleus.* This hypothalamic pathway courses in the *medial forebrain bundle* (Figure 15–12B), located laterally in the hypothalamus, and its caudal extension in the lateral tegmentum of the brain stem (Figure 15–13) and the lateral column of the spinal cord (Figure 15–15A). Disruption of axons of this pathway at any level can produce *Horner syndrome* (Figure 15–16). The hypothalamus also projects to other sites important in visceral sensory and motor function: the *parabrachial nucleus,* the *solitary nucleus, raphe nuclei, ventrolateral medulla,* and the *reticular formation* (Figure 15–13).

Circadian Rhythms and Sleep and Wakefulness

The *suprachiasmatic nucleus* (Figures 15–2 and 15–9) is the brain's master clock, receiving retinal input to entrain brain functions to the circadian cycle. Other hypothalamic nuclei receive input from the suprachiasmatic nucleus to organize circadian control of neuroendocrine and autonomic functions (Figure 15–9). The *preoptic sleep center* (Figures 15–9 and 15–10) and *tuberomammillary nucleus* (Figure 15–12B) regulate brain stem arousal centers, which include the pedunculopontine nucleus, locus ceruleus, and dorsal raphe nucleus, and, in turn, are regulated by these centers. The *lateral pontine tegmentum* is key to atonia during REM sleep.

Selected Readings

Horn J, Swanson L. The autonomic nervous system and the hypothalamus. In: Kandel ER, Schwartz JH, Jessell TM, Siegelbaum SA, Hudspeth AJ, eds. *Principles of Neural Science.* 5th ed. New York, NY: McGraw-Hill; in press.

McCormick D, Westbrook G. Sleep and dreaming. In: Kandel ER, Schwartz JH, Jessell TM, Siegelbaum SA, Hudspeth AJ, eds. *Principles of Neural Science.* 5th ed. New York, NY: McGraw-Hill; in press.

References

Andrews ZB. The extra-hypothalamic actions of ghrelin on neuronal function. *Trends Neurosci.* 2011;34(1):31-40.

Appenzeller O. *Clinical Autonomic Failure: Practical Concepts.* New York, NY: Elsevier; 1986.

Bellinger LL, Bernardis LL. The dorsomedial hypothalamic nucleus and its role in ingestive behavior and body weight regulation: lessons learned from lesioning studies. *Physiol Behav.* 2002;76:432-442.

Bentivoglio M, Kristensson K. Neural-immune interactions in disorders of sleep-wakefulness organization. *Trends Neurosci.* 2007;30(12):645-652.

Blok BF, Holstege G. The central nervous system control of micturition in cats and humans. *Behav Brain Res.* 1998;92:119-125.

Blok BF, Sturms LM, Holstege G. Brain activation during micturition in women. *Brain.* 1998;121:2033-2042.

Blok BF, Willemsen AT, Holstege G. A PET study on brain control of micturition in humans. *Brain.* 1997;120:111-121.

Blouet C, Jo YH, Li X, Schwartz GJ. Mediobasal hypothalamic leucine sensing regulates food intake through activation of a hypothalamus-brainstem circuit. *J Neurosci.* 2009;29(26): 8302-8311.

Bourque CW. Central mechanisms of osmosensation and systemic osmoregulation. *Nat Rev Neurosci.* 2008;9(7):519-531.

Buijs RM, Van Eden CG. The integration of stress by the hypothalamus, amygdala and prefrontal cortex: balance between the autonomic nervous system and the neuroendocrine system. In:

Uylings HBM, Van Eden CG, DeBruin JPC, Feenstra MGP, Pennartz CMA, eds. *Progress in Brain Research.* Amsterdam: Elsevier Science; 2000:117-132.

Cechetto DF, Saper CB. Neurochemical organization of the hypothalamic projection to the spinal cord in the rat. *J Comp Neurol.* 1988;272:579-604.

Cirelli C, Tononi G. Is sleep essential? *PLoS Biology.* 2008;6(8):e216.

Dantzer R, O'Connor JC, Freund GG, Johnson RW, Kelley KW. From inflammation to sickness and depression: when the immune system subjugates the brain. *Nature Rev Neurosci.* 2008;9(1):46-56.

Ebstein RP, Israel S, Chew SH, Zhong S, Knafo A. Genetics of human social behavior. *Neuron.* 2010;65(6):831-844.

Elmquist JK, Maratos-Flier E, Saper CB, Flier JS. Unraveling the central nervous system pathways underlying responses to leptin. *Nat Neurosci.* 1998;1:445-450.

Elmquist JK, Scammell TE, Saper CB. Mechanisms of CNS response to systemic immune challenge: the febrile response. *Trends Neurosci.* 1997;20:565-570.

Fowler CJ. Neurological disorders of micturition and their treatment. *Brain.* 1999;122:1213-1231.

Fowler CJ, Griffiths D, de Groat WC. The neural control of micturition. *Nat Rev Neurosci.* 2008;9(6):453-466.

Gerendai I, Halasz B. Asymmetry of the neuroendocrine system. *News Physiol Sci.* 2001;16:92-95.

Gershon M. The enteric nervous system. *Annu Rev Neurosci.* 1981;4:227-272.

Gershon MD. Developmental determinants of the independence and complexity of the enteric nervous system. *Trends Neurosci.* 2010;33(10):446-456.

Guyenet PG. The sympathetic control of blood pressure. *Nat Rev Neurosci.* 2006;7(5):335-346.

Heanue TA, Pachnis V. Enteric nervous system development and Hirschsprung's disease: advances in genetic and stem cell studies. *Nat Rev Neurosci.* 2007;8(6):466-479.

Herzog ED. Neurons and networks in daily rhythms. Nature reviews. *Neuroscience.* 2007;8(10):790-802.

Hobson JA, Pace-Schott EF. The cognitive neuroscience of sleep: neuronal systems, consciousness and learning. *Nat Rev Neurosci.* 2002;3(9):679-693.

Holstege G. Some anatomical observations on the projections from the hypothalamus to brainstem and spinal cord: an HRP and autoradiographic tracing study in the cat. *J Comp Neurol.* 1987;260:98-126.

Holstege G. The emotional motor system in relation to the supraspinal control of micturition and mating behavior. *Behav Brain Res.* 1998;92:103-109.

Holstege G, Mouton LJ, Gerrits NM. Emotional motor systems. In: Paxinos G, Mai JK, eds. *The Human Nervous System.* London: Elsevier; 2004:1306-1324.

Imeri L, Opp MR. How (and why) the immune system makes us sleep. *Nat Rev Neurosci.* 2009;10(3):199-210.

Insel TR. The challenge of translation in social neuroscience: a review of oxytocin, vasopressin, and affiliative behavior. *Neuron.* 25 2010;65(6):768-779.

Inui A. Feeding and body-weight regulation by hypothalamic neuropeptides—mediation of the actions of leptin. *Trends Neurosci.* 1999;22:62–67.

Inui A. Ghrelin: an orexigenic and somatotrophic signal from the stomach. *Nat Rev Neurosci.* 2001;2:551-560.

Kerman IA. Organization of brain somatomotor-sympathetic circuits. *Exp Brain Res.* 2008;187(1):1-16.

Kilduff TS, Peyron C. The hypocretin/orexin ligand-receptor system: implications for sleep and sleep disorders. *Trends Neurosci.* 2000;23:359-365.

Leander P, Vrang N, Moller M. Neuronal projections from the mesencephalic raphe nuclear complex to the suprachiasmatic nucleus and the deep pineal gland of the golden hamster (Mesocricetus auratus). *J Comp Neurol.* 1998;399:73-93.

Lechan RM, Nestler JL, Jacobson S. The tuberoinfundibular system of the rat as demonstrated by immunohistochemical localization of retrogradely transported wheat germ agglutinin (WGA) from the median eminence. *Brain Res.* 1982;245:1-15.

Mifflin SW. What does the brain know about blood pressure? *News Physiol Sci.* 2001;16:266-271.

Mignot E. A commentary on the neurobiology of the hypocretin/orexin system. *Neuropsychopharmacology.* 2001;25 (5 Suppl):S5-13.

Moore RY. Neural control of the pineal gland. *Behav Brain Res.* 1996;73:125-130.

Moore RY, Speh JC, Card JP. The retinohypothalamic tract originates from a distinct subset of retinal ganglion cells. *J Comp Neurol.* 1995;352:351-366.

Mtui EP, Anwar M, Reis DJ, Ruggiero DA. Medullary visceral reflex circuits: local afferents to nucleus tractus solitarii synthesize catecholamines and project to thoracic spinal cord. *J Comp Neurol.* 1995;351:5-26.

Munch IC, Moller M, Larsen PJ, Vrang N. Light-induced c-Fos expression in suprachiasmatic nuclei neurons targeting the paraventricular nucleus of the hamster hypothalamus: phase dependence and immunochemical identification. *J Comp Neurol.* 2002;442:48-62.

Nathan PW, Smith RC. The location of descending fibres to sympathetic neurons supplying the eye and sudomotor neurons supplying the head and neck. *J Neurol Neurosurg Psychiatry.* 1986;49:187-194.

Nauta WJH, Haymaker W. Hypothalamic nuclei and fiber connections. In: Haymaker W, Anderson E, Nauta WJH, eds. *The Hypothalamus.* Springfield, IL: Charles C. Thomas; 1969:136-209.

Noda M. The subfornical organ, a specialized sodium channel, and the sensing of sodium levels in the brain. *Neuroscientist.* 2006;12(1):80-91.

Okumura T, Takakusaki K. Role of orexin in central regulation of gastrointestinal functions. *J Gastroenterol.* 2008;43(9):652-660.

Pace-Schott EF, Hobson JA. The neurobiology of sleep: genetics, cellular physiology and subcortical networks. *Nat Rev Neurosci.* 2002;3(8):591-605.

Price CJ, Hoyda TD, Ferguson AV. The area postrema: a brain monitor and integrator of systemic autonomic state. *Neuroscientist.* 2008;14(2):182-194.

Le Gros Clark WE, Beattie J, Riddoch G, McOmish Dott N. *The Hypothalamus: Morphological, Functional, Clinical and Surgical Aspects*. Edinburgh: Oliver & Boyd; 1938:2-68.

Rogers RC, Kita H, Butcher LL, Novin D. Afferent projections to the dorsal motor nucleus of the vagus. *Brain Res Bull*. 1980;5:365-373.

Rolls A, Schaich Borg J, de Lecea L. Sleep and metabolism: role of hypothalamic neuronal circuitry. *Best Pract Res Clin Endocrinol Metab*. 2010;24(5):817-828.

Ross HE, Young LJ. Oxytocin and the neural mechanisms regulating social cognition and affiliative behavior. *Front Neuroendocrinol*. 2009;30(4):534-547.

Ruggiero DA, Cravo SL, Arango V, Reis DJ. Central control of the circulation by the rostral ventrolateral reticular nucleus: anatomical substrates. In: Ciriello J, Caverson MM, Polosa C, eds. *Progress in Brain Research*. Amsterdam: Elsevier, 1989.

Ruggiero DA, Cravo SL, Golanov E, Gomez R, Anwar M, Reis DJ. Adrenergic and non-adrenergic spinal projections of a cardiovascular-active pressor area of medulla oblongata: quantitative topographic analysis. *Brain Res*. 1994;663: 107-120.

Sakurai T. The neural circuit of orexin (hypocretin): maintaining sleep and wakefulness. *Nat Rev Neurosci*. 2007;8(3):171-181.

Saper CB. Hypothalamic connections with the cerebral cortex. In: Uylings HBM, Van Eden CG, DeBruin JPC, Feenstra MGP, Pennartz CMA, eds. *Progress in Brain Research*. Amsterdam: Elsevier Science; 2000:39-47.

Saper CB, Chou TC, Elmquist JK. The need to feed: homeostatic and hedonic control of eating. *Neuron*. 2002;36(2):199-211.

Saper CB, Fuller PM, Pedersen NP, Lu J, Scammell TE. Sleep state switching. *Neuron*. 2010;68(6):1023-1042.

Saper CB, Loewy AD, Swanson LW, Cowan WM. Direct hypo-thalamo-autonomic connections. *Brain Res*. 1976;117: 305-312.

Saper CB. Hypothalamus. In: Paxinos G, Mai JK, eds. *The Human Nervous System*. London: Elsevier; 2004:513-550.

Saper CB, Scammell TE, Lu J. Hypothalamic regulation of sleep and circadian rhythms. *Nature*. 2005;437(7063): 1257-1263.

Sartor K. *MR Imaging of the Skull and Brain*. Berlin: Springer; 1992.

Siegel JM. Narcolepsy: a key role for hypocretins (orexins). *Cell*. 1999;98:409-412.

Siegel JM. Clues to the functions of mammalian sleep. *Nature*. 2005;437(7063):1264-1271.

Silverman AJ, Zimmerman EA. Magnocellular neurosecretory system. *Annu Rev Neurosci*. 1983;6:357-380.

Stefaneanu L, Kontogeorgos G, Kovacs K, Horvath E. Hypophy-sis. In: Paxinos G, Mai JK, eds. *The Human Nervous System*. London: Elsevier; 2004:551-561.

Sutcliffe JG, De Lecea L. The hypocretins: setting the arousal threshold. *Nat Rev Neurosci*. 2002;3:339-349.

Swaab DF, Fliers E, Hoogendijk WJG, Veltman DJ, Zhuo JN. Interaction of prefrontal cortical and hypothalamic systems in the pathogenesis of depression. In: Uylings HBM, ed. *Progress in Brain Research*. Amsterdam: Elsevier. 2000.

Swaab DF, Hofman MA. Sexual differentiation of the human hypothalamus in relation to gender and sexual orientation. *Trends Neurosci*. 1995;18:264-270.

Swanson LW. Organization of mammalian neuroendocrine system. In: Bloom FE, ed. *Intrinsic Regulatory Systems of the Brain*. Bethesda, MD: American Physiological Society; 1986:317-363.

Swanson LW, Kuypers HGJM. The paraventricular nucleus of the hypothalamus: cytoarchitectonic subdivisions and organiza-tion of projections to the pituitary, dorsal vagal complex, and spinal cord as demonstrated by retrograde fluorescence double-labeling methods. *J Comp Neurol*. 1980;1984: 555-570.

Szymusiak R, McGinty D. Hypothalamic regulation of sleep and arousal. *Ann NY Acad Sci*. 2008;1129:275-286.

Thannickal TC, Moore RY, Nienhuis R, et al. Reduced num-ber of hypocretin neurons in human narcolepsy. *Neuron*. 2000;27(3):469-474.

Thompson RH, Swanson LW. Organization of inputs to the dor-somedial nucleus of the hypothalamus: a reexamination with Fluorogold and PHAL in the rat. *Brain Res Brain Res Rev*. 1998;27:89-118.

Ulrich-Lai YM, Herman JP. Neural regulation of endocrine and autonomic stress responses. Nature reviews. *Neuroscience*. 2009;10(6):397-409.

Veazey RB, Amaral DG, Cowan MW. The morphology and con-nections of the posterior hypothalamus in the cynomolgus monkey (Macaca fascicularis). II. Efferent connections. *J Comp Neurol*. 1982;207:135-156.

Vizzard MA, Erickson VL, Card JP, Roppolo JR, De Groat WC. Transneuronal labeling of neurons in the adult rat brainstem and spinal cord after injection of pseudorabies virus into the urethra. *J Comp Neurol*. 1995;355:629-640.

Watson RE Jr., Hoffmann GE, Wiegand SJ. Sexually dimorphic opioid distribution in the preoptic area: manipulation by gonadal steroids. *Brain Res*. 1986;398:157-163.

Young KA, Gobrogge KL, Liu Y, Wang Z. The neurobiology of pair bonding: insights from a socially monogamous rodent. *Front Neuroendocrinol*. 2011;32(1):53-69.

Young LJ, Murphy Young AZ, Hammock EA. Anatomy and neurochemistry of the pair bond. *J Comp Neurol*. 2005;493(1):51-57.

1. A person has a pituitary gland tumor. Which of the following brain structures is most likely to become affected as the tumor enlarges?
   A. Oculomotor nerve
   B. Medial orbitofrontal cortex
   C. Mammillary body
   D. Optic chiasm

2. Complete the following analogy using the best choice:

   The parvocellular neurosecretory system is to the magnocellular neurosecretory system, as
   A. the anterior pituitary gland is to the posterior pituitary gland.
   B. the median eminence is to the adrenal gland.
   C. the paraventricular nucleus is to the lateral hypothalamus.
   D. the supraoptic nucleus is to the arcuate nucleus.

3. Which of the following statements best describes the median eminence?
   A. It contains the neurovascular contacts of magnocellular neurosecretory neurons.
   B. It contains the neurovascular contacts of parvocellular neurosecretory neurons.
   C. It is where descending hypothalamic pathways course.
   D. It is where ascending serotonergic and noradrenergic systems course from the brain stem to the forebrain.

4. Which of the following statements best describes how the central nervous system innervates smooth muscle and skeletal muscle?
   A. Smooth muscle is innervated by autonomic preganglionic neurons, whereas skeletal muscle is innervated by somatic motor neurons.
   B. Smooth muscle is innervated by autonomic postganglionic neurons, whereas skeletal muscle is innervated by somatic motor neurons.
   C. Preganglionic neurons innervate postganglionic neurons, which innervate smooth muscle; skeletal muscle is innervated by somatic motor neurons.
   D. Preganglionic neurons innervate postganglionic neurons and somatic motor neurons; postganglionic neurons innervate smooth muscle; somatic motor neurons innervate skeletal muscle.

5. The components of the autonomic nervous system in the spinal cord are regulated by which of the following brain structures?
   A. Mammillary body
   B. Supraoptic nucleus
   C. Paraventricular nucleus
   D. Arcuate nucleus

6. A man has difficulty staying awake during the day. He often falls asleep during meetings and in social interactions. When he falls asleep, he usually looses all muscle tone. Which of the following neurotransmitters/neuromodulatory agents is affected in this patient?
   A. Orexin
   B. Histamine
   C. GABA
   D. 5-HT

7. Some antihistamine medications used to treat allergic reactions can cause drowsiness. This is because
   A. they act directly on hypothalamic centers to trigger sleep.
   B. they shift the biological clock in the suprachiasmatic nucleus later in the day, so the brain thinks it is night time.
   C. they can block the central action of histamine, which activates forebrain neurons.
   D. they can block the actions of the retinal projection to the hypothalamus.

8. The hypothalamus receives viscerosensory information to regulate blood pressure and fluid intake. Which of the following statements best describes how this information is transmitted to the hypothalamus?
   A. It is relayed by the solitary and parabrachial nuclei.
   B. It is transmitted directly by axons in the anterolateral system.
   C. It is relayed from the insular and primary somatic sensory cortical areas.
   D. It is transmitted from the orbitofrontal and cingulate cortical areas.

9. A person has a stroke that produces the following signs: ipsilateral mild ptosis, dry skin on the ipsilateral face, vertigo, ataxia of the left leg, and hoarse voice. A single occlusion of which artery could produce all of these signs?
   A. Internal carotid artery
   B. Anterior choroidal artery
   C. Superior cerebellar artery
   D. Posterior inferior cerebellar artery

10. A person has the following neurological signs: constricted pupil in left eye, decreased sweating on left side of face, and reddening of the left side of the face. Which of the following statements does not describe a site of a single lesion that produces these signs?
    A. Dorsolateral midbrain
    B. Medial pons
    C. Lateral spinal cord white matter
    D. Damage to sympathetic postganglionic axons in the neck

Chapter 16

The Limbic System and Cerebral Circuits for Reward, Emotions, and Memory

CLINICAL CASE | Anterior Temporal Lobe Degeneration

A 67-year-old woman was dining with her family when she was not able to recognize a food she commonly ate. She had been an empathetic person but recently has begun to be self-centered and unconcerned about others' feelings, including those of her daughter, with whom she was close. She had been socially dominant and extraverted, but recently lost that dominance, and has become neurotic and introverted. She had been a successful travel agent and had visited many countries worldwide, but she was now unable to recall the names of many of the places she had visited multiple times.

Over the next 2 years, her condition progressed, so that she was unable to recognize familiar people, words, and objects. Despite having normal calculation abilities, she stopped controlling her own finances. Around this time, her eating behavior changed. She also expressed socially inappropriate behaviors. For example, she developed a preference for sweets and condiments, and sometimes she ate condiments as food. She also tried to eat nonfood items. Her sensory and motor functions were unaffected, as were her visuospatial functions and episodic memory. Her speech and language were grammatically correct and fluent.

Figure 16–1A is from the patient, showing clear and marked degeneration of the right anterior temporal lobe; Figure 16–1B is an MRI from a healthy person at a similar placement within the anterior temporal lobe. Degeneration is manifested both as a reduction in the gray and white matter of the anterior temporal lobe and insular region, as well as a corresponding expansion of the lateral sulcus and other temporal lobe sulci (eg, rostral superior temporal sulcus). Notice that other brain regions (eg, head of caudate nucleus) appear normal.

Answer the following question based on your reading of this chapter.

1. **Degeneration in which part of the temporal lobe accounts for the patient's impairments?**

—Continued next page

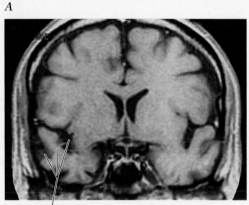
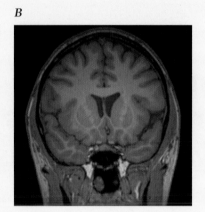

A   *B*

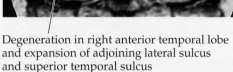

Degeneration in right anterior temporal lobe
and expansion of adjoining lateral sulcus
and superior temporal sulcus

FIGURE 16–1 Frontotemporal dementia. **A.** Coronal MRIs from a patient with frontotemporal dementia **B.** Coronal MRI from a healthy person. (**A,** Reproduced with permission from Gainotti G, Barbier A, Marra C. Slowly progressive defect in recognition of familiar people in a patient with right anterior temporal atrophy. *Brain*. 2003;126:792-803. **B,** Courtesy of Dr. Joy Hirsch, Columbia University.)

Key neurological signs and corresponding damaged brain structures

Frontotemporal dementia

The patient is suffering from frontotemporal dementia, a progressive degenerative disease characterized by loss of parts of the frontal and/or anterior temporal lobe; it can be lateralized. In this patient, it is primarily right-sided.

Brodmann's area 38, amygdala, and corticocortical connections

Brodmann's area 38, the cortex of the temporal pole (see Figure 2–19), has corticocortical interconnections with other limbic cortical areas, including orbitofrontal cortex;

it is interconnected with the amygdala, as well. These areas form a network, so that the personality changes, oral tendencies, and semantic impairments are difficult to attribute to a single structure.

References

Gainotti G, Barbier A, Marra C. Slowly progressive defect in recognition of familiar people in a patient with right anterior temporal atrophy. *Brain*. 2003;126:792-803.

Gorno-Tempini ML, Rankin KP, Woolley JD, Rosen HJ, Phengrasamy L, Miller BL. Cognitive and behavioral profile in a case of right anterior temporal lobe neurodegeneration. *Cortex*. 2004;40(4-5):631-644.

Mummery CJ, Patterson K, Price CJ, Ashburner J, Frackowiak RSJ, Hodges JR. A voxel-based morphometry study of semantic dementia: relationship between temporal lobe atrophy and semantic memory. *Ann Neurol*. 2000;47:36-45.

Olson IR, Plotzker A, Ezzyat Y. The enigmatic temporal pole: a review of findings on social and emotional processing. *Brain*. 2007;130 (Pt 7):1718-1731.

The limbic system is a diverse collection of cortical and subcortical regions that are crucial for normal human behavior. Who you are—your memories, your unique personality, your thoughts, your emotions—in large measure is determined by the functions of the diverse brain regions that comprise the limbic system. Virtually all psychiatric diseases involve dysfunction of these structures.

Nineteenth century neurologists and anatomists recognized that damage to particular parts of the human brain was associated with disorders of emotion and memory. These lesions, unlike those of the cerebellum, occipital lobe, or cortical regions around the central sulcus, for example, spared perception and movement. This research led to the understanding that the neural systems for reward, emotions, and memory are distinct from the sensory and motor systems and, hence, are grouped into a single system called the limbic system. The term *limbic* derives from the Latin word *limbus* for "border," because many of the structures engaged in these functions encircle the diencephalon on the medial brain surface and are at the border between subcortical nuclei and the cerebral cortex.

However, the more that is understood about the myriad functions of limbic system structures, the less helpful it is to adhere to the notion of a single system. It becomes more meaningful to consider the component functional systems. As a consequence, the term *limbic system* is gradually being abandoned in favor of a more functionally descriptive terminology. Nevertheless, the notion of the limbic system has some utility. Brain structures that comprise the limbic system have been conserved throughout much of vertebrate evolution, reflecting the common and important need for the functions they serve.

The basic organizational plan of the circuits for reward, emotions, and memory appears to be different from the sensory and motor systems. The different sensory and motor systems consist of structurally and functionally independent regions that are interconnected only at the highest levels of processing. This functional independence makes sense. For example, although perceptions are enriched when information from different modalities is combined, you can nevertheless identify an apple by touch alone or a dog by the sound of a bark. In contrast, circuits for reward, emotions, and memory are highly integrated from the start. This no doubt reflects the fact that reward and emotion depend on the concurrent analysis of diverse sensory information and actions, and therefore are highly integrated behaviors. So, too, are memories. The sight of an old house and children playing in the yard can evoke vivid recollection of times spent during childhood.

This chapter first considers the components of the limbic system in relation to their generalized roles in reward, emotions, and memory. Then the chapter reexamines the same structures from the perspective of their spatial interrelations, their tracts, and their connections.

Anatomical and Functional Overview of Neural Systems for Reward, Emotions, and Memory

The circuits for reward, emotions, and memory have tremendous anatomical and functional diversity, involving an interplay between cortical and subcortical structures (Table 16–1). Components of the limbic system are highly interconnected, just as their functions are interdependent. And not surprisingly, it is difficult to categorically assign one or another function to each component of the limbic system. Even so, major functional distinctions emerge after disturbance to one or another structure, such as after removal for intractable epilepsy or after stroke.

The **hippocampal formation** is central to memory and the **amygdala,** to emotions (Figure 16–2A). In addition, the amygdala participates in the acquisition, consolidation, and recall of emotional memories. Two other subcortical structures— the **ventral tegmental area** and the **ventral striatum** and other components of the **emotional loop of the basal**

Table **16–1**   Components of the limbic system

Major brain division	Structure	Component part
Cerebral hemisphere (telencephalon)	Limbic association cortex	Orbitofrontal
		Cingulate
		Entorhinal
		Temporal pole
		Perirhinal
		Parahippocampal
	Hippocampal formation	Hippocampus (Ammon's horn)
		Subiculum
		Dentate gyrus
	Amygdala	Corticomedial
		Basolateral
		Central nucleus[1]
	Ventral striatum	Nucleus accumbens
		Olfactory tubercle
		Ventromedial caudate and putamen
Diencephalon	Thalamus	Anterior nucleus
		Medial dorsal nucleus
		Midline nuclei
	Hypothalamus	Mammillary nuclei
		Ventromedial nucleus
		Lateral hypothalamic area
	Epithalamus[2]	Habenula
Midbrain	Portions of the periaqueductal gray matter and reticular formation	

[1]The bed nucleus of stria terminalis is largely included within the division of the central nucleus.

[2]In addition to the two major divisions of the diencephalon, there is a third division that includes the pineal gland, located along the midline, and the bilaterally paired habenula nuclei.

ganglia (see Figure 14–2)—are key to reward and other reward-related behaviors, punishment, and aspects of decision. Recall that the ventral striatum comprises the nucleus accumbens and adjoining parts of the ventral caudate nucleus and putamen. And all of these structures are interconnected with the **limbic association cortex** (Figures 16–3 and 16–4). These cortical areas receive information from integrative thalamic nuclei, higher-order sensory areas; and from the other cortical association areas. In turn, they project to the subcortical limbic system structures.

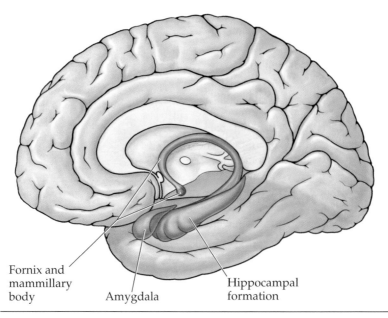

Fornix and
mammillary
body   Amygdala

Hippocampal
formation

FIGURE 16–2 Three-dimensional view of the amygdala and the hippocampal formation. The fornix, which is the output pathway of the hippocampal formation, and the mammillary body, a target to which it projects, are also illustrated.

The Limbic Association Cortex Is Located on the Medial Surface of the Frontal, Parietal, and Temporal Lobes

There are three major cortical association areas: (1) the parietal-temporal-occipital area, (2) the dorsolateral prefrontal association cortex (Figure 16–3, inset), and (3) the limbic association cortex. The limbic association cortex consists of morphologically and functionally diverse regions on four sets of gyri primarily on the medial and orbital surfaces of the cerebral hemisphere (Figures 16–3 and 16–4): the cingulate gyrus, the parahippocampal gyrus, the orbitofrontal and medial frontal gyri, and the gyri of the temporal pole. On the ventral brain surface (Figure 16–4), the lateral boundary of the limbic association cortex corresponds approximately to the **collateral sulcus.**

The **cingulate gyrus,** receiving its major thalamic input from the **anterior nucleus,** comprises three functional regions: rostral, middle, and posterior (Figure 16–3). The rostral portion of the cingulate gyrus is important in emotions, with connections with the amygdala, orbitofrontal, and insular cortex. We learned that a portion of this cortex receives information about physically painful stimuli. This portion is also involved in "emotional pain" of certain social situations (Figure 2–7). We also learned in Chapter 5 that the anterolateral system projects to the medial dorsal nucleus of the thalamus to convey physical pain information to the anterior cingulate gyrus. The portion under the genu of the corpus callosum, sometimes termed the **subgenual** region of the cingulate gyrus, is associated with the mood disorder, **depression.** This region is the target of therapeutic brain stimulation to ameliorate depression in patients who are refractory to pharmacological antidepressant therapy. The middle portion corresponds to the cingulate motor areas

(see Chapter 10; Figure 10–7B). This portion may be involved in aspects of movement control driven by emotions and reward. The posterior cingulate appears to be more related to higher-order sensory functions and memory. The **parahippocampal gyrus** contains several subdivisions that provide information to the hippocampal formation (Figure 16–4). These areas are discussed below. Together, the cingulate and parahippocampal gyri form a C-shaped ring of cortex that partially encircles the corpus callosum, diencephalon, and midbrain (Figure 16–2). The **cingulum** (or cingulum bundle) is a collection of axons that courses in the white matter deep within the cingulate and parahippocampal gyri. Cortical association fibers course in the cingulum and terminate in the parahippocampal gyrus.

Rostral to the cortical ring are the **medial frontal** and **orbitofrontal gyri.** These areas are central to reward and decision making. A famous case study called attention to the orbitofrontal cortex in emotions. Phineas Gage was a railway foreman who was seriously injured in an accident in which an explosion drove a metal rod through his skull, largely ablating the orbitofrontal cortex and adjoining prefrontal cortex on one side of the brain. He survived but was a changed man. He was no longer a responsible worker, he became "short-tempered, capricious, and profane;" he was "no longer Gage." These changes occurred without major defects in intellect. Frontal lobe research led to development of the prefrontal lobotomy—whereby physical removal of orbitofrontal cortex and adjacent areas or section of its connections—to quell the disruptive behaviors of psychiatric disease. The orbitofrontal cortex receives information from all sensory modalities, typically via higher-order sensory cortical regions, together with inputs from subcortical reward centers (see below). It is thought to integrate this information for decision making and to evaluate the hedonic value of stimulation.

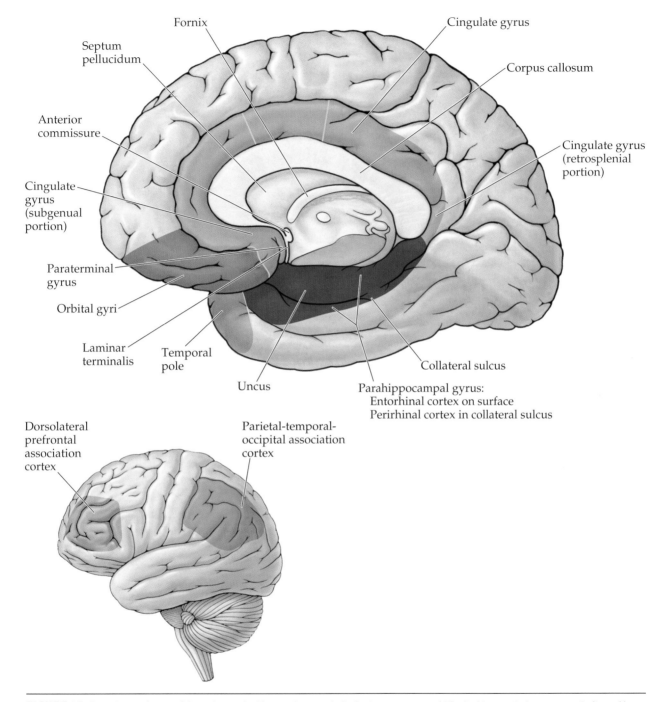

FIGURE 16–3 Midsagittal view of the right cerebral hemisphere, with the brain stem removed. The limbic association areas are indicated by the different shaded regions. The lines drawn on the cingulate cortex roughly divide it into anterior, middle, and posterior regions, as described in the text. The inset shows the prefrontal association cortex and the parietal-temporal-occipital association cortex.

The cortex of the **temporal pole**, corresponding to Brodmann's area 38 (Figures 16–3 and 16–4; see Figure 2–19) is interconnected with the orbitofrontal cortex and subcortically with the amygdala and hypothalamus. Lesion of this part of the temporal lobe can produce personality changes, such as social withdrawal. In this chapter's case study, the person with degeneration of the temporal pole changed from being highly extroverted and empathetic to introverted and cold. Indiscriminate eating habits also are reported.

The Hippocampal Formation Plays a Role in Consolidating Explicit Memories

Important insights into the function of the hippocampal formation have been obtained by studying the behavior of patients whose medial temporal lobe either was damaged because of a stroke or was ablated to ameliorate the serious symptoms of temporal lobe epilepsy. In one of the most extensively examined cases, this region was removed bilaterally from a

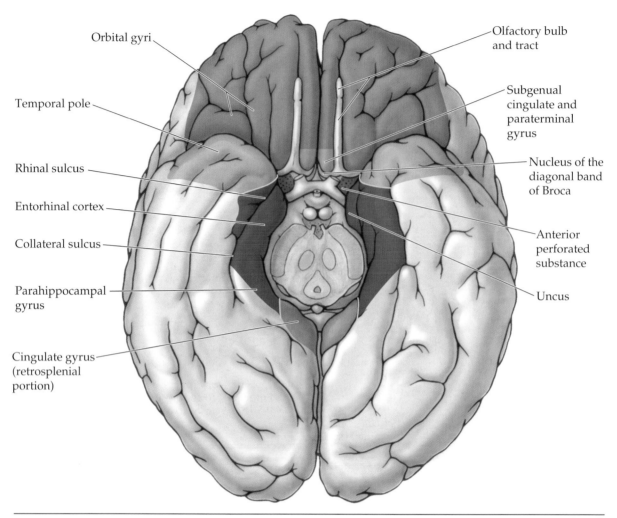

FIGURE 16–4 Ventral surface of the cerebral hemispheres, showing key components of the limbic association cortex (shaded area) as well as other basal forebrain structures. The collateral sulcus extends rostrally as the rhinal sulcus (sometimes termed fissure).

patient referred to as H.M. After surgery, H.M. lost the capacity for consolidating short-term memory into long-term memory, but he retained the memory of events that occurred before the lesion. This is termed **anterograde amnesia.** The impairment was selective for consolidating **explicit memories** (also termed **declarative memories**), such as the conscious recollection of facts. By contrast, H.M. and other patients with hippocampal (or medial temporal lobe) damage are capable of remembering procedures and actions (ie, **implicit or nondeclarative memory**), and they retain the capacity for a variety of simple forms of memory. More common than surgical ablation, sometimes after a severe heart attack, patients suffer bilateral damage to a key part of the hippocampal formation. During a heart attack, circulation of blood to the brain can become compromised because of insufficiency in the pumping action of the heart. This brain injury results because certain neurons in the hippocampal formation require consistently high circulating blood oxygen levels. What has emerged from this research is that the hippocampal formation is involved in

the long-term consolidation of explicit memory. It is thought that the memories themselves reside in the higher-order association areas of the cerebral cortex.

Whereas the hippocampal formation is best known for its role in memory consolidation, it has also been implicated in the body's response to stress and emotions. Interestingly, animal and human fMRI studies suggest that the posterior part of the hippocampal formation is more important for explicit memory, cognition, and spatial memory, while the anterior portion is more related to stress and emotions. Interestingly, London taxicab drivers, who must master the complex London street map, have a larger posterior hippocampal formation than control subjects. Located anteriorly, there is a division related to stress and emotions. Further, the size of the hippocampal formation is reduced in **schizophrenia,** linking it with human psychiatric disease.

The **hippocampal formation** comprises three anatomical components, each with distinctive morphologies and connections (Figure 16–5; Table 16–1; see Box 16–1): the

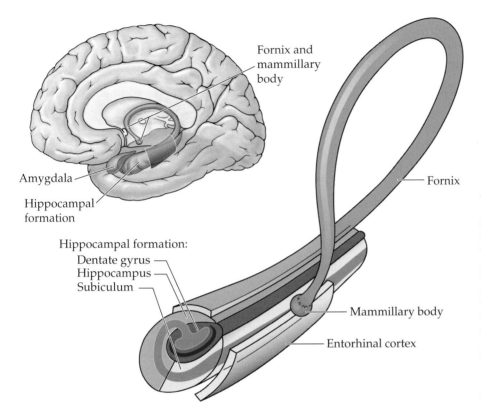

FIGURE 16–5 The general spatial relations of components of the hippocampal formation, its efferent pathway (fornix), and the entorhinal cortex are shown. The middle portion of the hippocampal formation is distinguished in the schematic view. A coronal slice through the hippocampal formation (cut end, anteriorly) reveals a cylindrical shape and circular sequence of component structures (i.e., dentate gyrus, hippocampus, and subiculum). These components are present at all anterior-to-posterior levels; each forming a longitudinal strip along the antero-posterior axis of the cylinder.

dentate gyrus, the **hippocampus** proper, and the **subiculum.** (The nomenclature of the hippocampal formation is variable, and exactly which components are considered to be part of this structure may differ, depending on the source.) The three components are organized roughly as parallel strips running antero-posteriorly within the temporal lobe and together forming a cylinder (Figure 16–5). These strips are initially a flattened sheet located on the brain surface, but during prenatal development they become buried within the cortex (see Figure 16–16A). The flat sheet also folds in a complex manner to assume its mature configuration, which resembles a jelly-roll pastry. The dentate gyrus—together with the subventricular zone of the lateral ventricle, which was discussed in Chapter 9 (see Box 9–1)—are the two brain sites for neurogenesis in the mature brain.

The hippocampal formation has serial and parallel circuits

The hippocampal formation receives complex sensory and cognitive information from a portion of the **limbic association cortex** termed the **entorhinal cortex** (Figures 16–3, 16–4, and 16–5). In fact, the hippocampal formation works so closely with the adjoining entorhinal cortex that the two are functionally inseparable. The entorhinal cortex, located on the parahippocampal gyrus adjacent to the hippocampal formation, collects information from other parts of the limbic association cortex (perirhinal and parahippocampal cortex) as well as from other association areas (Figure 16–6A). Extensive processing of information occurs within the hippocampal

formation, within a prominent **serial circuit,** in which information is projected in sequential steps (see Box 16–1). There is also a parallel circuit, in which information from the entorhinal cortex projects directly to each hippocampal component. Combined serial and parallel processing within neural circuits is also a feature of sensory and motor pathways.

The output neurons of the hippocampal formation are **pyramidal neurons,** similar to the neocortex covering most of the cerebral hemisphere, and they are located in the hippocampus and subiculum. The dentate gyrus contains neurons, termed granule cells, that make connections only within the hippocampal formation. Pyramidal neurons have axon branches that collect on the surface of the hippocampal formation. Eventually these axons form a compact fiber bundle, the **fornix** (Figures 16–2 and 16–5), which projects to other subcortical telencephalic and diencephalic structures. The hippocampal formation, together with the fornix, has a C-shape. Two output systems can be distinguished within the fornix, from the subiculum and the hippocampus (Figures 16–6B and 16–7B). Although these systems are involved in the cognitive aspects of memory, it is not yet understood how their functions differ.

From the subiculum, axons synapse mostly in the **mammillary bodies** of the hypothalamus (Figures 16–2 and 16–6B). This projection completes an anatomical loop: Via the **mammillothalamic tract,** the mammillary body projects to the **anterior nuclei** of the thalamus, which project to the **cingulate gyrus** (Figure 16–6B). The cingulate gyrus provides information to the entorhinal cortex, which projects to the hippocampal formation. In 1937, James Papez postulated that this

Box 16–1

Circuits of the Hippocampal Formation and Entorhinal Cortex Are Important for Memory

Memory impairment after damage to the hippocampal formation and certain adjoining cortical structures is selective for **explicit memories** (also termed **declarative memories**). Consolidation of both forms of explicit memories is impaired: **semantic memory,** such as knowledge of facts, people, and objects, including new word meaning, and the **episodic memory** of events that have a specific spatial and temporal context, such as meeting a friend last week. Formation of **spatial memories** is also impaired, such as being able to navigate around a familiar city. By contrast, patients with hippocampal (or medial temporal lobe) damage are capable of remembering procedures and actions (ie, **implicit** or **nondeclarative memory),** and they retain the capacity for a variety of simple forms of learning and memory.

The three divisions of the hippocampal formation—the dentate gyrus, hippocampus, and subiculum, and any component parts—each have a relatively simple circuit, compared with other cerebral cortical areas. Moreover, the basic circuit is the same from anterior in the temporal lobe, posteriorly. In this way, it is much like that of the cerebellum in which local circuits were the same for the different cerebellar cortical regions. In a slice through the hippocampal formation (Figure 16–17), we see that pyramidal cells of the entorhinal cortex send their axons to the dentate gyrus, roughly in the same coronal plane as the hippocampal formation, to synapse on granule cells. This is the **perforant pathway.** Granule cell axons, termed **mossy fibers,** synapse on pyramidal cells of one subregion of the hippocampus, termed the CA3 region, where neurons, in turn, send their axons (called the **Schaefer collaterals**) to neurons of the CA1 region.

(These axon collaterals spare the CA2 region.) The subiculum receives the next projection in the sequence, from the CA1 region, and it projects back to the entorhinal cortex. Both CA1 and the subiculum also project axons into the fornix, primarily to the septal nuclei and mammillary bodies, respectively. Additional parallel projections from entorhinal cortex to the hippocampus and subiculum are also important. It is not yet known how the myriad connections of the entorhinal cortex and hippocampal formation are organized to play a pivotal role in memory consolidation, spatial memory and navagation, and other aspects of cognition. However, an important clue exists: The strength of many synapses in the hippocampal formation can be modified under various experimental conditions.

A model for the functional organization of the hippocampal formation is based on its anatomical circuitry. Information that is first processed in the higher-order association areas on the lateral surface of the cerebral hemisphere, such as the parietal-temporal-occipital association area, is next processed in the limbic association cortex on the medial temporal lobe. This processing takes place in three key areas: the perirhinal cortex, the parahippocampal cortex, and the entorhinal cortex (Figure 16–3). From here, information is transmitted to the hippocampal formation (Figure 16–6), where further processing results in changes in the amount or timing of activity of certain populations of neurons. The complex neural responses comprise a "representation" of the memory, which unfortunately is not well understood. Finally, via two sets of return projections to the cortex—back to entorhinal cortex directly and, via the fornix, to the mammillary bodies and anterior thalamus to the cingulate cortex—this hippocampal memory representation enables consolidation of explicit and spatial memories in the association areas.

pathway plays an important role in emotion. It is now known that the circuit named in his honor is part of a complex network of bidirectional connections and that many components of this network play an important role in memory. Some fornix fibers from the subiculum project to the amygdala. This may be part of the circuit for consolidating emotional memories.

From the hippocampus, most axons do not synapse in the mammillary bodies, but rather, in several other locations, including the **septal nuclei,** located more rostrally in the forebrain in close apposition to the septum pellicudum (Figure 16–6B). Little is known about the function of septal nuclei. In a fascinating series of experiments in the early 1950s, laboratory rats, when given the choice of receiving either electrical stimulation of the septal nuclei or food and water, preferred the electrical stimulation. Investigators reasoned that this region is a so-called pleasure center that likely plays an important role in regulating highly motivated behaviors, such as reproductive behaviors or feeding. The septal nuclei give rise to a cholinergic (see Figure 2–3A) and GABAergic projection, via the fornix, back to the hippocampal formation. This return septal projection is important in regulating hippocampal activity during certain active behavioral states.

The hippocampal formation has diverse cortical projections

The fornix is an extremely large tract, with over one million heavily myelinated axons on each side. This number is comparable to the number of myelinated axons in one medullary pyramid or an optic nerve. Despite its size, a major target of axons of the fornix is the ipsilateral mammillary body, whose output is also highly focused, on the **anterior thalamic nuclei.** How can the hippocampal formation, with such a focused subcortical projection, have a generalized role in memory? One answer is that the fornix is not the only major output of the hippocampal formation. The subiculum and hippocampus also project back to the entorhinal cortex (Figure 16–6C), which, in turn, has diverse efferent corticocortical connections to the prefrontal cortex, orbitofrontal cortex, parahippocampal gyrus, cingulate gyrus, and insular cortex (Figure 16–6B). And collectively these cortical areas also have widespread projections. Through the divergence of connections emerging from the entorhinal cortex to cortical association areas, the hippocampal formation can influence virtually all association areas of the temporal, parietal, and frontal lobes, as

A

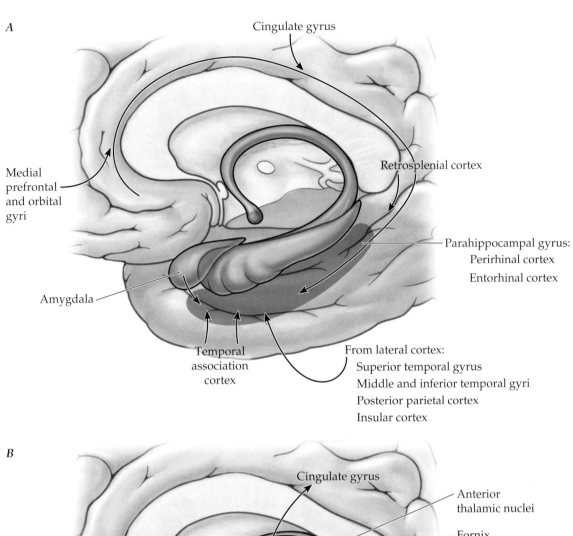

Cingulate gyrus

Retrosplenial cortex

Parahippocampal gyrus:
Perirhinal cortex
Entorhinal cortex

Medial prefrontal and orbital gyri

Amygdala

Temporal association cortex

From lateral cortex:
Superior temporal gyrus
Middle and inferior temporal gyri
Posterior parietal cortex
Insular cortex

B

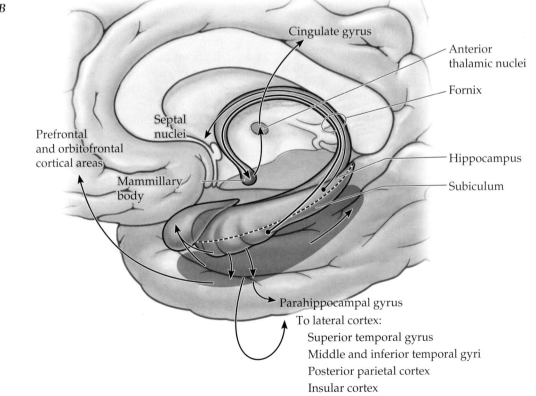

Cingulate gyrus

Anterior thalamic nuclei

Fornix

Septal nuclei

Prefrontal and orbitofrontal cortical areas

Mammillary body

Hippocampus

Subiculum

Parahippocampal gyrus

To lateral cortex:
Superior temporal gyrus
Middle and inferior temporal gyri
Posterior parietal cortex
Insular cortex

FIGURE 16–6 Serial and parallel hippocampal circuits. *A.* Cortical inputs to the hippocampal formation. *B.* Subcortical outputs via the fornix. There are also cortical projections from the hippocampal formation back to the entorhinal cortex, which projects back to the cortical areas from which it received input.

well as some higher-order sensory areas, after as few as three synapses. The divergence in the cortical output of the hippocampal formation parallels the widespread convergence of its inputs, also via the entorhinal cortex, from association areas.

The Amygdala Contains Three Major Functional Divisions for Emotions and Their Behavioral Expression

The **amygdala** (sometimes termed the amygdaloid complex) is a collection of morphologically, histochemically, and functionally diverse nuclei. Located largely within the rostral temporal lobe (Figure 16–2), the main portion of the amygdala is almond-shaped (*amygdala* is Greek for "almond"). One of its output pathways, however, the **stria terminalis,** and one of its component nuclei, the **bed nucleus of the stria terminalis,** are C-shaped (Figure 16–7). Axons of the other output pathway of the amygdala, the **ventral amygdalofugal pathway,** take a somewhat more direct route to their targets.

Amygdala circuits are preferentially involved in emotions and their overt behavioral expressions. The functions of amygdala circuits are therefore similar to the functions originally proposed for the entire limbic system. What stimuli are responded to, how overt responses to these stimuli are organized, and the internal responses of the body's organs are all dependent on this subcortical structure. Following damage to the amygdala, people lose the ability to recognize the affective meaning of facial expression, especially threatening faces. People also fail to recognize the emotional content of speech. Given the defects observed with its damage, it is not surprising that the amygdala is a central figure in emotion regulation, especially in relation to fear. For example, analysis of staring eyes, a vocalization, and body posture can lead to a set of potential emotional outcomes, such as fear or anxiety, and a set of possible actions, such as fleeing or attacking a potential foe. In animals, electrical stimulation of the amygdala, depending on the particular site, can evoke diverse defense reactions and visceral motor responses. The numerous nuclei of the amygdala can be divided into three principal nuclear groups (Figure 16–8): basolateral, central, and cortical. Each group has different connections and functions.

The basolateral nuclei are reciprocally connected with the cerebral cortex

The **basolateral nuclei** (Figure 16–7A) comprise the largest division of the amygdala. These nuclei are thought to attach emotional significance to a stimulus. The basolateral nuclei receive information about the particular characteristics of a stimulus from higher-order sensory cortical areas in the temporal and insular cortical areas and from association cortex. Limbic association cortex conveys this information to the amygdala to link particular stimuli, such as seeing a particular object or hearing a certain sound, with particular emotions. The amygdala is an important target of the **ventral stream** for object recognition (see Figures 7–15 and 7–16). Importantly,

the amygdala and hippocampal formation receive somewhat different kinds of sensory information. Whereas the amygdala receives highly processed sensory information, it retains its modality characteristics (eg, visual or auditory). On the other hand, the hippocampal formation receives more integrated sensory information that is thought to reflect complex features of the environment, such as spatial relationships and contexts. For example, when you see a snake, you may feel threatened and fearful. Visual pathways through the ventral portion of the temporal lobe convey information about the snake to the amygdala. The amygdala uses this information to organize your response, both the emotions you feel and your overt behavior to this potential danger. The hippocampal formation is thought to be important in learning the complex environmental setting, or context, in which the snake was seen.

The major efferent connections of the basolateral amygdala are directed back to the cerebral cortex, either directly or indirectly. The cortical areas receiving a direct projection from the basolateral amygdala are the limbic association cortex—which includes the cingulate gyrus, temporal pole, and medial orbitofrontal cortex—and the dorsolateral prefrontal cortex. The amygdala also projects directly to the hippocampal formation, which, as discussed earlier, is thought to be important in learning the emotional significance of complex stimuli or the context in which emotionally charged stimuli are experienced. In addition to direct cortical projections, the basolateral division has extensive subcortical projections that give rise, indirectly, to connections to the cortex. Via the **ventral amygdalofugal pathway,** the basolateral amygdala projects to the thalamic relay nucleus for association areas in the frontal lobe, the **medial dorsal nucleus.** It also has a major projection to cholinergic forebrain neurons located in the **basal nucleus** (of Meynert), which itself has widespread cortical projections (see next section and Figure 2–3A). Finally, neurons of the basolateral nuclei also project to the central amygdala nuclei (see section below on the basal forebrain), which are important in mediating behavioral responses to emotional stimuli.

The central nuclei project to autonomic control centers in the brain stem and hypothalamus

An important function of the **central nuclei** (Figure 16–7B) is to mediate emotional responses. In regulating the autonomic nervous system, the central nuclei receive viscerosensory input from brain stem nuclei, in particular the **solitary nucleus** and the **parabrachial nucleus** (see Chapter 6). In turn, the central nuclei project via the **ventral amygdalofugal pathway** to the **dorsal motor nucleus of the vagus** as well as to other brain stem parasympathetic nuclei and nearby portions of the reticular formation. The central nuclei also regulate the autonomic nervous system through projections to the lateral hypothalamus (see Chapter 15). As discussed earlier in this chapter, the central nuclei receive an input from the basolateral nuclei. This is the key path for fear conditioning, which helps to shape responses to emotional stimuli.

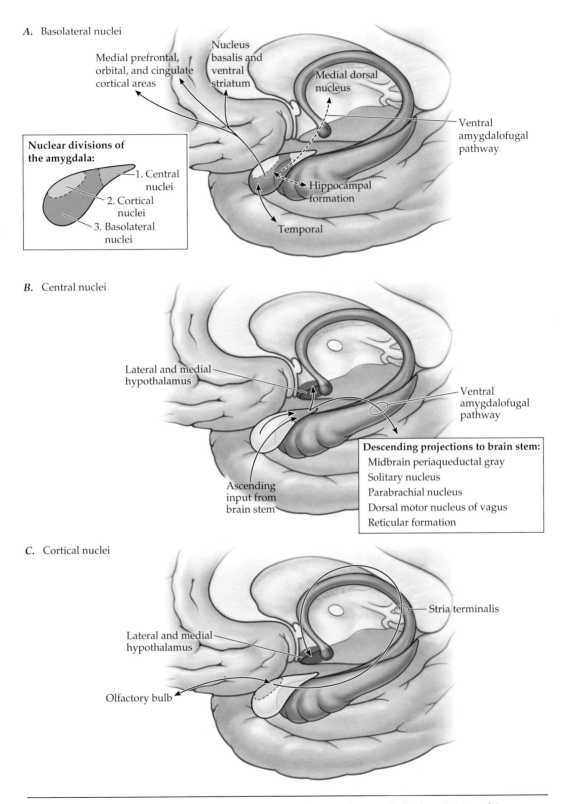

A. Basolateral nuclei

Medial prefrontal, orbital, and cingulate cortical areas

Nucleus basalis and ventral striatum

Medial dorsal nucleus

Ventral amygdalofugal pathway

Nuclear divisions of the amygdala:
1. Central nuclei
2. Cortical nuclei
3. Basolateral nuclei

Hippocampal formation

Temporal

B. Central nuclei

Lateral and medial hypothalamus

Ventral amygdalofugal pathway

Descending projections to brain stem:
Midbrain periaqueductal gray
Solitary nucleus
Parabrachial nucleus
Dorsal motor nucleus of vagus
Reticular formation

Ascending input from brain stem

C. Cortical nuclei

Stria terminalis

Lateral and medial hypothalamus

Olfactory bulb

FIGURE 16–7 Principal connections of the amygdala. The inset shows schematically the three divisions of the amygdala. **A.** The basolateral nuclei are reciprocally connected with the cortex of the temporal lobe, including higher-order sensory areas and association cortex. The basolateral amygdala also projects to the medial dorsal nucleus of the thalamus, the basal nucleus, and the ventral striatum. **B.** The central nuclei receive input from the brain stem, especially from visceral afferent relay nuclei (ie, solitary nucleus and parabrachial nucleus). The targets of its efferent projections include the hypothalamus and autonomic nuclei in the brain stem. **C.** The cortical nuclei have reciprocal connections with the olfactory bulb and efferent projections via the stria terminalis to the ventromedial nucleus of the hypothalamus.

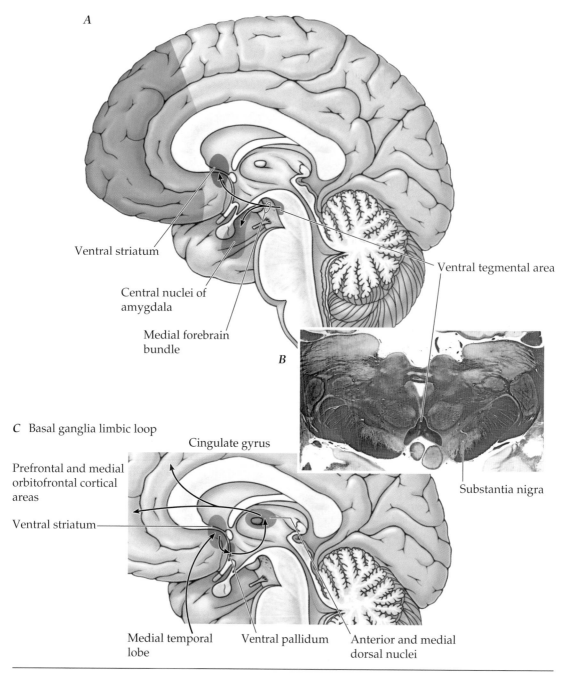

FIGURE 16–8 Brain regions important in addiction and reinforcement. **A.** The ventral tegmental area gives rise to a dopaminergic projection to the amygdala and ventral striatum that is important in various aspects of addiction. The ventral tegmental area also projects to the prefrontal cortex. **B.** Transverse section through the midbrain-diencephalon junction, showing the location of the ventral tegmental area and substantia nigra, both of which contain dopaminergic neurons. **C.** An expanded view of the region containing components of the limbic loop of the basal ganglia.

The central nuclei of the amygdala are part of the collection of nuclei that share morphological, histochemical, and connection characteristics, called the **extended amygdala.** These nuclei extend caudally within the basal forebrain and beneath the basal ganglia. Included in this group is the bed nucleus of the stria terminalis. Together with parts of the ventral striatal circuits, this is an important structure in substance abuse and dependence. They may help organize drug-seeking and drug-taking behaviors that are characteristics of addiction.

The cortical nuclei are reciprocally connected with olfactory structures

As discussed in Chapter 9, the cortical nuclei receive olfactory information from the olfactory bulb (Figure 16–7C; see

Figure 9–9). The piriform cortex, along with the lateral orbitofrontal cortex, is thought to be important in olfactory perception. In animals, the cortical nuclei play a role in behaviors triggered by olfactory stimuli, especially sexual responses.

The Mesolimbic Dopamine System and Ventral Striatum Are Important in Reward

The brain has two major dopamine systems. One originates from the **substantia nigra pars compacta** (Figure 16–8B) and projects primarily to two parts of the striatum, the caudate and the putamen, and less so to the nucleus accumbens. This is termed the **nigrostriatal dopaminergic system.** The other is the **mesolimbic (sometimes termed mesocorticolimbic) dopaminergic system,** which originates from the **ventral tegmental area** (Figure 16–8B). This system provides the principal dopaminergic innervation of the **nucleus accumbens** (Figure 16–8A; see Figures 16–10 and 16–11), the **amygdala,** and various parts of the cortex, especially the **prefrontal cortex.** The mesolimbic dopaminergic axons travel in the **medial forebrain bundle** (Figure 16–8A). Whereas dysfunction of the nigrostriatal system is associated with Parkinson disease, dysfunction of the mesolimbic dopaminergic system is implicated in schizophrenia and depression.

The dopaminergic systems are important in responding to natural rewarding stimuli for survival, such as feeding and reproduction. However, dopaminergic neurons do not simply signal the hedonic (ie, subjective experience of pleasure) value of events, because novel negative reinforcing stimuli can also activate the dopaminergic systems. Nevertheless, the mesolimbic dopaminergic system is central to the brain's reward circuit. Most drugs of abuse—like psychostimulants (such as cocaine, methamphetamine, and MDMA), sedative-hypnotics (including ethanol), nicotine, THC (tetrahydrocannabinol, the active compound in marijuana), and opiates—produce an increase in dopamine in several target areas of the mesocorticolimbic dopaminergic system. (Note that opiates also use nondopaminergic mechanisms.) Several substance-specific mechanisms account for this effect, including decreased reuptake of dopamine at synaptic sites and disinhibition of ventral tegmental neurons so that they can release more dopamine and, hence, have a stronger reinforcing effect. The nucleus accumbens, which is part of the ventral striatum, is a particularly important area because the reinforcing effects of drugs of abuse are greatly diminished or eliminated when dopamine transmission is blocked there. Another area important for the reinforcing actions of drugs, especially ethanol, is the central amygdala nuclei (see Figure 16–13).

The nucleus accumbens is also a key site for neural interactions responsible for drug reinforcement and the motivation to seek drugs. Release of dopamine in the nucleus accumbens is critically involved in forming the associations between drug-related cues and rewarding experiences. The nucleus accumbens is a striatal component of the limbic loop (see Chapter 14). This loop can provide an emotional context for planning motor behavior. The output nucleus of the limbic loop is the **ventral pallidum,** which projects to the **anterior** and **medial dorsal thalamic nuclei** and then to the **medial orbitofrontal** and **medial prefrontal cortex,** and **cingulate cortex** (Figure 16–8C). The various frontal association areas project to premotor areas to influence movements directly (see Figure 10–2B). This circuit could mediate the flexible responses to cues associated with drug use and abuse.

Connections Exist Between Components of the Limbic System and the Three Effector Systems

The limbic system is difficult to study partly because a bewilderingly large number of interconnections exist between its many structures. What might be the functions of these myriad interconnections? Many of the connections relate to the behavioral expression of emotions. Complex polysynaptic pathways ultimately link limbic system structures with the three effector systems for the behavioral expression of emotion: the endocrine, autonomic, and somatic motor systems (Figure 16–9).

Paths by which the limbic system may influence pituitary hormone secretion involve indirect connections between the amygdala and the periventricular hypothalamus (Figure 16–9A). One such path, for example, involves the projection from the cortical amygdala, via the **stria terminalis,** to the **ventromedial nucleus** (Figure 16–7C). This nucleus projects to a key component of the parvocellular neurosecretory system, the **arcuate nucleus** (see Chapter 15).

The visceral consequences of emotions are mediated by direct and indirect connections to brain stem and spinal nuclei of the autonomic nervous system (Figure 16–9B). As discussed earlier, the central nuclei of the amygdala project directly to brain stem autonomic centers (Figure 16–7B). The amygdala also affects autonomic function indirectly, through projections to the lateral hypothalamus, which influences autonomic function through neural circuits of the reticular formation and other parts of the hypothalamus. Recall that the hypothalamus, including part of the paraventricular nucleus and the lateral hypothalamus, gives rise to descending pathways that regulate autonomic function (see Figure 15–8).

The overt behavioral signs of emotion, such as flight or fight reactions, are mediated by the actions of the limbic system on the **somatic motor systems** (Figure 16–9C), especially the reticulospinal tracts (see Figure 10–5B). For example, projections from the hippocampus, septal nuclei, and amygdala to the lateral hypothalamus can influence the reticulospinal system (Figure 16–9C). These connections may be important in triggering stereotypic responses, such as defense reactions and reproductive behaviors. Experimental studies in animals have also shown that the periaqueductal gray matter mediates motor behaviors typical of particular species, such as growling and hissing in carnivores responding to environmental threats. The periaqueductal gray matter receives inputs from the central amygdala nuclei and the hypothalamus.

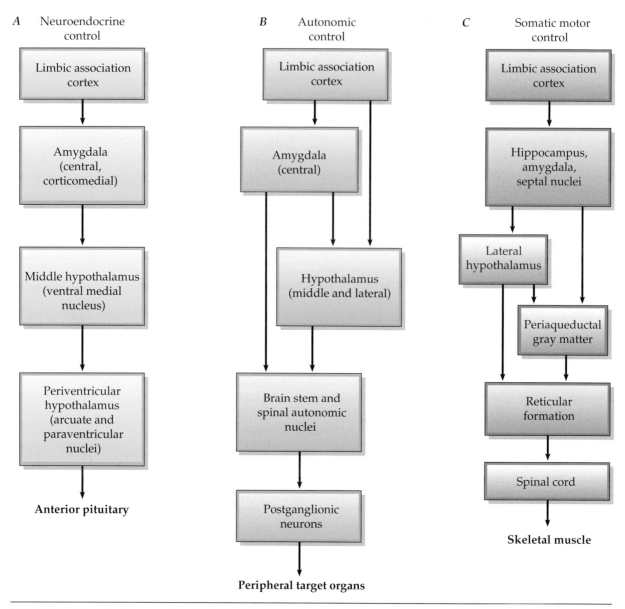

FIGURE 16–9 Relations between the limbic system and effector systems. **A.** Neuroendocrine control is mediated by the amygdala via the periventricular hypothalamus. **B.** Autonomic control is mediated by both the amygdala and the lateral hypothalamus, via descending pathways that originate from the central nucleus of the amygdala and the middle and lateral hypothalamus. **C.** Somatic motor control is mediated by relatively direct projections to the reticular formation, for stereotypic behaviors, and through more complex telencephalic and diencephalic circuitry (not shown), for more flexible control.

The limbic system can also influence somatic motor functions in more complex and behaviorally flexible ways through the **limbic loop of the basal ganglia,** which includes the ventral striatum, ventral pallidum, and thalamic medial dorsal nucleus (see Figure 16–15B; see Figure 14–8). Cortical inputs to this loop derive from the limbic association areas, hippocampal formation, and basolateral nuclei of the amygdala. As noted in Chapter 14, the output of the limbic loop is to the limbic association areas of the frontal lobe. These areas can influence the planning of movements through projections

to premotor areas and possibly the execution of movements through projections to the cingulate motor areas (see Figure 10–7B).

All Major Neurotransmitter Regulatory Systems Have Projections to the Limbic System

The innervation of the limbic system by the major neurotransmitter regulatory systems (see Chapter 2; Figure 2–3)

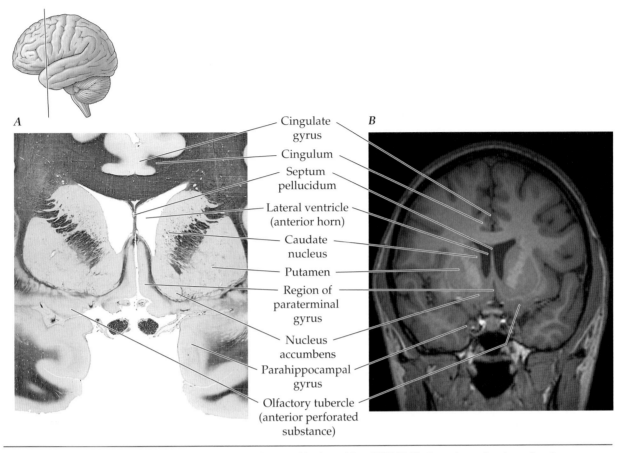

Cingulate
gyrus

Cingulum

Septum
pellucidum

Lateral ventricle
(anterior horn)

Caudate
nucleus

Putamen

Region of
paraterminal
gyrus

Nucleus
accumbens

Parahippocampal
gyrus

Olfactory tubercle
(anterior perforated
substance)

A

B

FIGURE 16–10 Myelin-stained coronal section through the rostral forebrain (*A*) and MRI (*B*). The inset shows the plane of section. (*B*, Courtesy of Dr. Joy Hirsch, Columbia University.)

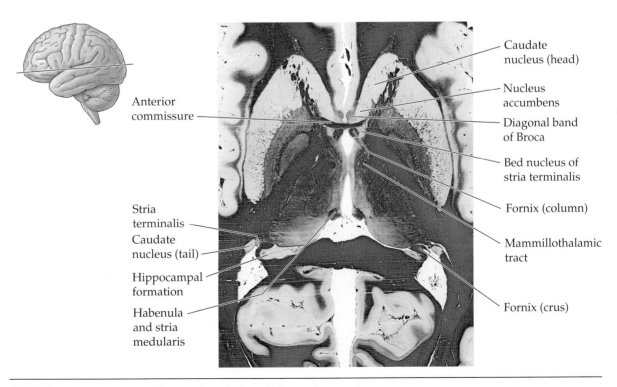

Caudate
nucleus (head)

Nucleus
accumbens

Diagonal band
of Broca

Bed nucleus of
stria terminalis

Fornix (column)

Mammillothalamic
tract

Fornix (crus)

Anterior
commissure

Stria
terminalis

Caudate
nucleus (tail)

Hippocampal
formation

Habenula
and stria
medularis

FIGURE 16–11 Myelin-stained horizontal section through the anterior commissure.

is particularly important for normal thoughts, moods, and behaviors. This conclusion is based on the observation that many of the drugs used to treat psychiatric illness—the disorders of thought, such as schizophrenia, and of mood, such as depression and anxiety—selectively affect one of the neurotransmitter systems. These neurotransmitter systems have direct and widespread connections with the limbic system:

- The **ventral tegmental area** influences many limbic system structures, as indicated earlier (Figure 16–8). Coursing through the **medial forebrain bundle,** the dopaminergic fibers synapse on neurons in the dorsolateral prefrontal association area, medial orbitofrontal cortex, cingulate gyrus, ventral striatum, amygdala, and hippocampal formation. An important hypothesis for the pathophysiology of schizophrenia is that an exaggerated dopamine response leads to prefrontal cortex dysfunction, which is a key region for organization of thoughts and behaviors.

- **Serotonergic** projections to limbic system structures of the telencephalon and diencephalon originate from the **dorsal and median raphe nuclei** (see Figure 16–19B, C). Coursing within three tracts—the medial forebrain bundle, the dorsal longitudinal fasciculus, and the medial longitudinal fasciculus—the ascending serotonergic projection synapses on neurons in the amygdala, hippocampal formation, all areas of the striatum, and cerebral cortex. Drugs that block serotonin reuptake mechanisms are effective in treating mood disorders, including anxiety and obsessive-compulsive disorders.

- The **noradrenergic** projection, which originates from the **locus ceruleus** (see Figure 16–19C), influences the entire cerebral cortex, including the limbic association areas, as well as limbic and other subcortical structures. This system, together with the serotonergic system, may play a role in depression because drugs that ameliorate depression result in elevations of these two monoamines.

- The **cholinergic** projection originates from large neurons in the **basal nucleus,** the **medial septal nucleus,** and the **nucleus of the diagonal band of Broca** (see Figure 16–12). Additional brain stem cholinergic cell groups with widespread cortical (and thalamic) projections are found near the **pedunculopontine nucleus** (see Figure 16–19B). As discussed in Chapter 14, the pedunculopontine nucleus is an important output nucleus of the basal ganglia, and is a target of deep brain electrical stimulation to ameliorate signs of Parkinson disease. Targets of the cholinergic projection include the entire neocortex (including the limbic association cortex), the amygdala, and the hippocampal formation. **Alzheimer disease,** characterized by progressive dementia, begins with a loss of these basal forebrain cholinergic neurons. As the disease progresses, other neurotransmitter systems are also affected.

Regional Anatomy of Neural Systems for Emotions, Learning, and Memory, and Reward

Knowledge of the three-dimensional configuration of individual limbic system structures is essential for understanding their location in two-dimensional slices. As noted earlier in this chapter, three components of the limbic system have a C-shape: (1) the hippocampal formation and its output pathway, the fornix (Figure 16–2), (2) part of the amygdala and one of its pathways, the stria terminalis (Figure 16–7), and (3) the limbic association cortex, especially the cingulate and parahippocampal gyri (Figure 16–3). As a consequence of their C-shape, a coronal section through the cerebral hemisphere may transect these structures twice: first dorsally and then ventrally. In horizontal sections, C-shaped structures are located rostrally and caudally.

The Nucleus Accumbens and Olfactory Tubercle Comprise Part of the Basal Forebrain

Sections through the rostral forebrain cut through components of the limbic loop of the basal ganglia. The input side of the loop (see Figures 14–5 and 14–8) is the **ventral striatum,** consisting of the **nucleus accumbens,** the olfactory tubercle, and the ventromedial parts of the caudate nucleus and putamen (Figures 16–10 and 16–12). The ventral striatum receives information from all of the nuclear divisions of the amygdala as well as from the hippocampal formation and limbic association cortex. The output nucleus of the limbic loop is the **ventral pallidum** (Figure 16–12), which projects to parts of the **medial dorsal nucleus** of the thalamus (see Figure 16–14B) and from there to the **dorsolateral prefrontal cortex, orbitofrontal cortex,** and **anterior cingulate gyrus.** The ventral striatum also has direct projections to the amygdala. Recall that the dorsal parts of the striatum are important in skeletal motor and oculomotor functions and cognition. Their outputs are focused on the internal and external segments of the globus pallidus and the substantia nigra pars reticulata. Nevertheless, as discussed in Chapter 14, there are ways the limbic and motor loops can interact, which allow the limbic loop to influence movement control.

Other than receiving olfactory input from the olfactory bulb and tract, little is known of the functions of the **olfactory tubercle.** The olfactory tubercle corresponds to the region on the ventral surface termed the **anterior perforated substance** (Figure 16–4). This is where penetrating branches of the middle and anterior cerebral arteries (the lenticulostriate arteries) enter the basal brain surface to supply parts of the basal ganglia and internal capsule. The slice shown in Figure 16–10 also cuts through the most anterior portions of the cingulate and parahippocampal gyri.

A

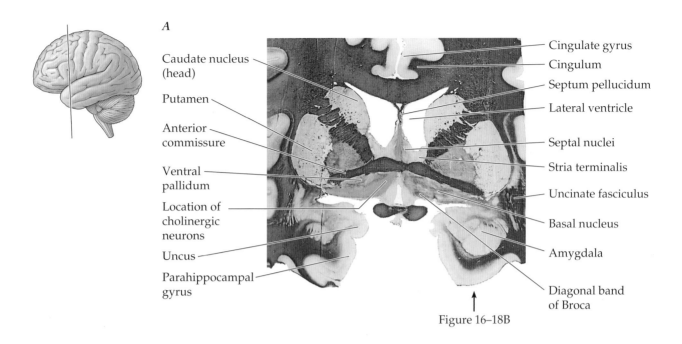

Caudate nucleus (head)

Putamen

Anterior commissure

Ventral pallidum

Location of cholinergic neurons

Uncus

Parahippocampal gyrus

Cingulate gyrus

Cingulum

Septum pellucidum

Lateral ventricle

Septal nuclei

Stria terminalis

Uncinate fasciculus

Basal nucleus

Amygdala

Diagonal band of Broca

Figure 16–18B

B

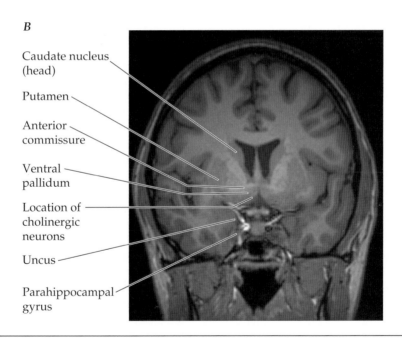

Caudate nucleus (head)

Putamen

Anterior commissure

Ventral pallidum

Location of cholinergic neurons

Uncus

Parahippocampal gyrus

FIGURE 16–12   Myelin-stained coronal section through the septal nuclei, basal nucleus, (**A**) and amygdala and MRI (**B**). The arrow points to the plane of section of this image in Figure 16-18B. The inset shows the plane of section. (**B,** Courtesy of Dr. Joy Hirsch, Columbia University.)

This is the level of the **temporal pole,** which has connections with orbitofrontal cortex and the amygdala; it also has direct projections to the hypothalamus. As discussed earlier, temporal pole cortex is important for personality. Connections with the orbitofrontal lobe are made by axons that travel within the **uncinate fasciculus** (Figure 16–12).

Basal Forebrain Cholinergic Systems Have Diffuse Limbic and Neocortical Projections

The **septal nuclei** are adjacent to the **septum pellucidum** (Figures 16–10 and 16–12), a nonneural structure that separates the anterior horns of the lateral ventricles of the two cerebral hemispheres. Animal studies have revealed that the septal nuclei consist of separate medial and lateral components. In humans, the lateral septal nucleus may correspond to neurons located near the ventricular surface, whereas the medial septal nucleus, to those near the septum pellucidum. Moreover, these medial cells are continuous with the gray matter on the medial surface of the cerebral hemisphere, just rostral to the **lamina terminalis.** This region, termed the **paraterminal gyrus** (Figure 16–3), merges with the **nucleus of the diagonal band of Broca,** which is located on the basal forebrain surface (Figures 16–4, 16–11, and 16–12).

The lateral septal nucleus is a target of the projection from the hippocampus, via the fornix. The medial septal nucleus receives its major input from the lateral septal nucleus and projects to three sites: (1) to the hippocampal formation, (2) to the periaqueductal gray matter and reticular formation, and (3) to the habenula, a portion of the diencephalon. The projection to the hippocampal formation, via the fornix, is important in regulating hippocampal neuronal activity. The projection to the periaqueductal gray matter and reticular formation, via the **medial forebrain bundle,** is thought to be important in evoking stereotypic behaviors in response to environmental stimuli. Finally, the projection to the **habenula,** located lateral and ventral to the pineal gland (Figure 16–11; see Figure AI–7), is part of a circuit with the midbrain medial dopaminergic and serotonergic systems. The habenulopeduncular tract (see Figure AII–15) is the highly myelinated output tract of the habenula.

The **basal forebrain** is located on the ventral surface of the cerebral hemisphere. It includes the paraterminal gyrus, nucleus of the diagonal band of Broca, and anterior perforated substance. The septal nuclei are continuous with many basal forebrain structures. On Figure 16–4, the basal forebrain is located approximately anterior to and beneath the optic chiasm and tracts. Large neurons are located here that use **acetylcholine** as their principal neurotransmitter. In addition to the medial septal nucleus, cholinergic neurons are located in the nucleus of the diagonal band of Broca and the **basal nucleus** (Figure 16–12). The various cholinergic neurons form a continuous band, from dorsomedially in the septal nuclei to ventrolaterally in the basal nucleus (Figure 16–12, orange shading). Other large cholinergic neurons are dispersed between the lamina of the globus pallidus and putamen and adjacent to the internal capsule. Some are present in the lateral hypothalamus. The basal forebrain cholinergic neurons (including those in the medial septal nucleus) excite their targets primarily through **muscarinic receptors;** such responses to acetylcholine are important in integrating information because they facilitate responses to other inputs. These cholinergic neurons, through widespread cortical projections, may also modulate overall cortical excitability.

The Cingulum Courses Beneath the Cingulate and Parahippocampal Gyri

Two cortical limbic areas, the cingulate and parahippocampal gyri, are seen in a series of coronal sections (Figures 16–10 and 16–12 to 16–16): The cingulate gyrus is located dorsally, and the parahippocampal gyrus is located ventrally. The pathway that connects regions of the dorsolateral prefrontal cortex, the orbitofrontal gyri and the cingulate gyrus with the parahippocampal gyrus, including the **entorhinal cortex,** is termed the **cingulum.** This pathway is located in the white matter beneath the cingulate gyrus (Figure 16–12). Unlike the cingulum, another limbic system cortical association pathway, the **uncinate fasciculus** (Figures 16–12 and 16–13), has a more direct trajectory for interconnecting anterior portions of the temporal lobe with medial orbital gyri of the frontal lobe.

The Three Nuclear Divisions of the Amygdala Are Revealed in Coronal Section

The amygdala is located in the rostral temporal lobe beneath the cortex of the parahippocampal gyrus (Figures 16–12 to 16–14A). The amygdala is rostral and slightly dorsal to the hippocampal formation. (Compare the parasagittal section in Figure 16–18B with the drawing in Figure 16–2.) The arrow in Figure 16–12 shows the approximate plane of section in Figure 16–18B. The amygdala and the rostral hippocampal formations form the **uncus** (Figures 16–3 and 16–14). Expanding space-occupying lesions above the tentorium cerebelli (see Figure 3–15), especially those of the temporal lobe, may displace the uncus medially. This **uncal herniation** compresses midbrain structures, ultimately resulting in coma and even death. Initially uncal herniation can compress the oculomotor nerves, which exit from the ventral midbrain surface. This results in third nerve dysfunction, including paralysis of extraocular muscles and loss of pupillary light reflexes.

The three nuclear divisions of the amygdala are schematically depicted in the inset to Figure 16–13. The **cortical** division of the amygdala merges with the overlying cortex of the medial temporal lobe. This division receives a major input directly from the **olfactory bulb.** The two other nuclear divisions, **basolateral** and **central,** are also shown. The **bed nucleus of the stria terminalis** is the C-shaped nuclear component of the amygdala. It has connections with brain stem autonomic and visceral afferent nuclei and thus has connections similar to those of the central nuclear division. Along with the central nucleus and several smaller nuclei, they form the extended amygdala. A portion of the bed nucleus of the stria terminalis is thought to be sexually dimorphic.

The stria terminalis and the ventral amygdalofugal pathway are the two output pathways of the amygdala

The **stria terminalis** carries output from the amygdala, predominantly from the cortical nuclei. The stria terminalis and its bed nucleus are located medial to the caudate nucleus, in a shallow groove formed at the junction of the thalamus and the caudate nucleus (Figures 16–11 and 16–14), termed the

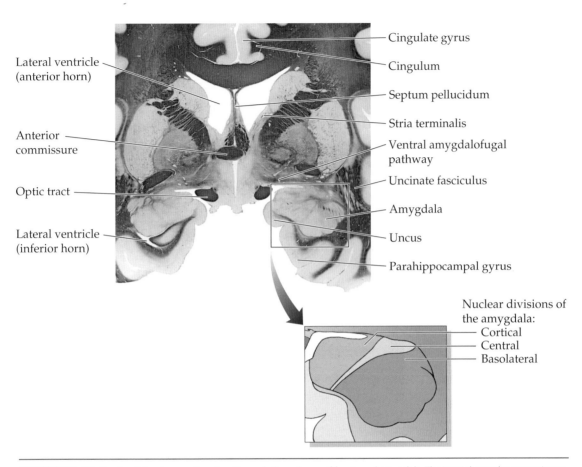

Cingulate gyrus

Cingulum

Septum pellucidum

Stria terminalis

Ventral amygdalofugal pathway

Uncinate fasciculus

Amygdala

Uncus

Parahippocampal gyrus

Lateral ventricle (anterior horn)

Anterior commissure

Optic tract

Lateral ventricle (inferior horn)

Nuclear divisions of the amygdala:
Cortical
Central
Basolateral

FIGURE 16–13 Myelin-stained coronal section through the column of fornix and amygdala. The inset shows the approximate location of the nuclear divisions in the amygdala.

terminal sulcus. Running along with the stria terminalis and bed nucleus is the **thalamostriate vein** (or terminal vein), which drains portions of the thalamus and caudate nucleus. The stria terminalis does not stain darkly because its axons are not heavily myelinated. A major target of the axons running in the stria terminalis is the **ventral medial nucleus of the hypothalamus,** which is important in feeding.

The other efferent pathway of the amygdala, the **ventral amygdalofugal pathway** (Figure 16–13), runs ventral to the anterior commissure and globus pallidus (see Chapter 14). The projections of the central and basolateral nuclei course primarily in this efferent pathway. The ventral pathway has four major targets:

1. The **medial dorsal nucleus** of the thalamus (Figures 16–15B and 16–16) links synaptically the basolateral amygdala indirectly with the frontal lobe. Separate portions of the medial dorsal nucleus project to the dorsolateral prefrontal and orbitofrontal cortical areas.

2. The ventral amygdalofugal pathway links the central nuclei of the amygdala with the lateral **hypothalamus** for autonomic nervous system control and with parvocellular neurons for neuroendocrine control. The central nuclei of the amygdala influence corticotropin

hormone release by parvocellular neurosecretory neurons of the paraventricular nucleus (Chapter 15). This control is exerted by disinhibition: GABAergic output neurons of the central nuclei synapse on GABAergic neurons in the hypothalamus that control the neurosecretory neurons. Disinhibition is an important feature of circuitry in the cerebellar cortex (Chapter 13) and basal ganglia (Chapter 14).

3. The **basal forebrain,** including the ventral striatum and the cholinergic neurons of the basal nucleus and nucleus of the diagonal band of Broca, links the amygdala synaptically with the cortex.

4. The **brain stem,** which contains parasympathetic preganglionic nuclei, receives a projection from the central nuclei.

The Hippocampal Formation Is Located in the Floor of the Inferior Horn of the Lateral Ventricle

Coronal sections through the temporal lobe, from rostral to caudal directions, slice first through the amygdala, then

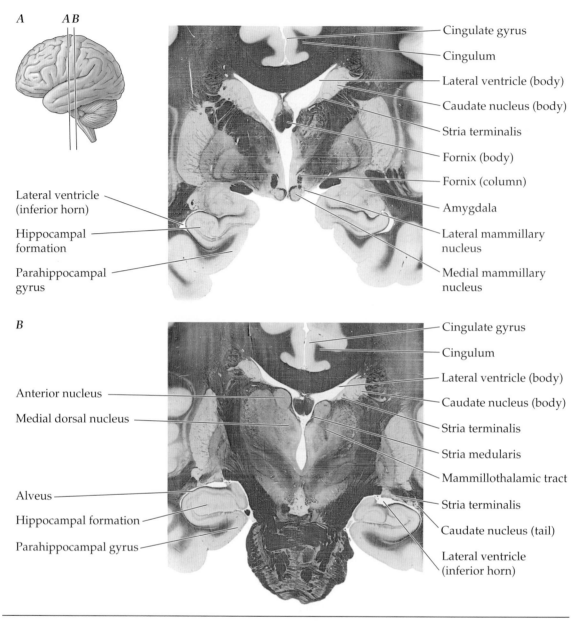

A   *A B*

A

Cingulate gyrus

Cingulum

Lateral ventricle (body)

Caudate nucleus (body)

Stria terminalis

Fornix (body)

Fornix (column)

Amygdala

Lateral mammillary nucleus

Medial mammillary nucleus

Lateral ventricle (inferior horn)

Hippocampal formation

Parahippocampal gyrus

B

Anterior nucleus

Medial dorsal nucleus

Alveus

Hippocampal formation

Parahippocampal gyrus

Cingulate gyrus

Cingulum

Lateral ventricle (body)

Caudate nucleus (body)

Stria terminalis

Stria medularis

Mammillothalamic tract

Stria terminalis

Caudate nucleus (tail)

Lateral ventricle (inferior horn)

FIGURE 16–14 Myelin-stained coronal section through the mammillary bodies (**A**) and through the mammillothalamic tract (**B**). In **B,** the mammillothalamic tract is seen on the right side only because the section is asymmetric. The inset shows the planes of section.

through both the amygdala and hippocampal formation, and finally through the hippocampal formation alone. (Figures 16–14 and 16–15 show these rostrocaudal relationships.) The hippocampal formation forms part of the floor of the inferior horn of the lateral ventricle. In coronal section (eg, Figure 16–15), the hippocampal formation is located ventrally and the fornix is located dorsally. In horizontal section (Figure 16–11), the hippocampal formation (which here is quite small) is caudal and the fornix is rostral. There is a minuscule portion of the hippocampal formation dorsal to the corpus callosum that is vestigial; in the mature brain, it is termed the indusium griseum (see Figure AII–16). Some schizophrenic individuals exhibit degeneration of the hippocampal formation and other medial temporal lobe neural structures.

In consequence, this produces an increase in the size of the lateral ventricle.

During development the hippocampal formation undergoes an infolding into the temporal lobe (Figure 16–16). The simple sequence of the component parts of the temporal lobe, from the parahippocampal gyrus on the lateral surface to the dentate gyrus on the medial surface, becomes more complex later in development. As the **hippocampal sulcus** forms, the dentate gyrus and the subiculum become apposed; the pial surfaces of these two structures fuse, and a hippocampal afferent pathway (the perforant pathway) courses through this fusion (Figure 16–17B).

The morphology of the hippocampal formation, as well as many of the limbic association areas, differs from that of

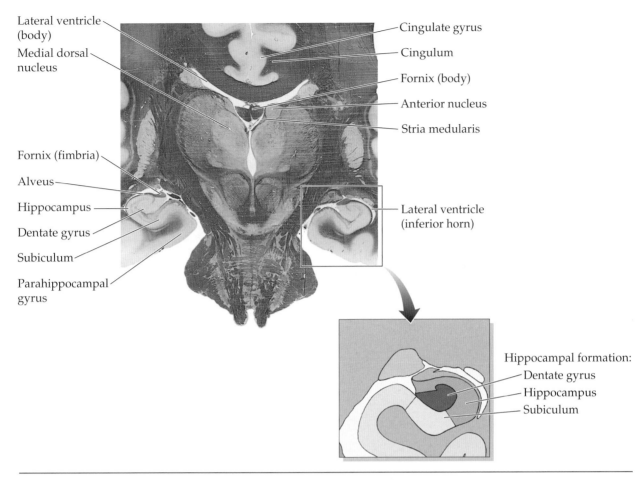

FIGURE 16–15 Myelin-stained coronal section through the medial dorsal nucleus of the thalamus. The divisions of the hippocampal formation are shown in the inset.

the rest of the cortex. As we learned in Chapter 9, the principal cortex is **neocortex** (eg, primary somatic sensory cortex or posterior parietal association cortex), which has six major cell layers (Figure 16–16B1). The other type of cortex is **allocortex** (Figure 16–16B2), which has fewer than six layers and is more variable. The hippocampal formation is a kind of allocortex termed **archicortex;** regions in the parahippocampal gyrus and the cingulate gyrus under the corpus callosum are the other kind of allocortex, termed **paleocortex.**

The three divisions of the hippocampal formation—the **dentate gyrus, hippocampus,** and **subiculum**—are shown in the inset in Figure 16–15. Each division has three principal cell layers, conforming to the common allocortex plan (Figure 16–16B). The pyramidal layer—or granule cell layer in the dentate gyrus—contains the projection neurons of the region. The other layers contain interneurons. Whereas the output neurons of the pyramidal layer (pyramidal neurons) in the hippocampus and subiculum can project outside the hippocampal formation (see Box 16–1), the granule cells of the dentate gyrus connect only within the hippocampal formation.

Pyramidal cells of the hippocampus and subiculum have extrinsic connections, sending their axons to cortical and subcortical targets (Figure 16–6B). The hippocampus and subiculum have extensive "back" projections to the entorhinal cortex that, in turn, project widely to other cortical regions (Figure 16–6). The principal subcortical targets are the mammillary bodies, which receive a projection from pyramidal cells mostly of the subiculum, and the lateral septal nucleus, which receives a projection primarily from the hippocampus. These axons course in the fornix. In addition to extrinsic connections, both sides of the hippocampal formation are interconnected through **commissural neurons** whose axons course in the ventral portion of the fornix.

A Sagittal Cut Through the Mammillary Bodies Reveals the Fornix and Mammillothalamic Tract

Structures that have a C-shape are oriented approximately in the sagittal plane. The sagittal section in Figure 16–18A is located close to the midline and transects the fornix, although not through its entire length. The sagittal section in Figure 16–18B is located farther laterally and cuts through the long axis of the hippocampal formation.

Pyramidal cell axons of the hippocampus and subiculum form the **alveus,** the myelinated envelope surrounding the hippocampal formation (Figure 16–18B). These axons collect on the medial side of the hippocampal formation to form the first

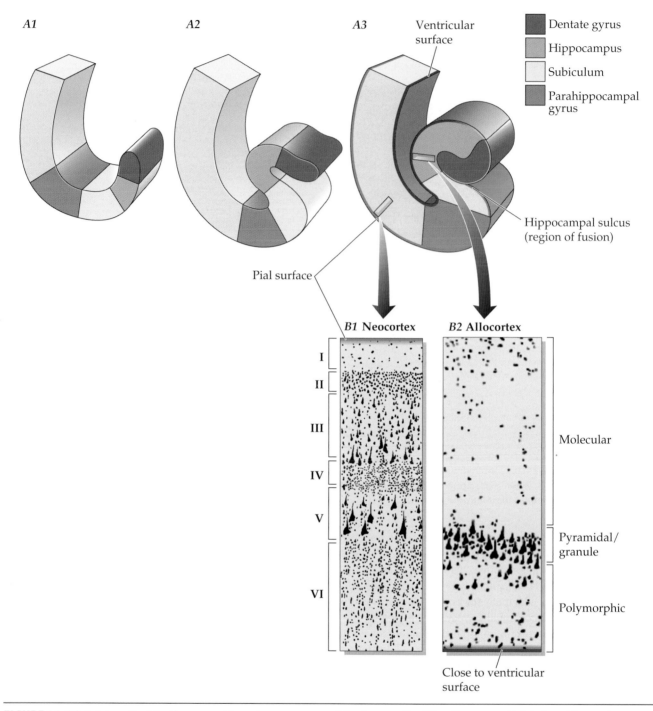

A1 *A2* *A3* Ventricular surface

Dentate gyrus
Hippocampus
Subiculum
Parahippocampal gyrus

Hippocampal sulcus (region of fusion)

Pial surface

B1 **Neocortex** *B2* **Allocortex**

I
II
III
IV
V
VI

Molecular

Pyramidal/ granule

Polymorphic

Close to ventricular surface

FIGURE 16–16 *A.* Schematic of the hippocampal formation at two stages of development (***A1, A2***) and in maturity (***A3***). (Adapted from Williams PL, Warwick R. *Functional Neuroanatomy of Man.* New York, NY: W. B. Saunders; 1975.) The neocortex (***B1***) on the lateral cortical surface has six cell layers, and the allocortex (***B2***), located medially, has fewer than six layers. The drawing of a Nissl-stained section through the neocortex of the human brain in ***B1*** is semischematic. The section through the allocortex is of a portion of the hippocampal formation, termed archicortex; it has only three cell layers. (Adapted from Brodmann K. *Vergleichende Lokalisationslehre der Grosshirnrinde in ihren Prinzipien Dargestellt auf Grund des Zellen-baues.* Barth, Germany; 1909.)

of the four anatomical parts of the fornix, termed the **fimbria.** The other three parts—the **crus** (where the axons are separate from the hippocampal formation), the **body** (where the axons from both sides join at the midline), and the **column** (where axons descend toward their targets)—bring the axons of the fornix to neurons in the diencephalon and rostral telencephalon.

The body and column of the fornix can be seen in Figure 16–18A. Note how the column of the fornix descends

caudal to the **anterior commissure** to terminate in the **mammillary body;** this is the **postcommissural fornix** (see also Figure 16–11, where the columns of the fornix are caudal to the anterior commissure). The mammillary body comprises the medial and lateral mammillary nuclei (Figure 16–14A), and the fornix terminates in both components. The major output, the **mammillothalamic tract,** originates from both the medial and lateral mammillary nuclei. Axons

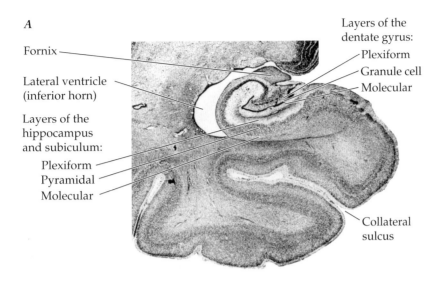

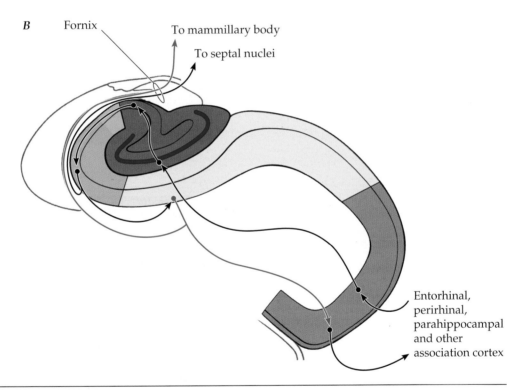

FIGURE 16–17 The hippocampal formation. **A.** Nissl-stained section through the human hippocampal formation, parahippocampal gyrus, and ventral temporal lobe. The hippocampus has three cytoarchitectonic divisions. These divisions are abbreviated CA for cornus ammonis, or Ammon's horn. (Early anatomists noted that the hippocampal formation, together with the fornix, looked like the horns of a ram.) **B.** The basic serial circuit of the hippocampal formation is superimposed on the cytoarchitecture of the hippocampal formation and entorhinal cortex. Additionally, entorhinal and association cortex projects in parallel to different hippocampal formation areas. (**A,** Courtesy of Dr. David Amaral, State University of New York at Stony Brook. **B,** Adapted from Zola-Morgan S, Squire LR, Amaral DG. Human amnesia and medial temporal lobe region: enduring memory impairment following a bilateral lesion limited to field CA1 of the hippocampus. *J Neurosci.* 1986;6[10]:2950-2967.)

of the mammillothalamic tract also can be seen leaving the mammillary body in Figure 16–18A. These axons are coursing toward the **anterior thalamic nuclei** (Figure 16–14B). The lateral mammillary nucleus (Figure 16–14A) also gives rise to the **mammillotegmental tract,** which descends to the midbrain and rostral pontine reticular formation. Degeneration

of the mammillary bodies, along with portions of the medial thalamus, occurs in **Korsakoff syndrome.** These patients have profound memory loss, attributable to impairment in expressin g the functions of the subiculum. This condition results from thimamine deficiency, typically accompanying alcoholism.

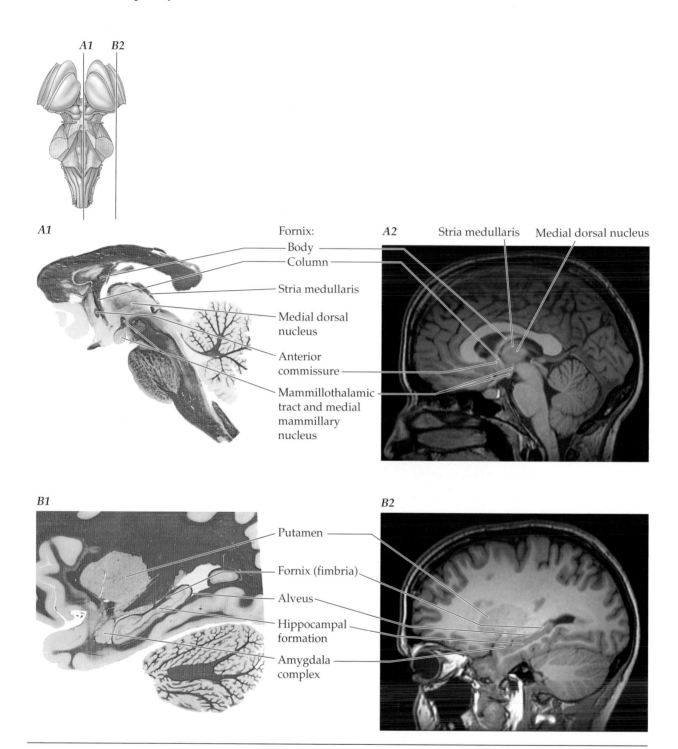

FIGURE 16–18 Sagittal views through the brain revealing portions of C-shaped limbic system structures. **A.** Myelin-stained midsagittal section through the cerebral hemisphere, diencephalon, and brain stem close to the midline (**A1**) and corresponding MRI (**A2**). Parasagittal section through the amygdaloid complex and hippocampal formation (**B1**) and corresponding MRI (**B2**). (**A2, B2,** Courtesy of Dr. Joy Hirsch, Columbia University.)

Fibers of the fornix also terminate in locations other than the mammillary bodies. Some of these fibers terminate directly in the anterior thalamic nuclei; others project to the amygdala and nucleus accumbens. Moreover, rostral to the anterior commissure, the **precommissural fornix,** which is smaller than the postcommissural portion, courses away from the midline. (It cannot be seen in the section in Figure 16–18A.) An important projection of the hippocampus is to the lateral septal nucleus through the precommissural fornix. A portion of the **stria medullaris,** which has a predominantly rostrocaudal course, is also revealed in this section (Figure 16–18A). As discussed earlier, the medial septal nucleus projects axons into the stria medullaris. These axons synapse in the habenula (see Figures AI–7 and AII–18).

Nuclei in the Brain Stem Link Telencephalic and Diencephalic Limbic Structures With the Autonomic Nervous System and the Spinal Cord

The **periaqueductal gray matter** and **reticular formation** (Figure 16–19) are thought to be important in the behavioral expression of emotions, such as stereotypic defense reactions or the body's response to stress. Septal neurons project to the midbrain reticular formation via neurons of the **lateral hypothalamus.** Neurons of the lateral hypothalamus are interspersed throughout the **medial forebrain bundle** (see Chapter 15). From these midbrain regions, the actions of neurons in wide areas of the reticular formation can be modified by the limbic system. The hypothalamus also projects to the periaqueductal gray matter. Chapter 5 considered the projection of the periaqueductal gray matter to the raphe nuclei (see Figure 5–8), which give rise to a spinal cord projection for regulating pain transmission.

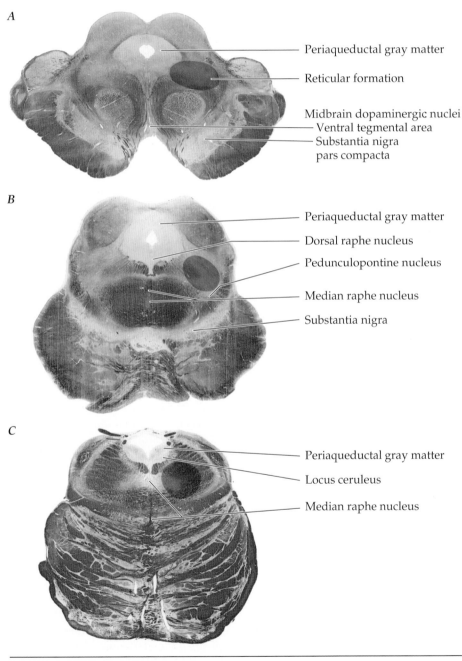

FIGURE 16–19 Components of the brain stem related to the limbic system. Myelin-stained sections through the rostral midbrain (**A**), caudal midbrain (**B**), and rostral pons (**C**). The reticular formation is indicated by green-shaded regions.

General Anatomy of the Limbic System

The limbic system comprises a set of structures located predominantly on the medial surface of the cerebral hemisphere (Figures 16–2 and 16–3). The diverse functions of the limbic system include important roles in *reward, memory, and emotions*—and their *behavioral* and *visceral consequences*. Many of the structures have a *C-shaped configuration*. The limbic system has three C-shaped components (Figures 16–2 to 16–5): (1) the *limbic association cortex,* (2) the *hippocampal formation* and *fornix,* and (3) part of the amygdala (*stria terminalis* and bed nucleus of the stria terminalis).

Limbic Association Cortex

The limbic cortical areas include the following structures (Figures 16–3 and 16–4): the *medial orbital gyri* of the frontal lobe, the *cingulate gyrus* in the frontal and parietal lobes, the *parahippocampal gyrus* in the temporal lobe, and the cortex of the *temporal pole*. The limbic cortical areas receive input from higher-order sensory areas in the temporal lobe and from the other cortical association areas, the *prefrontal association cortex* and the *parietal-temporal-occipital association area*. The two principal pathways carrying cortical association axons to and from other limbic system structures are the *cingulum* (located beneath the cingulate gyrus; Figure 16–12) and the *uncinate fasciculus* (Figure 16–12). The cytoarchitecture of limbic association cortex differs from that of other cortical regions. The cortex on the external surface of the parahippocampal gyrus lateral to the *collateral sulcus* (Figure 16–4) has at least six layers (neocortex), whereas the cortex medial to the sulcus is more variable and typically has fewer than six cell layers (*allocortex*) (Figure 16–16B). Cholinergic projections to limbic cortex, the hippocampal formation, and lateral cortical areas originate from the basal forebrain, including the *basal nucleus,* the *nucleus of the diagonal band of Broca,* and the *medial septal nucleus* (Figure 16–12).

Hippocampal Formation

The *hippocampal formation* (Figures 16–2 and 16–5) includes three cytoarchitectonically distinct subdivisions (Figures 16–5, 16–13, and 16–17): the *dentate gyrus,* the *hippocampus,* and the *subiculum*. The hippocampal formation plays an essential role in consolidation of explicit and spatial memory. The limbic association cortex provides the major input to the hippocampal formation. The *entorhinal cortex,* a specific portion of the rostral parahippocampal gyrus, projects directly to the hippocampal formation

(Figure 16–6A). Other portions of the limbic association cortex influence the hippocampal formation indirectly, via the entorhinal cortex. The dentate gyrus, hippocampus, and subiculum are separate processing stages in a sequence of intrinsic connections in the hippocampal formation (Figure 16–17). The flow of information through the hippocampal formation is largely unidirectional.

Hippocampal efferents originate from the subiculum and the hippocampus proper; the dentate gyrus projects only to part of the hippocampus. Cortical projections from the hippocampus and subiculum terminate in the entorhinal cortex, and from there information is widely distributed throughout the cerebral cortex (Figure 16–6B). Subcortical projections are via the *fornix*. Most of the axons in the fornix are those of *pyramidal cells* of the subiculum and hippocampus. Axons from the *subiculum* synapse in the *mammillary body* (Figures 16–6B, 16–14A, and 16–18A). These axons course in the postcommissural fornix (Figure 16–19A). The mammillary bodies project, via the *mammillothalamic tract* (Figures 16–14A and 16–18A), to the *anterior thalamic nuclei* (Figure 16–14B), which project to the *cingulate gyrus* (Figures 16–3 and 16–11). The hippocampus projects, via the precommissural fornix, to the *lateral septal nucleus* (Figures 16–6B and 16–12). The *medial septal nucleus,* which contains cholinergic and GABAergic neurons, projects back to the *hippocampal formation,* via the *fornix*.

Amygdala

The amygdala has three major nuclear divisions (Figures 16–7 and 16–13), which collectively are involved in *emotions* and their *behavioral expression:* the basolateral nuclei, the central nuclei, and the cortical nuclei. The *basolateral nuclei* receive a major input from the *cerebral cortex* and project to the *medial dorsal nucleus* of the thalamus, the *basal nucleus,* the *ventral striatum,* and back to the *cortex* (temporal, orbitofrontal, and prefrontal association areas). The *central nuclei,* important for the visceral expression of emotion and reward/addiction, are reciprocally connected with *viscerosensory* and *visceral motor nuclei* of the brain stem. They also project to the hypothalamus to regulate neuroendocrine functions. The *cortical nuclei* receive direct olfactory input. They may play a role in appetitive behaviors and neuroendocrine functions through their projections to the *ventromedial nucleus* of the hypothalamus.

The amygdala has two output pathways: (1) The *stria terminalis* (Figures 16–7C and 16–13), which is C-shaped, carries the efferent projection primarily from the *cortical nuclei,* and (2) the *ventral amygdalofugal pathway* (Figure 16–13) carries the efferents from the *central nuclei,* which descend to the brain stem, and those from the *basolateral nuclei,* which ascend to the *thalamus,* the *ventral striatum,* and the *basal nucleus* (Figures 16–12 and 16–13). The bed nucleus of the stria terminalis runs along with the stria.

Limbic Loop of the Basal Ganglia and Ventral Tegmental Area

The limbic loop of the basal ganglia comprises the *ventral striatum* (*nucleus accumbens,* and adjoining ventral portions of the caudate nucleus and putamen; Figures 16–8 and 16–10). Its output is directed to the *ventral pallidum* (Figure 16–12). The *medial dorsal nucleus* of the thalamus, which is a target of the ventral pallidum, projects to *orbitofrontal, medial frontal,* and *dorsolateral prefrontal cortex.* The *ventral tegmental area* (Figures 16–8 and 16–19A) contains *dopaminergic neurons* that project to the ventral striatum and prefrontal, medial frontal, and orbitofrontal cortex and is key to reward, punishment, and decision signaling in the brain.

Selected Readings

LeDoux J, Damasio A. Emotions and feelings. In: Kandel ER, Schwartz JH, Jessell TM, Siegelbaum SA, Hudspeth AJ, eds. *Principles of Neural Science.* 5th ed. New York, NY: McGraw-Hill; in press.

Shizgal P, Hyman SP. Homeostasis, motivation, and addictive states. In: Kandel ER, Schwartz JH, Jessell TM, Siegelbaum SA, Hudspeth AJ, eds. *Principles of Neural Science.* 5th ed. New York, NY: McGraw-Hill; in press.

References

Aggleton JP. The contribution of the amygdala to normal and abnormal emotional states. *Trends Neurosci.* 1993;16:328-333.

Albin RL, Mink JW. Recent advances in Tourette syndrome research. *TINS.* 2006;29(3):175-182.

Andy OJ, Stephan H. The septum of the human brain. *J Comp Neurol.* 1968;133:383-410.

Carlsen J, Heimer L. The basolateral amygdaloid complex as a cortical-like structure. *Brain Res.* 1988;441:377-380.

Corkin S. What's new with the amnesic patient H.M.? *Nat Rev Neurosci.* 2002;3:153-160.

Curtis MA, Kam M, Nannmark U, et al. Human neuroblasts migrate to the olfactory bulb via a lateral ventricular extension. *Science.* 2007;315(5816):1243-1249.

Dalgleish T. The emotional brain. *Nat Rev Neurosci.* 2004;5:582-589.

Dantzer R, O'Connor JC, Freund GG, Johnson RW, Kelley KW. From inflammation to sickness and depression: when the immune system subjugates the brain. *Nat Rev Neurosci.* 2008;9(1):46-56.

Davidson RJ, Putnam KM, Larson CL. Dysfunction in the neural circuitry of emotion regulation—a possible prelude to violence. *Science.* 2000;289:591-594.

de Olmos J. Amygdala. In: Paxinos G, Mai JK, eds. *The Human Nervous System.* Vol 738-868. London: Elsevier; 2004.

Drevets WC. Neuroimaging and neuropathological studies of depression: implications for the cognitive-emotional features of mood disorders. *Curr Opin Neurobiol.* 2001;11:240-249.

Duvernoy HM. *The Human Hippocampus: An Atlas of Applied Anatomy.* Berlin: Springer; 1998:213.

Fanselow MS, Dong HW. Are the dorsal and ventral hippocampus functionally distinct structures? *Neuron.* 2010;65(1):7-19.

Farnham FR, Ritchie CW, James DV, Kennedy HG. Pathology of love. *Lancet.* 1997;350:710.

Fisher H, Aron A, Brown LL. Romantic love: an fMRI study of a neural mechanism for mate choice. *J Comp Neurol.* 2005;493(1):58-62.

Fisher HE, Aron A, Brown LL. Romantic love: a mammalian brain system for mate choice. *Philos Trans R Soc Lond B Biol Sci.* 2006;361(1476):2173-2186.

Frackowiak RS. *Human Brain Function.* San Diego, CA: Elsevier; 2004.

Georgiadis JR, Kortekaas R, Kuipers R, et al. Regional cerebral blood flow changes associated with clitorally induced orgasm in healthy women. *Euro J Neurosci.* 2006;24(11):3305-3316.

Georgiadis JR, Reinders AA, Paans AM, Renken R, Kortekaas R. Men versus women on sexual brain function: prominent differences during tactile genital stimulation, but not during orgasm. *Human Brain Mapping.* 2009;30(10):3089-3101.

Gould E. How widespread is adult neurogenesis in mammals? *Nat Rev Neurosci.* 2007;8(6):481-488.

Grace AA. Gating of information flow within the limbic system and the pathophysiology of schizophrenia. *Brain Res Brain Res Rev.* 2000;31:330-341.

Grace AA, Bunney BS, Moore H, Todd CL. Dopamine-cell depolarization block as a model for the therapeutic actions of antipsychotic drugs. *Trends Neurosci.* 1997;20:31-37.

Haber SN. Integrative networks across basal ganglia circuits. In: Steiner H, Kuei T, eds. *Handbook of Basal Ganglia Structure and Function.* London: Elsevier; 2010:409-427.

Haber SN, Johnson Gdowski M. The basal ganglia. In: Paxinos G, Mai JK, eds. *The Human Nervous System.* London: Elsevier; 2004.

Haber SN, Knutson B. The reward circuit: linking primate anatomy and human imaging. *Neuropsychopharmacology.* 2010;35(1):4-26.

Hedren JC, Strumble RG, Whitehouse PJ, et al. Topography of the magnocellular basal forebrain system in the human brain. *J Neuropathol ExpNeurol.* 1984;43:1–21.

Holstege G, Huynh HK. Brain circuits for mating behavior in cats and brain activations and de-activations during sexual stimulation and ejaculation and orgasm in humans. *Horm Behav.* 2011;59:702-707.

Holstege G, Mouton LJ, Gerrits NM. Emotional motor systems. In: Paxinos G, Mai JK, eds. *The Human Nervous System.* London: Elsevier; 2004:1306-1324.

Hyman SE, Malenka RC. Addiction and the brain: the neurobiology of compulsion and its persistence. *Nat Rev Neurosci.* 2001;2:695-703.

Insausti R, Amaral D. Hippocampal formation. In: Paxinos G, Mai JK, eds. *The Human Nervous System.* London: Elsevier; 2004:871-914.

Krack P, Hariz MI, Baunez C, Guridi J, Obeso JA. Deep brain stimulation: from neurology to psychiatry? *TINS.* 2010;33(10):474-484.

Kringelbach ML. The human orbitofrontal cortex: linking reward to hedonic experience. *Nat Rev Neurosci.* 2005;6:691-702.

Kringelbach ML, Jenkinson N, Owen SL, Aziz TZ. Translational principles of deep brain stimulation. *Nat Rev Neurosci.* 2007;8(8):623-635.

Lazarini F, Lledo PM. Is adult neurogenesis essential for olfaction? *TINS.* 2010;34:20-30.

LeDoux JE. Emotion circuits in the brain. *Annu Rev Neurosci.* 2000;23:155-184.

Levitt P. A monoclonal antibody to limbic system neurons. *Science.* 1984;223:299-301.

Lledo PM, Alonso M, Grubb MS. Adult neurogenesis and functional plasticity in neuronal circuits. *Nat Rev Neurosci.* 2006;7(3):179-193.

Maguire EA, Gadian DG, Johnsrude IS, et al. Navigation-related structural change in the hippocampi of taxi drivers. *Proc Natl Acad Sci USA.* 2000;97(8):4398-4403.

Mayberg HS. Limbic-cortical dysregulation: a proposed model of depression. *J Neuropsychiatry Clin Neurosci.* 1997;9(3):471-481.

Meyer-Lindenberg A, Miletich RS, Kohn PD, et al. Reduced prefrontal activity predicts exaggerated striatal dopaminergic function in schizophrenia. *Nat Neurosci.* 2002;5:267-271.

Millhouse OE, DeOlmos J. Neuronal configurations in lateral and basolateral amygdala. *Neuroscience.* 1983;10:1269-1300.

Naidich TP, Daniels DL, Haughton VM, et al. Hippocampal formation and related structures of the limbic lobe: anatomical-MR correlations. Part I. Surface features and coronal sections. *Neuroradiology.* 1987;162:747-754.

Naidich TP, Daniels DL, Haughton VM, et al. Hippocampal formation and related structure of the limbic lobe: anatomical-MR correlations. Part II. Sagittal sections. *Neuroradiology.* 1987;162:755-761.

Nestler EJ, Barrot M, DiLeone RJ, Eisch AJ, Gold SJ, Monteggia LM. Neurobiology of depression. *Neuron.* 2002;34:13-25.

Olson IR, Plotzker A, Ezzyat Y. The enigmatic temporal pole: a review of findings on social and emotional processing. *Brain.* 2007;130(Pt 7):1718-1731.

Ortega-Perez I, Murray K, Lledo PM. The how and why of adult neurogenesis. *J Mol Histol.* 2007;38(6):555-562.

Papez JW. A proposed mechanism of emotion. *Arch Neurol Psychiatr.* 1937;38:725-743.

Paus T. Primate anterior cingulate cortex: where motor control, drive and cognition interface. *Nat Rev Neurosci.* 2001;2:417-424.

Perera TD, Park S, Nemirovskaya Y. Cognitive role of neurogenesis in depression and antidepressant treatment. *Neuroscientist.* 2008;14(4):326-338.

Pessoa L. On the relationship between emotion and cognition. *Nat Rev Neurosci.* 2008;9:148-158.

Petrides M, Pandya DN. The frontal lobe. In: Paxinos G, Mai JK, eds. *The Human Nervous System.* London: Elsevier; 2004:950-972.

Pfefferbaum A, Zipursky RB. Neuroimaging in schizophrenia. *Schizophr Res.* 1991;4:193-208.

Pierce RC, Kumaresan V. The mesolimbic dopamine system: the final common pathway for the reinforcing effect of drugs of abuse? *Neurosci Biobehav Rev.* 2006;30(2):215-238.

Pitkanen A, Savander V, LeDoux JE. Organization of intra-amygdaloid circuitries in the rat: an emerging frame-work for understanding functions of the amygdala. *Trends Neurosci.* 1997;20:517-523.

Price JL, Amaral DG. An autoradiographic study of the projections of the central nucleus of the monkey amygdala. *J Neurosci.* 1981;1:1242-1259.

Price JL, Russchen FT, Amaral DG. The limbic region. II: The amygdaloid complex. In: Björklund A, Hökfelt T, Swanson LW, eds. *Handbook of Chemical Neuroanatomy. Vol. 5. Integrated Systems of the CNS, Part I.* Amsterdam: Elsevier; 1987:279-388.

Saper CB. Hypothalamus. In: Paxinos G, Mai JK, eds. *The Human Nervous System.* London: Elsevier; 2004:513-550.

Talairach J, Tournoux P. *Co-planar Stereotaxic Atlas of the Human Brain.* New York, NY: Georg Thieme Verlag; 1988.

Vogt BA, Hof PR, Vogt LJ. Cingulate gyrus. In: Paxinos G, Mai JK, eds. *The Human Nervous System.* London: Elsevier; 2004:915-949.

Whitman MC, Greer CA. Adult neurogenesis and the olfactory system. *Prog Neurobiol.* Oct 2009;89(2):162-175.

Wiebe S, Blume WT, Girvin JP, Eliasziw M. A randomized, controlled trial of surgery for temporal-lobe epilepsy. *N Engl J Med.* 2001;345:311-318.

Williams PL, Warwick R. *Functional Neuroanatomy of Man.* New York, NY: W. B. Saunders; 1975.

Yin HH, Knowlton BJ. The role of the basal ganglia in habit formation. *Nat Rev Neurosci.* 2006;7(6):464-476.

Young KA, Gobrogge KL, Liu Y, Wang Z. The neurobiology of pair bonding: insights from a socially monogamous rodent. *Front Neuroendocrinol.* 2011;32(1):53-69.

Young LJ, Murphy Young AZ, Hammock EA. Anatomy and neurochemistry of the pair bond. *J Comp Neurol.* 2005;493(1):51-57.

Zola-Morgan S, Squire LR, Amaral DG. Human amnesia and the medial temporal region: enduring memory impairment following a bilateral lesion limited to field CA1 of the hippocampus. *J Neurosci.* 1986;6:2950-2967.

Study Questions

1. A patient with a rare memory disorder has an MRI. The neuroradiologist notes that the only significant change is that the hippocampal formation is degenerated. Which of the following statements best describes the most likely effect this would have on the image of the ventricular system?
   A. There would be no change to the ventricular system because the degeneration is localized to the hippocampal formation.
   B. This would be accompanied by shrinkage of the lateral ventricle.
   C. This would be accompanied by enlargement of the lateral ventricle.
   D. This would be accompanied by enlargement of the ventral, or temporal, horn of the lateral ventricle system.

2. Limbic cortical areas do not engage in primary sensory or motor functions. Rather, they integrate information, often from several cortical regions that are interconnected with the hippocampal formation, amygdala, or both. Which of the following is not considered a limbic cortical area?
   A. Anterior cingulate cortex
   B. Orbitofrontal cortex
   C. Posterior insular cortex
   D. Temporal pole

3. Which of the following best indicates a function of the orbitofrontal cortex?
   A. Integration of olfactory and gustatory messages important for deciding to ingest something
   B. Localization of stimuli in the space around us
   C. Identification of familiar faces
   D. Sensing emotional content in speech

4. Which part of the hippocampal formation is noted for receiving its input?
   A. Parahippocampal gyrus
   B. Subiculum
   C. Hippocampus
   D. Dentate gyrus

5. A fictitious patient has a disorder of brain connectivity in which the amygdala does not develop the proper connections from higher-order sensory areas. Which part of the amygdala would be primarily affected?
   A. Basolateral nuclei
   B. Central nucleus

   C. Extended amygdala/bed nucleus of the stria terminalis
   D. Corticomedial amygdala

6. After sustaining a small temporal lobe stroke, a patient fails to express an increase in his heart rate when he sees a threatening image. Which nuclear group of the amygdala is most likely affected by the stroke?
   A. Basolateral nuclei
   B. Central nucleus
   C. Extended amygdala/bed nucleus of the stria terminalis
   D. Corticomedial amygdala

7. The ventral tegmental area is thought to be important in reward. Which of the following choices lists the correct neurotransmitter used by the ventral segmental area and the brain region that is the key site of action?
   A. 5-HT; orbitofrontal cortex
   B. Dopamine; locus ceruleus
   C. Norepinephrine; thalamus
   D. Dopamine; ventral striatum

8. The _____ is the principal output tract of the corticomedial amygdala.
   A. uncinate fasciculus
   B. fornix
   C. ventral amygdalofugal pathway
   D. stria terminalis

9. Which of the following choices best describes the difference between neocortex and allocortex function and organization?
   A. Neocortex mediates aspects of olfaction, whereas allocortex mediates vision.
   B. Neocortex is located ventrally, on the base of the brain, and allocortex is located laterally.
   C. Typically, neocortex has six layers and allocortex has three layers.
   D. Allocortex, not neocortex, is susceptible to degeneration.

10. Which of the following statements best indicates how hippocampal formation neurons influence the rest of the brain?
   A. Via the fornix
   B. Via the fornix and back projections to the entorhinal cortex
   C. Via the fornix and back projections to the entorhinal cortex and the uncinate fasciculus
   D. Via the fornix and back projections to the entorhinal cortex, uncinate fasciculus, and stria terminalis

ATLAS

V

Atlas

Surface Topography of the Central Nervous System

T*he surface topography atlas is a collection of* drawings of the brain and rostral spinal cord. The various views are based on specimens and brain models. Key features are labeled on an accompanying line drawing of each view.

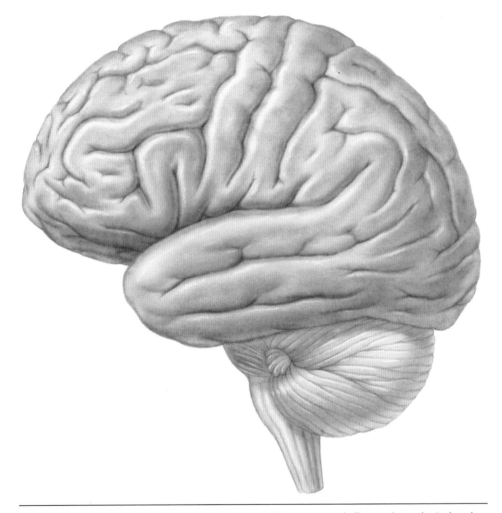

FIGURE AI–1 Lateral surface of the cerebral hemisphere, brain stem, cerebellum, and rostral spinal cord.

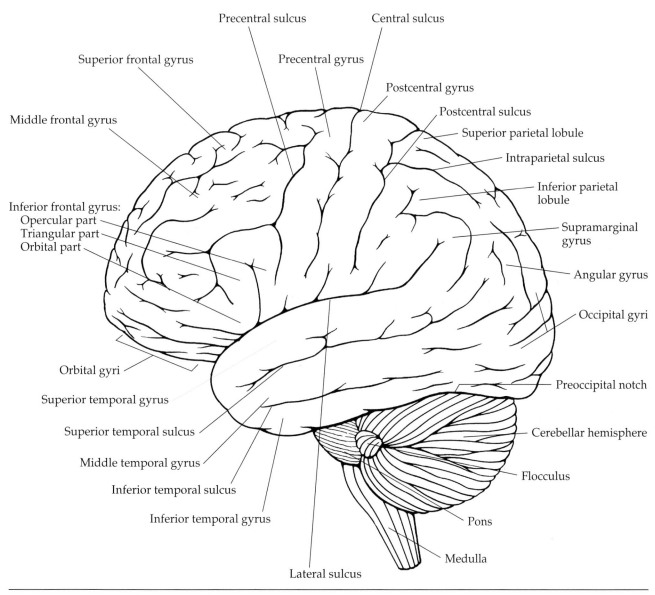

Continued—**FIGURE AI–1**

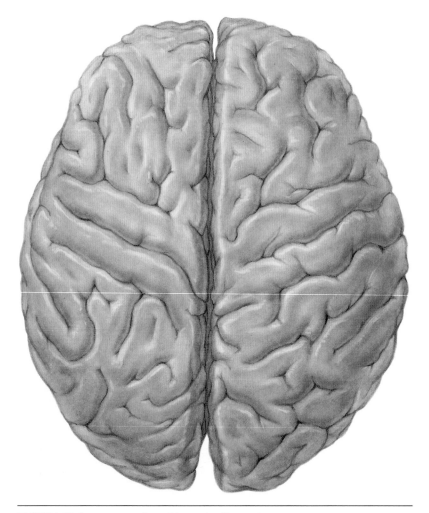

FIGURE AI-2 Superior surface of the cerebral hemisphere.

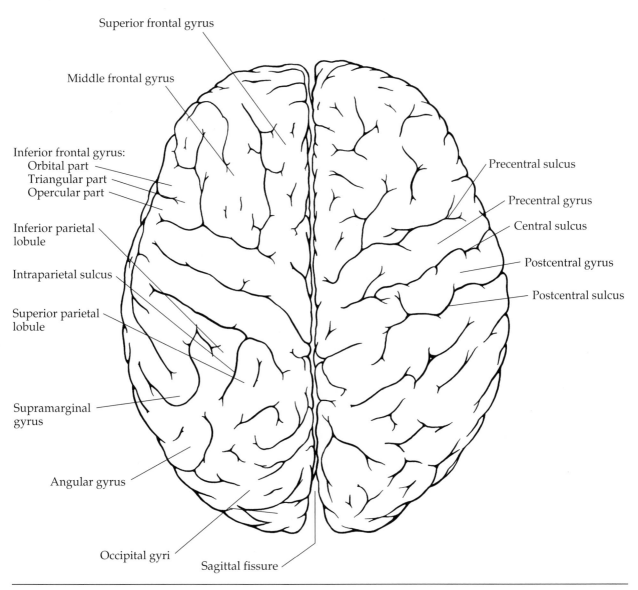

Superior frontal gyrus

Middle frontal gyrus

Inferior frontal gyrus:
 Orbital part
 Triangular part
 Opercular part

Inferior parietal lobule

Intraparietal sulcus

Superior parietal lobule

Supramarginal gyrus

Angular gyrus

Occipital gyri

Sagittal fissure

Precentral sulcus

Precentral gyrus

Central sulcus

Postcentral gyrus

Postcentral sulcus

Continued—**FIGURE AI–2**

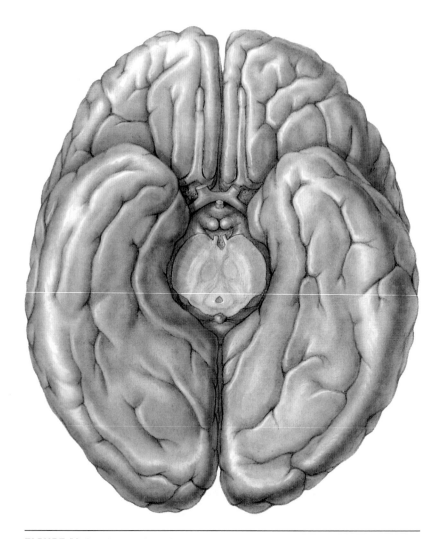

FIGURE AI–3 Inferior surface of the cerebral hemisphere and diencephalon. The brain stem is transected at the rostral midbrain.

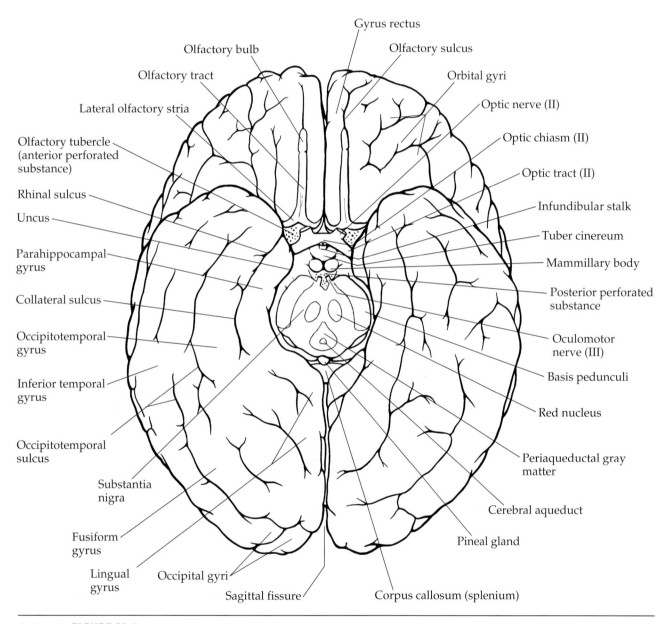

Gyrus rectus
Olfactory bulb
Olfactory sulcus
Olfactory tract
Orbital gyri
Lateral olfactory stria
Optic nerve (II)
Optic chiasm (II)
Olfactory tubercle
(anterior perforated
substance)
Optic tract (II)
Rhinal sulcus
Infundibular stalk
Uncus
Tuber cinereum
Parahippocampal
gyrus
Mammillary body
Collateral sulcus
Posterior perforated
substance
Occipitotemporal
gyrus
Oculomotor
nerve (III)
Inferior temporal
gyrus
Basis pedunculi
Red nucleus
Occipitotemporal
sulcus
Periaqueductal gray
matter
Substantia
nigra
Cerebral aqueduct
Fusiform
gyrus
Pineal gland
Lingual
gyrus
Occipital gyri
Sagittal fissure
Corpus callosum (splenium)

Continued—**FIGURE AI–3**

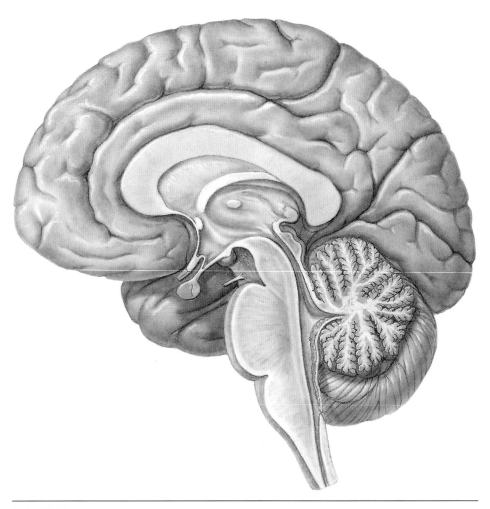

FIGURE AI–4 Medial surface of the cerebral hemisphere and midsagittal section through the diencephalon, brain stem, cerebellum, and rostral spinal cord.

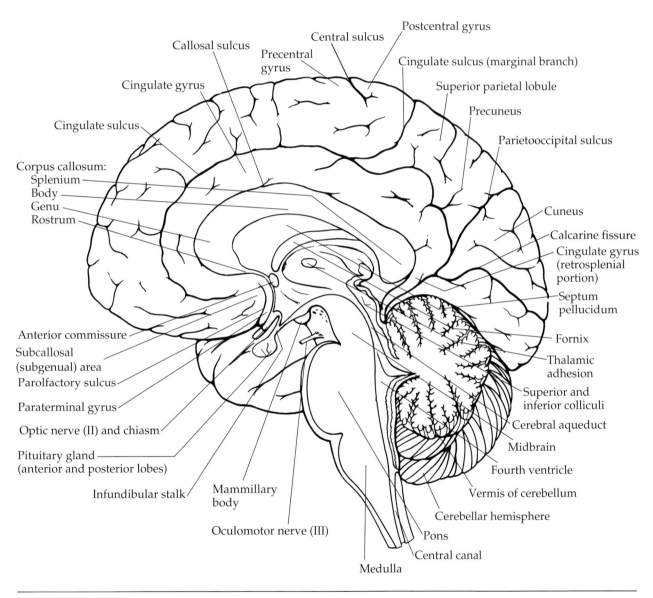

Continued—**FIGURE AI–4**

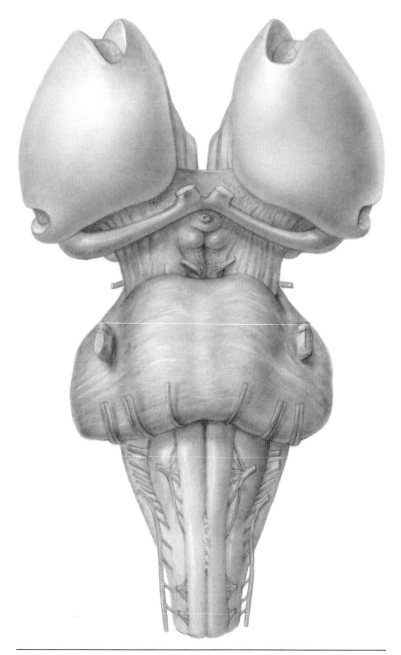

FIGURE AI–5 Ventral surface of the brain stem and rostral spinal cord. The striatum and diencephalon are also shown.

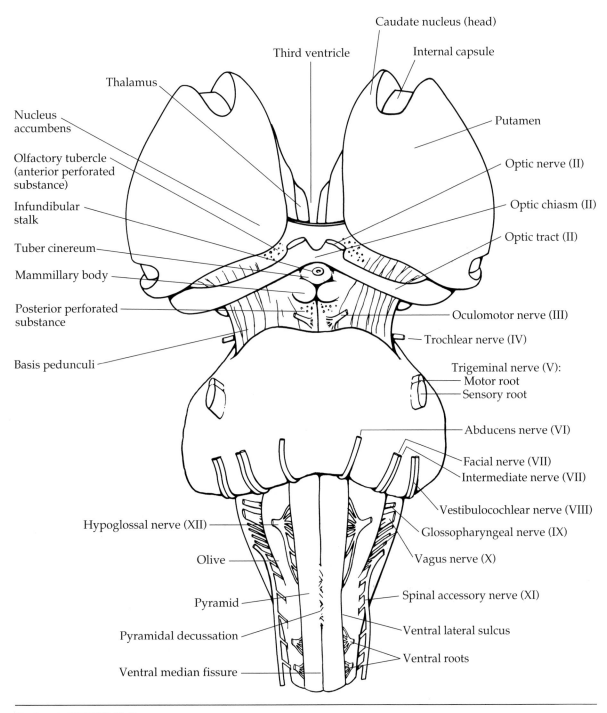

Caudate nucleus (head)

Third ventricle

Internal capsule

Thalamus

Nucleus accumbens

Putamen

Olfactory tubercle (anterior perforated substance)

Optic nerve (II)

Infundibular stalk

Optic chiasm (II)

Optic tract (II)

Tuber cinereum

Mammillary body

Posterior perforated substance

Oculomotor nerve (III)

Trochlear nerve (IV)

Basis pedunculi

Trigeminal nerve (V):
Motor root
Sensory root

Abducens nerve (VI)

Facial nerve (VII)
Intermediate nerve (VII)

Vestibulocochlear nerve (VIII)

Hypoglossal nerve (XII)

Glossopharyngeal nerve (IX)

Vagus nerve (X)

Olive

Spinal accessory nerve (XI)

Pyramid

Ventral lateral sulcus

Pyramidal decussation

Ventral roots

Ventral median fissure

*Continued—***FIGURE AI–5**

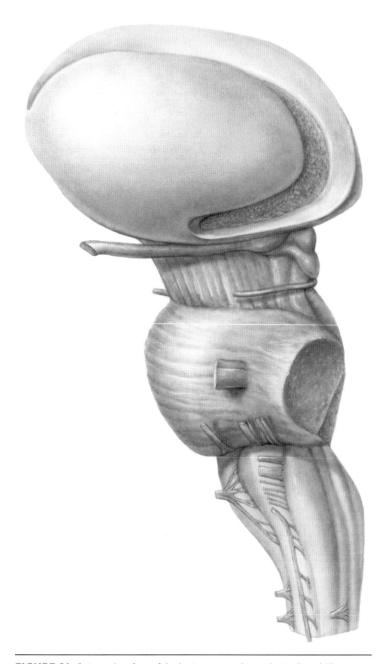

FIGURE AI–6 Lateral surface of the brain stem and rostral spinal cord. The striatum and diencephalon are also shown.

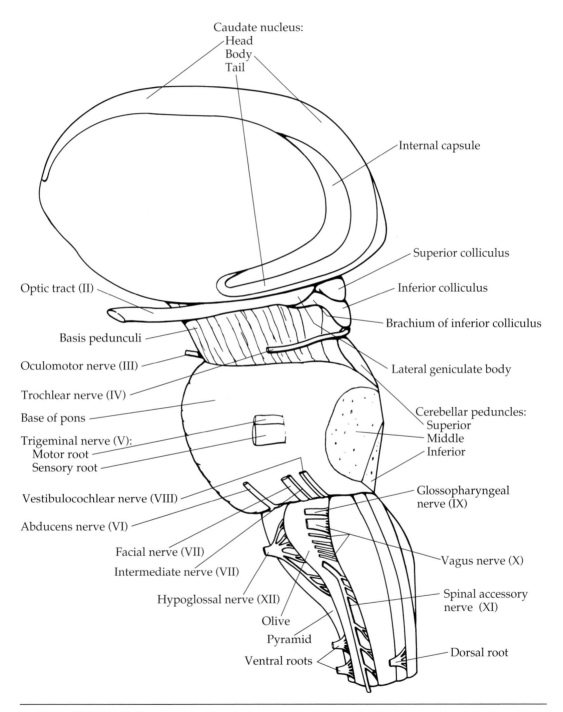

Caudate nucleus:
Head
Body
Tail

Internal capsule

Superior colliculus

Inferior colliculus

Optic tract (II)

Brachium of inferior colliculus

Basis pedunculi

Lateral geniculate body

Oculomotor nerve (III)

Trochlear nerve (IV)

Cerebellar peduncles:
Superior
Middle
Inferior

Base of pons

Trigeminal nerve (V):
Motor root
Sensory root

Vestibulocochlear nerve (VIII)

Glossopharyngeal
nerve (IX)

Abducens nerve (VI)

Facial nerve (VII)

Vagus nerve (X)

Intermediate nerve (VII)

Hypoglossal nerve (XII)

Spinal accessory
nerve (XI)

Olive

Pyramid

Dorsal root

Ventral roots

Continued—**FIGURE AI–6**

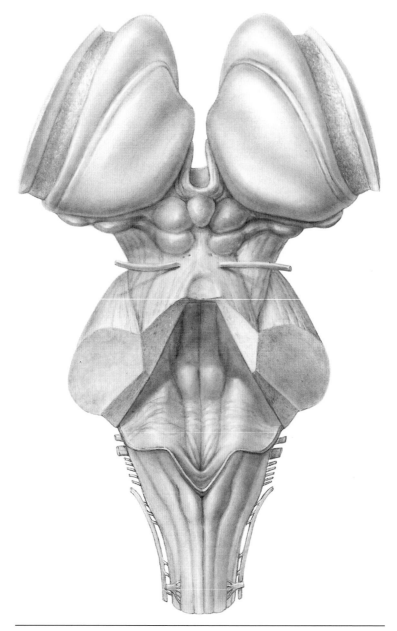

FIGURE AI–7 Dorsal surface of the brain stem and rostral spinal cord. The striatum and diencephalon are also shown. The cerebellum was removed to reveal the structures located on the floor of the fourth ventricle.

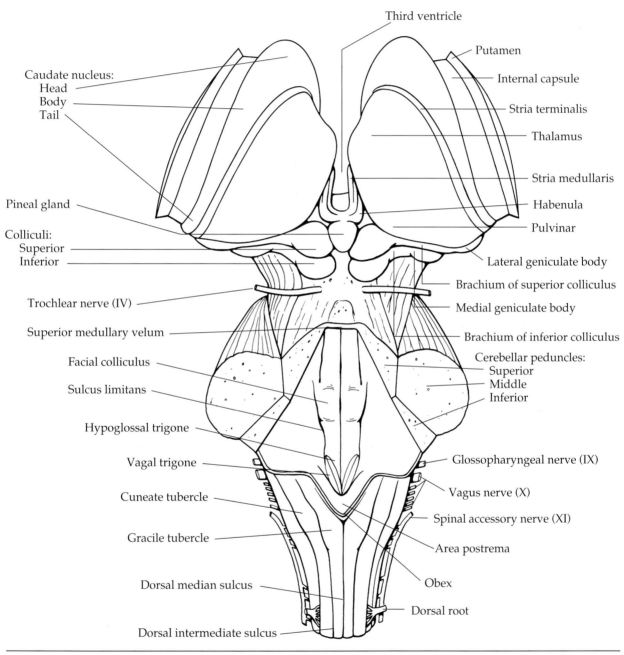

Continued—**FIGURE AI-7**

References

Braak H, Braak E. *Architectonics of the Human Telen cephalic Cortex.* Berlin, Germany: Springer-Verlag, 1976.

Carpenter MB, Sutin J. *Human Neuroanatomy.* Baltimore, MD: The Williams and Wilkins Company, 1983.

Crosby EC, Humphrey T, Lauer EW. *Correlative Anatomy of the Nervous System.* New York, NY: Macmillan, 1962.

Ferner H, Staubesand J. *Sobotta Atlas of Human Anatomy.* Baltimore, MD: Urban & Schwartzenberg, 1983.

Nieuwenhuys R, Voogd J, van Huijzen C. *The Human Central Nervous System,* 3rd ed. Berlin, Germany: Springer-Verlag, 1988.

Williams PL, Warwick R. *Functional Neuroanatomy of Man.* Philadelphia, PA: W. B. Saunders, 1975.

Zilles K. Cortex. In: Paxinos G, ed. *The Human Central Nervous System.* San Diego, CA: Academic Press, 1990.

Myelin-Stained Sections Through the Central Nervous System

The atlas of myelin-stained sections through the central nervous system is in three planes: transverse, horizontal, and sagittal. (See Figure 1–17 for schematic views of these planes of sections.) Transverse sections through the cerebral hemispheres and diencephalon are termed coronal sections because they are approximately parallel to the coronal suture. These sections also cut the brain stem, but parallel to its long axis. In addition, three sections are cut in planes oblique to the transverse and horizontal sections.

In this atlas, each level through the central nervous system is printed without labeled structures as well as with labels on an accompanying photograph (printed at reduced contrast to preserve the essence of the structure). Typically, the border of a structure is indicated either when the structure's location is extremely important for understanding the functional consequences of brain trauma or when the structure is clearly depicted on the section and it is didactically important to emphasize the border. Axons of cranial nerves and primary afferent fibers are indicated by bold lines to distinguish them from the other fibers.

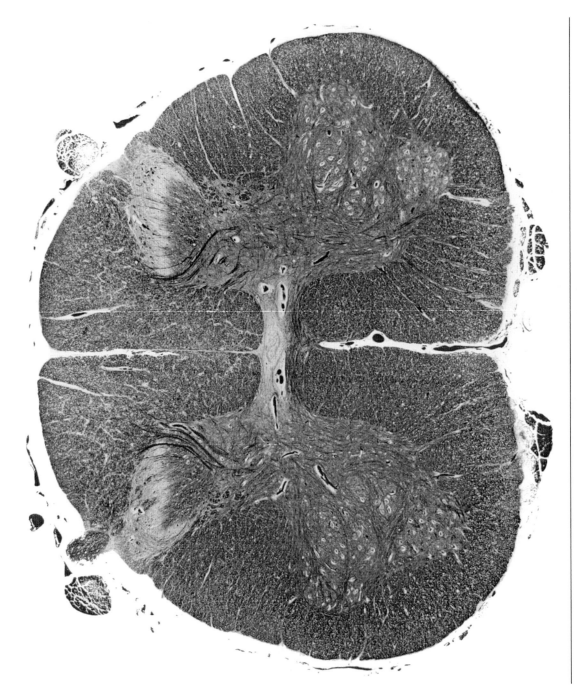

FIGURE AII–1 Transverse section of the first sacral segment (S1) and of the spinal cord (×20).

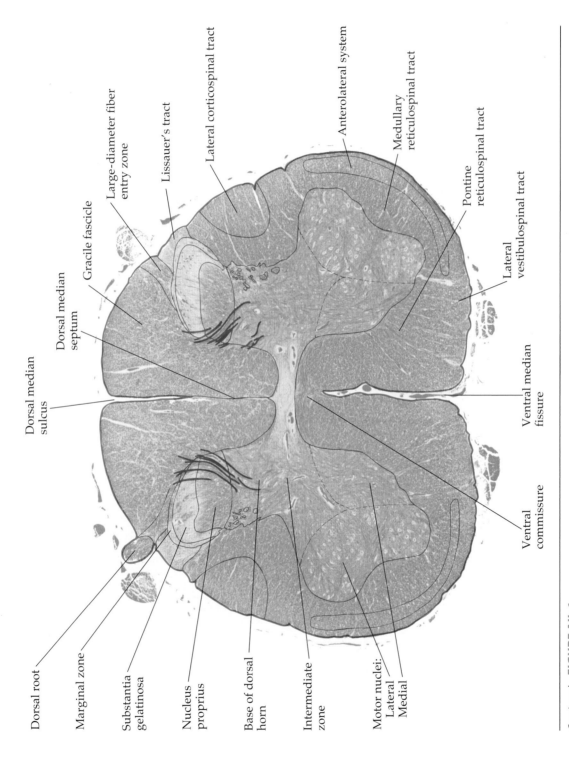

Dorsal median sulcus

Dorsal median septum

Gracile fascicle

Large-diameter fiber entry zone

Lissauer's tract

Lateral corticospinal tract

Anterolateral system

Medullary reticulospinal tract

Pontine reticulospinal tract

Lateral vestibulospinal tract

Ventral median fissure

Dorsal root

Marginal zone

Substantia gelatinosa

Nucleus proprius

Base of dorsal horn

Intermediate zone

Motor nuclei:
Lateral
Medial

Ventral commissure

Continued—**FIGURE AII–1**

435

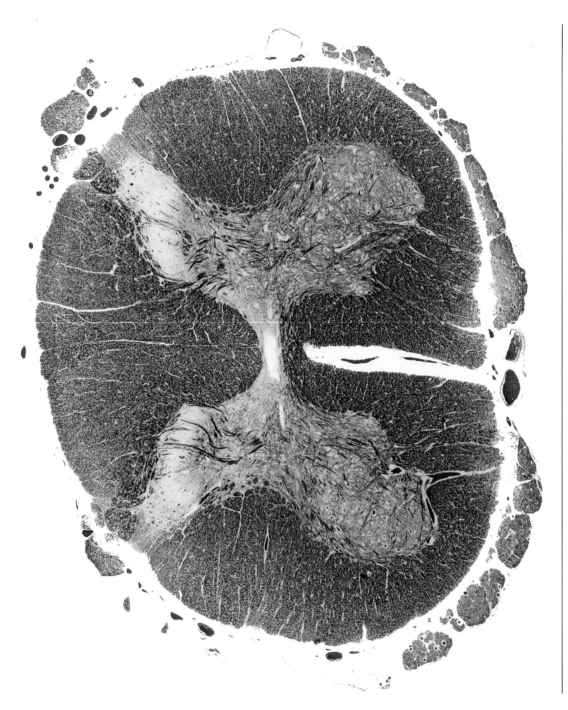

FIGURE AII–2 Transverse section of the second lumbar segment (L2) of the spinal cord. (×18)

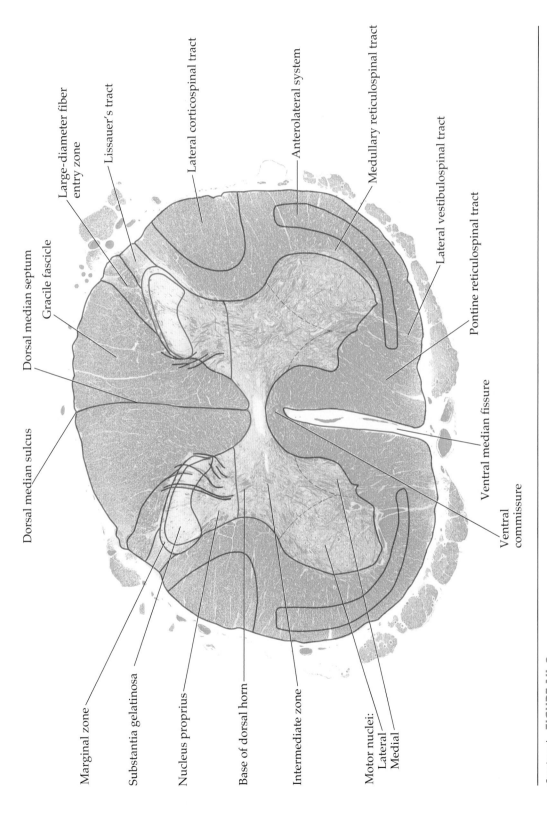

Dorsal median sulcus

Marginal zone

Substantia gelatinosa

Nucleus proprius

Base of dorsal horn

Intermediate zone

Motor nuclei:
Lateral
Medial

Dorsal median septum

Gracile fascicle

Large-diameter fiber entry zone

Lissauer's tract

Lateral corticospinal tract

Anterolateral system

Medullary reticulospinal tract

Lateral vestibulospinal tract

Pontine reticulospinal tract

Ventral median fissure

Ventral commissure

Continued—**FIGURE AII–2**

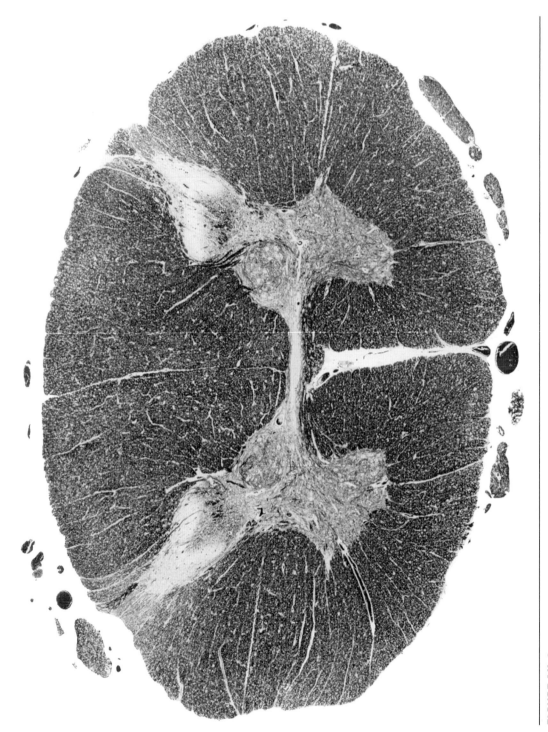

FIGURE AII–3 Transverse section of the first lumbar segment (L1) of the spinal cord. (×21)

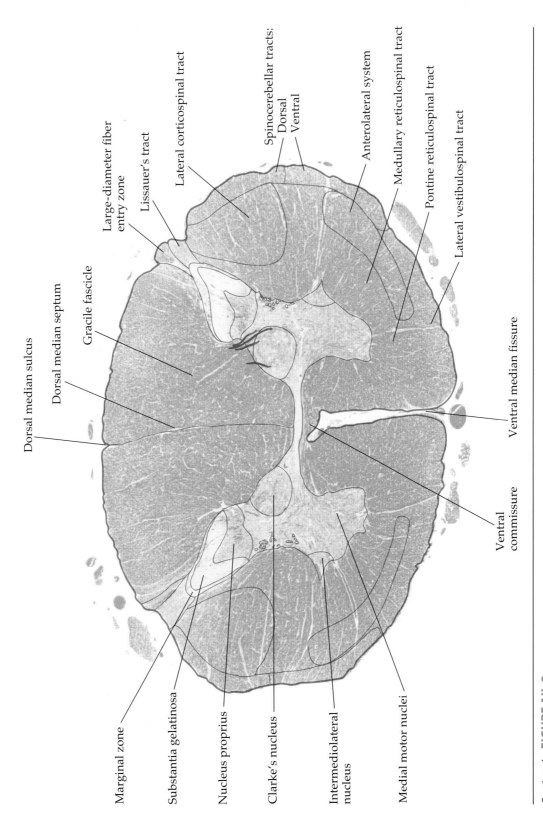

Dorsal median sulcus

Dorsal median septum

Gracile fascicle

Large-diameter fiber entry zone

Lissauer's tract

Lateral corticospinal tract

Spinocerebellar tracts:
Dorsal
Ventral

Anterolateral system

Medullary reticulospinal tract

Pontine reticulospinal tract

Lateral vestibulospinal tract

Ventral median fissure

Ventral commissure

Medial motor nuclei

Intermediolateral nucleus

Clarke's nucleus

Nucleus proprius

Substantia gelatinosa

Marginal zone

Continued—**FIGURE AII-3**

439

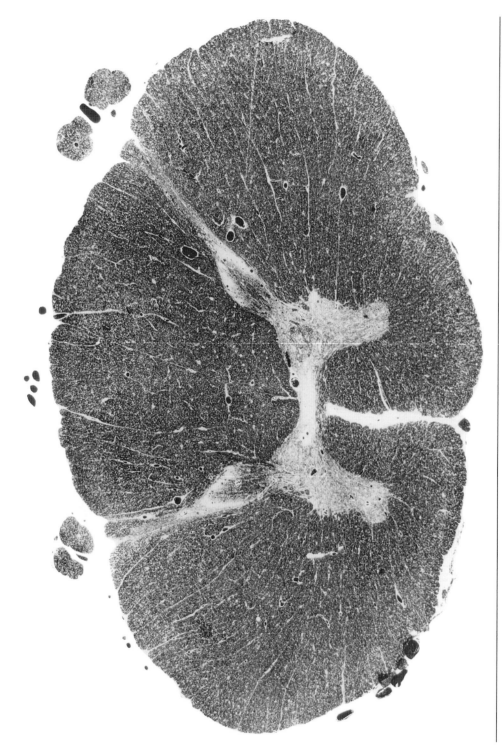

FIGURE AII–4 Transverse section of the third thoracic segment (T3) of the spinal cord. (×23)

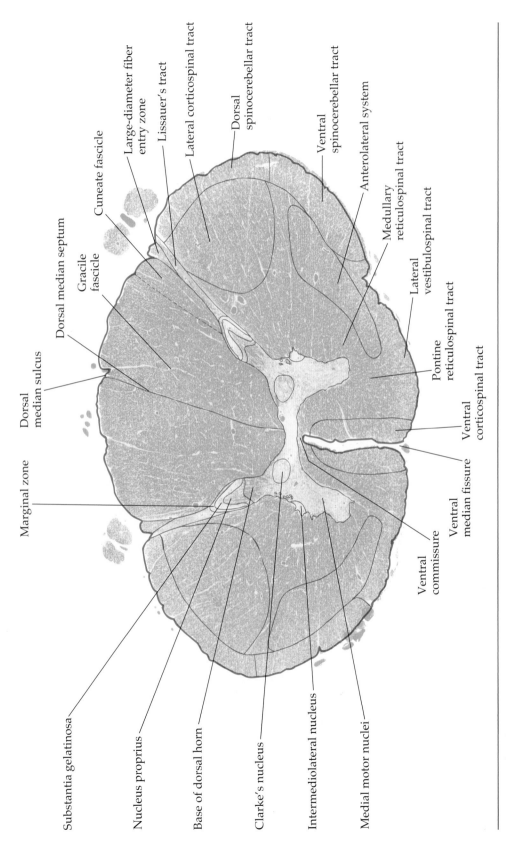

Substantia gelatinosa

Nucleus proprius

Base of dorsal horn

Clarke's nucleus

Intermediolateral nucleus

Medial motor nuclei

Marginal zone

Dorsal median sulcus

Dorsal median septum

Gracile fascicle

Cuneate fascicle

Large-diameter fiber entry zone

Lissauer's tract

Lateral corticospinal tract

Dorsal spinocerebellar tract

Ventral spinocerebellar tract

Anterolateral system

Medullary reticulospinal tract

Lateral vestibulospinal tract

Pontine reticulospinal tract

Ventral corticospinal tract

Ventral median fissure

Ventral commissure

Continued—**FIGURE AII–4**

441

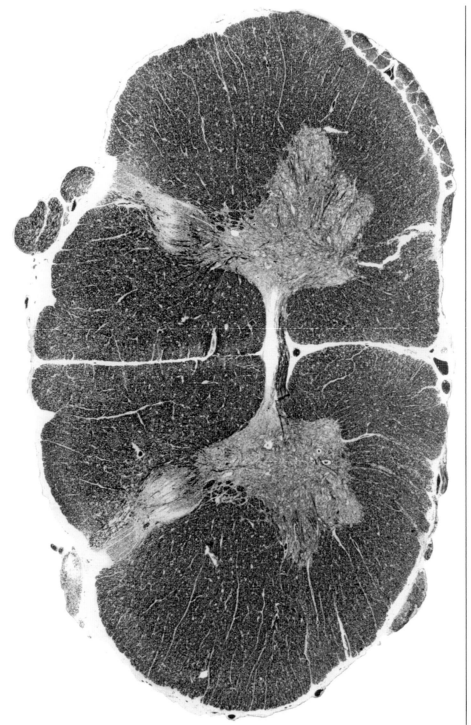

FIGURE AII–5 Transverse section of the seventh cervical segment (C7) of the spinal cord. (×16)

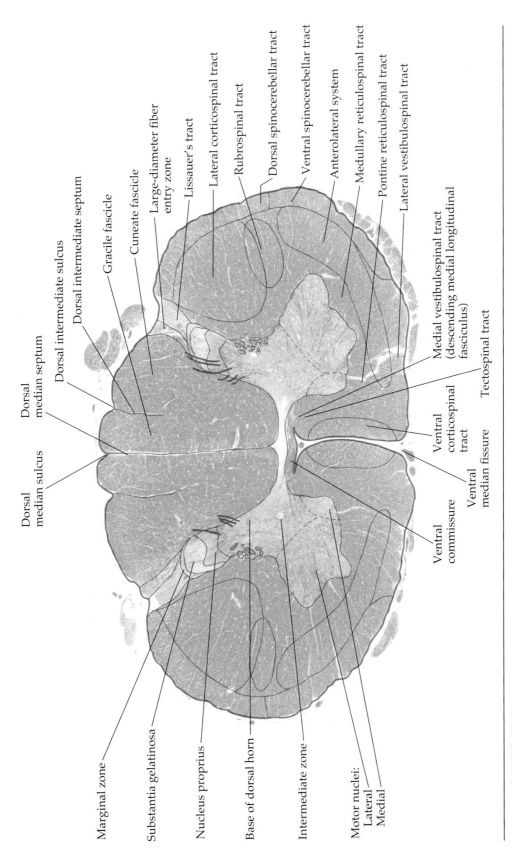

Marginal zone

Substantia gelatinosa

Nucleus proprius

Base of dorsal horn

Intermediate zone

Motor nuclei:
Lateral
Medial

Dorsal median sulcus

Dorsal median septum

Dorsal intermediate sulcus

Dorsal intermediate septum

Gracile fascicle

Cuneate fascicle

Large-diameter fiber entry zone

Lissauer's tract

Lateral corticospinal tract

Rubrospinal tract

Dorsal spinocerebellar tract

Ventral spinocerebellar tract

Anterolateral system

Medullary reticulospinal tract

Pontine reticulospinal tract

Lateral vestibulospinal tract

Medial vestibulospinal tract (descending medial longitudinal fasciculus)

Tectospinal tract

Ventral corticospinal tract

Ventral median fissure

Ventral commissure

Continued—**FIGURE AII–5**

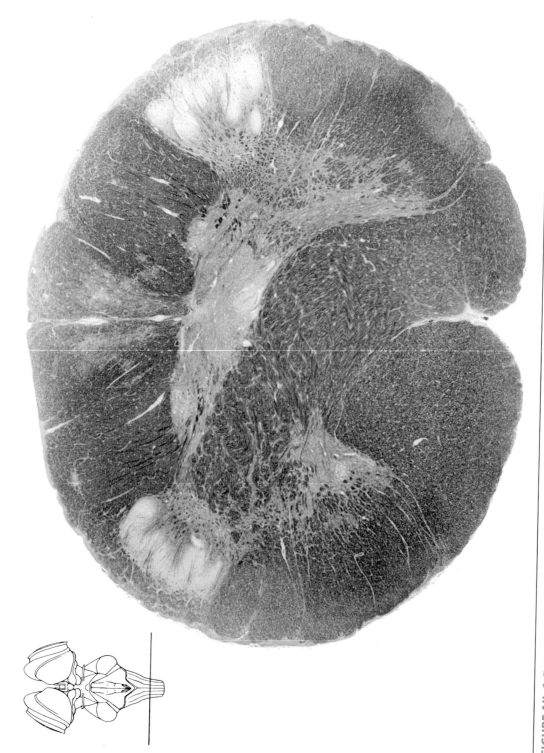

FIGURE AII–6 Transverse section of the caudal medulla at the level of the pyramidal (motor) decussation and the spinal (caudal) trigeminal nucleus. (×17)

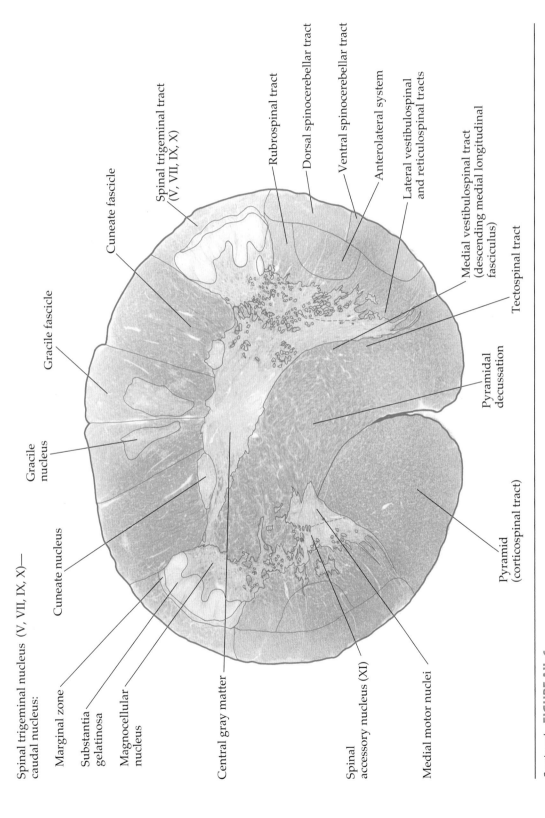

Spinal trigeminal nucleus (V, VII, IX, X)—caudal nucleus:

Marginal zone

Substantia gelatinosa

Magnocellular nucleus

Gracile nucleus

Cuneate nucleus

Gracile fascicle

Cuneate fascicle

Spinal trigeminal tract (V, VII, IX, X)

Rubrospinal tract

Dorsal spinocerebellar tract

Ventral spinocerebellar tract

Anterolateral system

Lateral vestibulospinal and reticulospinal tracts

Medial vestibulospinal tract (descending medial longitudinal fasciculus)

Tectospinal tract

Pyramidal decussation

Pyramid (corticospinal tract)

Medial motor nuclei

Spinal accessory nucleus (XI)

Central gray matter

Continued—**FIGURE AII–6**

445

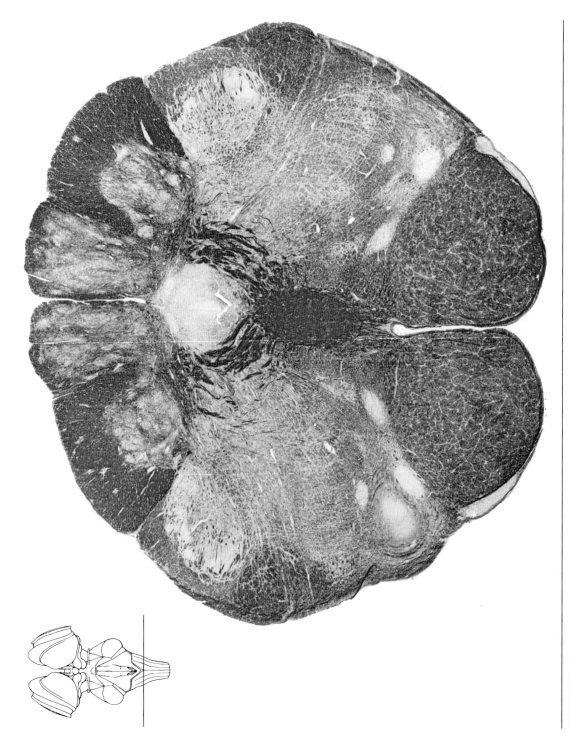

FIGURE AII–7 Transverse section of the medulla at the level of the dorsal column nuclei and the somatic sensory decussation. (×12)

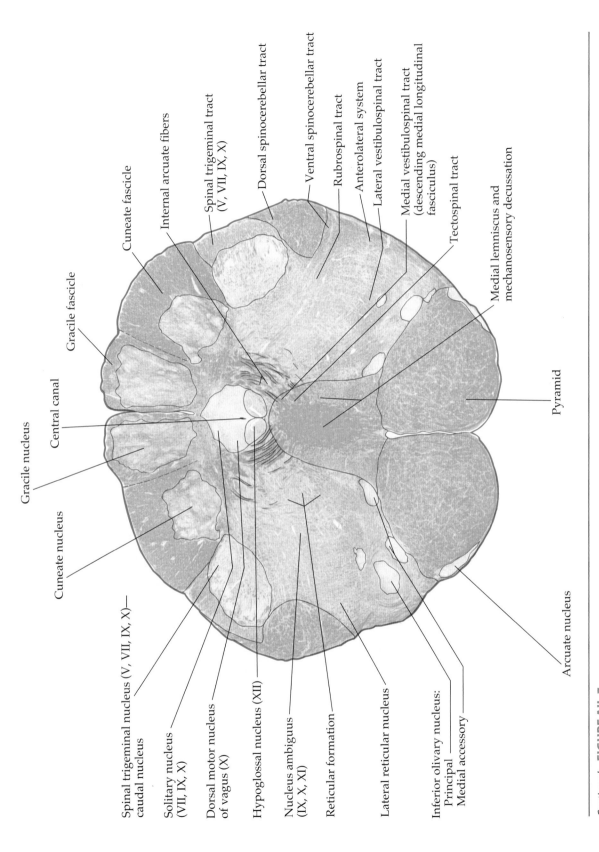

Gracile nucleus

Cuneate nucleus

Central canal

Gracile fascicle

Cuneate fascicle

Internal arcuate fibers

Spinal trigeminal tract (V, VII, IX, X)

Dorsal spinocerebellar tract

Ventral spinocerebellar tract

Rubrospinal tract

Anterolateral system

Lateral vestibulospinal tract

Medial vestibulospinal tract (descending medial longitudinal fasciculus)

Tectospinal tract

Medial lemniscus and mechanosensory decussation

Pyramid

Arcuate nucleus

Spinal trigeminal nucleus (V, VII, IX, X)—caudal nucleus

Solitary nucleus (VII, IX, X)

Dorsal motor nucleus of vagus (X)

Hypoglossal nucleus (XII)

Nucleus ambiguus (IX, X, XI)

Reticular formation

Lateral reticular nucleus

Inferior olivary nucleus:
Principal
Medial accessory

Continued—**FIGURE AII-7**

447

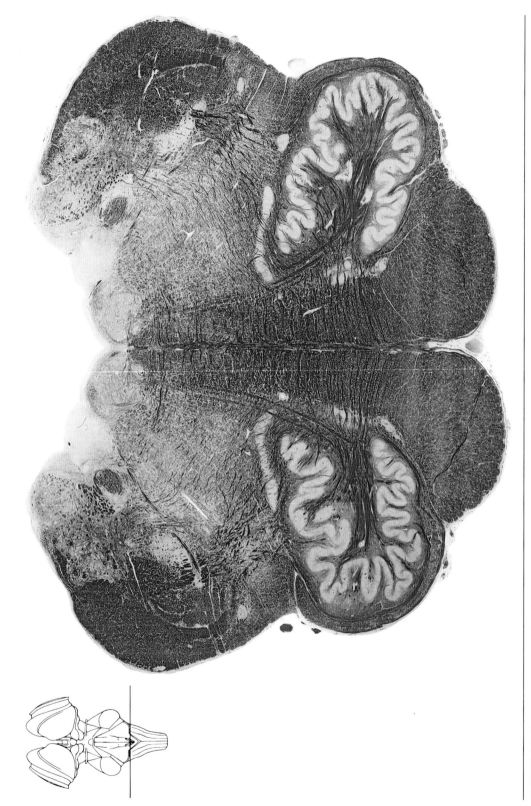

FIGURE AII–8 Transverse section of the medulla through the hypoglossal nucleus. (×9)

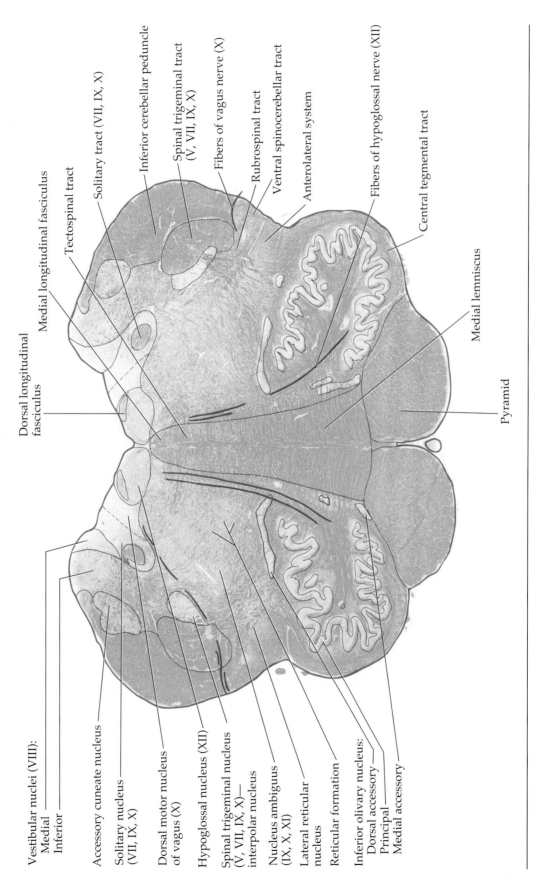

Vestibular nuclei (VIII):
Medial
Inferior

Accessory cuneate nucleus

Solitary nucleus
(VII, IX, X)

Dorsal motor nucleus
of vagus (X)

Hypoglossal nucleus (XII)

Spinal trigeminal nucleus
(V, VII, IX, X)—
interpolar nucleus

Nucleus ambiguus
(IX, X, XI)

Lateral reticular
nucleus

Reticular formation

Inferior olivary nucleus:
Dorsal accessory
Principal
Medial accessory

Dorsal longitudinal
fasciculus

Medial longitudinal fasciculus

Tectospinal tract

Solitary tract (VII, IX, X)

Inferior cerebellar peduncle

Spinal trigeminal tract
(V, VII, IX, X)

Fibers of vagus nerve (X)

Rubrospinal tract

Ventral spinocerebellar tract

Anterolateral system

Fibers of hypoglossal nerve (XII)

Central tegmental tract

Medial lemniscus

Pyramid

Continued—**FIGURE AII–8**

449

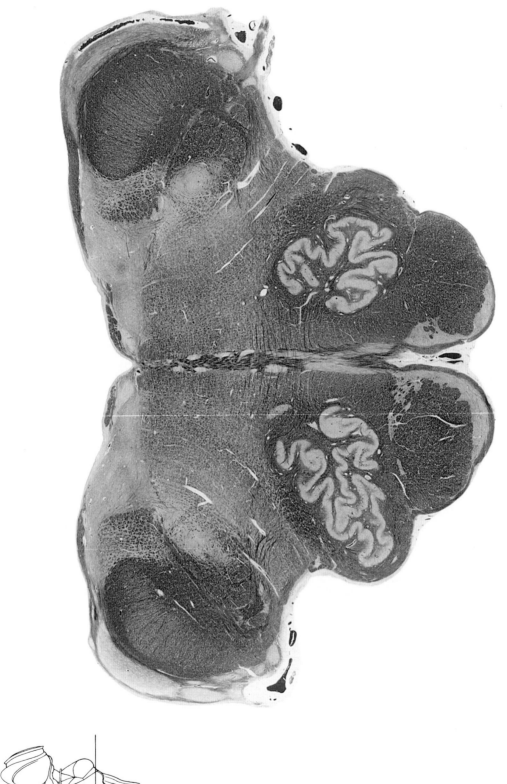

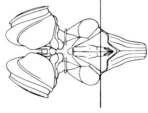

FIGURE AII–9 Transverse section of the rostral medulla through the cochlear nuclei. (×9)

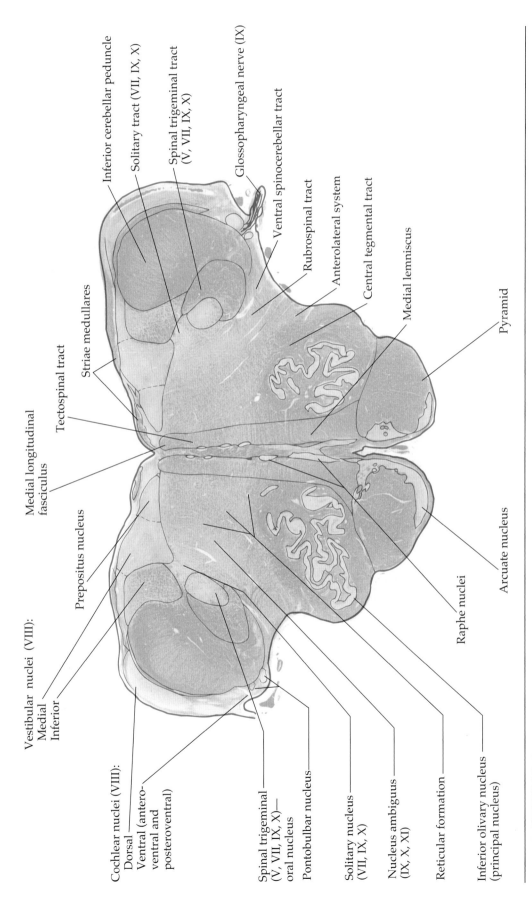

Vestibular nuclei (VIII):
Medial
Inferior

Medial longitudinal
fasciculus

Tectospinal tract

Striae medullares

Prepositus nucleus

Cochlear nuclei (VIII):
Dorsal
Ventral (antero-
ventral and
posteroventral)

Spinal trigeminal
(V, VII, IX, X)—
oral nucleus

Pontobulbar nucleus

Solitary nucleus
(VII, IX, X)

Nucleus ambiguus
(IX, X, XI)

Reticular formation

Inferior olivary nucleus
(principal nucleus)

Inferior cerebellar peduncle

Solitary tract (VII, IX, X)

Spinal trigeminal tract
(V, VII, IX, X)

Glossopharyngeal nerve (IX)

Ventral spinocerebellar tract

Rubrospinal tract

Anterolateral system

Central tegmental tract

Medial lemniscus

Pyramid

Arcuate nucleus

Raphe nuclei

Continued—**FIGURE AII–9**

451

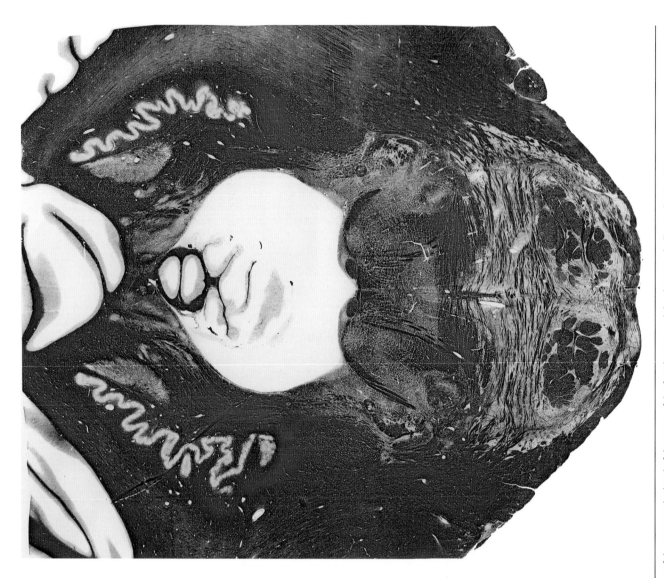

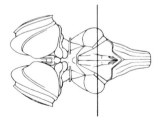

FIGURE AII–10 Transverse section of the pons at the level of the genu of the facial nerve and the deep cerebellar nuclei. (×4.3)

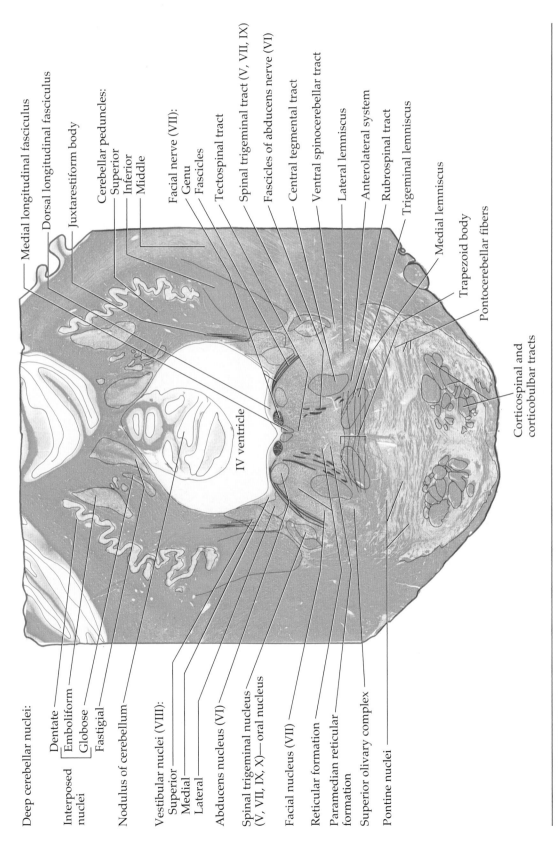

Deep cerebellar nuclei:
Interposed nuclei — Dentate / Emboliform / Globose
Fastigial
Nodulus of cerebellum

Vestibular nuclei (VIII):
Superior
Medial
Lateral

Abducens nucleus (VI)

Spinal trigeminal nucleus (V, VII, IX, X)—oral nucleus

Facial nucleus (VII)

Reticular formation

Paramedian reticular formation

Superior olivary complex

Pontine nuclei

Medial longitudinal fasciculus

Dorsal longitudinal fasciculus

Juxtarestiform body

Cerebellar peduncles:
Superior
Inferior
Middle

Facial nerve (VII):
Genu
Fascicles

Tectospinal tract

Spinal trigeminal tract (V, VII, IX)

Fascicles of abducens nerve (VI)

Central tegmental tract

Ventral spinocerebellar tract

Lateral lemniscus

Anterolateral system

Rubrospinal tract

Trigeminal lemniscus

Medial lemniscus

Trapezoid body

Pontocerebellar fibers

IV ventricle

Corticospinal and corticobulbar tracts

Continued—**FIGURE AII–10**

453

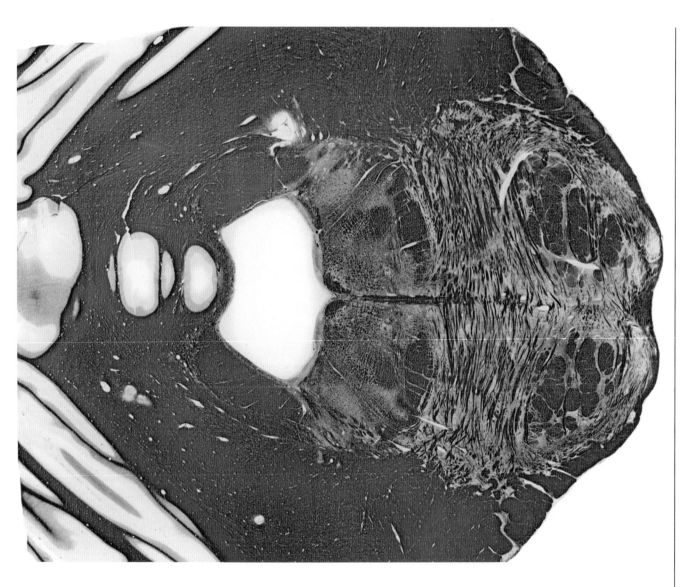

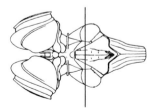

FIGURE AII–11 Transverse section of the pons through the main trigeminal sensory nuclei. (×10)

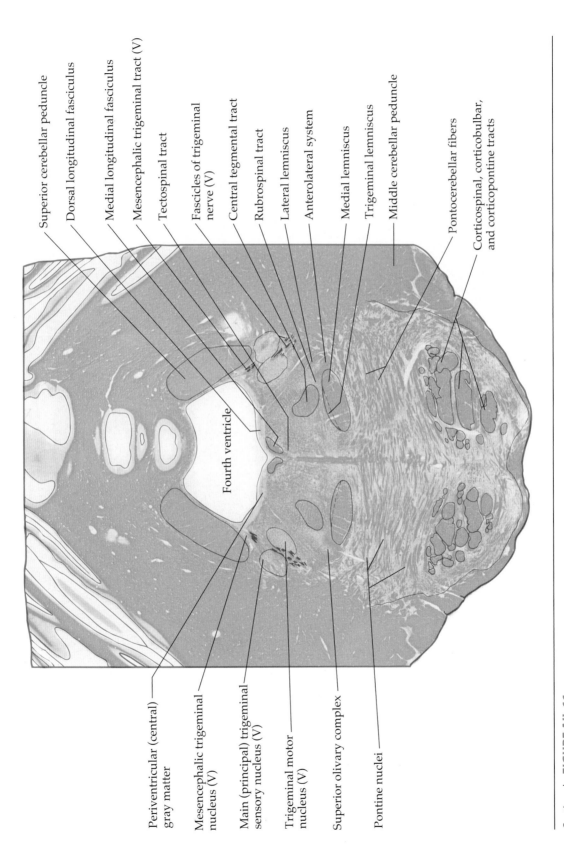

Superior cerebellar peduncle
Dorsal longitudinal fasciculus
Medial longitudinal fasciculus
Mesencephalic trigeminal tract (V)
Tectospinal tract
Fascicles of trigeminal nerve (V)
Central tegmental tract
Rubrospinal tract
Lateral lemniscus
Anterolateral system
Medial lemniscus
Trigeminal lemniscus
Middle cerebellar peduncle
Pontocerebellar fibers
Corticospinal, corticobulbar, and corticopontine tracts

Fourth ventricle

Periventricular (central) gray matter
Mesencephalic trigeminal nucleus (V)
Main (principal) trigeminal sensory nucleus (V)
Trigeminal motor nucleus (V)
Superior olivary complex
Pontine nuclei

Continued—**FIGURE AII–11**

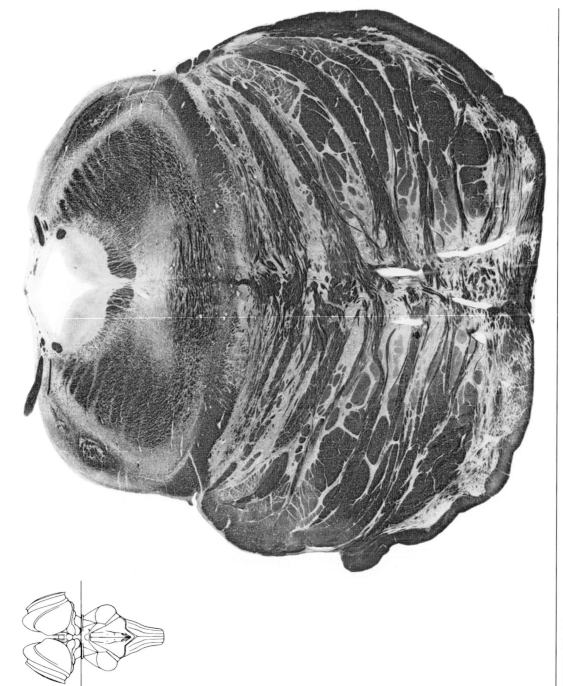

FIGURE AII–12 Transverse section through the rostral pons (isthmus) at the level of the decussation of the trochlear nerve. (×6)

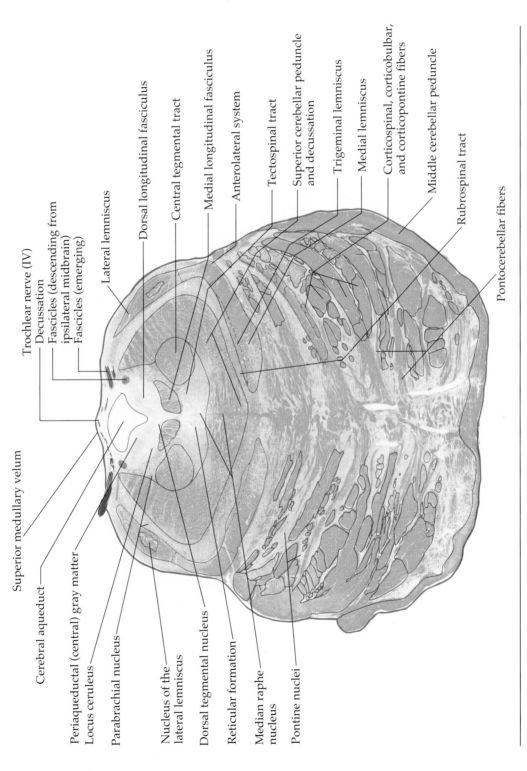

Superior medullary velum

Trochlear nerve (IV)
Decussation
Fascicles (descending from ipsilateral midbrain)
Fascicles (emerging)

Lateral lemniscus

Dorsal longitudinal fasciculus

Central tegmental tract

Medial longitudinal fasciculus

Anterolateral system

Tectospinal tract

Superior cerebellar peduncle and decussation

Trigeminal lemniscus

Medial lemniscus

Corticospinal, corticobulbar, and corticopontine fibers

Middle cerebellar peduncle

Rubrospinal tract

Pontocerebellar fibers

Cerebral aqueduct

Periaqueductal (central) gray matter
Locus ceruleus

Parabrachial nucleus

Nucleus of the lateral lemniscus

Dorsal tegmental nucleus

Reticular formation

Median raphe nucleus

Pontine nuclei

Continued—**FIGURE AII–12**

457

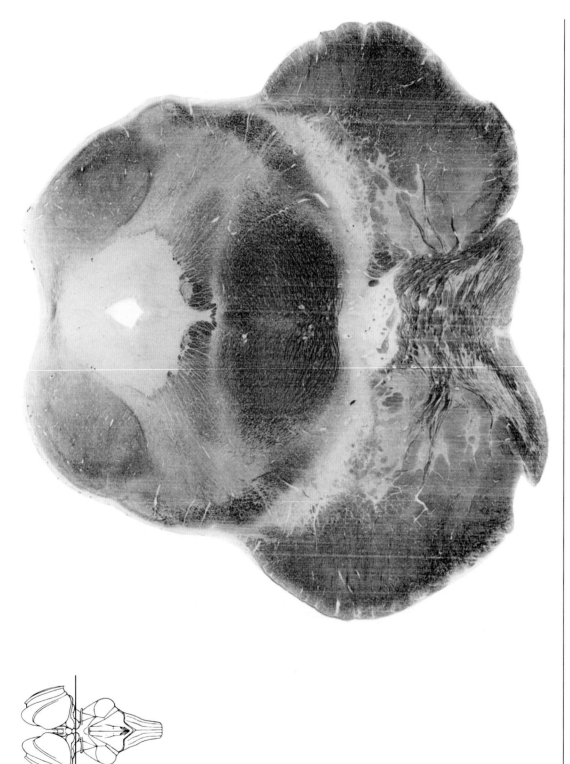

FIGURE AII–13 Transverse section of the caudal midbrain at the level of the inferior colliculus. (×5.6)

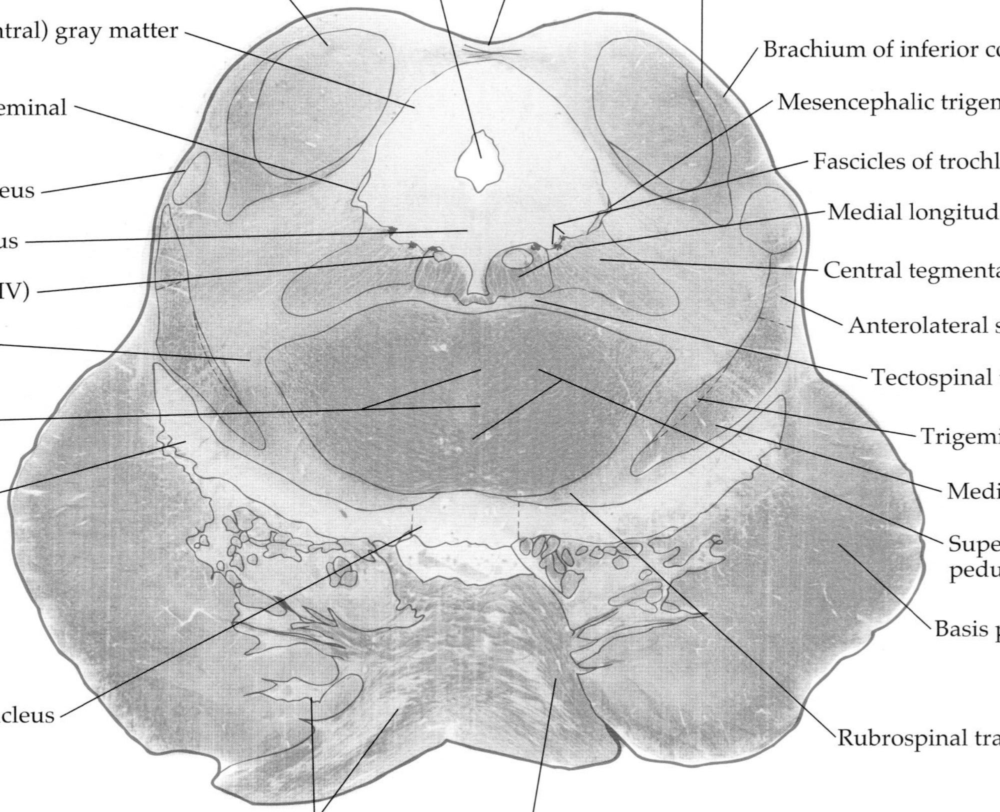

Periaqueductal (central) gray matter

Mesencephalic trigeminal nucleus (V)

Parabigeminal nucleus

Dorsal raphe nucleus

Trochlear nucleus (IV)

Pedunculopontine nucleus

Median raphe nucleus

Substantia nigra

Interpeduncular nucleus

Inferior colliculus (central nucleus)

Cerebral aqueduct

Commissure of inferior colliculus

Lateral lemniscus

Periaqueductal (central) gray matter

Brachium of inferior colliculus

Mesencephalic trigeminal tract (V)

Fascicles of trochlear nerve (IV)

Medial longitudinal fasciculus

Central tegmental tract

Anterolateral system

Tectospinal tract

Trigeminal lemniscus

Medial lemniscus

Superior cerebellar peduncle and decussation

Basis pedunculi

Rubrospinal tract

Pontocerebellar fibers

Pontine nuclei

Continued—**FIGURE AII–13**

459

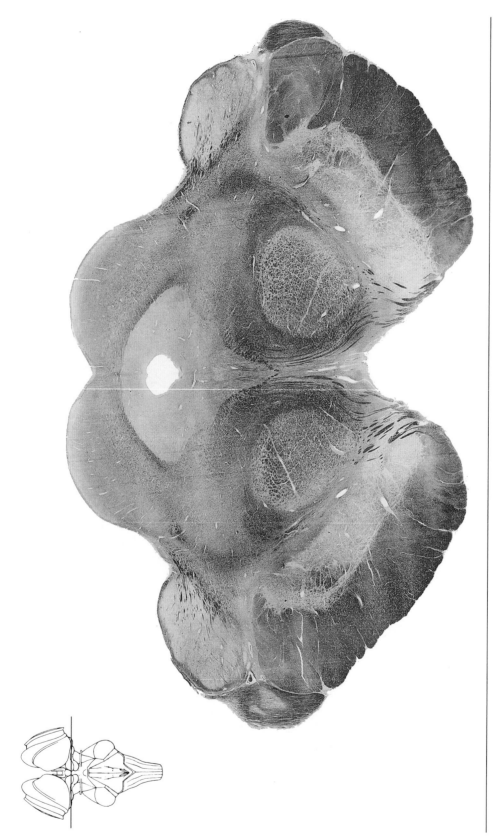

FIGURE AII–14 Transverse section of the rostral midbrain at the level of the superior colliculus. (×5.0)

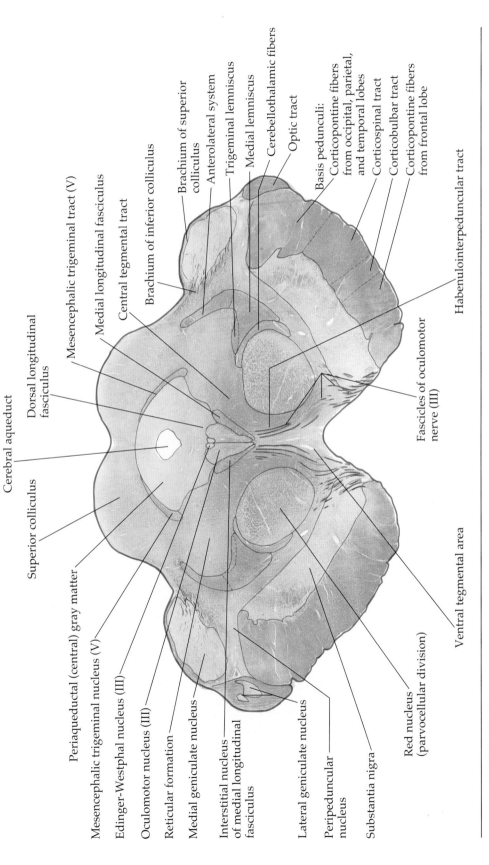

Cerebral aqueduct

Dorsal longitudinal fasciculus

Mesencephalic trigeminal tract (V)

Medial longitudinal fasciculus

Central tegmental tract

Brachium of inferior colliculus

Brachium of superior colliculus

Anterolateral system

Trigeminal lemniscus

Medial lemniscus

Cerebellothalamic fibers

Optic tract

Basis pedunculi:
Corticopontine fibers from occipital, parietal, and temporal lobes

Corticospinal tract

Corticobulbar tract

Corticopontine fibers from frontal lobe

Habenulointerpeduncular tract

Periaqueductal (central) gray matter

Mesencephalic trigeminal nucleus (V)

Edinger-Westphal nucleus (III)

Oculomotor nucleus (III)

Reticular formation

Medial geniculate nucleus

Interstitial nucleus of medial longitudinal fasciculus

Lateral geniculate nucleus

Peripeduncular nucleus

Substantia nigra

Red nucleus (parvocellular division)

Ventral tegmental area

Fascicles of oculomotor nerve (III)

Superior colliculus

Continued—**FIGURE AII–14**

461

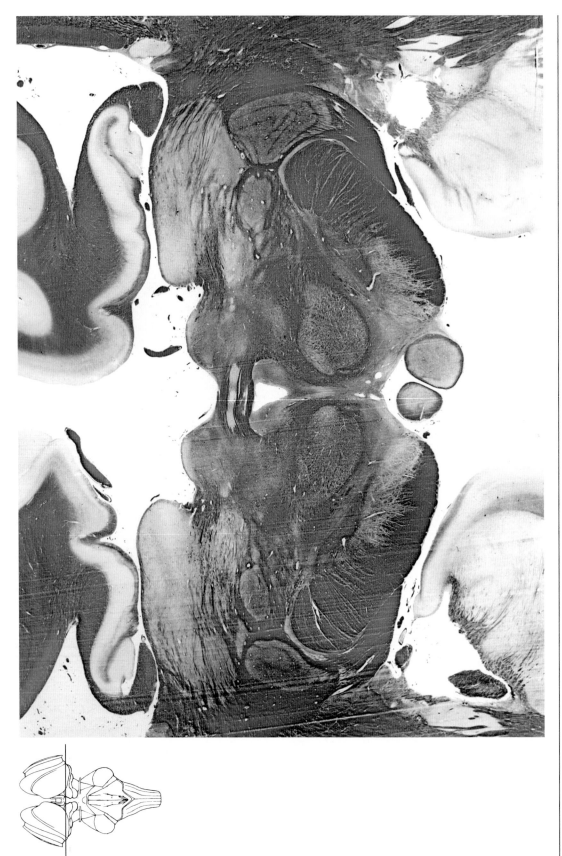

FIGURE AII–15 Transverse section of the juncture of the midbrain and diencephalon. (×3.3)

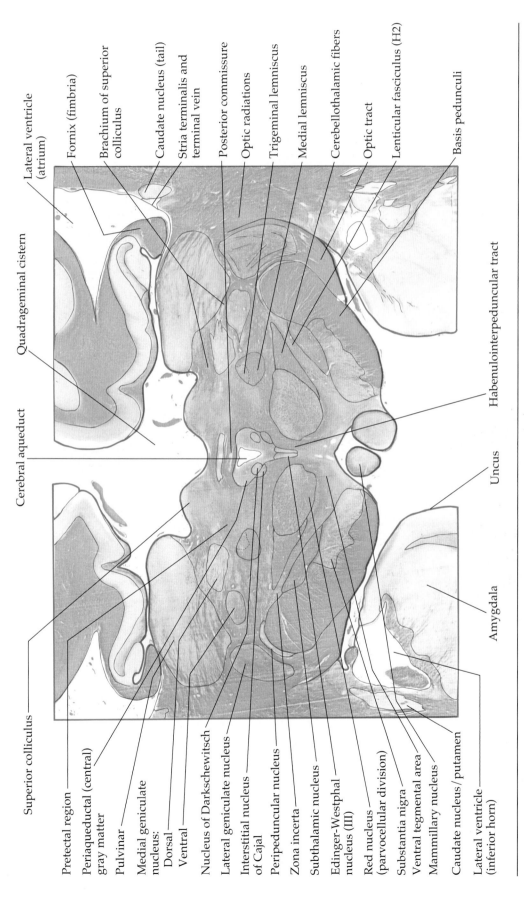

Superior colliculus

Quadrageminal cistern

Lateral ventricle (atrium)

Fornix (fimbria)

Brachium of superior colliculus

Caudate nucleus (tail)

Stria terminalis and terminal vein

Posterior commissure

Optic radiations

Trigeminal lemniscus

Medial lemniscus

Cerebellothalamic fibers

Optic tract

Lenticular fasciculus (H2)

Basis pedunculi

Cerebral aqueduct

Habenulointerpeduncular tract

Uncus

Amygdala

Pretectal region

Periaqueductal (central) gray matter

Pulvinar

Medial geniculate nucleus:
Dorsal
Ventral

Nucleus of Darkschewitsch

Lateral geniculate nucleus

Interstitial nucleus of Cajal

Peripeduncular nucleus

Zona incerta

Subthalamic nucleus

Edinger-Westphal nucleus (III)

Red nucleus (parvocellular division)

Substantia nigra

Ventral tegmental area

Mammillary nucleus

Caudate nucleus / putamen

Lateral ventricle (inferior horn)

Continued—**FIGURE AII–15**

463

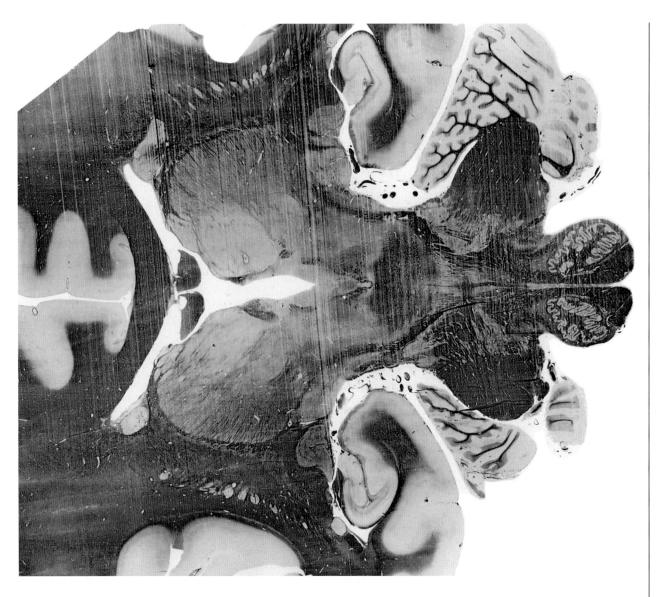

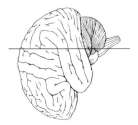

FIGURE AII–16 Coronal section of the diencephalon and cerebral hemisphere through the posterior limb of the internal capsule and the medial and lateral geniculate nuclei. The midbrain and pontine tegmentum, lateral cerebellum, and ventral medulla are also shown. (×2.1)

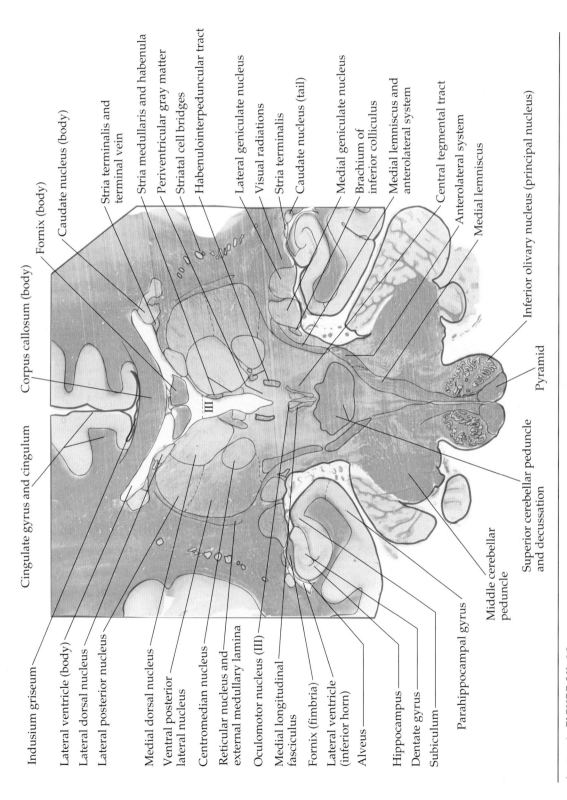

Indusium griseum

Lateral ventricle (body)
Lateral dorsal nucleus
Lateral posterior nucleus

Medial dorsal nucleus
Ventral posterior
lateral nucleus
Centromedian nucleus
Reticular nucleus and
external medullary lamina
Oculomotor nucleus (III)
Medial longitudinal
fasciculus
Fornix (fimbria)
Lateral ventricle
(inferior horn)
Alveus
Hippocampus
Dentate gyrus
Subiculum
Parahippocampal gyrus

Cingulate gyrus and cingulum

Corpus callosum (body)

Fornix (body)

Caudate nucleus (body)

Stria terminalis and
terminal vein
Stria medullaris and habenula
Periventricular gray matter
Striatal cell bridges
Habenulointerpeduncular tract

Lateral geniculate nucleus
Visual radiations
Stria terminalis
Caudate nucleus (tail)

Medial geniculate nucleus
Brachium of
inferior colliculus
Medial lemniscus and
anterolateral system
Central tegmental tract
Anterolateral system
Medial lemniscus

Inferior olivary nucleus (principal nucleus)

Pyramid

III

Superior cerebellar peduncle
and decussation

Middle cerebellar
peduncle

Continued—**FIGURE AII–16**

465

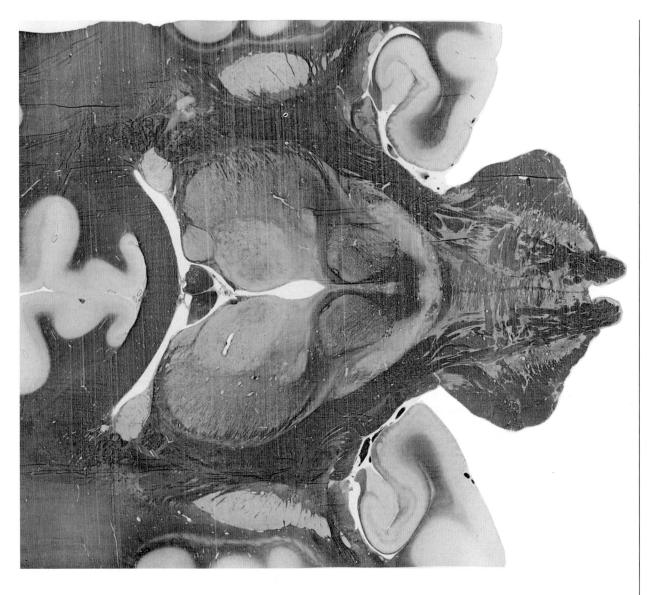

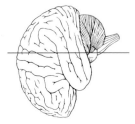

FIGURE AII–17 Coronal section of the diencephalon and cerebral hemisphere through the posterior limb of the internal capsule and ventral posterior nucleus. The midbrain tegmentum and base of the pons are also shown. (×2.3)

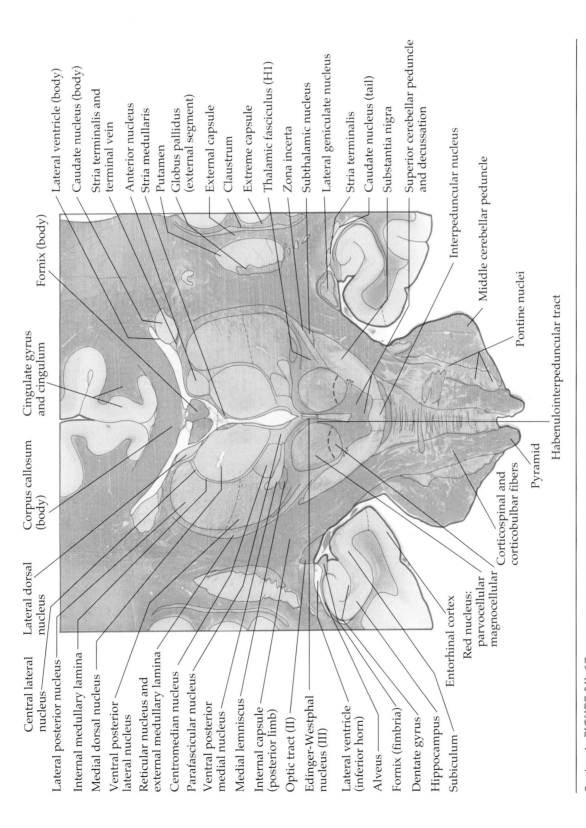

Central lateral nucleus

Lateral dorsal nucleus

Corpus callosum (body)

Cingulate gyrus and cingulum

Fornix (body)

Lateral ventricle (body)
Caudate nucleus (body)
Stria terminalis and terminal vein
Anterior nucleus
Stria medullaris
Putamen
Globus pallidus (external segment)
External capsule
Claustrum
Extreme capsule
Thalamic fasciculus (H1)
Zona incerta
Subthalamic nucleus
Lateral geniculate nucleus
Stria terminalis
Caudate nucleus (tail)
Substantia nigra
Superior cerebellar peduncle and decussation

Interpeduncular nucleus
Middle cerebellar peduncle
Pontine nuclei
Habenulointerpeduncular tract
Pyramid
Corticospinal and corticobulbar fibers
Red nucleus: parvocellular magnocellular
Entorhinal cortex
Subiculum
Hippocampus
Dentate gyrus
Fornix (fimbria)
Alveus
Lateral ventricle (inferior horn)
Edinger-Westphal nucleus (III)
Optic tract (II)
Internal capsule (posterior limb)
Medial lemniscus
Ventral posterior medial nucleus
Parafascicular nucleus
Centromedian nucleus
Reticular nucleus and external medullary lamina
Ventral posterior lateral nucleus
Medial dorsal nucleus
Internal medullary lamina
Lateral posterior nucleus

Continued—**FIGURE AII–17**

467

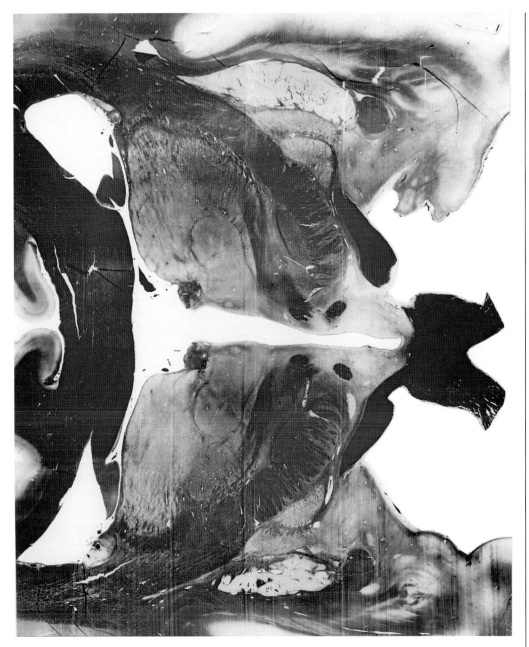

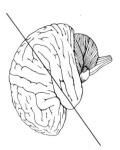

FIGURE AII–18 Oblique section of the cerebral hemisphere and diencephalon through the optic chiasm and tracts. (×2.3)

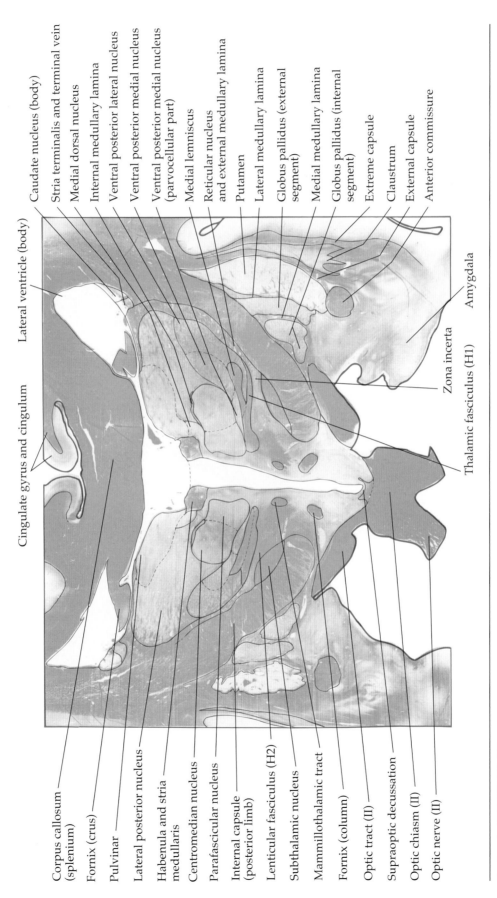

Corpus callosum (splenium)
Fornix (crus)
Pulvinar
Lateral posterior nucleus
Habenula and stria medullaris
Centromedian nucleus
Parafascicular nucleus
Internal capsule (posterior limb)
Lenticular fasciculus (H2)
Subthalamic nucleus
Mammillothalamic tract
Fornix (column)
Optic tract (II)
Supraoptic decussation
Optic chiasm (II)
Optic nerve (II)

Cingulate gyrus and cingulum
Lateral ventricle (body)

Caudate nucleus (body)
Stria terminalis and terminal vein
Medial dorsal nucleus
Internal medullary lamina
Ventral posterior lateral nucleus
Ventral posterior medial nucleus
Ventral posterior medial nucleus (parvocellular part)
Medial lemniscus
Reticular nucleus and external medullary lamina
Putamen
Lateral medullary lamina
Globus pallidus (external segment)
Medial medullary lamina
Globus pallidus (internal segment)
Extreme capsule
Claustrum
External capsule
Anterior commissure

Zona incerta
Thalamic fasciculus (H1)
Amygdala

Continued—**FIGURE AII–18**

469

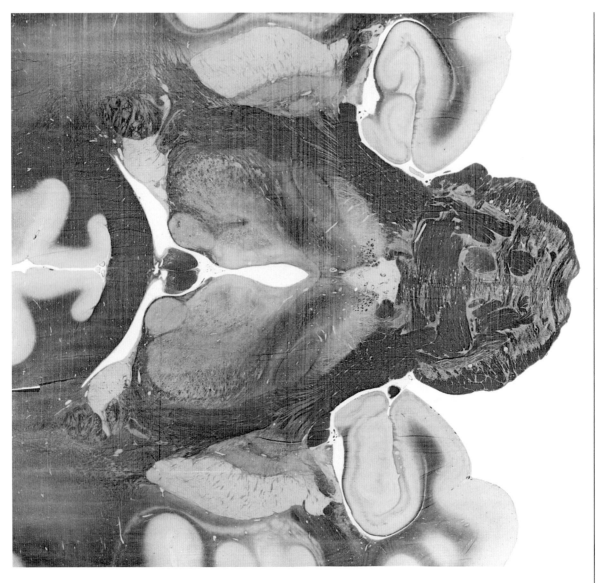

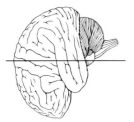

FIGURE AII–19 Coronal section of the diencephalon and cerebral hemisphere through the posterior limb of the internal capsule and anterior thalamic nuclei. The ventral midbrain and ventral pons are also shown. (×2.2)

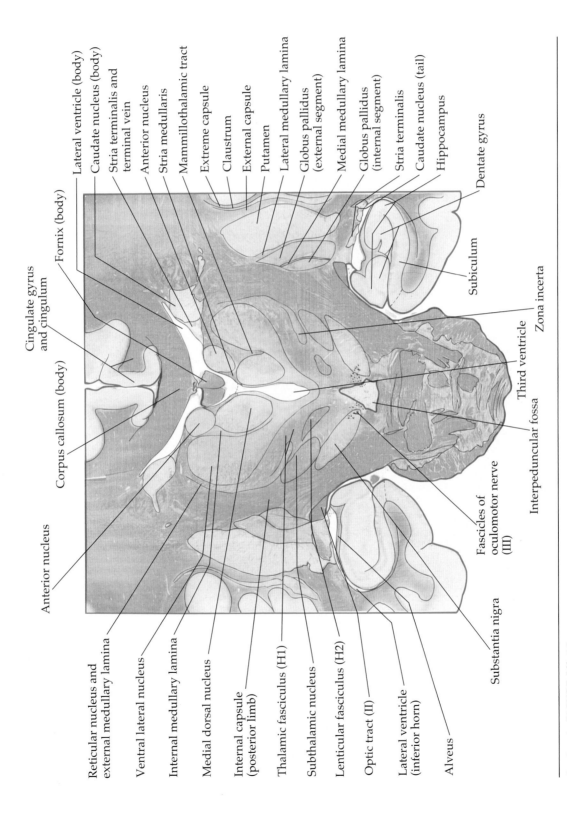

Anterior nucleus

Cingulate gyrus
and cingulum

Fornix (body)

Corpus callosum (body)

Lateral ventricle (body)
Caudate nucleus (body)
Stria terminalis and
terminal vein
Anterior nucleus
Stria medullaris
Mammillothalamic tract
Extreme capsule
Claustrum
External capsule
Putamen
Lateral medullary lamina
Globus pallidus
(external segment)
Medial medullary lamina
Globus pallidus
(internal segment)
Stria terminalis
Caudate nucleus (tail)
Hippocampus
Dentate gyrus

Subiculum

Zona incerta

Third ventricle

Interpeduncular fossa

Fascicles of
oculomotor nerve
(III)

Substantia nigra

Alveus

Lateral ventricle
(inferior horn)

Optic tract (II)

Lenticular fasciculus (H2)

Subthalamic nucleus

Thalamic fasciculus (H1)

Internal capsule
(posterior limb)

Medial dorsal nucleus

Internal medullary lamina

Ventral lateral nucleus

Reticular nucleus and
external medullary lamina

Continued—**FIGURE AII–19**

471

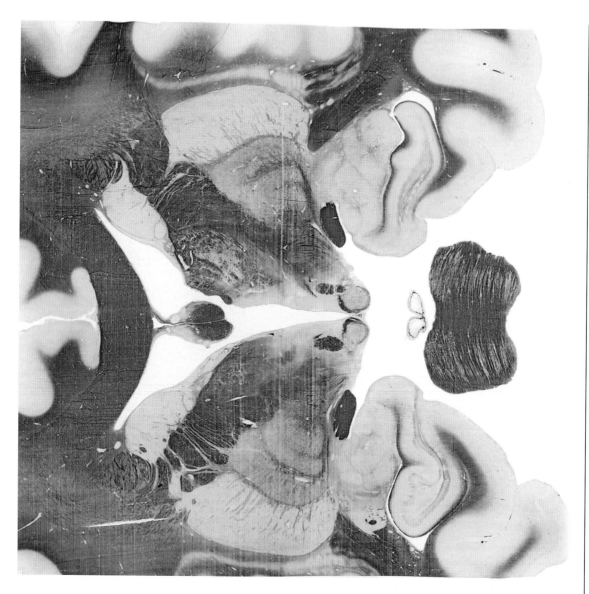

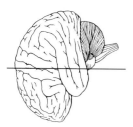

FIGURE AII–20 Coronal section of the cerebral hemisphere and diencephalon through the intraventricular foramen. The base of the pons is also shown. (×2.1)

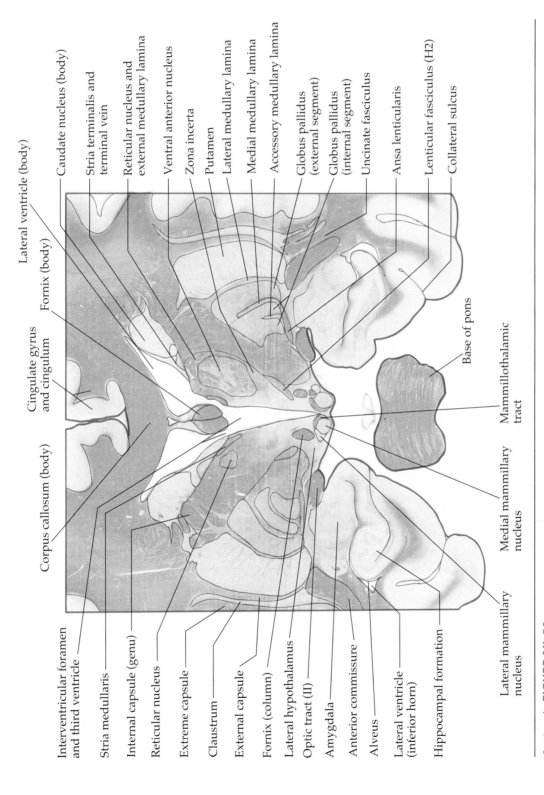

Interventricular foramen and third ventricle

Stria medullaris

Internal capsule (genu)

Reticular nucleus

Extreme capsule

Claustrum

External capsule

Fornix (column)

Lateral hypothalamus

Optic tract (II)

Amygdala

Anterior commissure

Alveus

Lateral ventricle (inferior horn)

Hippocampal formation

Corpus callosum (body)

Cingulate gyrus and cingulum

Lateral ventricle (body)

Fornix (body)

Caudate nucleus (body)

Stria terminalis and terminal vein

Reticular nucleus and external medullary lamina

Ventral anterior nucleus

Zona incerta

Putamen

Lateral medullary lamina

Medial medullary lamina

Accessory medullary lamina

Globus pallidus (external segment)

Globus pallidus (internal segment)

Uncinate fasciculus

Ansa lenticularis

Lenticular fasciculus (H2)

Collateral sulcus

Base of pons

Mammillothalamic tract

Medial mammillary nucleus

Lateral mammillary nucleus

*Continued—***FIGURE AII–20**

473

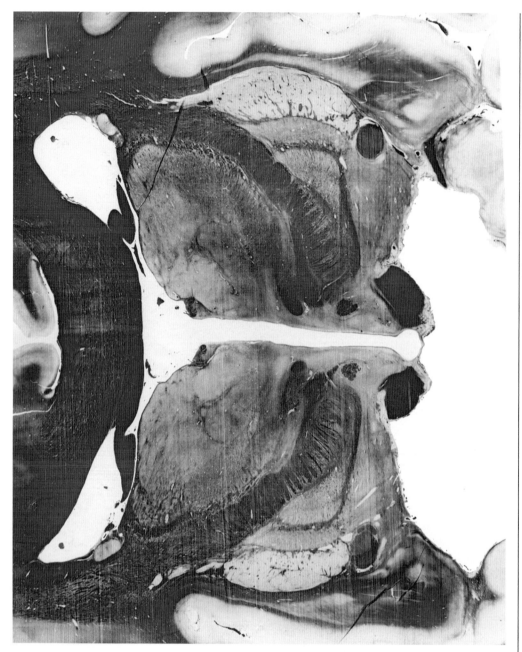

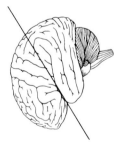

FIGURE AII–21 Oblique section of the cerebral hemisphere and diencephalon through the ansa lenticularis and optic tract. (×2.4)

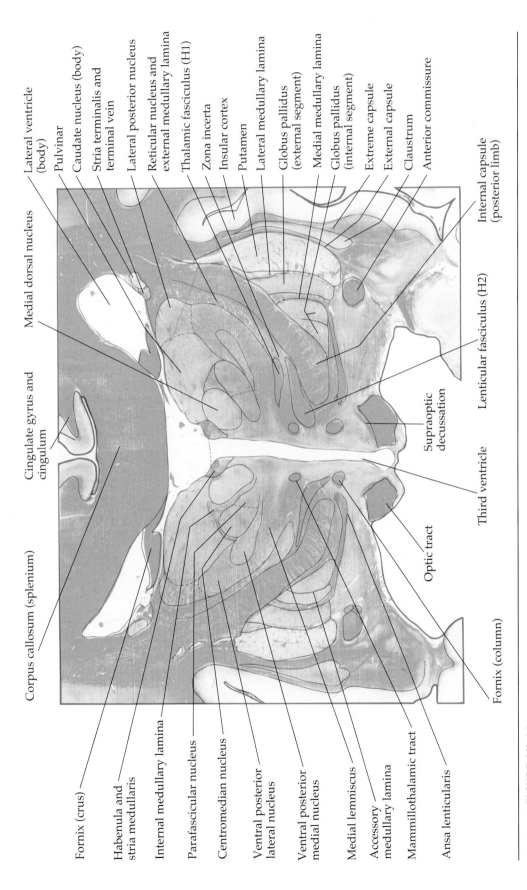

Corpus callosum (splenium)

Cingulate gyrus and
cingulum

Medial dorsal nucleus

Lateral ventricle
(body)

Pulvinar

Caudate nucleus (body)

Stria terminalis and
terminal vein

Lateral posterior nucleus

Reticular nucleus and
external medullary lamina

Thalamic fasciculus (H1)

Zona incerta

Insular cortex

Putamen

Lateral medullary lamina

Globus pallidus
(external segment)

Medial medullary lamina

Globus pallidus
(internal segment)

Extreme capsule

External capsule

Claustrum

Anterior commissure

Internal capsule
(posterior limb)

Fornix (crus)

Habenula and
stria medullaris

Internal medullary lamina

Parafascicular nucleus

Centromedian nucleus

Ventral posterior
lateral nucleus

Ventral posterior
medial nucleus

Medial lemniscus

Accessory
medullary lamina

Mammillothalamic tract

Ansa lenticularis

Optic tract

Third ventricle

Supraoptic
decussation

Lenticular fasciculus (H2)

Fornix (column)

*Continued—***FIGURE AII–21**

475

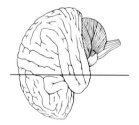

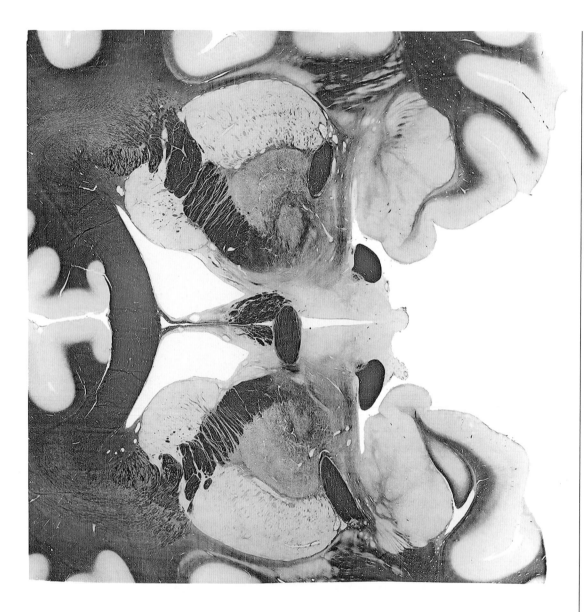

FIGURE AII–22 Coronal section of the cerebral hemisphere through the anterior limb of the internal capsule, column of the fornix, and amygdala. (×2.2)

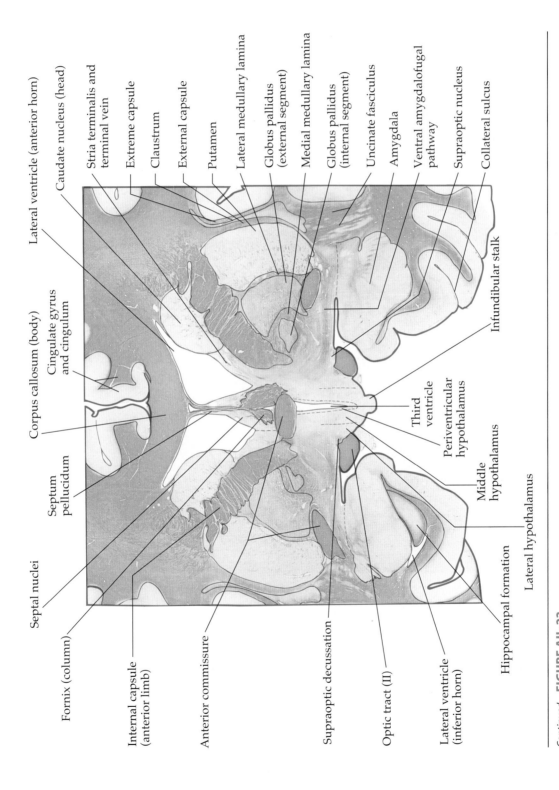

Septal nuclei

Corpus callosum (body)

Cingulate gyrus
and cingulum

Septum
pellucidum

Fornix (column)

Internal capsule
(anterior limb)

Anterior commissure

Supraoptic decussation

Optic tract (II)

Lateral ventricle
(inferior horn)

Hippocampal formation

Lateral hypothalamus

Lateral ventricle (anterior horn)

Caudate nucleus (head)

Stria terminalis and
terminal vein

Extreme capsule

Claustrum

External capsule

Putamen

Lateral medullary lamina

Globus pallidus
(external segment)

Medial medullary lamina

Globus pallidus
(internal segment)

Uncinate fasciculus

Amygdala

Ventral amygdalofugal
pathway

Supraoptic nucleus

Collateral sulcus

Infundibular stalk

Third
ventricle

Periventricular
hypothalamus

Middle
hypothalamus

Continued—**FIGURE AII–22**

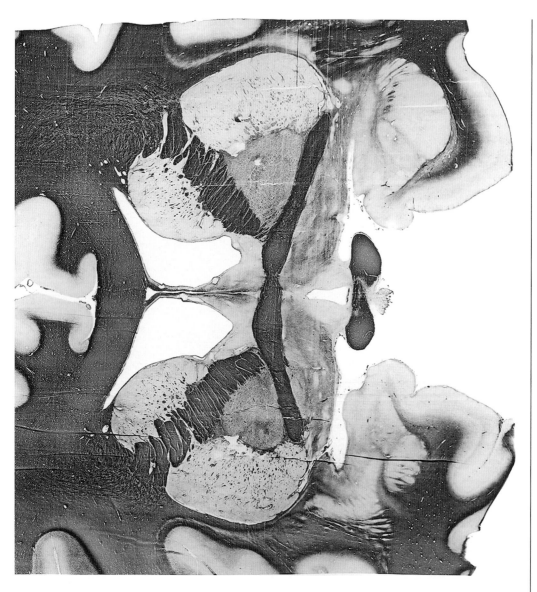

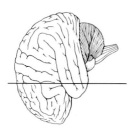

FIGURE AII–23 Coronal section of the cerebral hemisphere through the anterior limb of the internal capsule, anterior commissure, and optic chiasm. (×2.2)

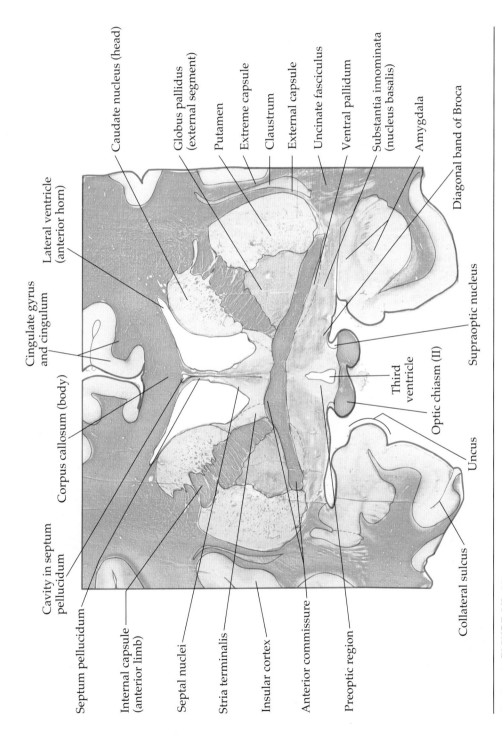

Septum pellucidum

Cavity in septum pellucidum

Internal capsule (anterior limb)

Septal nuclei

Stria terminalis

Insular cortex

Anterior commissure

Preoptic region

Collateral sulcus

Cingulate gyrus and cingulum

Lateral ventricle (anterior horn)

Corpus callosum (body)

Caudate nucleus (head)

Globus pallidus (external segment)

Putamen

Extreme capsule

Claustrum

External capsule

Uncinate fasciculus

Ventral pallidum

Substantia innominata (nucleus basalis)

Amygdala

Diagonal band of Broca

Supraoptic nucleus

Third ventricle

Optic chiasm (II)

Uncus

Continued—**FIGURE AII–23**

479

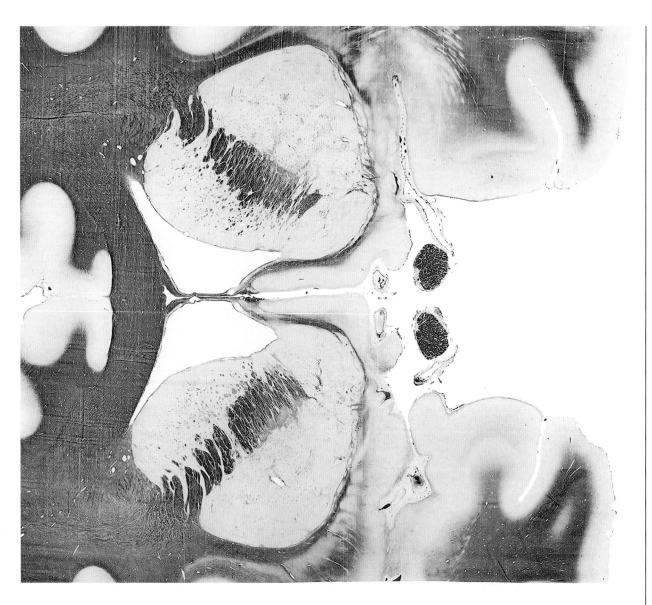

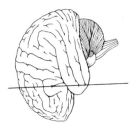

FIGURE AII–24 Coronal section of the cerebral hemisphere through the anterior limb of the internal capsule and the head of the caudate nucleus. (×2.4)

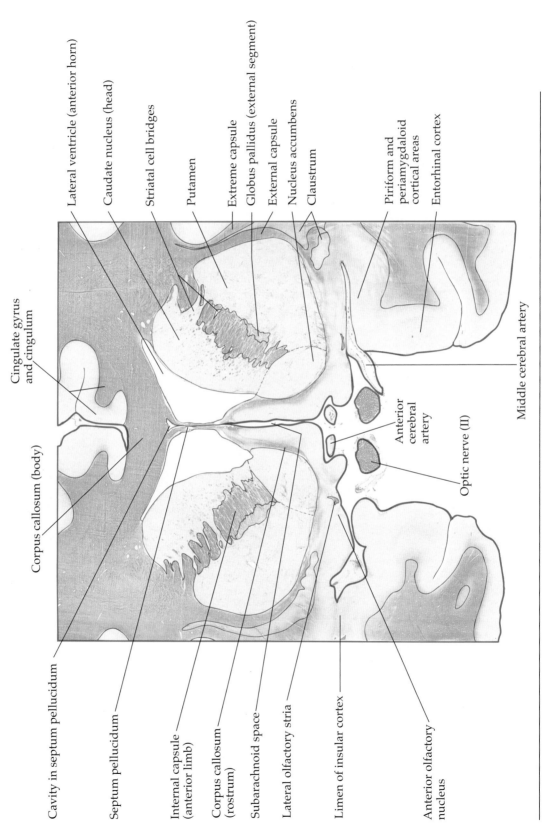

Cingulate gyrus
and cingulum

Lateral ventricle (anterior horn)

Caudate nucleus (head)

Striatal cell bridges

Putamen

Extreme capsule

Globus pallidus (external segment)

External capsule

Nucleus accumbens

Claustrum

Piriform and
periamygdaloid
cortical areas

Entorhinal cortex

Corpus callosum (body)

Cavity in septum pellucidum

Septum pellucidum

Internal capsule
(anterior limb)

Corpus callosum
(rostrum)

Subarachnoid space

Lateral olfactory stria

Limen of insular cortex

Anterior olfactory
nucleus

Anterior
cerebral
artery

Optic nerve (II)

Middle cerebral artery

Continued—**FIGURE AII–24**

481

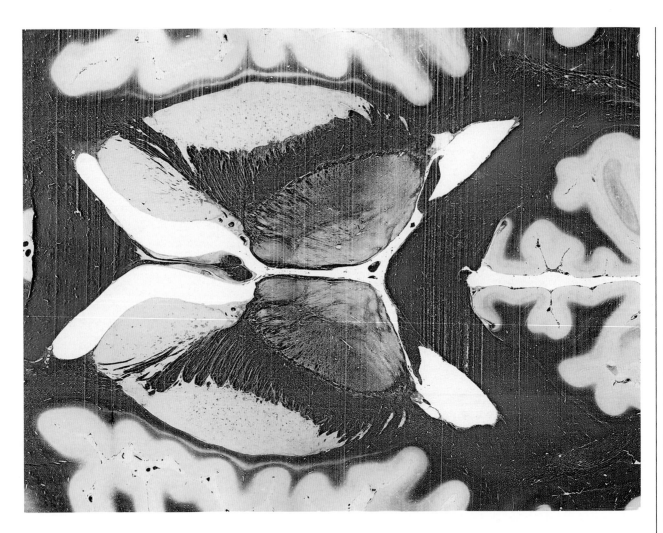

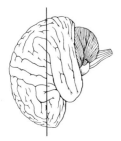

FIGURE AII–25 Horizontal section of the cerebral hemisphere and diencephalon through the anterior thalamic nuclei. (×1.9)

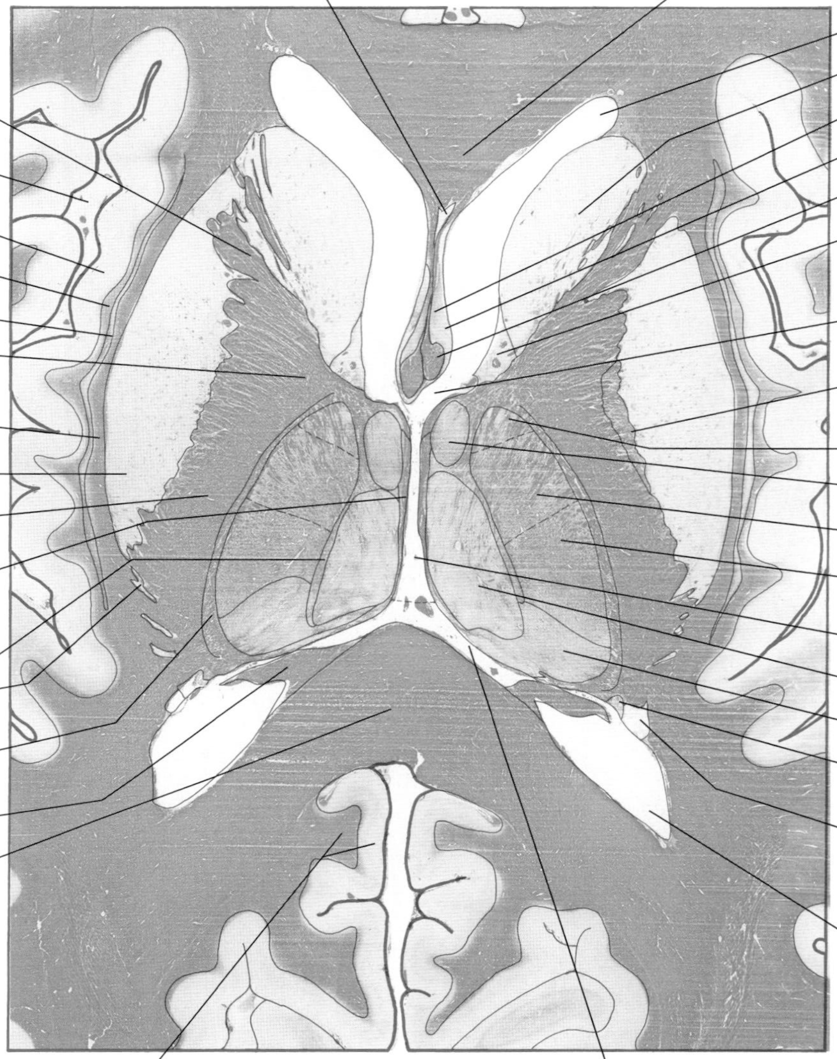
Cavity in septum pellucidum
Corpus callosum (genu)
Internal capsule (anterior limb)
Lateral sulcus
Insular cortex
Extreme capsule
Claustrum
Internal capsule (genu)
External capsule
Putamen
Internal capsule (posterior limb)
Stria medullaris
Internal medullary lamina
Striatal cell bridges
Reticular nucleus and external medullary lamina
Fornix (crus)
Corpus callosum (splenium)
Lateral ventricle (anterior horn)
Caudate nucleus (head)
Septum pellucidum
Septal nuclei
Fornix (body)
Stria terminalis and terminal vein
Interventricular foramen (of Monro)
Globus pallidus (external segment)
Ventral anterior nucleus
Anterior nucleus
Ventral lateral nucleus
Lateral posterior nucleus
Third ventricle
Medial dorsal nucleus
Pulvinar
Stria terminalis and terminal vein
Caudate nucleus (tail)
Lateral ventricle (atrium)
Cingulate gyrus and cingulum
Subarachnoid space

Continued—**FIGURE AII–25**

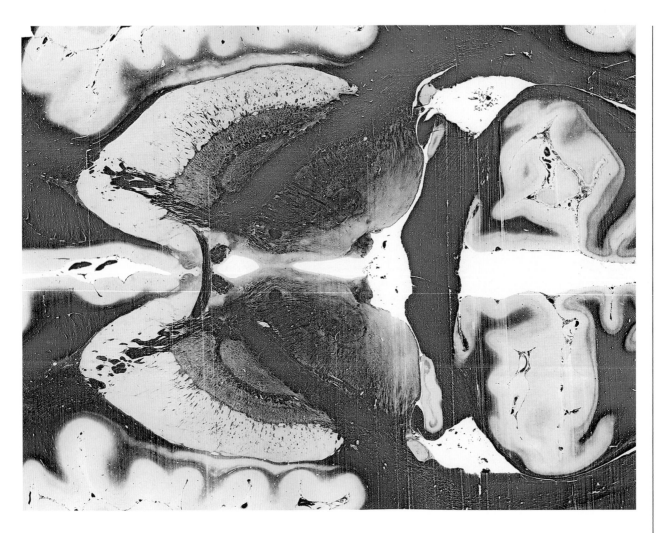

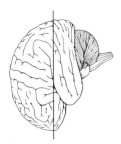

FIGURE AII–26 Horizontal section of the cerebral hemisphere and diencephalon at the level of the anterior commissure. (×1.9)

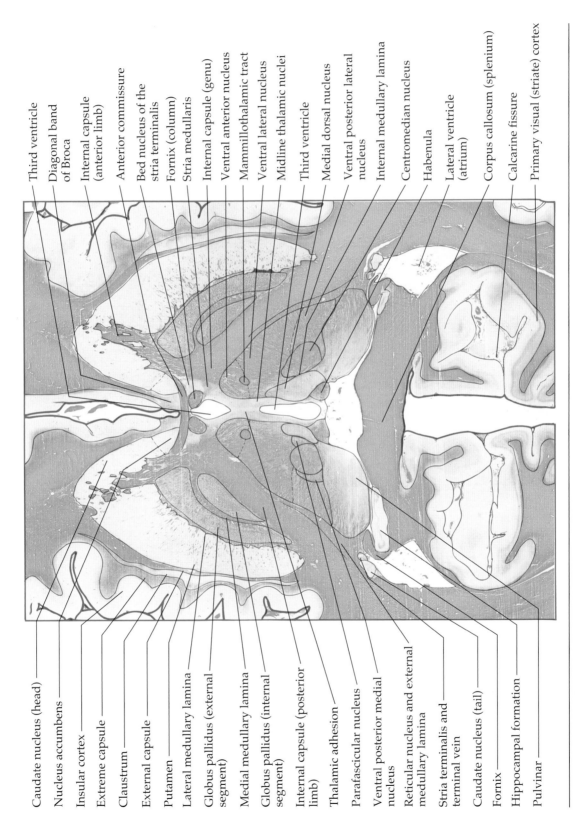

Caudate nucleus (head)

Nucleus accumbens

Insular cortex

Extreme capsule

Claustrum

External capsule

Putamen

Lateral medullary lamina

Globus pallidus (external segment)

Medial medullary lamina

Globus pallidus (internal segment)

Internal capsule (posterior limb)

Thalamic adhesion

Parafascicular nucleus

Ventral posterior medial nucleus

Reticular nucleus and external medullary lamina

Stria terminalis and terminal vein

Caudate nucleus (tail)

Fornix

Hippocampal formation

Pulvinar

Third ventricle

Diagonal band of Broca

Internal capsule (anterior limb)

Anterior commissure

Bed nucleus of the stria terminalis

Fornix (column)

Stria medullaris

Internal capsule (genu)

Ventral anterior nucleus

Mammillothalamic tract

Ventral lateral nucleus

Midline thalamic nuclei

Third ventricle

Medial dorsal nucleus

Ventral posterior lateral nucleus

Internal medullary lamina

Centromedian nucleus

Habenula

Lateral ventricle (atrium)

Corpus callosum (splenium)

Calcarine fissure

Primary visual (striate) cortex

Continued—**FIGURE AII–26**

485

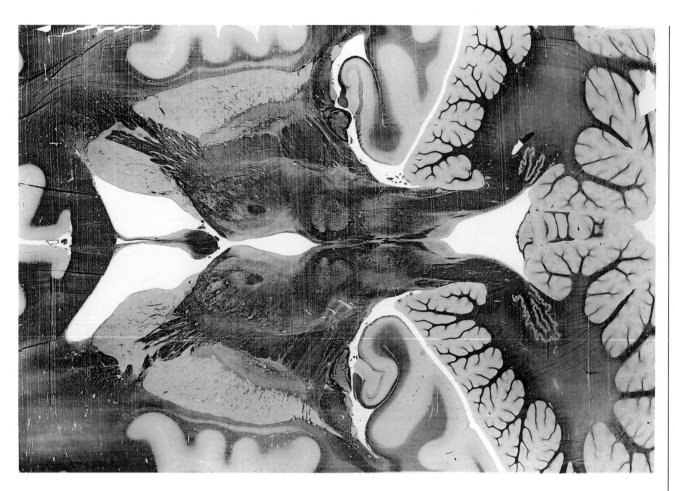

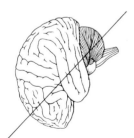

FIGURE AII–27 Oblique section of the cerebral hemisphere, diencephalon, brain stem, and cerebellum. (×1.6)

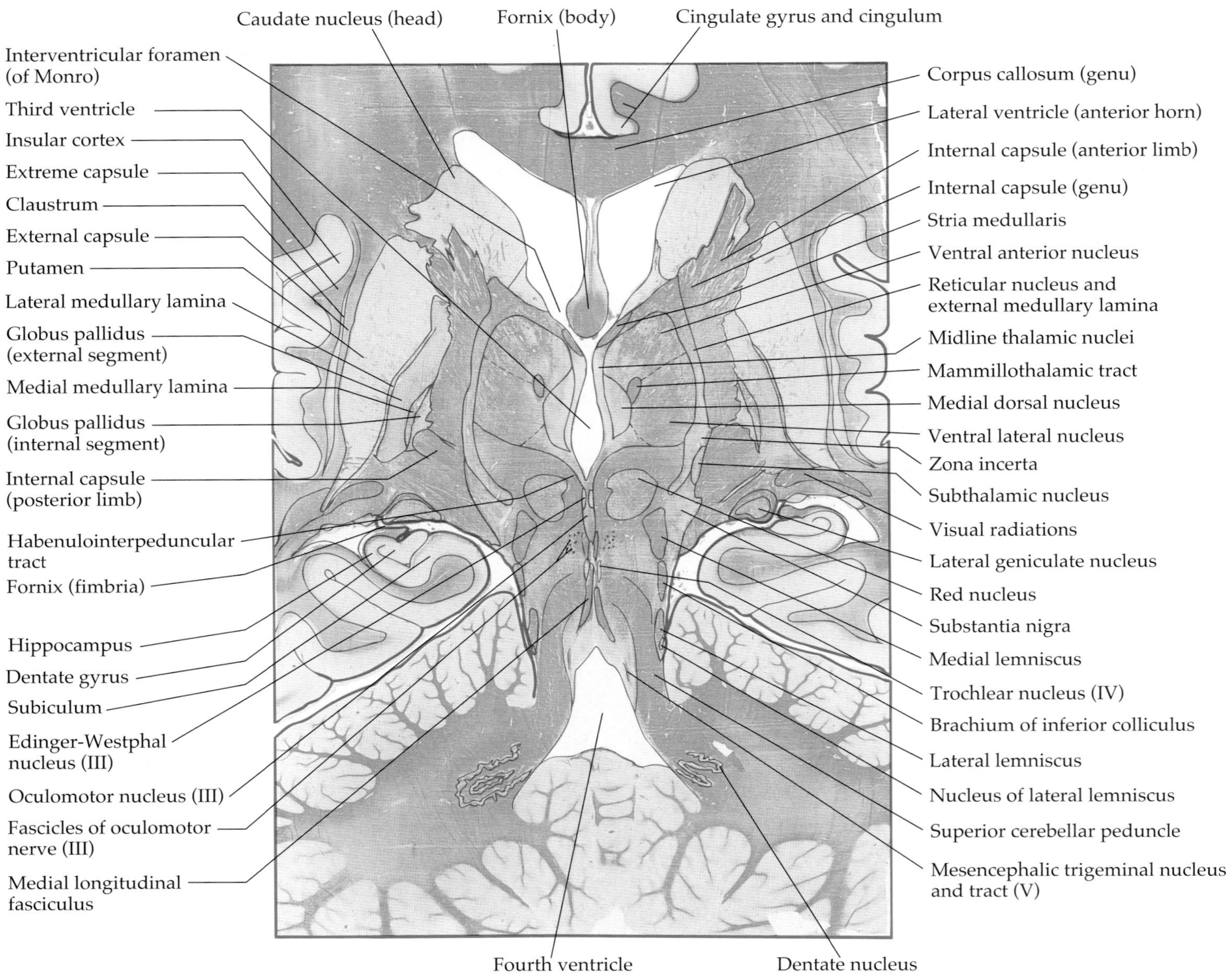

Caudate nucleus (head)

Cingulate gyrus and cingulum

Fornix (body)

Corpus callosum (genu)
Lateral ventricle (anterior horn)
Internal capsule (anterior limb)
Internal capsule (genu)
Stria medullaris
Ventral anterior nucleus
Reticular nucleus and external medullary lamina
Midline thalamic nuclei
Mammillothalamic tract
Medial dorsal nucleus
Ventral lateral nucleus
Zona incerta
Subthalamic nucleus
Visual radiations
Lateral geniculate nucleus
Red nucleus
Substantia nigra
Medial lemniscus
Trochlear nucleus (IV)
Brachium of inferior colliculus
Lateral lemniscus
Nucleus of lateral lemniscus
Superior cerebellar peduncle
Mesencephalic trigeminal nucleus and tract (V)

Dentate nucleus

Fourth ventricle

Interventricular foramen (of Monro)
Third ventricle
Insular cortex
Extreme capsule
Claustrum
External capsule
Putamen
Lateral medullary lamina
Globus pallidus (external segment)
Medial medullary lamina
Globus pallidus (internal segment)
Internal capsule (posterior limb)
Habenulointerpeduncular tract
Fornix (fimbria)
Hippocampus
Dentate gyrus
Subiculum
Edinger-Westphal nucleus (III)
Oculomotor nucleus (III)
Fascicles of oculomotor nerve (III)
Medial longitudinal fasciculus

Continued—**FIGURE AII-27**

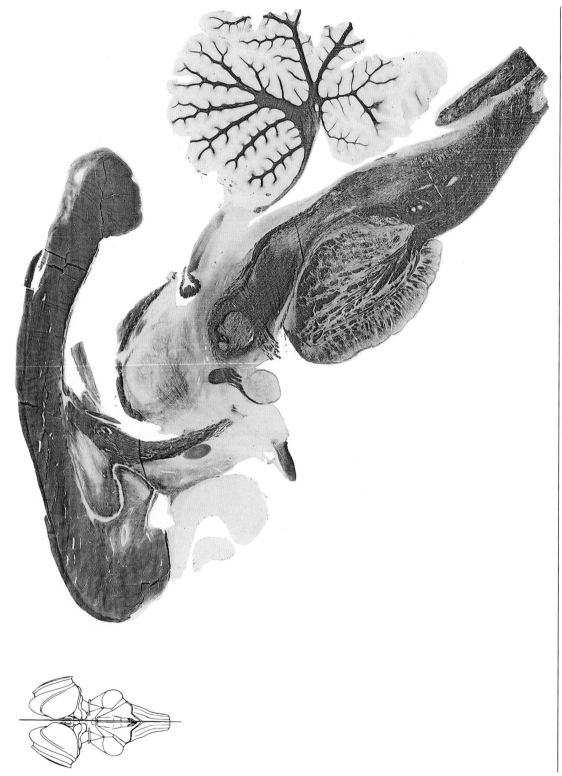

FIGURE AII–28 Sagittal section of the cerebral hemisphere, diencephalon, brain stem, and cerebellum close to the midline. (×1.9)

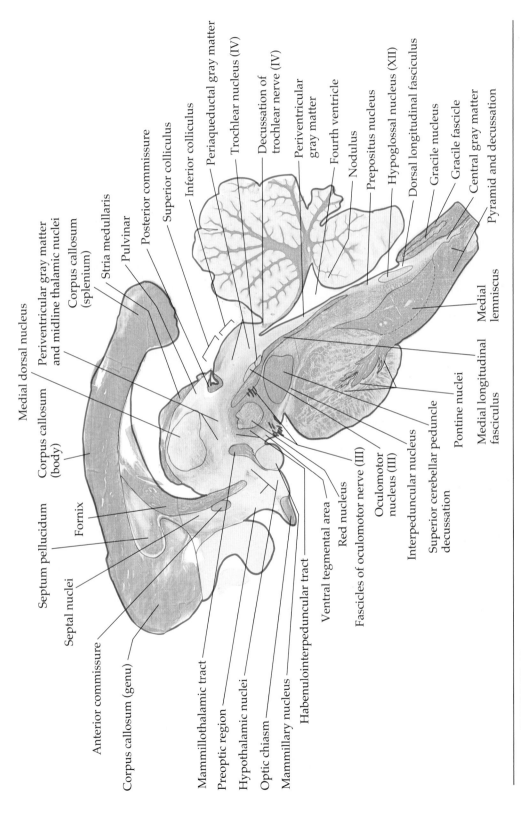

Medial dorsal nucleus

Periventricular gray matter
and midline thalamic nuclei

Corpus callosum
(splenium)

Stria medullaris

Pulvinar

Posterior commissure

Superior colliculus

Inferior colliculus

Periaqueductal gray matter

Trochlear nucleus (IV)

Decussation of
trochlear nerve (IV)

Periventricular
gray matter

Fourth ventricle

Nodulus

Prepositus nucleus

Hypoglossal nucleus (XII)

Dorsal longitudinal fasciculus

Gracile nucleus

Gracile fascicle

Central gray matter

Pyramid and decussation

Medial
lemniscus

Corpus callosum
(body)

Medial longitudinal
fasciculus

Pontine nuclei

Septum pellucidum

Fornix

Septal nuclei

Interpeduncular nucleus

Superior cerebellar peduncle
decussation

Anterior commissure

Corpus callosum (genu)

Oculomotor
nucleus (III)

Fascicles of oculomotor nerve (III)

Red nucleus

Ventral tegmental area

Mammillothalamic tract

Preoptic region

Hypothalamic nuclei

Optic chiasm

Mammillary nucleus

Habenulointerpeduncular tract

Continued—**FIGURE AII–28**

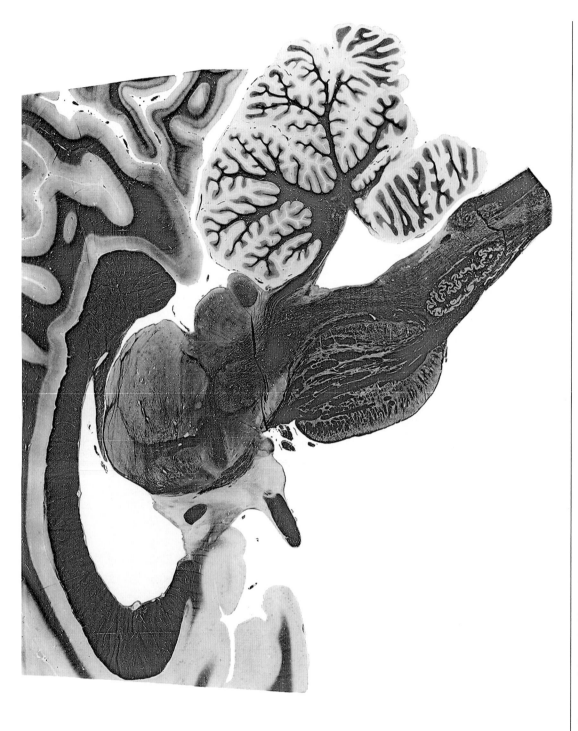

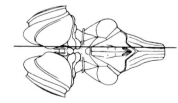

FIGURE AII–29 Sagittal section of the cerebral hemisphere, diencephalon, brain stem, and cerebellum through the mammillothalamic tract and anterior thalamic nucleus. (×1.8)

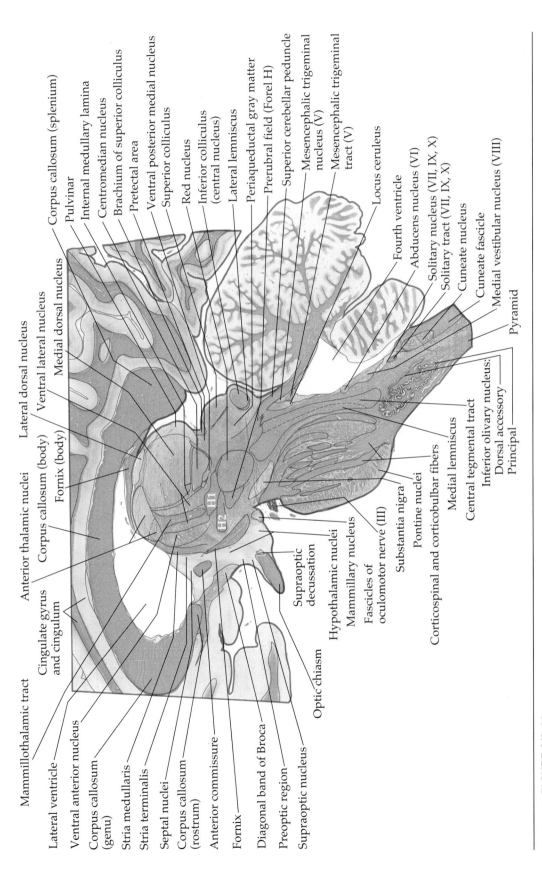

Continued—**FIGURE AII–29**

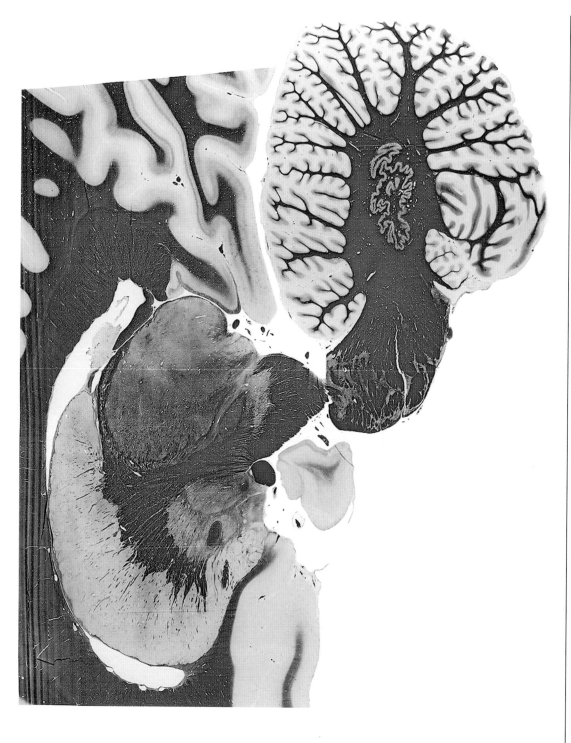

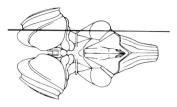

FIGURE AII–30 Sagittal section of the cerebral hemisphere, diencephalon, brain stem, and cerebellum through the ventral posterior lateral nucleus and the dentate nucleus. (×1.9)

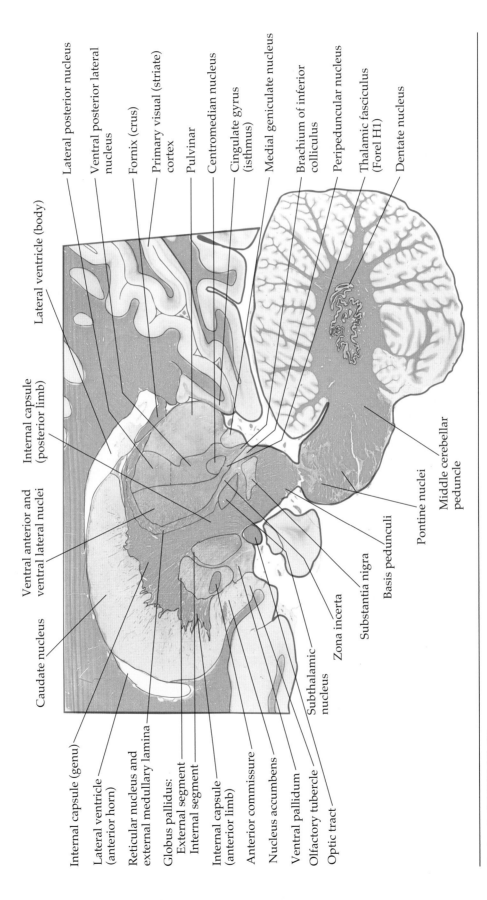

Lateral posterior nucleus

Ventral posterior lateral nucleus

Fornix (crus)

Primary visual (striate) cortex

Pulvinar

Centromedian nucleus

Cingulate gyrus (isthmus)

Medial geniculate nucleus

Brachium of inferior colliculus

Peripeduncular nucleus

Thalamic fasciculus (Forel H1)

Dentate nucleus

Lateral ventricle (body)

Internal capsule (posterior limb)

Ventral anterior and ventral lateral nuclei

Caudate nucleus

Middle cerebellar peduncle

Pontine nuclei

Basis pedunculi

Substantia nigra

Zona incerta

Subthalamic nucleus

Optic tract

Olfactory tubercle

Ventral pallidum

Nucleus accumbens

Anterior commissure

Internal capsule (anterior limb)

Globus pallidus:
External segment
Internal segment

Reticular nucleus and external medullary lamina

Lateral ventricle (anterior horn)

Internal capsule (genu)

Continued—**FIGURE AII–30**

493

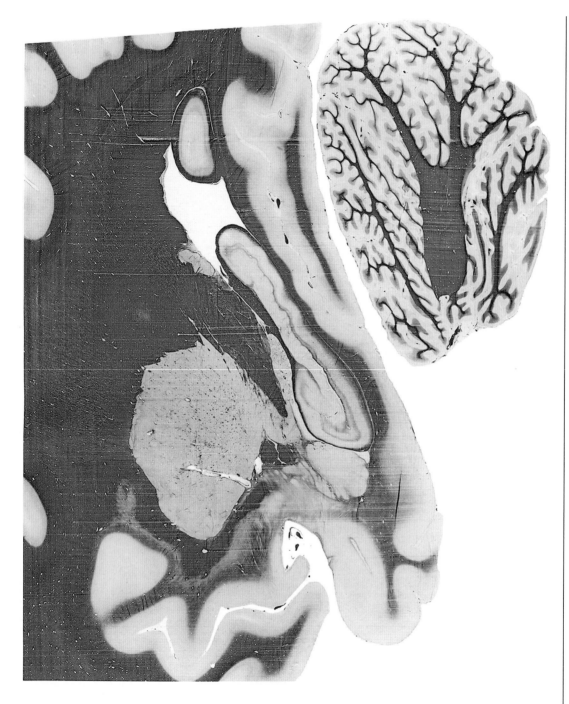

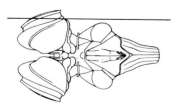

FIGURE AII–31 Sagittal section of the cerebral hemisphere and cerebellum through the amygdala and hippocampal formation. (×1.9)

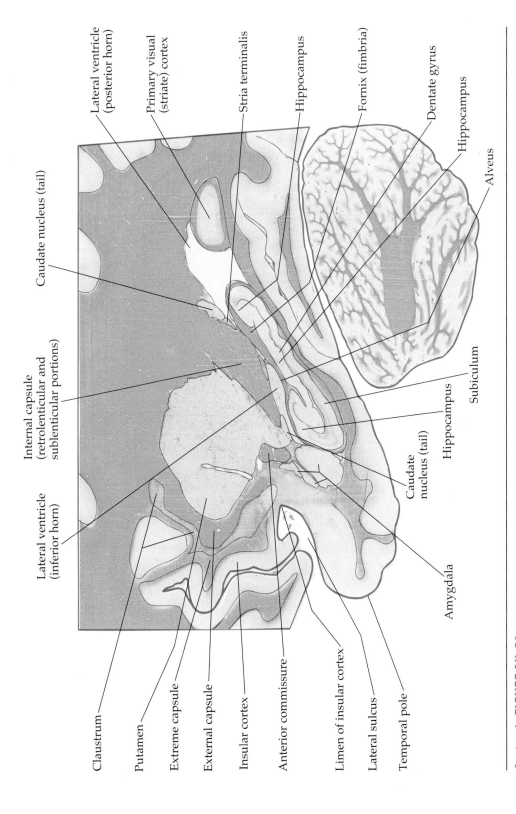

Caudate nucleus (tail)

Lateral ventricle (posterior horn)

Primary visual (striate) cortex

Stria terminalis

Hippocampus

Fornix (fimbria)

Dentate gyrus

Hippocampus

Alveus

Internal capsule (retrolenticular and sublenticular portions)

Subiculum

Hippocampus

Caudate nucleus (tail)

Lateral ventricle (inferior horn)

Claustrum

Putamen

Extreme capsule

External capsule

Insular cortex

Anterior commissure

Limen of insular cortex

Lateral sulcus

Temporal pole

Amygdala

Continued—**FIGURE AII–31**

495

References

Alheld GF, Heimer L, Switzer RC III. Basal ganglia. In: Paxinos G, ed. *The Human Central Nervous System*. San Diego, CA: Academic Press, 1990:483-582.

Andy OJ, Stephan H. The septum of the human brain. *J Comp Neurol*. 1968;133:383-410.

Bruce A. *A Topographical Atlas of the Spinal Cord*. Baltimore, MD: The Williams and Norgate, 1901.

Carpenter MB, Sutin J. *Human Neuroanatomy*. Williams & Wilkins Company, 1983.

Crosby EC, Humphrey T, Lauer EW. *Correlative Anatomy of the Nervous System*. Macmillan, 1962.

DeArmond SJ, Fusco MM, Dewey MM. *Structure of the Human Brain*. Oxford University Press, 1976.

de Olmos J. Amygdala. In: Paxinos G, Mai JK, eds. *The Human Nervous System*. Vol 738-868. London: Elsevier, 2004.

Haines D. *Neuroanatomy: An Atlas of Structures, Sections, and Systems*. Urban & Schwarzenberg, 1983.

Hirai T, Jones EG. A new parcellation of the human thalamus on the basis of histochemical staining. *Brain Res Rev*. 1989;14:1-34.

Insausti R, Amaral D. Hippocampal formation. In: Paxinos G, Mai JK, eds. *The Human Nervous System*. London: Elsevier, 2004:871-914.

Martin GF, Holstege G, Mehler WR. Reticular formation of the pons and medulla. In: Paxinos G, ed. *The Human Central Nervous System*. San Diego, CA: Academic Press, 1990.

Nathan PW, Smith MC. Long descending tracts in man. I. Review of present knowledge. *Brain*. 1955;78:248-303.

Nathan PW, Smith MC. The rubrospinal and central tegmental tracts in man. *Brain*. 1982;105:223-269.

Olszewski J, Baxter D, ed. *Cytoarchitecture of the Human Brain Stem. Vol. I: Head, Neck, Upper Extremities*. S. Karger, 1982.

Paxinos G, Törk I, Halliday G, Mehler WR. Human homologs to brainstem nuclei identified in other animals as revealed by acetylcholinesterase activity. In: Paxinos G, ed. *The Human Central Nervous System*. San Diego, CA: Academic Press, 1990:149-202.

Price JL. Olfactory system. In: Paxinos G, ed. *The Human Central Nervous System*. Academic Press, 1990:979-998.

Riley HA. *An Atlas of the Basal Ganglia, Brain Stem and Spinal Cord*. Baltimore, MD: The Williams and Wilkins Company, 1943.

Schaltenbrand G, Wahren W. *Atlas for Stereotaxy of the Human Brain*. Stuttgart, Germany: Georg Thieme, 1977.

Williams PL, Warwick R. *Functional Neuroanatomy of Man*. Philadelphia, PA: W. B. Saunders, 1975.

Answers to Clinical Cases

Chapter 1

1. Ventricular enlargement is a consequence of loss of neural tissue. Because the volume of the skull is fixed, as brain tissues decrease in volume due to a neurodegenerative process, there is a corresponding increase in ventricular volume.

2. The cerebral cortex and hippocampal formation are severely affected. By contrast, brain stem structures are not.

Chapter 2

1. Both the dorsal column-medial lemniscal pathway and the corticospinal tract decussate within the ventral portion of the medulla. Without these decussations, the two sides of the ventral medulla become somewhat separated. CSF is present where the decussating axons should be. Axons important for coordinating eye movements normally decussate in the dorsal pons. Without this decussation, the two sides of the dorsal pons also become somewhat separate, as revealed by the presence of CSF and the formation of a shallow sulcus.

2. No, the corpus callosum is an example of a structure with intact decussating axons.

Chapter 3

1. The proximal portion of the middle cerebral artery became occluded. This affected both deep branches to subcortical white matter and superficial branches supplying the cerebral cortex.

2. Since all descending motor control axons converge within the internal capsule, damage to this structure alone can produce the major limb and facial motor signs seen in this patient.

Chapter 4

1. Mechanoreceptive axons ascend within the dorsal columns, including those for touch, vibration sense, and limb proprioception. It is unclear why the patient's touch sense was spared.

2. The ability to maintain an upright posture depends, in part, on lower limb proprioception. Without limb proprioception, vision can partially substitute. Therefore, when this patient closes his eyes, he is deprived of this compensating modality and, in consequence, he looses his balance.

Chapter 5

1. Anterolateral system axons decussate just ventral to the central canal, where the syrinx originates. This is why they are damaged first. Mechanoreceptive axons are located farther dorsally, affording them some protection initially.

2. Limb motor neurons are located ventrolateral to the syrinx. As with the dorsal mechanoreceptive axons, motor neurons are initially afforded protection by their distance from the initial site of syrinx development. Eventually the syrinx expands to affect a significant portion of the ventral horn.

Chapter 6

1. The posterior inferior cerebellar artery, or PICA, supplies the dorsolateral medulla. This was infarcted in the patient. The territory supplied by PICA receives little or no collateral circulation from other arteries, which makes this region of the medulla particularly vulnerable to ischemia. Whereas only a wedge-shaped infarcted region is revealed on the MRI, it is likely that the entire territory is affected because of the paucity of collateral circulation.

2. PICA occlusion destroys the spinal trigeminal tract and nucleus at this level and caudal. These structures carry information about trigeminal protective senses on the ipsilateral side. By contrast, PICA occlusion damages the ascending anterolateral system fibers, which carry information from the contralateral limbs and trunk.

Chapter 7

1. See Figure 7–17C.

2. The infarction involved more than only the primary visual cortex on the medial occipital lobe surface. The optic radiations were also damaged.

3. The posterior parietal lobe, necessary for attending to stimuli, and the lateral occipital cortex, important for visual spatial function, were not affected by occlusion of the posterior cerebral artery.

Chapter 8

1. Unilateral hearing loss occurs because the acoustic neuroma impedes conduction of signals from auditory structures to the brain stem. Impairment in pons and cerebellar function, due to compression by the neuroma, likely explains the gait instability. Impairment in conduction of facial muscle control signals by the seventh (facial) nerve, because of compression by the neuroma, leads to mild flattening of the left nasolabial fold.

2. There is no impairment of the middle ear ossicles with an acoustic neuroma, hence preservation of air conduction.

Chapter 9

1. Taste buds in different locations on each side of the tongue are innervated by different peripheral nerves. Damage to multiple nerves, with very different peripheral locations, must occur for complete taste loss on one side of the tongue. By contrast, a single central lesion can disrupt taste information transmission to the thalamus and cortex.

2. The taste pathway, unlike other sensory pathways, is ipsilateral.

3. The central tegmental tract transmits taste information to the thalamus. A nearby structure, the parabrachial nucleus, is also involved in visceral and chemical sensations. The function of this nucleus also could be affected.

Chapter 10

1. Because the ascending pain pathway, the anterolateral system, decussates caudal to the lesion, the affected axons originated from the contralateral side. The ascending tactile pathway, the dorsal column, is an ipsilateral spinal path; it decussates in the medulla. The affected axons are on the same side as the lesion.

2. The anterolateral system decussates as it ascends. Neurons contributing to this pathway at the level of the lesion do not reach the affected side until 1-2 segments rostrally. Therefore, they bypass the injury.

3. The key motor pathway damaged by the lesion, the corticospinal tract, decussates rostral to the lesion, in the medulla. The damaged axons control muscles on the side of the spinal injury. This same side is also affected by damaged to the dorsal columns.

Chapter 11

1. Based on changes in signal on the MRIs, the location of the infarction is in the ventral pons, close to the midline. This is within the territory of paramedian and short circumferential branches of the basilar artery (see Figure 3–3B2).

2. Lower facial muscle control is mediated by a contralateral corticobulbar projection, as is limb muscle control. Therefore, after unilateral lesion of the corticobulbar and corticospinal tracts, there is loss of control of these muscles. By contrast, upper facial muscles and trunk muscles receive more bilateral control, so that after unilateral lesion, there is some residual, redundant, control.

3. After damage to the corticospinal tract, there are plastic changes that result in increased contralateral deep tendon reflexes. This results in abnormal limb posture, increased muscle tone, and difficulty in controlling the weakened limb. Usually these changes present weeks after the injury, but in this patient they occurred immediately after the injury. Further, these changes are most common after damage to the corticospinal tract during development, such as in cerebral palsy, and after spinal cord injury, and less frequent after adult stroke.

Chapter 12

1. This is due to a lesion of the left abducens nucleus. Abducens motor neurons are lesioned, which prevents left eye abduction. Further, there may be a slight adduction because of the unopposed action of the medial rectus muscle (Figure 12–1A, top). The right eye fails to adduct because internuclear neurons connecting the left abducens nucleus with the right oculomotor nucleus are lesioned.

2. This is due to a lesion of the MLF on the left side. This interrupts the signal to activates the right medial rectus muscle; hence, the right eye does not adduct.

Chapter 13

1. Romberg sign (see Chapter 4) is the inability of a person to stand upright when his or her eyes closed. There is swaying and a lost balance. It is due to loss of lower extremity proprioceptive. In Friedreich ataxia there is a loss of lower extremity proprioceptive because of degeneration of large-diameter mechanoreceptive afferents.

2. This is a classical posture use by patients with cerebellar disease. It is likely a strategy to provide better stability in maintaining an upright posture, in the face of impaired limb proprioception and motor control.

Chapter 14

1. The action of the basal ganglia on each side is to influence control on contralateral musculature. Basal ganglia output is directed to ipsilateral thalamus and motor cortex, which, in turn, controls contralateral muscles. Brain stem output would also be expected to primarily affect contralateral limb control, likely by contralateral reticulospinal projections.

2. Lenticulostriate branches of the middle cerebral artery supply the subthalamic nucleus.

Chapter 15

1. A branch of the posterior inferior cerebral artery (PICA) was affected. Since the total territory of PICA was not infarcted, the occlusion was most likely that of a more distal branch.
2. (1) loss of ipsilateral facial pain: spinal trigeminal tract and nucleus; (2) contralateral pain loss: anterolateral system; and (3) ataxia: climbing fibers from the olive, dorsal spinocerebellar tract, cuneocerebellar tract, and other fibers of the inferior cerebellar peduncle; (4) hoarse voice: nucleus ambiguus and consequent paralysis of ipsilateral laryngeal muscles; (5) ipsilateral ptosis: descending hypothalamic fibers that regulate the sympathetic nervous system control of the tarsal muscle.

Chapter 16

1. The temporal lobe serves diverse functions. The superior temporal gyrus is key to audition and language. The middle and inferior temporal gyri are important for visual perception. The temporal pole and medial temporal lobe contain limbic association cortex. The temporal pole, corresponding to Brodmann's area 38, is important in personality. This is the part damaged in the patient. This area has extensive interconnections with other limbic system cortical regions as well as the amygdala.

Answers to Study Questions

Chapter 1

1. A

Comment: The dendrite is the input side of a neuron, where postsynaptic neurotransmitter receptors are located; the cell body integrates synaptic information and provides support; the axon initiates and conducts action potentials; the axon terminal is the presynaptic site, where neurotransmitter is released at the synapse

3. D

Comment: Whereas a nucleus contains mostly cell bodies, incoming axons to the nucleus synapse on the dendrites of neurons in the nucleus. Neurons in the nucleus give rise to axons that project from the nucleus. Axons make synaptic connections within the nucleus.

8. C

Comment: The autonomic nervous innervates smooth muscle of blood vessels within muscle but not somatic striated muscle cells, which are innervated by somatic motor neurons.

2. C	4. B	5. B	6. B
7. A	9. C	10. A	11. C
12. A	13. C	14. C	15. B

Chapter 2

1. B

Comment: Because most pathways decussate in the brain; left body, right brain. Peripheral nerve damage on the left side could produce somatic sensory and motor disturbances, but it is unlikely that this damage would be so extensive, to affect the entire left side. If he had a systemic disease that affected nerve function, it would be likely that there would be some bilateral impairment or not symmetrical sensory and motor involvement.

2. D

Comment: Whereas the injury could have damaged astrocytes and the central canal of the ventricular system, this would not necessarily produce paralysis. The injury would certainly have extensively damaged axons within the lateral white matter. This would cause a loss of connections between the brain and the spinal cord.

10. B

Comment: Parietal cortex is on the surface; the insular cortex is beneath the surface cortex. Choice A is not correct because it places the anterior limb of the internal capsule lateral to the thalamus; it should be the posterior limb.

3. A	4. C	5. B	6. D
7. A	8. B	9. A	

Chapter 3

9. B

Comment: The anterior cerebral artery has a C-shape. It is located on the medial surface of the cerebral hemispheres. Thus, a view from the side of the brain is best to reveal its shape.

12. C

Comment: The foramina of Luschka and Magendie are located in the 4th ventricle. CSF exits here and then passes into the subarachnoid space. From the subarachnoid space, CSF flows into the dural sinuses through arachnoid granulations, which are small unidirectional valves.

1. B	2. A	3. A	4. D
5. C	6. D	7. A	8. B
10. A	11. C	13. C	14. A
15. D			

Chapter 4

3. B

Comment: At the level of the caudal medulla, where there is little or no inferior olivary nucleus, the anterior spinal artery supplies blood to the medial lemniscus.

6. A

Comment: Note that primary muscle spindle receptors synapse on motor neurons in the ventral horn

10. A

Comment: Response D has the correct somatotopy to explain the seizure progression, like the correct response (A). However, this seizure progression is classically within the postcentral gyrus. It progresses because of local connections within the cortex. Connectivity within the thalamus does not support this kind progression.

1. A	2. D	4. B	5. D
7. D	8. C	9. B	

Chapter 5

1. B
Comment: Second-order pain fibers ascend as they decussate. As a consequence, right-side lesion at T10 (umbilical level), which is what the patient suffered, will spare pain sensation up to a few sensations caudally on the left side.

2. D	3. A	4. B
5. B	6. A	7. B
8. D	9. A	10. A

Chapter 6

7. A
Comment: PICA supplies the portion of the trigeminal complex within the mid-medulla. This includes the upper part of the caudal nucleus and the interpolar nucleus. Occlusion of PICA will damage descending trigeminal afferents in the spinal trigeminal tract.

8. B
Comment: This is a classical sign; dissociation of the laterality of facial and limb pain. PICA occlusion spares facial and limb touch. It can produce taste loss—although this is not commonly tested—but this is on the ipsilateral side.

9. A
Comment: Mechanosensory information from the mucous membranes is processed in the solitary, not trigeminal, nuclei.

1. B	2. A	3. C	4. D
5. C	6. A	10. A	

Chapter 7

1. C	2. A	3. A

Comment: The visual field of each eye normally extends beyond the midline, so that there is a central region of binocular overlap when the visual fields of each are are considered together. The monocular crescents of each eye are independent; they do not overlap with the other. That is why they are called monocular.

4. C	5. A	6. C	7. B
8. A	9. C	10. D	11. C
12. D	13. A		

Chapter 8

1. A
Comment: Unilateral damage to the auditory pathway after the first synapse in central nervous system does not lead to unilateral deafness because of the extensive crossing of information. The only sites where a lesion can produce deafness in one ear are the peripheral auditory apparatus, eighth nerve, or cochlear nuclei.

2. B
Comment: Whereas the lateral superior olivary nucleus is important for localizing high-frequency sounds, this does not imply that it is where high-frequency sounds are selectively processed for perception. Indeed, there is a parallel path for all frequencies through the dorsal cochlear nucleus, which does not synapse in the lateral superior olivary nucleus. By contrast, when hair cells of the base of the cochlea have degenerated all transductive machinery for high-frequency sounds is lost.

3. D
Comment: The superior olivary nucleus contributes a small number of axons to the trapezoid body. But by far, most axons come from the anteroventral cochlear nucleus.

4. B
Comment: Neurons of the nucleus of the trapezoid body synapse with the lateral, not medial, superior olivary nucleus. This is part of the mechanism for localizing high-frequency sounds. The medial superior olivary nucleus is part of the circuitry for localizing low-frequency sounds.

5. D
Comment: Whereas afferent and efferent are often used interchangeably for sensory and motor, this is not true. Afferent means to bring information—whether sensory or motor in function—to a structure, whereas efferent means to bring information away from that structure.

6. A	7. A	8. D
9. A	10. C	

Chapter 9

1. C
Comment: The ascending gustatory pathway is ipsilateral.

2. A
Comment: The XIIth nerve innervates tongue muscles.

3. D

4. B
Comment: The thalamic gustatory nucleus is the parvocellular division of the ventral posterior medial nucleus. Whereas the medial dorsal nucleus transmits taste information to the orbitofrontal cortex for integrating tastes and smells, it does not receive direct input from the ascending taste pathway.

5. D

6. B
Comment: The axons of primary olfactory neurons regenerate; they are thought to be the only example of maintained capacity for axon regeneration in the adult mammalian brain. These axons are vulnerable to being transected (termed axotomy) by shearing forces during head trauma.

7. C

8. A
Comment: Each olfactory receptor gene is expressed in one, or at best only a few, glomeruli.

9. D

10. C
Comment: The orbitofrontal cortex receives olfactory information from the piriform cortex, either directly or relayed via the medial dorsal nucleus of the thalamus.

Chapter 10

1. D
Comment: The patient has a highly selective lesion because the impairment is restricted to the left arm. White matter lesions in the brain stem and spinal cord are unlikely to produce a single limb motor impairment because axons from all body parts intermingle within very small regions. Among the choices, only the precentral gyrus has a clear somatotopic organization. Moreover, occlusion of a small cortical branch of the middle cerebral artery could selectively damage the arm area of primary motor cortex, in the precentral gyrus.

2. A
Comment: Both the medial and lateral motor cortex represent limb muscles. The territories supplied by the middle cerebral and basilar arteries also contain pathways or nuclei for both limb and trunk control.

3. C
4. B
5. A
Comment: The rubrospinal tract is a lateral path and thus descends laterally in the spinal cord. As with other motor pathways, it synapses both on interneurons and motor neurons.

6. D
7. A
Comment: In the motor cortex, the foot representation is supplied by the anterior cerebral artery.

8. B
9. C
10. B

Chapter 11

1. C
Comment: Unlike the spinal cord, where the motor nuclei are located ventral to sensory nuclei, it is different in the caudal brain stem. This is because as the fourth ventricle develops, it displaces the sensory nuclei laterally. In the midbrain, the only cranial nerve sensory nucleus, the mesencephalic trigeminal nucleus, is located dorsal to the oculomotor nucleus, a dorsoventral organization like the spinal cord. Here in the midbrain, development of the narrow cerebral aqueduct does not displace the sensory nuclei.

2. A	3. D	4. B	5. D
6. B	7. A		

Comment: Facial motor neurons migrate from the ventricular surface ventrally, and possibly caudally, during development. This results in the unusual trajectory of facial motor axons as they leave the facial motor nucleus (Figure 11–9). Failure to migrate (in this fictitious condition) would result in retaining a position close to the ventricular floor, thus dorsal to the normal location. Ventral is not expected; this would mean farther migration. Caudal is not expected; this would

also mean more migration. Finally, lateral would mean misdirected migration.

8. B
Comment: Nucleus ambiguus has a rostrocaudal organization; motor neurons rostrally innervate pharyngeal muscles and caudally, laryngeal muscles. The tongue is innervated by motor neurons in the hypoglossal nucleus. Blood pressure regulation is more the function of the solitary nucleus and dorsal motor nucleus of the vagus.

9. C
10. A
Comment: Loss of pain on the contralateral limbs and trunk is because PICA supplies the ascending axons of the anterolateral system. Loss of ipsilateral facial pain is due to the damage to the trigeminal spinal tract, as well as the nucleus. There is no loss of facial touch. This is mediated by the main trigeminal sensory nucleus, which is located in the pons.

Chapter 12

1. B
Comment: The posterior spinal artery supplies the dorsolateral medulla, but caudal to the vestibular nuclei. The anterior inferior cerebellar artery supplies more rostral portions of the vestibular complex.

2. A
3. B
Comment: Despite its name, the lateral vestibulospinal tract is a medial pathway.

4. D
5. D
Comment: Eye position after third nerve lesion is considered "down and out."

6. A
Comment: The contribution of the superior oblique muscle, which is innerved by the trochlear nucleus, to downward gaze is greater when looking at the nose, hence greater vertical diplopia. Intortion—the other mechanical action of the superior oblique muscle—is weakened, hence double vision when you tilt your head sideways, termed tortional diplopia. This is often compensated by tilting the head in the other direction. Finally, horizontal diplopia is produced by a palsy involving control of the lateral or medial rectus muscles.

7. C
Comment: The vertical gaze center is the interstitial nucleus of the MLF; the paramedial pontine reticular formation is the horizontal gaze center and acts on the abducens nucleus.

8. C
9. A
10. D

Comment: The left abducens nucleus is spared, or else the left eye would not be abducted. The left medial rectus muscle is not paralyzed because vergence is normal.

Chapter 13

1. D

Comment: The tentorium separates the cerebellum from the overlying occipital and temporal lobes. Because of this, the tumor does not contact either lobe.

2. A
3. D
4. B

Comment: Limb motor signs are classically ipsilateral to cerebellar lesions. This is because the circuit is double crossed—once as the output of the cerebellum, and the second as the decussation of the motor pathway. The principal input paths to the cerebellum, the dorsal and cuneocerebellar tracts, are ipsilateral.

5. A

Comment: Routing information through the pontine nuclei adds one additional decussation to the cerebellar control circuit. Since the double crossing of the cerebellar output results in ipsilateral control, we see that the cortico-pontocerebellar circuit restores the typical decussated control by the cortex.

6. D
7. B
8. C

Comment: This condition would primarily produce loss of climbing fibers from the inferior olivary nucleus and mossy fibers from the pontine nuclei. Climbing fibers synapse on Purkinje cells, not granule cells. Mossy fibers synapse on granule cells, not Purkinje or basket cells.

9. B

Comment: The red nucleus is the recipient of cerebellar output; it provides no direct input to the cerebellum.

10. C

Comment: Virtually all cortical regions—motor, premotor, and association areas—project to the pontine nuclei, which provide mossy fiber inputs to the cerebellar cortex (more the cortex than the dentate nucleus). This provides both a route for cortical areas important in cognition and emotion to influence movement, via the cerebellum, as well as contributing to the nonmotor functions of the cerebellum.

Chapter 14

1. Dots correspond, from left (lateral) to right (medial): Insular cortex (sensory representations of pain, visceral sensations, and taste), claustrum (connects with cerebral cortex; may play role in consciousness), putamen (motor functions), external segment of the globus pallidus (part of indirect path; receives striatal input and projects to subthalamic nucleus), internal segment of the globus pallidus (direct path; basal ganglia

output to thalamus and brain stem), posterior limb of the internal capsule (ascending thalamocortical axons; descending cortical projections), thalamus (relay subcortical inputs to cortex), thalamic adhesion in the third ventricle (point of contact of two halves of thalamus).

2. D
3. B
4. A

Comment: In Parkinson's disease, the loss of dopamine results in less drive to the direct path, and bradykinesia results.

5. C

Comment: The lenticular fasciculus contains axons from the internal segment of the globus pallidus, not the substantial nigra pars reticulata.

6. B
7. C
8. A

Comment: Huntington's disease is an autosomal dominant disorder. The father has signs of advanced Huntington's disease, not the other three listed. The son may be showing early signs of Huntington's disease. These are hyperkinetic motor signs.

9. B
10. A

Chapter 15

1. D

Comment: The pituitary gland is located in the sella turcica. The optic chiasm is located directly above the sella turcica. As the tumor enlarges, because it is located with the bony sella, it can only expand dorsally, thereby impinging on the optic chiasm.

2. A
3. B

Comment: The descending autonomic pathway from the hypothalamus courses through the median forebrain bundle, en route to the brain stem.

4. C
5. C
6. A

Comment: The man likely has narcolepsy. The loss of muscle tone accompanying sleep is cataplexy, which is often associated with narcolepsy. Orexin-containing neurons in the lateral hypothalamus have been found to be diminished in number in the brains of people with narcolepsy.

7. C

Comment: The tuberoinfundibular nucleus releases histamine, as its neurotransmitter, throughout the forebrain. Histamine activates the target neurons. Antihistamines that cross the blood-brain barrier can block this action of histamine, and make the person drowsy.

8. A

9. D

10. B

Comment: These are signs of loss of sympathetic control of cranial structures on the left side. They can be produced by damage to the left: hypothalamus, descending hypothalamic projection, spinal cord, superior cervical ganglion, or sympathetic fibers in the neck. Localization of the lesion is determined by other signs. For example, if there is also ataxia, the lesion is likely in the dorsolateral medulla, or if there is limb paralysis, it is in the spinal cord.

Chapter 16

1. D

Comment: Cerebral degenerative disorders generally result in loss of neurons without concomitant replacement with more glia, or glial scaring. As a consequence, the affected brain regions shrink in size. Because the cranial cavity is of a fixed volume, this is accompanied by an increase in the nearby ventricle/aqueduct. Recall in Chapters 1 and 14, we viewed MRIs of patients with Alzheimer disease and Huntington's disease, where neural degeneration was associated with clear increases in the volume of the lateral ventricles.

2. C

Comment: The posterior insular cortex is the primary cortical area for aspects of pain and visceral sensation.

3. A

Comment: Face identification is more a function of the caudal-medial temporal lobe. Stimulation localization is mediated by the posterior parietal lobe. Emotional content in speech is a function of the right frontal lobe, opposite to where Broca's area is on the left.

4. D

Comment: The parahippocampal gyrus is formally not part of the hippocampal formation. It does receive input from many different association areas of the cortex.

5. A	6. B	7. D
8. D	9. C	10. B

Glossary

abducens (VI) nerve: cranial nerve; axons innervate the lateral rectus muscle

abducens nucleus: contains lateral rectus motor neurons and internuclear neurons; located in pons

accessory cuneate nucleus: relays somatic sensory information from upper trunk, arm, and neck to the cerebellum; located in medulla

accessory (XI) nerve: cranial nerve that innervates the sternocleidomastoid muscle and the upper part of the trapezius muscle

accessory optic system: transmits visual information to brain stem nuclei for eye movement control

accommodation-convergence reaction: a complex response that prepares the eyes for near vision by (1) increasing lens curvature, (2) constricting the pupils, and (3) coordinating convergence of the eyes

accommodation reflex: increase in lens curvature that occurs during near vision

acetylcholine: neurotransmitter used by motor neurons and neurons in several nuclei, including the basal nucleus and the pedunculopontine nucleus

acetylcholinesterase: enzyme that inactivates acetylcholine

acousticomotor function: motor behavioral response triggered or controlled by sound such as orienting towards a sound

adrenergic: neuron that uses adrenalin as a neurotransmitter or neuromodulator

afferent: axons that transmit information toward a particular structure; *afferent* is not synonymous with *sensory*, which means related to processing information from a receptor sheet (eg, body surface or retina)

airway protective reflex: closure of the larynx to prevent fluid and food from entering the trachea

akinesia: impairment in initiating voluntary movement

alar plate: dorsal portion of the neuroepithelium that gives rise to sensory nuclei of the spinal cord and brain stem

allocortex: cortex having a variable number of layers, but always fewer than six

alveus: thin sheet of myelinated axons covering hippocampal formation; axons of pyramidal neurons in the hippocampus and subiculum

Alzheimer disease: presenile dementia

amacrine cells: retinal interneuron

amygdala: telencephalic structure that plays an essential role in emotions and their behavioral expression; has three component nuclear divisions: basolateral, central, and corticomedial

amygdaloid nuclear complex: another name for the amygdala

anastomosis: a network of interconnected arteries

aneurysm: an abnormal ballooning of a part of an artery due to weakening of the arterial wall

angiogram: radiological image of vasculature

anosmia: absence of the sense of smell

ansa lenticularis: output pathway of the internal segment of the globus pallidus; axons terminate in the thalamus

anterior: toward the abdomen; synonymous with *ventral*

anterior cerebral artery: supplies blood to the medial frontal lobes and underlying deep structures

anterior choroidal artery: supplies blood to the choroid plexus in the lateral ventricle and several deep structures

anterior cingulate gyrus: portion of the cingulate important for emotions; activated while experiencing painful stimuli; a major target of the limbic loop of the basal ganglia

anterior circulation: arterial supply provided by the internal carotid artery

anterior commissure: tract that interconnects the anterior temporal lobes and olfactory structures on the two sides of the brain

anterior communicating artery: interconnects anterior cerebral arteries on the two sides of the brain; part of the circle of Willis

anterior inferior cerebellar artery (AICA): supplies the caudal pons and parts of the cerebellum

anterior limb of the internal capsule: subcortical tract between the anterior portions of the caudate nucleus and putamen; rostral to the thalamus

anterior lobe of the pituitary gland: contains epithelial cells that release hormones for controlling a variety of target glands in the periphery

anterior nuclei of the thalamus: receive input from the mammillary bodies and project to the cingulate gyrus

anterior nucleus of the thalamus: receives input from the mammillothalamic tract and projects to the cingulate cortex

anterior olfactory nucleus: relays information from the olfactory nucleus to other parts of the central nervous system

anterior perforated substance: basal forebrain region where branches of the anterior and middle cerebral arteries (lenticulostriate) penetrate and supply deep structures

anterior spinal arteries: branches of the vertebral artery that supply the ventral half of the spinal cord; courses within the ventral sulcus of the spinal cord; also receives arterial blood from radicular arteries

anterior temporal lobes: involved in emotions, especially during anxiety states

anterior thalamic nuclei: participate in aspects of learning and memory; principal target of the mammillary bodies

anterograde: away from a neuron's cell body and toward the axon terminal; typically related to the pattern of degeneration (*see* Wallerian degeneration) or axonal transport

anterograde amnesia: failure to remember new events

anterolateral system: spinal pathways for pain, temperature, and itch; includes spinothalamic, spinomesencephalic (spinotectal), and spinoreticular tracts

anteroventral cochlear nucleus: portion of the cochlear nucleus important for sound localization in the horizontal plane; located in the rostral medulla

antidiuretic hormone: released by the posterior lobe of the pituitary; acts on the kidney to concentrate urine

aphasia: impairment in language; characterized by reduced ability of a person to read, write, or speak their intentions

apraxia: inability to perform a movement when asked, even though the person has the physical ability to contract the muscles, is willing to perform the movement, and has already learned to make the movement

aortic arch: site of arterial blood pressure sensor

arachnoid granulations: unidirectional valves for cerebrospinal fluid to flow from the subarachnoid space to the circulatory system

arachnoid mater: middle meningeal layer

arachnoid villi: *see* arachnoid granulations

arbor vitae: appearance of cerebellar white matter on sagittal section

archicortex: primitive three-layered cortex; primarily in hippocampal formation

arcuate nucleus: hypothalamic nucleus important for control of neuroendocrine function and feeding

area 3a: Brodmann's cytoarchitectonic area; part of the primary somatic sensory cortex that receives information from muscle receptors; involved in balance sense

area postrema: portion of caudal medulla where there is no blood-brain barrier; important for sensing blood-borne toxins and in control of vomiting

Argyll Robertson pupils: pupil sign characterized by a small diameter and unreactive to light but which gets smaller to accommodation; associated with neurosyphilis

ascending pathway: pathway transmitting information from lower levels of the central nervous system to higher levels; typically used to describe somatic sensory pathways of the spinal cord and brain stem

association cortex: areas of cortex that serve diverse mental processes but that are not engaged in basic stimulus processing or control of muscle contractions; formally those areas that associate sensory events with motor responses and perform mental processes that intervene between sensory inputs and motor outputs

associative loop (of basal ganglia): the basal ganglia circuit that receives input primarily from association cortex of the frontal, parietal, and temporal lobes and projects to prefrontal and premotor cortical areas

astrocytes: class of glial cell that serve diverse support functions, including axonal guidance during development and helping to maintain the blood-brain barrier

ataxia: uncoordinated and highly inaccurate movements; typically associated with cerebellar damage

athetosis: slow, writhing involuntary movements

autism spectrum disorder: a condition presenting with deficits in social interactions, impaired verbal and nonverbal communication, and expression of stereotyped patterns of behavior

autonomic motor column: formation of sympathetic and parasympathetic preganglionic neurons into rostrocaudal columns in the spinal cord and brain stem

autonomic nervous system: part of peripheral nervous system engaged in the control of body organs; consists of separate sympathetic and parasympathetic divisions

axial muscles: muscles located close to the body midline; control neck and back

axon: portion of neuron specialized for conducting information encoded in the form of action potentials

axon terminal: presynaptic component of the synapse; where neurotransmitters are released

β-endorphin: an endogenous opiate cleaved from the large peptide proopiomelanocortin; plays a role in opiate analgesia

Babinski's sign: extension (also termed dorsiflexion) of the big toe in response to scratching the lateral margin and then the ball of the foot (but not the toes); associated with lesions of the corticospinal system in adults; present normally in children until about two years of age

ballistic movement: movement with high initial velocity

bare nerve endings: sensitive to noxious and thermal stimuli as well as itch-producing agents

baroreceptor: blood pressure receptor

basal cells: cells that differentiate to become taste receptor cells; thought to be stem cells

basal forebrain: portion of the ventral telencephalon caudal to the frontal lobes; contains the basal nucleus (of Meynert) and structures for emotions and olfaction

basal ganglia: telencephalic nuclei with strong interconnections with the cerebral cortex; serve diverse motor, cognitive, and emotional functions

basal hair cells: auditory hair cells located near the cochlear base

basal nucleus (of Meynert): contains neurons that use acetylcholine as their neurotransmitter and project widely throughout the cerebral cortex; neurons are among the first to degenerate in Alzheimer disease

basal plate: portion of the ventral neuroepithelium that gives rise to motor nuclei of the spinal cord and brain stem

base (midbrain): the most ventral portion of the midbrain; also termed basis pedunculi

base of the pons: ventral portion of the pons; contains primarily pontine nuclei and descending cortical axons

basilar artery: supplies pons and parts of the cerebellum and midbrain

basilar membrane: component of the organ of Corti that oscillates in response to sounds; mechanical displacement of the membrane stimulates auditory hair cells

basis pedunculi: ventral portion of the midbrain; contains descending cortical axons

basket neurons: inhibitory interneurons of the cerebellar cortex; make dense and strong synaptic connections on cell body of Purkinje neuron

basolateral nuclei (of the amygdala): division of amygdala that receives information from sensory systems and cortical association areas

bed nucleus of the stria terminalis: C-shaped component of the amygdala; related in function to the central nucleus

benign positional vertigo: most common form of vertigo, or the sudden sensation of spinning; can be evoked for testing purposes by placement of the head in a particular position and then quickly lying down backwards over a table

bilateral control: form of somatic or visceromotor control in which a cranial nerve or spinal motor nucleus receives projections from both sides of the cortex; typically provides a measure of redundancy, so that if one projection becomes damaged, the other projection can provide basic control

bilateral projection: one structure sends axons to both sides of the central nervous system

bilateral temporal visual field defect: *see* bitemporal heteronymous hemianopia

bipolar morphology: neuron shape characterized by a pair of axon-like processes emerging from opposite sides of a neuron's cell body; bipolar neuron

bipolar neurons: one of three major morphological types of neuron; characterized by a pair of axon-like processes emerging from opposite sides of the neuron's cell body; most commonly sensory relay neurons

bitemporal heteronymous hemianopia: loss of peripheral vision; common with lesions involving the optic chiasm

blind spot: blind portion of visual field; corresponds on the retina to the exit point of the optic nerve, where there are no photoreceptors

blobs: location of color-sensitive neurons in primary visual cortex; primarily in layers II and III

blood-brain barrier: cellular specializations that prevent blood-borne materials from gaining access to the central nervous system

blood-cerebrospinal fluid barrier: specializations that prevent blood-borne materials from gaining access to the cerebrospinal fluid

border zone infarct: loss of arterial supply at the peripheral borders of the territories supplied by major cerebral vessels

border zones: peripheral borders of the territories supplied by major cerebral vessels

brachium of inferior colliculus: output pathway from the inferior colliculus to the medial geniculate nucleus

brachium of superior colliculus: input pathway to the superior colliculus from the retina

bradykinesia: movement disorder in which movements are slowed or absent

brain: cerebral hemispheres, diencephalon, cerebellum and brain stem

brain stem: medulla, pons, and midbrain

branchial arches: also known as gill arches; territory of developing head and neck; many cranial nerves develop in association with the branchial arches

branchiomeric: derived from the branchial arches

branchiomeric motor column: motor neurons that innervate muscles that develop from the branchial arches

branchiomeric skeletal motor fibers: *see* branchiomeric motor column

Broca's area: portion of the inferior frontal lobe important for articulation of speech

Brodmann's areas: divisions of the cerebral cortex based on the size and shapes of neurons in the different laminae and their packing densities; named after Korbinian Brodmann, a German neuroanatomist who worked during the late 19th and early 20th centuries

Brown-Séquard syndrome: set of signs associated with spinal cord hemisection; include ipsilateral loss of motor functions, ipsilateral loss of mechanical sensations, and contralateral loss of pain, temperature, and itch; all caudal to the lesion

bulb: archaic term for medulla and pons; commonly used to describe a cortical projection system (*see* corticobulbar tract)

C-shaped: description of the shape of many telencephalic structures

calcarine fissure: located in the primary visual cortex; occipital lobe

callosal connections: connections made by callosal neurons

callosal neurons: class of cortical projection neuron

capillary endothelium: inner layer of a capillary in brain and spinal cord contributes to the blood brain barrier

carotid circulation: *see* anterior circulation

carotid sinus: blood-pressure-sensing organ

carotid siphon: segment of the internal carotid artery

cataplexy: transient loss of muscle tone without loss of consciousness

cauda equina: spinal nerves within the vertebral canal caudal to the last spinal segment

caudal: toward the tail or coccyx

caudal nucleus (of the spinal trigeminal nucleus): important for facial pain, temperature sense, and itch; located in the caudal medulla; rostral extension of the dorsal horn

caudal solitary nucleus: important for viscerosensory function; located in the caudal medulla

caudate nucleus: input nucleus of the basal ganglia; comprised of the head, body and tail

cell body: where the nucleus is located and from which the axon and dendrites emerge

cell bridges: *see* striatal cell bridges

cell stains: method of revealing neuronal cell bodies; an example is the Nissl stain

central canal: portion of the ventricular system located in the spinal cord and caudal medulla

central nervous system: division of the nervous system located within the skull and vertebral column

central nucleus (of the amygdala): nuclear division of the amygdala important for the visceral expression of emotions, such as changes in blood pressure and gastrointestinal function during anxiety

central sulcus: separates frontal and parietal lobes

central tegmental tract: contains the ascending gustatory projection from the solitary nucleus to the thalamus and descending axons from the parvocellular red nucleus to the inferior olivary nucleus

centromedian nucleus: thalamic diffuse-projecting nucleus with widespread projections to the frontal lobe and striatum

cephalic flexure: bend in neuraxis at the level of the midbrain

cerebellar glomerulus: basic processing unit of the cerebellum; comprises one mossy fiber axon terminal (presynaptic), and many granule cell dendrites and several Golgi axons (postsynaptic)

cerebellar tentorium: rigid dural flap dorsal to the cerebellum; separates the cerebellum from the cerebral cortex and defines the posterior fossa

cerebellopontine angle: where the cerebellum joins the brain stem

cerebellothalamic tract: output pathway from the deep cerebellar nuclei to the thalamus

cerebellum: portion of the hindbrain; important for automatic control of movements and thought to play a role in automating many complex sensory and cognitive functions

cerebral angiography: radiological technique for imaging brain vasculature

cerebral aqueduct (of Sylvius): portion of the ventricular system in the midbrain

cerebral cortex: portion of the telencephalon; important for diverse sensory, motor, cognitive, emotional, and integrative functions

cerebral hemispheres: major brain division

cerebral peduncle: ventral portion of midbrain, formally corresponds to the tegmentum and base

cerebral segment (of internal carotid artery): immediately proximal to the bifurcation into the middle and anterior cerebral arteries

cerebrocerebellum: comprises the lateral cerebellar cortex and dentate nucleus; important for motor planning

cerebrospinal fluid: watery fluid contained within the ventricular system and subarachnoid space

cervical: spinal cord segment; there are eight in total

cervical flexure: bend in the developing nervous system; located in the midbrain; persists into maturity

cervical segment (of internal carotid artery): the most proximal portion of the internal carotid; from the carotid bifurcation to the point of entrance to the carotid canal of the skull

cholinergic: a neuron that uses acetylcholine as its neurotransmitter

chorda tympani nerve: a branch of cranial nerve VII; carries taste afferents

chorea: disordered movement characterized by involuntary rapid and random movements of the limbs and trunk

choroid epithelium: cells of the choroid plexus specialized to secrete cerebrospinal fluid

choroid plexus: intraventricular organ that contains cells that secrete cerebrospinal fluid

ciliary ganglion: peripheral ganglion containing parasympathetic postganglionic neurons

ciliary muscle: intraocular muscle that increases lens curvature

cingulate cortex: comprises anterior, middle and posterior divisions; diverse behavioral functions, including role in emotional valance and movement control

cingulate gyrus: C-shaped gyrus on medial brain surface spanning the frontal and parietal lobes; surrounds the corpus callosum

cingulate motor areas: premotor cortical area located in the cingulate gyrus

cingulum: C-shaped tract located within the white matter of the cortex beneath the cingulate gyrus

circle of Willis: anastomotic network of arteries on the ventral surface of the diencephalon

circumventricular organs: a set of eight structures lying near the ventricular surface that do not have a blood-brain barrier

cisterna magna: the portion of the subarachnoid space, dorsal to the medulla and caudal to the cerebellum, where cerebrospinal fluid pools

cisterns: portions of the subarachnoid space where cerebrospinal fluid pools

Clarke's nucleus: contains neurons that project to the ipsilateral cerebellum via the dorsal spinocerebellar tract

claustrum: telencephalic nucleus located beneath the insular cortex

climbing fibers: axons of the inferior olivary nucleus that synapse on Purkinje neurons in the cerebellar cortex; forms one of the strongest excitatory synapses in the central nervous system

cochlea: inner ear organ for hearing

cochlear apex: portion of the cochlea sensitive to low-frequency tones

cochlear division (of the vestibulocochlear nerve): cranial nerve sensitive to sounds

cochlear nuclei: first relay site for axons of the cochlear division of the vestibulocochlear nerve; located in the medulla

collateral circulation: redundant arterial supply for a given structure

collateral sulcus: separates the parahippocampal gyrus from more lateral temporal lobe regions

colliculi: set of four structures on the dorsal midbrain; superior colliculi are important for saccadic eye movement control, and inferior colliculi are important for hearing

color columns: collections of neurons in the primary visual cortex, predominantly located in layers II and III; also termed color blobs

columnar organization (of the cerebral cortex): vertical arrays of neurons that serve similar functions

commissural neurons: class of cortical neuron that contains an axon that projects to the contralateral cortex via the corpus callosum

commissure: tract through which axons cross the midline

computerized tomography: a technique for producing images of a single plane of tissue

conditioned taste aversion: rapid and very robust form of learning in which an individual avoids foods that made it ill

cone bipolar cells: class of retinal interneuron that transmits control signals from cone cells to ganglion neurons

cones: photoreceptor class sensitive to light wavelength (ie, color)

constrictor muscles of the iris: produce pupillary constriction

contralateral: relative spatial term related to the opposite side of the body

contralateral homonymous hemianopia with macular sparing: visual field defect in which there is a loss of vision in the contralateral visual field but preservation of foveal (or macular) vision; can be produced with visual system lesions affecting a portion of the primary visual cortex

contralateral homonymous hemianopia: visual field defect characterized by the loss of sight of the contralateral visual field; can be produced with visual system lesions affecting the optic tract, lateral geniculate nucleus, optic radiations, or primary visual cortex

cornea: transparent avascular portion of the sclera

corona radiata: portion of the subcortical white matter superior (or dorsal) to the internal capsule

coronal: plane of section or imaging plane; parallel to the coronal suture; equivalent to transverse plane for cerebral hemispheres and diencephalon

corpus callosum: commissure connecting the two cerebral hemispheres; contains four major subdivisions: rostrum, genu, body, and splenium

corpus striatum: subcortical telencephalic nuclei comprised of the caudate nucleus, putamen, and nucleus accumbens; generally synonymous with the striatum

cortex: thin sheet of neuronal cell bodies and afferent and efferent axons

cortical column: collection of radially oriented neurons that have similar functions and anatomical connections; basic functional unit of the cerebral cortex

cortical nucleus (of the amygdala): receives input from olfactory structures; projects to the hypothalamus via the stria terminalis

corticobulbar fibers: axons that originate in the cerebral cortex and project to the brain stem; primarily terminating in the cranial nerve motor nuclei of the pons and medulla; projections to specific nuclei and to the reticular formation usually have more specific terms (eg, corticoreticular)

corticobulbar tract: cortical projections that terminate on cranial nerve motor nuclei in the medulla and pons

corticocortical association connections: connections between cortical areas on the same side

corticocortical association neurons: cortical neurons that project axons to cortical areas on the same side

corticomedial nuclei: nuclei of the amygdala that play a role in visceral motor control

corticopontine pathway: descending projection from the cerebral cortex to the pontine nuclei; major input to the cerebrocerebellum

corticoreticular fibers: axons that originate from neurons in layer V of the cortex that project to the reticular formation

cortico-reticulo-spinal pathway: indirect cortical pathway to the spinal cord via neurons of the reticulospinal tract

corticospinal tract: projection from the cerebral cortex to the spinal cord

cranial and spinal roots: nerves that enter and exit the spinal cord and brain stem

cranial nerve II: optic nerve; contains axons of retinal ganglion cells; major targets are the lateral geniculate nucleus, rostral midbrain, nuclei at the midbrain-diencephalon junction, and hypothalamus

cranial nerve motor nuclei: location of motor neurons whose axons are located in the cranial nerves

cranial nerves: sensory and motor nerves containing axons that enter and exit the brain stem, diencephalon, and telencephalon; analogous to the spinal nerves

cribriform plate: part of the ethmoid bone; contains tiny foramina through which olfactory nerve fibers course from the olfactory epithelium to the olfactory bulb

crude touch: a nondiscriminative form of tactile sensation that remains after damage to the dorsal column-medial lemniscal pathway or to large-diameter afferent fibers; may be mediated by unmyelinated C-fiber mechanoreceptors

crus (of the fornix): posterior portion of fornix where it has a flattened appearance

cuneate fascicle: tract containing ascending axons of dorsal root ganglion neurons that innervate the upper trunk (rostral to T6), arm, neck, and back of the head; mediates mechanosensations

cuneate nucleus: termination of axons in the cuneate fascicle; neurons project axons to contralateral ventral posterior nucleus of the thalamus; mediates mechanosensations

cuneocerebellar tract: pathway from the lateral cuneate nucleus to the cerebellum; courses through the inferior cerebellar peduncle

cytoarchitecture: characterization of the morphology of the cerebral cortex based on the density of neuronal cell bodies

cytochrome oxidase: mitochondrial enzyme; marker for neuronal metabolism

declarative memory: memory such as the conscious recollection of facts

decussate: crossing the midline

decussation: a site where axons cross the midline

deep brain stimulation (DBS): use of electrodes to electrically stimulate an area of the brain; most commonly used in the basal ganglia to treat movement disorders

deep cerebellar nuclei: sets of nuclei located beneath the cerebellar cortex; fastigial, interposed (comprising the globose and emboliform), and dentate nuclei

deep cerebral veins: veins that drain the diencephalon and parts of the brain stem

Deiters' nucleus: lateral vestibular nucleus; origin of the lateral vestibulospinal tract

dendrites: receptive portion of a neuron

dentate gyrus: component of the hippocampal formation; receives input from the entorhinal cortex and contains neurons that project to the hippocampus proper

dentate nucleus: one of the deep cerebellar nuclei; transmits the output of the lateral cerebellar hemisphere

depression: a psychiatric disorder characterized by the persistent feeling of hopelessness and dejection; can be associated with poor concentration, lethargy, and sometimes suicidal tendencies

dermatome: area of skin innervated by sensory axons within a single dorsal root

descending motor pathways: connections between the cerebral cortex or brain stem to the spinal cord; densest to the intermediate zone and ventral horn

descending pain inhibitory system: neural circuit for modulating transmission of information about pain from nociceptors, through the dorsal horn, and to the brain stem; primarily originates from serotonergic neurons in the raphe nuclei and noradrenergic neurons in the reticular formation; projects to the spinal cord dorsal horn

descending projection neurons: neurons that give rise to descending pathways

detached retina: pathological condition in which portions of the retina separate from the pigment epithelium

diabetes insipidus: condition in which the kidneys are unable to concentrate urine because of the absence of vasopressin (or antidiuretic hormone); the individual produces copious amounts of urine

diencephalon: one of the secondary brain vesicles; major brain division in maturity, containing primarily the thalamus and hypothalamus; means "between brain"

diffuse-projecting neurons: thalamic neurons that project widely to several cortical areas

diffuse-projecting nuclei: location of thalamic diffuse-projecting neurons

diffusion-weighted magnetic resonance imaging: type of magnetic resonance imaging that can distinguish axonal orientation, especially axons within tracts

direct path: pathway through the basal ganglia from the striatum to the internal segment of the globus pallidus; promotes the production of movements

disinhibition: removal of inhibition; net effect is similar to excitation

distal muscles: muscles that innervate the limbs, especially distal to the elbow; controlled principally by the lateral descending motor pathways

dopamine: neurotransmitter

dopaminergic: neurons that use dopamine as their neurotransmitter

dorsal: close to the back; also termed posterior

dorsal cochlear nucleus: auditory relay nucleus located in the pons; receives input from primary auditory receptors and projects to the contralateral inferior colliculus; implicated in vertical localization of sounds

dorsal column nuclei: cuneate and gracile nuclei; receive input from mechanoreceptor axons in the dorsal columns

dorsal column–medial lemniscal system: tracts, nuclei, and cortical areas collectively involved in mechanosensations (touch, vibration sense, pressure, and limb position sense)

dorsal columns: located on the dorsal spinal cord surface; contain ascending axons of mechanoreceptors; gracile fascicle (or tract) carries axons that originate from receptors on the leg and lower back, whereas the cuneate tract carries axons that originate from receptors on the upper back, arm, neck, and back of the head

dorsal cortex (of inferior colliculus): portion of the surface of the inferior colliculus

dorsal horn: laminae I–VI of the spinal gray matter; processes incoming somatic sensory information, especially about pain, temperature, and itch

dorsal intermediate septum: separates the cuneate and gracile fascicles

dorsal longitudinal fasciculus: pathway to and from the hypothalamus; located in the periventricular and aqueductal gray matter

dorsal median septum: divides the dorsal columns into right and left halves

dorsal motor nucleus of the vagus: contains parasympathetic preganglionic neurons whose axons course in the vagus nerve (cranial nerve X); located in the medulla

dorsal raphe nucleus: located in the rostral pons and caudal midbrain; most neurons in the nucleus use serotonin as their neurotransmitter; projects widely to telencephalic and diencephalic structures

dorsal root: spinal sensory root

dorsal root ganglia: contains cell bodies of primary sensory neurons that innervate skin and deep tissues of the back of the head, neck, limbs, and trunk

dorsal root ganglion neurons: cell bodies of primary sensory neurons that innervate skin and deep tissues of the back of the head, neck, limbs, and trunk

dorsal spinocerebellar tract: an ipsilateral pathway to the cerebellum; originates in Clarke's nucleus

dorsolateral prefrontal cortex: cortical region important for organizing behavior, working memory, and a variety of higher mental processes

dorsoventral axis: between the back and abdomen

dura mater: outermost and toughest meningeal layer; contains an outer periosteal layer and an inner meningeal layer

dural sinus: channel for returning venous blood to the systemic circulation; also a path for flow of cerebrospinal fluid into the venous circulation

dural sinuses: channels within the meningeal layer of the dura, through which venous blood and cerebrospinal fluids are returned to the systemic circulation

dynorphin: neurotransmitter/neuromodulator

dysphagia: impairment in ability to swallow

ectoderm: outermost layer of the embryo

Edinger-Westphal nucleus: contains parasympathetic preganglionic neurons that innervate smooth muscle in the eye to control pupil diameter and lens curvature

efferent: axons transmit information away from a particular structure, efferent is not synonymous with *motor,* which means related to muscle or glandular function

eighth cranial nerve (VIII): vestibulocochlear nerve; separate cochlear division for hearing and vestibular division for balance

electrical synapses: site of communication between neurons that does not use a neurotransmitter; usually associated with a gap junction, where ions and other small and intermediate-sized molecules can pass

emboliform nucleus: one of the deep cerebellar nuclei; together with the globose nucleus is termed the interposed nucleus

encapsulated axon terminals: specialized tissue surrounding the terminal of certain mechanoreceptors; helps to determine the sensitivity and duration of the response of the receptor to a mechanical stimulus

endocrine hormones: biologically active chemicals released by endocrine cells into the blood; regulate metabolism, growth, and other cellular and bodily functions

endoderm: innermost layer of the embryo

endolymph: fluid that fills most of the membranous labyrinth; resembles intracellular fluid in its ionic constituents; has a high potassium concentration and low sodium concentration

enkephalin: neurotransmitter

enteric nervous system: nervous system division that controls the functions of the large intestine

enteroendocrine cells: specialized cells located in the gastrointestinal tract; ghrelin, which promotes feeding, is secreted by enteroendoendocrine cells in the stomach

entorhinal cortex: portion of the medial temporal lobe; major input to the hippocampal formation

ependymal cells: epithelial cell type that lines the ventricles

epiglottis: pharyngeal structure that, during swallowing, helps to prevent passage of fluids and food into the trachea

episodic memory: memory of events that have a specific spatial and temporal context (such as meeting a friend last week)

ethmoid bone: cranial bone; contains the cribriform plate, through which olfactory sensory axons course en route from the olfactory mucosa to the olfactory bulb

explicit memory: conscious recollection of facts; also termed declarative memory

extended amygdala: collection of basal forebrain nuclei that share morphological, histochemical, and connection characteristics; includes central nuclei of the amygdala and the bed nucleus of the stria terminalis; participates in reward and substance abuse along with the ventral striatum

external capsule: white matter region between the putamen and the claustrum; contains primarily cortical association fibers

external nucleus: component of the inferior colliculus that participates in ear reflexes in animals, such as when a cat orients its ears to a sound source

external segment of the globus pallidus: contains neurons that project to the subthalamic nucleus; part of the indirect basal ganglia path

extrastriate cortex: visual cortical areas excluding the primary (or striate) cortex

extreme capsule: white matter region between the claustrum and insular cortex; contains primarily cortical association fibers

facial (VII) nerve: contains axons of motor neurons that innervate muscles of facial expression, as well as the stapedius muscle and part of the digastric muscle; exits from the pontomedullary junction

facial colliculus: surface landmark on ventricular (dorsal) surface of the pons; overlies the genu of the facial nerve and the abducens nucleus

facial motor nucleus: located in the pons, it contains motor neurons whose axons course within the facial nerve to innervate muscles of facial expression, the posterior belly of the digastric muscle, and the stapedius muscle

facial nucleus: contains motor neurons that innervate muscles of facial expression, as well as the stapedius muscle and part of the digastric muscle; located in the pons

falx cerebri: dural flap between the two cerebral hemispheres; extension of the meningeal layer of the dura

fastigial nucleus: one of the deep cerebellar nuclei; transmits the output of the vermis to the medial descending motor pathways

fenestrated capillaries: contain pores through which substances can diffuse from within the capillary to surrounding tissue

fimbria: portion of the fornix that covers part of the hippocampal formation

first lumbar vertebra: marks the approximate location of the caudal end of the spinal cord within the vertebral canal

fissure: groove in the cortical surface; more consistent in shape and depth than a sulcus

flaccid paralysis: inability to contract a muscle, together with a profound loss of muscle tone

FLAIR: MRI pulse sequence that suppresses signal related to cerebrospinal fluid; abbreviation for fluid attenuated inversion recovery

flexure: bend in the axis of the central nervous system or axis of the embryo

flocculonodular lobe: portion of the cerebellar cortex involved in eye movement control and balance

flocculus: *see* flocculonodular lobe

floor plate: ventral surface of the developing central nervous system; key site for organizing the dorsoventral patterning of the spinal cord during development

folia: thin folds of the cerebellar cortex

foramen of Magendie: opening in the fourth ventricle where cerebrospinal fluid can pass into the subarachnoid space; located on the midline

foramina of Luschka: openings in the fourth ventricle where cerebrospinal fluid can pass into the subarachnoid space; located at the lateral recesses of the ventricle

forebrain: most rostral primary brain vesicle; divides into the telencephalon and diencephalon

Forel's field H2: another name for the lenticular fasciculus; region of the white matter though which axons from the internal segment of the globus pallidus course en route to the thalamus

form pathway (for vision): circuit specialized for discriminating features of the shapes of visual stimuli; information in this path is used for object recognition

fornix: a major output tract from the hippocampal formation

fourth ventricle: portion of the ventricular system located in the brain stem; separates medulla and pons from the cerebellum

fovea: portion of the retina with the greatest visual acuity, where only cone receptors are located; located in the center of the macula

fractionate movements: ability to isolate one movement from another, such as move one finger while keeping the other fingers still

fractionation (of movement): ability to move one finger or limb segment independent of the other fingers or limb segments; often termed individuation

fractured somatotopy: characteristic of a central sensory or motor representation in which the somatotopic plan is disorganized and a single body part becomes represented at multiple sites

Friedreich's ataxia: an autosomal recessive disease that results in progressive spinocerebellar ataxia; chromosome 9 mutation; expansion of a GAA trinucleotide repeat within the gene that codes for the mitochondrial protein frataxin

frontal: close to the forehead

frontal association cortex: major association area located rostral to the premotor cortical regions on the lateral and medial brain surfaces and on the orbital surface

frontal eye fields: portion of the lateral frontal lobe important in the control of eye movements

frontal lobe: one of the lobes of the cerebral hemisphere

functional localization: identification of brain regions that participate in particular functions

functional magnetic resonance imaging (fMRI): a form of magnetic resonance imaging that can monitor blood oxygenation, which correlates with neuronal activity

functional neuroanatomy: examines those parts of the nervous system that work together to accomplish a particular task

GABA: γ-aminobutyric acid; principal inhibitory neurotransmitter in the central nervous system

gag reflex: stereotypic contraction of pharyngeal muscles in response to stimulation of the posterior oral cavity; the afferent limb is the glossopharyngeal nerve, and the efferent limb is the vagus nerve primarily

ganglion: collections of neuronal cell bodies outside the central nervous system

ganglion cell layer: innermost retinal cell layer; contains cell bodies of ganglion cells

ganglion cells: retinal projection neurons; axons course in the optic nerve and terminate in the diencephalon and midbrain

geniculate ganglion: location of cell bodies of primary sensory neurons that project in the intermediate nerve (cranial nerve VII)

genu: Latin for knee; used to describe structures with an acute bend, such as the corpus callosum and facial nerve

genu of the internal capsule: separates the anterior and posterior limbs of the internal capsule

ghrelin: protein secreted by enteroendocrine cells of the stomach; promotes food intake

girdle muscles: striated muscles that insert proximally and attach on parts of the shoulder or hip

glial cells: major cell type in the nervous system; outnumber neurons about 10 to 1; also termed glia

globose nucleus: deep cerebellar nucleus; together with the emboliform nucleus comprise the interposed nuclei, which transmit information from the intermediate cerebellar hemisphere

globus pallidus: basal ganglia nucleus; comprises distinct internal and external divisions

glomerulus: collection of neuronal cell bodies and processes surrounded by glial cells; structures within the glomerulus are physically isolated from surrounding neurons; typically corresponds to a basic functional processing unit

glossopharyngeal (IX) nerve: cranial nerve; located in the medulla

glutamate: principal excitatory neurotransmitter of neurons in the central nervous system

Golgi neurons: inhibitory interneurons of the cerebellar cortex

Golgi tendon organ (or receptor): stretch receptors in muscle tendon that signals active muscle force; afferent component of the golgi tendon reflex; distal receptive portion of group Ib axons

gracile fascicle: medial component of the dorsal column; transmits mechanoreceptive information from the legs and lower trunk to the ipsilateral gracile nucleus

gracile nucleus: target of the axons of the gracile fascicle; transmits information to the contralateral thalamus via the medial lemniscus

granular layer: innermost cell layer of the cerebellum; primarily contains granule and Golgi neurons and the axon terminals of mossy fibers

granule cell: cerebellar excitatory interneuron; cell of origin of parallel fibers

granule neurons: the only excitatory interneuron of the cerebellar cortex

gray matter: portions of the central nervous system that contain predominantly neuronal cell bodies

great cerebral vein (of Galen): major vein; carries venous drainage from the diencephalon and deep telencephalic structures

gyri: grooves in the cerebral cortex

gyrus rectus: located on the inferior frontal lobe; runs parallel to the olfactory tract

habenula: portion of the diencephalon; located lateral and ventral to the pineal gland; part of a circuit with the midbrain medial dopaminergic and the serotonergic systems

hair cells: auditory receptor neurons

hearing: one of the five major senses

hemiballism: movement disorder produced by damage to the subthalamic nucleus; characterized by involuntary rapid (ballistic) limb movements

hemiplegic cerebral palsy: an acquired condition characterized by perinatal damage to brain circuits; commonly affects sensory and motor cortical areas; damage to the corticospinal tract produces motor signs that include spasticity and incoordination

hemorrhagic stroke: condition following the rupture of an artery; tissue around the hemorrhage can become damaged because blood leaks out of the artery under high pressure

Heschl's gyri: location of primary auditory cortex

hierarchical organization: property of neural systems in which individual components comprise distinct functional levels with respect to one another

higher-order auditory areas: regions of the temporal lobe that process complex aspects of sounds; major input from lower-order auditory areas (eg, primary and secondary)

hindbrain: most caudal portion of the brain; includes the medulla, pons, and cerebellum

hippocampal formation: telencephalic structure located primarily within the temporal lobe; comprises the dentate gyrus, hippocampus, and subiculum; involved in learning and memory

hippocampal sulcus: separates the dentate gyrus from the subiculum; largely obscured in the mature brain

hippocampus: component of the hippocampal formation

histamine: neuroactive compound; generally excitatory; important in hypothalamic circuits for regulating sleep and wakefulness

Hoffmann's sign: thumb adduction in response to flexion of the distal phalanx of the third digit; an upper limb equivalent of the Babinski sign

horizontal cells: retinal interneuron

horizontal localization of sound: ability to identify the position of the source of a sound in the horizontal plane

Horner syndrome: constellation of neurological signs associated with dysfunction of the sympathetic innervation of the head

Huntington disease: genetic autosomal dominant disorder; produces hyperkinetic motor signs

hydrocephalus: buildup of cerebrospinal fluid within the brain

hyperkinetic signs: set of abnormal involuntary motor behaviors characterized by increased rate of occurrence and inability to control; examples include tremor, tics, chorea, and athetosis

hypoglossal motor neurons: innervate intrinsic tongue muscles

hypoglossal (XII) nerve: cranial nerve located in the medulla

hypoglossal nucleus: location of hypoglossal motor neurons

hypokinetic signs: set of abnormal involuntary motor behaviors characterized by decreased rate of occurrence or slowing; examples include bradykinesia (slowing of movements) and failure to initiate a motor behavior in a timely manner

hypothalamic sulcus: roughly separates the hypothalamus and thalamus on the medial brain surface

hypothalamus: major brain division; part of diencephalon

immunocytochemistry: process in which antibodies to a particular molecule are used to label that molecule in tissue

implicit memory: memory of procedures and actions; also termed nondeclarative memory

incus: one of the middle ear ossicles (bones); essential for conducting changes in air pressure from the tympanic membrane to the oval window; located between the other two ossicles

indirect cortical pathways: motor pathway from the cerebral cortex that synapses first in the brain stem before synapsing on spinal neurons

indirect path: pathway through the basal ganglia from the striatum, to the external segment of the globus pallidus, to the subthalamic nucleus, and then to the internal segment of the globus pallidus; functions to retard the production of movements

infarction: death of tissue because of cessation of blood flow

inferior cerebellar peduncle: predominantly an input pathway to the cerebellum

inferior colliculus: located in the caudal midbrain, on its dorsal surface; contains neurons that are part of the ascending auditory pathway

inferior ganglia: location of primary somatic sensory cell bodies of vagus and glossopharyngeal nerves that innervate visceral tissues

inferior oblique muscle: extraocular muscle that depresses the eye, mostly when the eye is adducted

inferior olivary nuclear complex: collection of nuclei in the medulla that give rise to the climbing fibers of the cerebellum; forms the olive, a surface landmark on the ventral medullar surface

inferior parietal lobule: located dorsal to the lateral sulcus; important for a variety of higher brain functions, including language and perception

inferior petrosal sinus: major dural sinus

inferior rectus muscle: extraocular muscle that depresses the eye, especially when eye is abducted

inferior sagittal sinus: major dural sinus

inferior salivatory nuclei: location of parasympathetic preganglionic neurons that innervate cranial glands

inferior temporal gyrus: important in visual form perception

inferior vestibular nucleus: receives direct input from the vestibular organs; projects to various brain stem and spinal targets for eye movement control and balance

infundibular stalk: interconnects hypothalamus and pituitary gland; also termed the infundibulum

initial segment: junction of the neuronal cell body and axon; important site for integration of electrical signals and for initiating action potentials conducted along the axon

inner hair cells: principal auditory receptor neuron

inner nuclear layer: retinal layer that contains the cell bodies and proximal processes of the retinal interneurons: bipolar, horizontal, and amacrine cells

inner synaptic (or plexiform) layer: where synaptic connections between the bipolar cells and the ganglion cells are made

input nuclei (of basal ganglia): consisting of the striatum; receive input from cerebral cortex

insular cortex: portion of the cerebral cortex buried beneath the frontal, parietal, and temporal lobes; several sensory representations are located there, including those for taste, balance, and pain

insulin: hormone secreted by the pancreatic islet cells; can inhibit food intake through hypothalamic circuits

intention tremor: slow oscillatory movement of the distal limb as it approaches the endpoint of the movement; results from cerebellar dysfunction or damage

interaural intensity difference: a mechanism for determining the horizontal location of high-frequency sounds

interaural time difference: a mechanism for determining the horizontal location of low-frequency sounds

intermediate hemisphere: portion of the cerebellar cortex involved in limb and trunk control

intermediate horn: the lateral intermediate zone of the spinal cord; location of sympathetic preganglionic neurons

intermediate nerve: sensory and parasympathetic branch of cranial nerve VII

intermediate zone: portion of spinal gray matter located between the dorsal and ventral horns

intermediolateral cell column: *see* intermediolateral nucleus

intermediolateral nucleus: location of sympathetic preganglionic neurons; present from about T1 to about L2

internal arcuate fibers: decussating fibers of the dorsal column nuclei

internal capsule: location of axons coursing to and from the cerebral cortex; present between the thalamus and parts of the basal ganglia

internal carotid artery: major cerebral artery; supplies blood to the cerebral cortex and many deep structures excluding the brain stem and cerebellum

internal medullary laminae: bands of white matter that divide the thalamus into several nuclear divisions

internal segment of the globus pallidus: one of the principal output nuclei of the basal ganglia

interneurons: neurons with an axon that remains locally within the nucleus or cortical region where the cell body is located

internuclear neurons: neurons located in the abducens nucleus that project to the contralateral oculomotor nucleus to transmit control signals for horizontal saccadic eye movements

internuclear ophthalmoplegia: produced by lesion of the medial longitudinal fasciculus between the levels of the abducens and oculomotor nuclei; interrupts axons of internuclear neurons; inability to adduct the ipsilateral eye when looking to the side opposite the lesion

interpeduncular cistern: where cerebrospinal fluid collects between the cerebral peduncles

interpeduncular fossa: space between the cerebral peduncles

interpolar nucleus: component of the spinal trigeminal nucleus; important for facial pain, especially within the mouth and teeth

interposed nuclei: deep cerebellar nuclei; comprises the globose and emboliform nuclei

intersegmental neurons: spinal interneurons that interconnect neurons in different segments; also termed propriospinal neurons

interstitial nucleus of Cajal: involved in eye and head control; located in rostral midbrain; gives rise to a small descending motor pathway

interstitial nucleus of the MLF: center for control of vertical eye movements; located in rostral midbrain

interventricular foramen (of Monro): conduit through which cerebrospinal fluid and choroid plexus passes from the lateral ventricles to the third ventricle

interventricular foramina: *see* interventricular foramen

intracavernous segment: portion of internal carotid artery as it passes through the cavernous sinus

intralaminar nuclei: set of thalamic nuclei that have diffuse cortical projections and may play a role in regulating the level of cortical activity and arousal

intrapetrosal segment: portion of the carotid artery as it travels through the petrous bone

intrasegmental neurons: local spinal interneurons; their axons remain with the segment of the cell body

intrinsic nuclei (of basal ganglia): include the external part of the globus pallidus, part of the ventral pallidum, subthalamic nucleus, substantia nigra pars compacta, ventral tegmental area

ipsilateral: on the same side; term used relative to a particular landmark or event

ischemia: decreased delivery of oxygenated blood to the tissue

ischemic stroke: occlusion of an artery that results in downstream cessation of blood flow

isthmus: narrow portion of the developing brain stem between the pons and midbrain; in maturity the isthmus is typically included as part of the rostral pons

itch: sensory experience produced by histamine

itch-sensitive receptors: activation leads to the sensation itch; also termed pruritic receptor

jaw-jerk (or closure) reflex: automatic closure of the jaw upon stimulation of muscle spindle afferents in jaw muscles; analogous to the knee-jerk reflex

jaw proprioception: the ability to sense jaw angle; more commonly used to describe the sensory events signaled by primary sensory neurons whose cell bodies are located within the mesencephalic trigeminal nucleus

juxtarestiform body: efferent pathway from the cerebellum to the caudal brain stem; principal location of axons from the fastigial nucleus to vestibular and other brain stem neurons

knee-jerk reflex: automatic extension of the leg upon stimulation of the patella tendon; the stimulus stretches muscle spindle receptors in the quadriceps muscle

Korsakoff syndrome: a form of memory loss in patients with alcoholism or thiamine deficiency; produced by degeneration of the mammillary bodies and parts of the medial thalamus

lacrimal gland: tear gland

lamina terminalis: rostral wall of the third ventricle; marks location of most anterior portion of the neural tube

laminated: morphological feature in which neuronal cell bodies or axons form discrete layers

large-diameter axon: mechanoreceptive sensory axons

large-diameter fiber entry zone: site at which large-diameter axons enter the spinal cord; located medial to Lissauer's tract

laryngeal closure reflex: automatic contraction of laryngeal adductor muscles to prevent food and fluids from entering the trachea

lateral cerebellar hemisphere: cortical component of the cerebrocerebellum; involved primarily in motor planning

lateral column: portion of the spinal white matter; contains diverse somatic sensory, cerebellar, and motor control pathways

lateral corticospinal tract: pathway in which descending axons for voluntary limb control descend; originates primarily from the motor areas of the frontal lobe

lateral descending pathways: motor pathways for controlling limb muscles

lateral gaze palsy: *see* internuclear ophthalmoplegia

lateral geniculate nucleus: thalamic visual relay nucleus

lateral hypothalamus (or hypothalamic zone): important for feeding and sleep-wakefulness; orexin-containing neurons are unique to this brain region

lateral intermediate zone: portion of spinal gray matter that plays a role in limb muscle control

lateral lemniscus: ascending brain stem auditory pathway

lateral medullary lamina: band of axons that separates the external segment of the globus pallidus and the putamen

lateral medullary syndrome: set of neurological signs associated with occlusion of the posterior inferior cerebellar artery; signs include difficulty in swallowing, vertigo, loss of pain and temperature sense on the ipsilateral face and contralateral limbs and trunk, ataxia, and Horner syndrome

lateral olfactory stria: pathway by which axons from the olfactory tract project to the olfactory cortical areas

lateral posterior nucleus: thalamic nucleus with projections to the posterior parietal lobe

lateral rectus muscle: ocular abductor muscle; moves eye laterally

lateral reticular nucleus: precerebellar nucleus; transmits information from the cerebral cortex and spinal cord to the intermediate cerebellum

lateral septal nucleus: telencephalic nucleus; part of limbic system

lateral sulcus: separates the temporal lobe from the frontal and parietal lobes

lateral superior olivary nucleus: contains neurons sensitive to interaural intensity differences; plays role in horizontal localization of high-frequency sounds

lateral ventral horn: contains motor neurons that innervate limb muscles

lateral ventricle: telencephalic component of the ventricular system; bilaterally paired, with four components (anterior horn, body, atrium, posterior horn, and inferior horn)

lateral vestibular nucleus: key brain stem nucleus for control of proximal muscles; important in balance; gives rise to the lateral vestibulospinal tract

lateral vestibulospinal tract: ipsilateral pathway; component of the medial descending pathways

laterality: pertains to one side or the other

L-dopa: precursor to dopamine; used in the treatment of Parkinson disease

lenticular fasciculus: region of the white matter through which axons from the internal segment of the globus pallidus course en route to the thalamus

lenticular nucleus: globus pallidus (both internal and external segments) and putamen

lenticulostriate arteries: branches of the middle cerebral artery and anterior cerebral artery that supply deep structures of the cerebral hemispheres, including parts of the internal capsule and basal ganglia; originate from the proximal portions of the arteries

leptin: hormone produced by adipocytes in proportion to the amount of body fat; suppresses feeding

levator palpebrae superioris muscle: principal eyelid elevator

limb position sense: ability to judge the position of one's limbs without using vision

limbic association cortex: diverse regions of primarily the frontal and temporal lobes; involved in emotions, learning, and memory

limbic loop (of basal ganglia): the basal ganglia circuit that receive input from limbic cortical areas, basolateral amygdala, and the hippocampal formation and projects to the orbitofrontal cortex and anterior cingulate cortex

limbic system: brain structures and their interconnections that collectively mediate emotions, learning, and memory

Lissauer's tract: location of central branches of small-diameter afferent fibers prior to termination in the superficial dorsal horn

lobe: major division of the cerebral cortex

lobule: a division of a lobe

locus ceruleus: principal noradrenergic brain stem nucleus; located in the rostral pons

long circumferential branches: brain stem arterial branches that supply the most dorsolateral portions; also supply the cerebellum

longitudinal axis: the head-to-tail (or head-to-coccyx) axis of the nervous system

lumbar: spinal cord segment; there are five in total

lumbar cistern: space within the vertebral canal where cerebrospinal fluid pools; commonly used for withdrawing cerebrospinal fluid from patients

lumbar tap: process of removing cerebrospinal fluid from the lumbar cistern; needle is inserted into the intervertebral space between the third and fourth (or the fourth and fifth) lumbar vertebrae

M cell: retinal ganglion neuron with a large dendritic arbor; plays a preferential role in sensing of visual motion; magnocellular

macroglia: glial cell class that comprises oligodendrocytes, Schwann cells, astrocytes, and ependymal cells; serve a variety of support and nutritive functions; contrast with microglia

macula lutea: portion of the central retina that contains the fovea

macular region: portion of the retina surrounding the macula lutea

macular sparing: maintenance of vision around the fovea after visual cortex damage that produces a loss of parafoveal and peripheral vision

magnetic resonance angiography: application of magnetic resonance imaging to study vasculature by monitoring motion of water molecules in blood vessels

magnetic resonance imaging: radiological technique to examine brain structure; uses primarily the water content of tissue to provide a structural image

magnocellular division (of red nucleus): component of the red nucleus that contains large neurons that project to the spinal cord as the rubrospinal tract

magnocellular neurosecretory system: hypothalamic neurons in the supraoptic and paraventricular nuclei that project their axons to the posterior lobe of the pituitary, where they release oxytocin and vasopressin

magnocellular visual system: components of the visual system in the retina, lateral geniculate, and visual cortical areas that originate from M-type ganglion cells; sensitive primarily to moving stimuli

main (or principal) trigeminal sensory nucleus: brain stem relay nucleus for mechanosensory information from the face and oral cavity

malleus: one of the middle ear ossicles (bones); essential for conducting changes in air pressure from the tympanic membrane to the oval window; attaches to the tympanic membrane

mammillary bodies: hypothalamic nuclear complex; contains the medial and lateral mammillary nuclei; the mammillary bodies give rise to the mammillothalamic and mammillotegmental tracts

mammillotegmental tract: originates from the lateral mammillary nucleus; terminates in the pontine tegmentum

mammillothalamic tract: originates from both the medial and lateral mammillary nuclei; terminates in the anterior thalamic nuclei

mandibular division: trigeminal sensory nerve root that innervates primarily the lower face and parts of the oral cavity

marginal zone: outermost layer of the dorsal horn

mastication: chewing

maxillary division: trigeminal sensory nerve root that innervates primarily the lips, cheek, and parts of the oral cavity

mechanoreceptive afferent fibers: sensory axons that have mechanoreceptive terminals

mechanoreceptors: sensory receptors sensitive to mechanical stimulation

medial descending pathways: motor pathways for controlling axial and other proximal muscles

medial dorsal nucleus (of the thalamus): principal thalamic nucleus projecting to the frontal lobe

medial forebrain bundle: pathway that carries functionally diverse brain stem pathways to subcortical nuclei and the cerebral cortex, including the monoaminergic pathways

medial geniculate nucleus: thalamic auditory relay nucleus

medial lemniscus: brain stem tract that contains axons traveling from the dorsal column nuclei to the thalamus

medial longitudinal fasciculus: brain stem tract that contains axons from the vestibular nuclei, extraocular motor nuclei, and various brain stem nuclei; primarily for control of eye movements

medial mammillary nucleus: principal nucleus of the mammillary body; projects to the anterior nuclei of the thalamus

medial medullary lamina: band of myelinated axons that separates the internal and external segments of the globus pallidus

medial olfactory stria: small tract that contains axons from other brain regions that project to the olfactory bulb

medial orbital gyri: *see* medial orbitofrontal gyri

medial orbitofrontal gyri: part of the limbic association cortex

medial prefrontal cortical areas: portion of the prefrontal cortex one function of which is object recognition

medial preoptic area: portion of the anterior hypothalamus that contains parvocellular neurosecretory neurons; sexually dimorphic

medial rectus muscle: extraocular muscle that adducts eye (ie, moves toward the nose); innervated by the oculomotor nerve (cranial nerve III)

medial septal nucleus: telencephalic nucleus; important projections to the hippocampal formation; gives rise to cholinergic and GABA-ergic projections

medial superior olivary nucleus: contains neurons sensitive to interaural timing differences; plays role in horizontal localization of low-frequency sounds

medial ventral horn: contains motor neurons that innervate proximal limb and axial muscles; controlled by the medial descending pathways

medial vestibular nucleus: part of the vestibular nuclear complex; gives rise to the medial vestibulospinal tract for head and eye coordination

medial vestibulospinal tract: motor pathway for coordinating head and eye movements

median eminence: contains the primary capillaries of the hypophyseal portal system; located in the proximal portion of the infundibular stalk; lacks blood-brain barrier

median raphe nuclei: located along or close to the brain stem midline; use serotonin as neurotransmitter

medium spiny neurons: major class of striatal neuron; projects to the globus pallidus

medulla: major brain division; part of hindbrain

medullary dorsal horn: extension of dorsal horn into the medulla; also termed caudal nucleus

Meissner's corpuscle: mechanoreceptor

melanin-concentrating hormone: peptide that affects food intake

membranous labyrinth: cavity within which the vestibular apparatus are located; contains endolymph

meninges: membranes that cover the central nervous system; comprises dura, arachnoid, and pia

Merkel's receptor: mechanoreceptor

mesencephalic trigeminal nucleus: contains cell bodies of jaw muscle stretch receptors; only site in the central nervous system that contains cell bodies of sensory receptor neurons; more similar to a ganglion than a nucleus

mesencephalic trigeminal tract: contains the axons of jaw muscle stretch receptors

mesencephalon: secondary brain vesicle; major brain division; also termed midbrain

mesocorticolimbic dopaminergic system: dopaminergic projection to the frontal lobe and ventral striatum; primarily originates from the ventral tegmental area

mesoderm: middle layer of the embryo

mesolimbic dopaminergic system: originates from the ventral tegmental nucleus; supplies dopamine to nucleus accumbens and parts of frontal lobe; sometimes termed mesocorticolimbic dopaminergic system

metencephalon: secondary brain vesicle; gives rise to the pons and cerebellum

Meyer's loop: component of the optic radiation from the lateral geniculate nucleus to the occipital lobe that courses through the rostral temporal lobe; axons transmit visual information from the contralateral upper visual field

microglia: class of glial cell that subserves a phagocytic or scavenger role; responds to nervous system infection or damage; contrasts with macroglia

microzones (of cerebellum): small clusters of Purkinje neurons receive climbing fiber inputs that have similar physiological characteristics, such as processing somatic sensory information from the same body part

midbrain: major brain division

midbrain dopaminergic neurons: correspond to dopaminergic neurons in the substantia nigra pars compacta and the ventral tegmental area

midbrain tectum: region dorsal to the cerebral aqueduct; corresponds to the superior and inferior colliculi

middle cerebellar peduncle: major input pathway to the cerebrocerebellum; consists of axons of pontine nuclei

middle cerebral artery: supplies blood to the lateral surface of the cerebral cortex and deep structures of the cerebral hemisphere and diencephalon

middle ear ossicles: three bones that conduct sound pressure waves from the tympanic membrane to the oval window

middle temporal gyrus: located on the lateral temporal lobe; important in higher visual functions, especially object recognition

midline thalamic nuclei: diffuse-projecting nuclei; one of its major targets is the hippocampal formation

midsagittal: anatomical or imaging plane through the midline that is parallel both to the longitudinal axis of the central nervous system and to the midline, between the dorsal and ventral surfaces

miosis: pupillary constriction

mirror neurons: discharge when an animal preforms a movement or sees movements being performed by another

mitral cells: projection neuron of the olfactory bulb

mixed nerve: peripheral nerve composed of somatic sensory and motor axons

modality: sensory attribute that corresponds to quality (eg, pain)

molecular layer: outermost cerebellar layer; contains stellate and basket neurons, Purkinje cell dendrites, climbing fibers, and parallel fibers

mossy fiber terminal: enlarged axon terminal; one of the principal components of the cerebellar glomerulus

mossy fibers: in the cerebellum, major input to the cortex that originates from diverse structures, including the spinal cord and pontine nuclei; in the hippocampus, axon branch of granule cells in the dentate gyrus that synapse on neurons in the CA3 region

motion pathway (for vision): circuit specialized for discriminating the speed and direction of moving visual stimuli

motor cranial nerve nuclei: contain cell bodies of somatic and branchiomeric motor neurons; nuclei containing parasympathetic preganglionic motor neurons are typically termed autonomic motor nuclei or columns

motor homunculus: representation of body musculature in the primary motor cortex; organization is similar to the form of the body

motor neurons: central nervous system neurons that have an axon that projects to the periphery, to synapse on striated muscles (somatic or branchiomeric motor neurons) or autonomic postganglionic neurons and adrenal cells (autonomic motor neurons)

motor unit: a single alpha-motor neuron and all of the muscle fibers that it innervates

Müller cell: retinal glial cell that stretches from the outer to the inner limiting membranes; have important structural and metabolic functions

multipolar neurons: neurons with a complex dendritic array and a single axon; principal neuron class in the central nervous system

muscarinic receptors: membrane proteins that transduce acetylcholine into neuronal depolarization; named for agonist muscarine

muscle spindle receptor: stretch receptor in muscle; has efferent sensitivity control

myelencephalon: secondary brain vesicle; forms the medulla of the mature brain

myelin: fatty substance that contains numerous myelin proteins

myelin sheath: covering around peripheral and central axons to speed action potential conduction; formed by Schwann cells in the periphery and oligodendrocytes in the central nervous system

myelin stains: methods to reveal the presence of the myelin sheath

myotatic reflexes: mechanoreceptors in muscle excite or inhibit motor neurons at short latency with only one or just a few synapses (eg, the knee-jerk [stretch] reflex)

narcolepsy: disease in which the patient experiences persistent daytime sleepiness; often associated with cataplexy, which is the transient loss of muscle tone without a loss of consciousness

nasal hemiretina: portion of the retina medial to a vertical line that runs through the macula

nasal mucosal glands: located in the nasal cavity, secrete mucous, which is rich in glycoproteins; protects the nasal epithelium

neocortex: phylogenetically most recent portion of the cerebral cortex; most abundant form of cortex; has six or more layers

neural crest: collection of dorsal neural tube cells that migrate peripherally and give rise to all of the neurons whose cell bodies are outside of the central nervous system; also gives rise to Schwann cells and the arachnoid and pial meningeal layers

neural degeneration: deterioration in neuron structure and function

neural groove: midline region of the neural tube where neurons and glial cells do not proliferate; where the floor plate forms

neural induction: process by which a portion of the dorsal ectoderm of the embryo becomes committed to form the nervous system

neural plate: dorsal ectoderm region from which the nervous system forms

neural tube: embryonic structure that gives rise to the central nervous system; cells in the walls of the neural tube form neurons and glial cells, whereas the cavity within the tube forms the ventricular system

neuraxis: principal axis of the central nervous system

neuroactive compounds: chemicals that alter neuronal function

neuroectoderm: portion of the ectoderm that gives rise to the nervous system; corresponds to the neural plate

neurohypophysis: portion of the pituitary that develops from the neuroectoderm; where vasopressin and oxytocin are released into the systemic circulation

neuromelanin: polymer of the catecholamine precursor dihydroxyphenylalanine (or dopa), which is contained in the neurons in the pars compacta

neuromeres: segments of the developing hindbrain

neuron: nerve cell

neurophysins: protein that derives from the prohormone that gives rise to oxytocin and vasopressin; coreleased with oxytocin and vasopressin

neurotransmitter: typically small molecular weight compounds (eg, glutamate and γ-aminobutyric acid, and acetylcholine) that excite or inhibit neurons

nigrostriatal dopaminergic system: originates from the substantia nigra pars compacta and terminates primarily in the dorsal and lateral portions of the putamen and caudate nucleus

nigrostriatal tract: pathway in which nigrostriatal axons course

nociceptors: somatic sensory receptors that are selectively activated by noxious or damaging stimuli

nodulus: portion of the cerebellum critical for vestibular control of eye and head movements

nondeclarative memory: memory of procedures and actions

noradrenalin: neurotransmitter; also termed norepinephrine

noradrenergic: neuron that uses noradrenalin as a neurotransmitter

notochord: releases substances important for organizing the ventral neural tube, such as determining whether a developing neuron becomes a motor neuron; located ventral to the developing nervous system

noxious: tissue damaging

noxious stimuli: a tissue-damaging stimulus; can be mechanical, thermal, or in response to various forms of trauma

nucleus: collection of neuronal cell bodies within the central nervous system

nucleus accumbens: component of the striatum located ventrally and medially; key structure in drug addiction

nucleus ambiguus: contains primarily motor neurons that innervate the pharynx and larynx; also contains parasympathetic preganglionic neurons; located in the medulla

nucleus of the diagonal band of Broca: cholinergic telencephalic nucleus with diverse cortical projections; located in the basal forebrain

nucleus of the lateral lemniscus: auditory projection nucleus; located in the rostral pons

nucleus of the trapezoid body: contains inhibitory neurons that receive input from the anteroventral cochlear nucleus and project to the lateral superior olivary nucleus; may participate in shaping the interaural timing sensitivity of neurons in the lateral superior olivary nucleus located in the pons

nucleus proprius: contains neurons that process somatic sensory information; corresponds to laminae III–IV of the dorsal horn

nystagmus: rhythmical oscillations of the eyeball

occipital lobe: one of the lobes of the cerebral hemisphere

occipital somites: somites from which neck and cranial structures develop

ocular dominance columns: clusters of neurons in the primary visual cortex that receive and process information predominantly from either the ipsilateral or the contralateral eye

oculomotor (III) nerve: motor cranial nerve; contains axons that innervate the medial rectus, superior rectus, inferior rectus, inferior oblique, and levator palpebrae muscles, as well as axons of parasympathetic preganglionic neurons

oculomotor loop: basal ganglia circuit that engages frontal eye movement control areas

oculomotor nucleus: contains motor neurons that innervate the medial rectus, superior rectus, inferior rectus, inferior oblique, and levator palpebrae muscles

odorants: chemicals that produce odors

olfactory bulb: telencephalic structure that receives input from olfactory sensory neurons and projects to the olfactory cortical areas

olfactory discrimination: ability to discriminate one odorant from another

olfactory epithelium: portion of the olfactory mucosa that contains olfactory sensory neurons

olfactory (I) nerve: central branches of olfactory sensory neurons; travels the short distance between the olfactory. mucosa, through the cribriform plate, to synapse in the olfactory bulb

olfactory receptor: transmembrane protein complex in an olfactory sensory neuron; transduces a particular set of odorants into a neural potential; any given olfactory sensory neurons contains a single (or just a few) olfactory receptor types

olfactory sulcus: groove on the inferior frontal lobe surface in which the olfactory bulb and tract course

olfactory tract: contains axons that interconnect the olfactory bulb with the other olfactory nuclear regions of the brain

olfactory tubercle: region on the ventral brain surface that receives input from the olfactory tract; may play a role in emotions in addition to olfaction

oligodendrocytes: class of glial cell that forms the myelin sheath around axons within the central nervous system

olive: landmark on ventral surface of the medulla under which the inferior olivary nucleus is located

olivocochlear bundle: efferent projection from the inferior olivary nucleus to hair cells in the cochlea

olivocochlear projection: *see* olivocochlear bundle

Onuf's nucleus: located in sacral spinal cord; contains motor neurons that innervate anal and urethral sphincters

operculum: portions of frontal, parietal, and temporal lobes that overlie the insular cortex

ophthalmic artery: supplies the eye; can be a pathway for collateral brain circulation after occlusion of the internal carotid artery

ophthalmic division: trigeminal sensory nerve root that innervates primarily the upper face

optic chiasm: site of decussation of ganglion cell axons from the nasal hemiretinae

optic disk: site on retina where ganglion cell axons exit from the eye

optic (II) nerve: sensory cranial nerve that contains axons of retinal ganglion cells; major projections are to the lateral geniculate nucleus, superior colliculus, and pretectal nuclei

optic radiations: pathway from the lateral geniculate nucleus to the primary visual cortex; forms the lateral wall of the posterior horn of the lateral ventricle

optic tectum: also termed the superior colliculus

optic tract: retinal ganglion cell axon pathway between the optic chiasm and the lateral geniculate nucleus

optokinetic reflexes: ocular reflexes that use visual information; supplements the actions of vestibulo-ocular reflexes

oral nucleus: rostral component of the spinal trigeminal nucleus

orbitofrontal (or orbital) gyri: portion of the inferior frontal lobe that contains the orbital gyri; overlie the bony orbits

orbitofrontal cortex: part of prefrontal cortex; important for emotion and personality

orexin: peptide that is essential for the proper maintenance of the aroused state; loss of orexin is implicated in the sleep disorder narcolepsy; may also participate in feeding; also termed hypocretin

organ of Corti: component of the inner ear for transducing sound into neural signals

organum vasculosum of the lamina terminalis: one of the circumventricular organs; region in which the bloodbrain barrier is absent; axons project to magnocellular neurons of the paraventricular nucleus

orientation column: cluster of neurons in the primary visual cortex that processes information about the orientation of a visual stimulus

orthonasal olfaction: when molecules travel from the external environment, through the nostrils (nares), to activate olfactory neurons in the olfactory epithelium

orthostatic hypotension: sudden reduction in systemic blood pressure upon standing upright; sometimes termed postural hypotension

otic ganglion: contains parasympathetic postganglionic neurons that innervate the parotid gland, which secretes saliva

otolith organs: the utricle and saccule; sensitive to linear acceleration

outer hair cells: class of auditory receptor neurons; may be more important in regulating the sensitivity of the organ of Corti than in auditory signal transduction

outer nuclear layer: retinal layer that contains the cell bodies of photoreceptors (rods and cones)

outer synaptic (or plexiform) layer: retinal layer in which connections are made between photoreceptors and two classes of retinal interneurons (horizontal cells and bipolar neurons)

output nuclei (of basal ganglia): consisting of the globus pallidus-internal part, part of the ventral pallidum, and the substantia nigra pars reticulata

oxytocin: peptide released by magnocellular neurons in the paraventricular and supraoptic nuclei

P cell: retinal ganglion neurons with a small dendritic arbor; plays a preferential role in sensing of form and color; parvocellular

pacinian corpuscle: rapidly adapting mechanoreceptor sensitive to high-frequency vibration

pain: sensation evoked by noxious stimulation

palate: arch-shaped portion of the superior oral cavity

paleocortex: type of cerebral cortex with fewer than six layers; commonly associated with processing of olfactory stimuli; located on the basal surface of the cerebral hemispheres, in part of the insular cortex, and caudally along the parahippocampal gyrus and retrosplenial cortex

pallidotomy: therapeutic lesion of a portion of the globus pallidus to alleviate dyskinesias

parabrachial nucleus: transmits viscerosensory information from the solitary nucleus to the diencephalon; located in the rostral pons

parafascicular nucleus: thalamic diffuse-projecting nucleus with widespread projections to the frontal lobe and striatum

parahippocampal gyrus: located on medial temporal lobe; contains cortical association areas that project to the hippocampal formation

parallel fibers: axons of cerebellar granule cells that course along the long axis of the folia; a single parallel fiber makes synapses with many Purkinje cells

parallel organization: property of neural systems in which pathways with similar anatomical organizations serve distinct functions

parallel sensory pathways: two or more sensory pathways that have similar anatomical projections and overlapping sets of functions

paramedian arterial branches: supply the most medial portions of the brain stem; originate primarily from the basilar artery

paramedian pontine reticular formation: transmits control signals from the contralateral cerebral cortex to brain stem centers for controlling horizontal saccades; major target of neurons in this structure is the abducens nucleus

parasagittal: anatomical or imaging plane off the midline that is parallel both to the longitudinal axis of the central nervous system and to the midline, between the dorsal and ventral surfaces

parasympathetic nervous system: component of the autonomic nervous system; originates from the brain stem and the caudal sacral spinal cord

parasympathetic preganglionic neurons: autonomic neurons located in the central nervous system; project to parasympathetic postganglionic neurons, which are located in the periphery

paraterminal gyrus: located anterior to the rostral wall of the third ventricle and ventral to the rostrum of the corpus callosum

paraventricular nucleus: hypothalamic nucleus that contains magnocellular neurosecretory neurons, parvocellular neurosecretory neurons, and descending projection neurons that regulate the functions of the autonomic nervous system

paravertebral ganglia: contain sympathetic postganglionic neurons

parietal lobe: one of the lobes of the cerebral hemisphere

parietal-temporal-occipital association area: association cortex at the junction of the parietal, temporal, and occipital lobes; important for linguistics, perception, and other higher brain functions

parietooccipital sulcus: separates the parietal and occipital lobes

Parkinson disease: results from loss of dopaminergic neurons in the substantia nigra pars compacta; characterized by slowing or absence of movement (bradykinesia) and tremor

parotid gland: salivary gland; innervated by axons of the glossopharyngeal (IX) nerve

parvocellular division (of red nucleus): component of the red nucleus that contains small neurons that project to the inferior olivary nucleus as the rubroolivary tract

parvocellular neurosecretory system: hypothalamic neurons located predominantly in the periventricular zone; neurons project to the median eminence where they make neurovascular contacts with capillaries and release factors into the blood that are carried to the anterior lobe by the portal veins

parvocellular visual system: components of the visual system in the retina, lateral geniculate, and visual cortical areas that originate from P-type ganglion cells; sensitive primarily to color, size, and the shapes of stimuli

peduncles: a large collection of axons

pedunculopontine nucleus: a pontine nucleus that receives a projection from the internal segment of the globus pallidus; participates in diverse functions, including regulating arousal and movement control; contains cholinergic neurons

perforant pathway: projection from the entorhinal cortex to the dentate gyrus

periamygdaloid cortex: one of the olfactory cortical areas; receives a direct projection from the olfactory tract; located on the rostromedial temporal lobe

periaqueductal gray matter: central region of the midbrain that surrounds the cerebral aqueduct; participates in diverse functions, including pain suppression

periglomerular cell: an inhibitory interneuron in the olfactory bulb that receives input from olfactory sensory neurons and inhibits mitral cells in the same and adjacent glomeruli

perilymph: fluid that fills the space between the membranous labyrinth and the temporal bone; resembles extracellular fluid and cerebrospinal fluid

peripheral autonomic ganglia: clusters of sympathetic and parasympathetic postganglionic neurons

peripheral nervous system: contains the axons of motor neurons, the peripheral axons and cell bodies of dorsal root ganglion neurons, the axon of autonomic preganglionic neurons, and the cell body and axon of autonomic postganglionic neurons

periventricular nucleus: contains parvocellular neurosecretory neurons; located in the hypothalamus, beneath the walls of the third ventricle

periventricular zone: portion of the hypothalamus that contains most of the parvocellular neurosecretory neurons; located beneath the walls and floor of the third ventricle

pharynx: the portion of the digestive tube between the esophagus and mouth; the throat

pheromones: a chemical produced and secreted by an animal that influences the behavior and development of other members of the same species

pia mater: inner meningeal layer; adheres closely to the surface of the central nervous system

pigment epithelium: external to the photoreceptor layer; it serves a phagocytic role during renewal of rod outer segment disks

pineal gland: endocrine gland located dorsal to the superior colliculus that is involved in the sleep/wake cycle; secretes melatonin

piriform cortex: one of the olfactory cortical areas; receives a direct projection from the olfactory tract; located on the rostromedial temporal lobe

pituitary portal circulation: connects capillary beds of the median eminence and anterior lobe of the pituitary; portal vein

pons: one of the major brain divisions; Latin for bridge

pontine cistern: site of accumulation of cerebrospinal fluid at the pontomedullary junction

pontine flexure: bend in the developing nervous system at the pons

pontine nuclei: relay information from the ipsilateral cerebral cortex to the contralateral cerebellar cortex and deep nuclei, principally the lateral cerebellar cortex and the dentate nucleus

pontomedullary junction: where the pons and medulla join

pontomedullary reticular formation: contains diverse motor, sensory, and integrative nuclei; especially important in arousal and visceral and skeletal muscle control

portal circulation: contains two capillary beds joined by portal veins; present in the pituitary gland and the liver

portal veins: join the two capillary beds of a portal circulation

positron emission tomography: functional imaging technique based on the emission of positively charged unstable subatomic particles (positrons); PET

postcentral gyrus: important for mechanical sensations, including position sense; located in the parietal lobe

postcommissural fornix: principal division of the fornix; contains axons principally from the subiculum that terminate in the mammillary bodies

posterior: toward the abdomen

posterior cerebellar incisure: shallow groove in the posterior lobe of the cerebellum

posterior cerebral artery: supplies portions of the occipital and temporal lobes as well as the diencephalon

posterior circulation: arterial supply provided by the vertebral and basilar arteries

posterior commissure: interconnects midbrain structures in the two halves of the brain stem; axons that mediate the pupillary light reflex in the nonilluminated eye course within the anterior commissure

posterior communicating artery: branch of the internal carotid artery that joins the posterior cerebral arteries; connects the anterior and posterior circulations, thereby providing a pathway for collateral circulation; part of the circle of Willis

posterior inferior cerebellar artery (PICA): supplies the dorsolateral medulla and portions of the inferior (posterior) cerebellum

posterior limb of the internal capsule: component of the internal capsule that lies lateral to the thalamus; carries axons from various sources including those coursing to and from the primary motor and somatic sensory cortical areas

posterior lobe of cerebellum: portion of cerebellar cortex between the anterior and flocculonodular lobes; comprises lobules VI–IX

posterior lobe (of pituitary gland): contains axons and terminations of the paraventricular and supraoptic nuclei of the hypothalamus; axon terminations release vasopressin (ADH) and oxytocin at neurovascular contacts with systemic capillaries

posterior parietal lobe (or cortex): caudal to the primary somatic sensory cortex; important for proprioception, spatial awareness, attention and visually guided limb and eye movements; part of the where pathway for visual motion and actions

posterior spinal arteries: supply blood to the dorsal columns and dorsal horn predominantly

posterolateral fissure: separates the posterior and flocculonodular cerebellar lobes

posteroventral cochlear nucleus: contributes to a system of connections that regulate hair cell sensitivity

postganglionic neuron: autonomic neuron that projects to a peripheral motor target, such as a smooth muscle or a gland

postsynaptic neuron: component of a synapse; contacted by a presynaptic neuron

precentral gyrus: contains the primary motor cortex and the caudal portion of the premotor cortex; located in the frontal lobe

precommissural fornix: small division of the fornix that contains axons primarily from the hippocampus that terminate in the septal nuclei

prefrontal association cortex: involved in diverse functions, including thought and working memory

prefrontal cortex loop: circuit of the basal ganglia that projects to the prefrontal cortex; involved in higher brain functions, such as thought and working memory

prefrontal cortex: *see* prefrontal association cortex

preganglionic neuron: autonomic neuron located in the central nervous system

premotor areas: participate in the planning of movements; located in the frontal lobe, in areas 6, 23, and 24

premotor cortex: specific premotor region located in the lateral portion of area 6

preoccipital notch: surface landmark that forms part of the boundary between the temporal and occipital lobes on the lateral surface

preoptic area: serves diverse functions including the control of sex hormone release from the anterior pituitary gland and regulation of sleep and wakefulness; located in the most rostral part of the hypothalamus

preoptic sleep center: hypothalamic center that regulates transition from wakefulness to sleep

prepositus nucleus: participates in eye position control; receives abundant inputs from the vestibular nuclei; located in the medulla

presynaptic neuron: component of the synapse; transmits information to the postsynaptic neuron

presynaptic terminal: axon terminal

pretectal nuclei: involved in pupillary light reflex; located in the junction between the midbrain and diencephalon

prevertebral ganglia: sympathetic ganglia that lie along the vertebral column

primary auditory cortex: first cortical processing site for auditory information; located in the transverse temporal gyri (of Heschl) in the temporal lobe; corresponds to cytoarchitectonic area 41

primary fissure: separates the anterior and posterior lobes of the cerebellum

primary motor cortex: contains neurons that participate in the control of limb and trunk movements; contains neurons that synapse directly on motor neurons; consists of area 4

primary olfactory cortex: defined as the target areas of olfactory tract axons; located in the rostromedial temporal lobe and the basal surface of the frontal lobes; corresponds to the paleocortex

primary olfactory neurons: transduce odorant molecules into neural signals; located within the olfactory epithelium

primary sensory (or afferent) fibers: somatic sensory receptor; dorsal root ganglion neuron

primary somatic sensory cortex: participates in somatic sensations, principally mechanical sensations and limb position sense; corresponds to cytoarchitectonic areas 1, 2, and 3; located in the postcentral gyrus

primary vestibular afferents: innervate vestibular hair cells; terminate primarily in the vestibular nuclei and cerebellum

primary visual cortex: participates in visual perceptions; located in the occipital lobe

projection neurons: cortical pyramidal neurons that project their axons to subcortical sites

proopiomelanocortin: a large peptide from which β-endorphin is cleaved

proprioception: sense of the position of the body; usually that of a limb or one limb segment relative to another

propriospinal neurons: spinal interneurons that interconnect neurons in different segments; also termed intersegmental neurons

prosencephalon: most rostral brain vesicle; gives rise to the telencephalon and diencephalon, which are the forebrain structures

prosopagnosia: inability to recognize faces

proximal limb muscles: muscles that innervate the shoulder or hip

pruritic: related to itch

pruritic receptor: sensory receptors responsible for the sensation of itch; activated by histamine

pseudoptosis: partial dropping of the eyelid

pseudounipolar neurons: neuron type that has a single axon and few or no dendrites in maturity (eg, the dorsal root ganglion neuron)

pterygopalatine ganglion: peripheral ganglion containing the cell bodies of parasympathetic postganglionic neurons that innervate nasal and oropharyngeal mucosal glands and lacrimal glands

pulmonary aspiration: the presence of food or consumed fluids in the lungs

pulvinar nucleus: major thalamic nucleus that has diverse projections to the parietal, temporal, and occipital lobes; involved in perception and linguistic functions

pupillary constriction: reduction in pupil diameter

pupillary dilation: increase in pupil diameter

pupillary light reflex: closure of the pupil with visual stimulation of the retina; used to test midbrain function in comatose patients

pupillary reflexes: changes in pupil diameter that occur without voluntary control; usually occur together with other ocular reflexes

Purkinje layer: location of Purkinje cell bodies

Purkinje neuron (or cell): output neuron of the cerebellar cortex; makes GABAergic inhibitory synapses on neurons of deep cerebellar nuclei and vestibular nuclei

putamen: component of the striatum; important in limb and trunk control

pyramid: tract on ventral surface of medial medulla; contains descending cortical axons, including the corticobulbar and corticospinal tracts

pyramidal neuron (or cell): cortical projection neuron class with characteristic pyramidal-shaped cell body

pyramidal decussation: where pyramidal cell axons from the motor and premotor areas cross the midline; located in the medulla

pyramidal signs: motor impairments that follow lesion of the corticospinal system

pyramidal tract: location of descending motor control pathway that originates in the motor and somatic sensory areas

quadrigeminal bodies: another name for the superior and inferior colliculi

quadrigeminal cistern: portion of the subarachnoid space that overlies the superior and inferior colliculi

radial glia: type of astrocyte that plays a role in organizing neural development; form scaffold for neuron growth and migration

radicular arteries: segmental arteries that supply the spinal cord, together with anterior and posterior spinal arteries

radicular pain: pain localized to the distribution of a single dermatome or several adjoining dermatomes

raphe nuclei: contain serotonin; located along the midline throughout most of the brain stem

rapidly adapting: response characteristic of neurons to a sudden stimulus in which a brief series of action potentials decrement rapidly to few or no action potentials

Rathke's pouch: an ectodermal diverticulum in the roof of the developing oral cavity from which the anterior and intermediate lobes of the pituitary develop

receptive membrane: portion of a neuron's membrane that contains receptors sensitive to neuroactive compounds or a particular stimulus

red nucleus: plays a role in limb movement control; gives rise to the rubrospinal and rubroolivary tracts

reduced myotatic reflexes: a condition in which the strength of muscle stretch or tendon reflexes are diminished

regional neuroanatomy: examines the spatial relations between brain structures within a portion of the nervous system

relaxation times: in magnetic resonance imaging, the times it takes protons to return to the energy state they were in before excitation by electromagnetic waves

relay nuclei: contain neurons that transmit (or relay) incoming information to other sites in the central nervous system

release-inhibiting hormones: chemicals that inhibit the release of a hormone from the anterior pituitary gland; usually neuroactive compounds secreted into the portal circulation at the median eminence

releasing hormones: chemicals that promote the release of a hormone from the anterior pituitary gland; usually neuroactive compounds secreted into the portal circulation at the median eminence

REM sleep: abbreviation for rapid eye movement characterized by dreaming, low limb and trunk muscle tone, and low-amplitude high-frequency electroencephalographic activity

reproductive behaviors: relatively stereotypic behaviors between members of the same species that lead to a reproductive act; in animals, the hypothalamus plays an important role in promoting reproductive behaviors, often in response to pheromones

restless legs syndrome: a disorder in which patients experience abnormal sensations in their legs that prompt the urge to move their legs to quell the sensation; abnormal sensations and movements are more common during rest and sleep than during activity

reticular formation: a diffuse collection of nuclei in the central (medial) portion of the brain stem that play a role in a variety of functions, including regulation of arousal, motor control and vegetative functions

reticular nucleus: a thalamic nucleus that projects to other thalamic nuclei; plays a role in regulating thalamic neuronal activity

reticulospinal tract: descending motor pathway that originates from the reticular formation, primarily in the pons and medulla, and synapses in the spinal cord

retina: peripheral portion of the visual system that contains photoreceptors as well as interneurons and projection neurons for the initial processing of visual information and transmission to several brain structures; develops from the diencephalon

retinitis pigmentosa: disease in which breakdown products accumulate at the pigment epithelium of the retina

retinohypothalamic tract: axons of retinal ganglion cells that project to the suprachiasmatic nucleus; information in this tract is used to synchronize circadian rhythms to the day-night cycle

retroinsular cortex: location of a vestibular cortical area; junction of the posterior insular cortex with the cortex on the lateral brain surface.

retronasal olfaction: when molecules travel from the oropharynx to activate olfactory neurons in the olfactory epithelium

Rexed's laminae: thin sheets of neurons in the spinal cord, which are clearest in the dorsal horn; they are significant because neurons in different layers receive input from different afferent and brain sources and, in turn, project to different targets

rhinal sulcus: rostral extension of the collateral sulcus, which separates the parahippocampal gyrus from more lateral temporal lobe regions

rhodopsin: photopigment in rod cells

rhombencephalon: most caudal primary brain vesicle; gives rise to the pons and medulla

rhombic lip: portion of the developing pons that gives rise to most of the cerebellum

rhombomeres: segments in the developing pons and medulla; eight in total

rigidity: condition in patients with Parkinson disease in which there is resistance to passive movement about a joint; sometimes there are phasic decreases in this resistance, termed cog-wheel rigidity

rod bipolar cells: retinal interneurons that transmit signals from rod cells to ganglion cells

rods: photoreceptors for vision under low light conditions (scotopic vision); located away from the macula portion of the retina

rostral: toward the nose

rostral interstitial nucleus of the medial longitudinal fasciculus: plays a role in control of vertical saccades

rostral spinocerebellar tract: transmits information about the level of activation in cervical spinal interneuronal systems to the cerebellum; thought to relay internal signals from motor pathways, via spinal interneurons, to the cerebellum

rostrocaudal axis: from the nose to the coccyx; the long axis of the central nervous system

rubrospinal tract: projection from the magnocellular portion of the red nucleus to the spinal cord

Ruffini's corpuscle: type of mechanoreceptor; distal process of large-diameter myelinated afferent fibers (A-β)

saccades: rapid, darting movements of the eye from one site of gaze to another

saccadic eye movements: *see* saccades

saccule: vestibular sensory organ (or otolith organ) sensitive to linear acceleration

sacral: spinal cord segment; there are five in total

sagittal: anatomical or imaging plane that is parallel both to the longitudinal axis of the central nervous system and to the midline, between the dorsal and ventral surfaces

scala media: inner ear fluid compartment

scala tympani: inner ear fluid compartment

scala vestibuli: inner ear fluid compartment; conducts pressure waves from the tympanic membrane to the other fluid compartments

Schaefer collaterals: collateral axon branch of neurons in the CA3 region of the hippocampus that synapse on neurons in the CA1 region

schizophrenia: psychiatric disease characterized by disordered thoughts, often associated with hallucinations

Schwann cells: glial cells that form the myelin sheath around peripheral axons

sclera: nonneural cover over the eye

scotoma: blind spot

seasonal affective disorder (SAD): form of depression during periods when days are short and nights are long

secondary auditory areas: cortical areas that process auditory information from the primary area

secondary somatic sensory cortex: cortical areas that process somatic sensory information from the primary area

segmental interneurons: neurons whose axons remain within a single spinal cord segment

segmental: pertaining to the segmental organization of the spinal cord

semantic memory: memory and knowledge of facts, people, and objects, including new word meaning

semicircular canals: vestibular organs sensitive to angular acceleration; there are three semicircular canals, each sensitive to acceleration in a different plane

semilunar ganglion: contains cell bodies of primary trigeminal sensory neurons

sensory: related to any of a wide range of stimuli from the environment or from within the body

sensory cranial nerve nuclei: process sensory information from the cranial nerves

sensory homunculus: form of somatic sensory representation in the postcentral gyrus (primary somatic sensory cortex)

septal nuclei: may participate in assessing the reward potential of events; receives input from the hippocampus and projects to the hypothalamus and other areas; located in rostral portion of the cerebral hemispheres

septum pellucidum: forms the medial walls of the anterior horn and part of the body of the lateral ventricle

serotonergic: neurons that use serotonin as a neurotransmitter

serotonin: neuroactive compound; also termed 5-HT (5-hydroxytryptamine)

short circumferential branches: supply ventral portions of the brain stem away from the midline; primarily from the basilar artery

sigmoid: S-shaped

sigmoid sinus: dural blood sinus that drains the transverse sinus and flows into the inferior petrosal sinus; located bilaterally

six layers: describes laminar pattern of neocortex

skeletal somatic motor: neuron class in which axons synapse on skeletal muscle that derives from the somites

skeletomotor loop: basal ganglia circuit that engages the motor and premotor areas

slowly adapting: response characteristic of neurons to an enduring stimulus in which a prolonged series of action potentials decrement slowly or not at all

small-diameter axons: afferent fibers that are sensitive to pain, temperature, and itch (ie, histamine)

smell: one of the five major senses

smooth pursuit eye movements: slow eye movements that follow visual stimuli

soft palate: caudal, arch-shaped, portion of superior oral cavity formed by muscle

solitary nucleus: contains neurons that receive and process gustatory and viscerosensory information and project to other brain stem and diencephalic nuclei, including the parabrachial nucleus and the thalamus

solitary tract: where the central branches of gustatory and viscerosensory axons collect before synapsing in the solitary nucleus

somatic: related to the body

somatic motor systems: pathways and neurons that participate in limb and trunk muscle control

somatic sensory: body sense; includes pain, temperature sense, itch, touch, and limb position sense

somatic skeletal motor column: motor nuclei in the spinal cord that contain motor neurons that innervate somatic skeletal muscle

somatotopy: organization of central sensory and motor representations based on the shape and spatial characteristics of the body

somites: para-axial mesoderm that organizes development of muscles, bones, and other structures of the neck, limbs, and trunk

spastic paralysis: condition in which the presence of spasticity produces an inability to voluntarily control striated muscle

spasticity: velocity-dependent increase in muscle tone; occurs after damage to the corticospinal system during development or in maturity

spina bifida: neural tube defect; failure of the caudal neural tube to close, producing impairments in lumbosacral spinal cord functions

spinal accessory (XI) nerve: cranial motor nerve that innervates the sternocleidomastoid muscle and parts of the trapezius muscle

spinal accessory nucleus: contains motor neurons whose axons course in the spinal accessory (XI) nerve to innervate the sternocleidomastoid muscle and parts of the trapezius muscle

spinal border cells: neurons that contribute axons to the ventral spinocerebellar tract

spinal cord: major division of the central nervous system

spinal nerves: mixed nerves present at each spinal segment

spinal tap: colloquial term for lumber puncture in which a needle is inserted into the lumbar cistern to collect a sample of cerebral spinal fluid; most commonly used for diagnostic testing

spinal trigeminal nucleus: portion of the trigeminal sensory nuclear complex within the medulla and caudal pons; contains the caudal, interposed, and oral subnuclei; involved in diverse trigeminal functions, the most important of which are pain, temperature, and itch

spinal trigeminal tract: pathway in which trigeminal afferent fibers course before synapsing in the spinal trigeminal nucleus

spinocerebellar tracts: paths transmitting somatic sensory information from the limbs and trunk to the cerebellum for movement control

spinocerebellum: portion of the cerebellum that plays a key role in limb and trunk control; includes the vermis and intermediate hemisphere of the cortex and the fastigial and interposed nuclei

spinomesencephalic tract: transmits somatic sensory information from the limbs and trunk to the midbrain

spinoreticular tract: transmits somatic sensory information from the limbs and trunk to the reticular formation

spinotectal tract: transmits somatic sensory information from the limbs and trunk to the dorsal midbrain; term often used interchangeably with spinomesencephalic tract

spinothalamic tract: transmits somatic sensory information from the limbs and trunk to the thalamus

spiral ganglion: where the cell bodies of auditory primary sensory neurons are located

stapes: one of the middle ear ossicles (bones); essential for conducting changes in air pressure from the tympanic membrane to the oval window; attaches to the oval window

stellate cells: in the cerebellum, inhibitory interneurons located in the molecular layer; more generally, a class of small multipolar neuron in the central nervous system

stem cells: multipotential cell that can develop into nerve, glial, or other cell types

sternocleidomastoid muscle: flexes the head and rotates head to opposite side

straight sinus: drains the inferior sagittal sinus and certain veins; empties into the confluence of sinuses; located where the falx cerebri and tentorium cerebelli meet; located on midline

stria (or stripe) of Gennari: band of myelinated axons in layer 4B of the primary visual cortex; axons interconnect local areas of cortex for visual stimulus processing

stria medullaris: pathway that courses along the lateral walls of the third ventricle; contains axons from the septal nuclei to the habenula

stria terminalis: C-shaped pathway from the amygdala to portions of the diencephalon and cerebral hemispheres; also contains neurons

striasome: an anatomical compartment of the striatum that contains patch-like distributions of particular neurochemicals (eg, acetylcholinesterase; encephalin)

striatal cell bridges: places of continuity of the caudate nucleus and putamen that span the internal capsule

striate cortex: another term for the primary visual cortex based on the location of the stria of Gennari

striatum: component of the basal ganglia; comprises the caudate nucleus, putamen, and nucleus accumbens

subarachnoid space: between the outer portion of the arachnoid and the pia; where cerebrospinal fluid accumulates over the surface of the brain and spinal cord

subcommissural organ: a circumventricular organ; located near the posterior commissure

subdural hematoma: hemorrhage of blood into the potential space between the dura and the arachnoid

subdural space: potential space between the dura and the arachnoid

subfornical organ: one of the circumventricular organs; region in which the blood-brain barrier is absent; axons project to magnocellular neurons of the paraventricular nucleus

subgenual cortex: located ventral to the genu of the corpus callosum; associated with clinical depression and is a target of brain stimulation for intractable depression

subiculum: component of the hippocampal formation

submandibular ganglion: contain postganglionic neurons that innervate the oral mucosa and the submandibular and sublingual glands

submodality: category of a sensory modality, such as color vision, bitter, or pain

substance P: neuroactive compound; present in neurons that process painful stimuli

substantia gelatinosa: laminae II and III of the dorsal horn; process pain, temperature, and itch

substantia nigra pars compacta: portion of the substantia nigra where neurons contain dopamine and project widely to the striatum

substantia nigra pars reticulata: portion of the substantia nigra where neurons contain GABA and project to the thalamus primarily

substantia nigra: component of the basal ganglia; comprises the pars reticulata and the pars compacta

subthalamic nucleus: basal ganglia nucleus involved in limb control; when damaged, can produce hemiballism; part of the indirect basal ganglia circuit

sulci: grooves

sulcus limitans: groove that separates developing sensory and motor structures in the spinal cord and brain stem

sulcus: groove

superior cerebellar artery: supplies rostral pons and cerebellum; long circumferential branch of the basilar artery

superior cerebellar peduncle: tract that primarily carries axons from the deep cerebellar nuclei to the brain stem and thalamus

superior colliculus: plays a key role in controlling saccades; located in the rostral midbrain

superior ganglion: of the vagus and glossopharyngeal nerves, contains cell bodies of somatic sensory afferent fibers

superior oblique muscle: depresses the eye when the eye is adducted and intorts the eye when it is abducted

superior olivary nuclear complex: involved in processing incoming auditory signals; especially important for horizontal localization of sounds

superior olivary nuclei: auditory relay nuclei predominantly important in the horizontal localization of sounds

superior parietal lobule: important for spatial localization

superior petrosal sinus: dural sinus; drains into the sigmoid sinus

superior rectus muscle: elevates the eye

superior sagittal sinus: dural sinus; drains into the straight sinus

superior salivatory nucleus: contains parasympathetic preganglionic neurons whose axons course in the intermediate (VII) nerve

superior temporal gyrus: involved in hearing and speech

superior vestibular nucleus: one of four vestibular nuclei; located in the pons

supplementary eye field: cortical eye movement control center located primarily on the medial wall of the frontal lobe; involved in more cognitive aspects of saccadic eye movement control

supplementary motor area: portion of the medial frontal lobe important in the control of eye movements

supporting cells: provide structural and possibly trophic support for taste buds

suprachiasmatic nucleus: hypothalamic nucleus important for circadian rhythms; center of the biological clock

supraoptic nucleus: contains magnocellular neurosecretory neurons; secretes oxytocin and vasopressin into the systemic circulation in the posterior pituitary gland

Sylvian fissure: separates the temporal lobe from the parietal and frontal lobes; also termed the lateral sulcus

sympathetic nervous system: component of the autonomic nervous system

sympathetic preganglionic neurons: sympathetic nervous system neurons that are located in the central nervous system and synapse on sympathetic postganglionic neurons and cells in the adrenal medulla

synapses: specialized sites of contact where neurons communicate and where neurotransmitters are released; comprise three components—presynaptic axon terminal, synaptic cleft, and postsynaptic membrane

synaptic cleft: narrow intercellular space between the neurons at synapses

syringomyelia: cavity

T1 relaxation time: proton relaxation time related to the overall tissue environment; also termed spin-lattice relaxation time

T2 relaxation time: proton relaxation time related to interactions between protons; also termed spin-spin relaxation time

tabes dorsalis: degenerative loss of large-diameter mechanoreceptive fibers; associated with end-stage neurosyphilis

tarsal muscle: a smooth muscle that assists the actions of the levator palpebrae muscle; under control of the sympathetic nervous system

tastants: chemicals that produce tastes

taste: one of the five major senses

taste buds: gustatory organ, which consists of taste receptor cells, support cells, and basal cells, which may be stem cells for replenishing taste receptor cells

taste receptor cells: component of taste buds; transduce oral chemicals into gustatory signals

tectorial membrane: component of the organ of Corti; stereocilia of hair cells embed within the tectorial membrane

tectospinal tract: projection from the deep layers of the superior colliculus to the spinal cord

tectum: most dorsal portion of the brain stem; present only in midbrain in maturity

tegmentum: portion of the brain stem between the tectum and the base; present throughout the brain stem; Latin for cover

telencephalon: secondary brain vesicle that gives rise to structures of the cerebral hemisphere; derives from the prosencephalon

temporal hemiretina: temporal hall of the retina

temporal lobe: one of the lobes of the cerebral hemisphere

temporal pole: most rostral portion of the temporal lobe

tentorium cerebelli: dural flap between the occipital lobes and the cerebellum

terminal ganglia: parasympathetic ganglia that contain postganglionic neurons; receive input from the vagus nerve; located on the structure their axons innervate

thalamic adhesion: site of adhesion of the two halves of the thalamus; said to be present in approximately 80% of individuals; in humans, no axons decussate in the thalamic adhesion

thalamic fasciculus: tract in which axons from the deep cerebellar nuclei and part of the internal segment of the globus pallidus course to the thalamus

thalamic radiations: axons of thalamic nuclei that project to the cerebral cortex

thalamostriate vein: follows C-shaped course of caudate nucleus and stria terminalis

thalamus: major site of relay nuclei that transmit information to the cerebral cortex; component of the diencephalon

thermoreceptors: primary sensory neurons sensitive to thermal changes

third ventricle: component of the ventricular system; located between the two halves of the diencephalon

thoracic: spinal cord segment; there are 12 in humans

tonotopic organization: or tonotopy; where sounds of different frequencies are processed by different brain regions; sounds of similar frequencies are processed by neighboring brain regions, while sounds of very different frequencies are processed by brain regions that are farther apart

touch: one of the five major senses

tractography: an MRI approach (diffusion MRI) to identify the locations of tracts based on information about the local directions of brain water diffusion; a commonly used tractography method is diffusion tensor imaging (DTI)

transcranial magnetic stimulation (TMS): noninvasive brain stimulation technique in which a pulse of magnetic energy is use to activate neurons; repetitive TMS (rTMS) uses a series of pulses

transient ischemic attack (TIA): brief cessation of cerebral blood flow to a local brain region that produces transient dysfunction of the area; dysfunction lasts for a period of minutes to hours

tract: collection of axons within the central nervous system

transverse plane: perpendicular to the longitudinal axis of the central nervous system, between the dorsal and ventral surfaces

transverse sinus: dural sinus that carries blood into the systemic circulation

trapezius muscle: contains several functional regions that support the weight of the arm and act on the scapula

trapezoid body: site of decussation of auditory fibers

tremor: trembling or shaking movement

trigeminal ganglion: location of cell bodies of all trigeminal afferent fibers except those afferents innervating muscle spindle receptors; also termed semilunar ganglion

trigeminal lemniscus: tract in which axons from the main trigeminal sensory nucleus ascend to the thalamus

trigeminal mesencephalic nucleus: contains cell bodies of primary sensory neurons innervating stretch receptors in jaw muscles

trigeminal motor nucleus: contains motor neurons that innervate jaw muscles

trigeminal (V) nerve: mixed cranial nerve containing sensory axons that innervate much of the head and oral cavity and motor axons that innervate jaw muscles

trigeminocerebellar pathways: projection from spinal trigeminal nuclei to the cerebellum

trigeminothalamic tract: projection from spinal trigeminal nuclei to the thalamus

trochlear (IV) nerve: cranial nerve that contains the axons of trochlear motor neurons, which innervate the superior oblique muscle

trochlear nucleus: contains motor neurons that innervate the superior oblique muscle

tubercles: a round nodule or eminence that marks the location of an underlying nucleus or cortical region; cuneate and gracile tubercles are located on the dorsal medulla and the olfactory tubercle is located on the ventral surface of the basal forebrain

tuberomammillary nucleus: hypothalamic nucleus; contains neurons that use histamine as a neurotransmitter; diverse projections to activate forebrain neurons

tufted cells: olfactory bulb projection neurons

tympanic membrane: ear drum; oscillates in response to environmental pressure changes associated with sounds; coupled to middle ear ossicles

uncal herniation: displacement of the uncus medially due to an expanding space-occupying lesion above the cerebellar tentorium

uncinate fasciculus: association pathway interconnecting frontal and anterior temporal cortical areas

uncus: bulge on the medial temporal lobe; overlies the anterior hippocampal formation and amygdala

unipolar neuron: neuron with a cell body and axon but few dendrites

urination: release of urine from the bladder

utricle: vestibular sensory organ (or otolith organ) sensitive to linear acceleration

vagus (X) nerve: mixed cranial nerve; contains axons of branchiomeric motor neurons that innervate laryngeal and pharyngeal muscles, parasympathetic preganglionic fibers, gustatory and visceral afferent fibers, and somatic sensory afferents; located in the medulla

vascular organ of the lamina terminalis: a circumventricular organ; located in the rostral wall of the third ventricle

vasopressin: neuroactive peptide that also acts on peripheral structures, including promoting fluid reabsorption in the kidney; also termed antidiuretic hormone (ADH)

venogram: radiological image of veins

ventral: toward the abdomen; synonymous with anterior

ventral (anterior) commissure: *see* ventral spinal commissure

ventral (or anterior) corticospinal tract: pathway for control of axial and proximal limb muscles of the neck and upper body

ventral amygdalofugal pathway: output pathway from the basolateral and central nuclei of the amygdala

ventral anterior thalamic nucleus: part of the motor thalamus; receiving primarily information from the internal segment of the globus pallidus of the basal ganglia; projects to cortical motor and premotor areas

ventral cochlear nucleus: concerned with processing the horizontal sound localization; division of cochlear nucleus

ventral column: portion of spinal cord white matter medial to the ventral horn; contains primarily descending fibers for controlling axial and proximal limb musculature

ventral horn: laminae VIII and IX of the spinal gray matter; location of neurons for somatic motor control

ventral lateral thalamic nucleus: part of the motor thalamus; receiving primarily information from the deep cerebellar nuclei; projects to cortical motor and premotor areas

ventral medial nucleus (of the hypothalamus): participates in appetitive behaviors, such as feeding

ventral pallidum: output nucleus of the limbic circuit of the basal ganglia; located ventral to the anterior commissure

ventral posterior lateral nucleus: division of the ventral posterior nucleus where information from the dorsal column nuclei is processed

ventral posterior medial nucleus: division of the ventral posterior nucleus where trigeminal information is processed

ventral posterior nucleus: thalamic nucleus for processing somatic sensory information; projects to the primary somatic sensory cortex

ventral root: where motor axons leave the spinal cord

ventral spinal commissure: where axons of the anterolateral system decussate; located ventral to lamina X and the central canal

ventral spinocerebellar tract: transmits information about the level of activation in thoracic, lumbar, and sacral spinal interneuronal systems to the cerebellum; thought to relay internal signals from motor pathways, via spinal interneurons, to the cerebellum

ventral striatum: consists of the ventromedial portions of the caudate nucleus and putamen and the nucleus accumbens

ventral tegmental area: contains dopaminergic neurons that project to the ventromedial portion of the striatum and the prefrontal cortex; located in the rostral midbrain

ventricles: dilated channels within the ventricular system; contain choroid plexus

ventricular system: cavities within the central nervous system that contain cerebrospinal fluid

ventricular zone: innermost layer of the developing central nervous system; layer from which nerve cells are generated

ventrolateral medulla: contains neurons that participate in blood pressure regulation through projections to the intermediolateral cell column

ventrolateral nucleus: principal motor control nucleus of the thalamus; receives cerebellar input and projects to primary and premotor cortical areas

ventrolateral preoptic area: important in promoting REM and non-REM sleep, through inhibitory connections with other hypothalamic nuclei and brain stem nuclei that promote wakefulness

ventromedial hypothalamic nucleus: important in regulating appetite and other consummatory behaviors; receives input from limbic system structures

ventromedial posterior nucleus: thalamic nucleus important for processing noxious stimuli; projects to the posterior insular cortex; caudal to the thalamic region that processes viscerosensory information

vergence movements: convergent or divergent eye movements; ensure that the image of an object of interest falls on the same place on the retina of each eye

vermis: midline portion of the cerebellar cortex; plays a role in axial and proximal limb control

vertebral arteries: branch from the subclavian artery; two vertebral arteries converge to form the basilar artery

vertebral canal: cavity within the vertebral column within which the spinal cord is located

vertebral-basilar circulation: arterial supply to the brain stem and parts of the temporal and occipital lobes

vertigo: the sense of the world spinning around or that of an individual whirling around

vestibular ganglion: location of cell bodies of primary vestibular neurons; also termed Scarpa's ganglion

vestibular labyrinth: fluid-filled cavities within the temporal bone within which the vestibular organs are located

vestibular division of CN VIII: component of CN VIII that supplies the semicircular canals, utricle, and saccule

vestibular nuclei: major termination site of vestibular sensory fibers

vestibulocerebellum: portion of the cerebellum that receives a monosynaptic projection from primary vestibular axons; processes this information for eye movement control and balance; includes primarily the flocculonodular lobe

vestibulocochlear (VIII) nerve: contains afferent fibers that innervate the auditory and vestibular structures of the inner ear

vestibuloocular reflex: automatic control of eye position by vestibular sensory information

vestibulospinal tract: axons that originate from the vestibular nuclei and project to the brain stem

vibration sense: the capacity to detect and distinguish mechanical vibration of the body

visceral: related to the internal organs of the body

visceral (autonomic) motor fibers: axons of autonomic preganglionic or postganglionic neurons as they course in the periphery

visceral motor nuclei: contain autonomic preganglionic neurons

viscerosensory: related to the sensory innervation of the internal organs of the body

vision: one of the five major senses

visual field: the total area that is seen

visual field defect: loss of vision within a portion of the visual field

visual motion pathway: originates primarily from the magnocellular ganglion cells of the retina and projects to V5 and ultimately to regions of the posterior parietal cortex

vomeronasal organ: peripheral olfactory organ important for detecting pheromones; well-documented as a functional structure in animals, but its function in humans is controversial

Wallenberg syndrome: *see* lateral medullary syndrome

Wallerian degeneration: deterioration of the structure and function of the distal portion of an axon, when cut; also termed anterograde generation

Wernicke's area: important for understanding speech; located in the posterior superior temporal gyrus (area 22)

what pathway: corticocortical circuits important for identifying an object using vision, touch, or sound

where-how pathway: corticocortical circuits important for identifying the location of an object using vision, touch, or sound and use of that information to help direct limb or eye movements

white matter: location of predominantly myelinated axons

working memory: the temporary storing of information used to plan and shape upcoming behaviors

zona incerta: contains GABA-ergic neurons that project widely to the cerebral cortex; nuclear region of the diencephalon

Index

A

Abducens nerve, 132, 150, 259, 272, 284, 427, 429
  fascicles of, 453
  lesion, 292
  in pons, 288f
Abducens nucleus, 257, 265, 272, 278f, 284, 453, 491
  extraocular muscle control and, 284f
  lesion, 292
  in pons, 290
Accessory cuneate nucleus, 304, 311–312, 313f, 449
Accessory medullary lamina, 473, 475
Accessory nerve, 259
Accessory optic system, 157–159
Accommodation reflex, 292
Accommodation-convergence reaction, 292
Acetylcholine, 7, 35f, 54, 333, 404
  basal forebrain and, 34
  diencephalon and, 34
  in modulatory systems, 34
  olivocochlear system and, 189–190
  pedunculopontine nucleus and, 346, 371
Acetylcholinesterase, 344f
Acoustic neuroma, 181–183, 182f
Acousticomotor function, 191
Addiction, 395f, 396
Adenohypophysis, 358
ADH. See Antidiuretic hormone
Adipocytes, 372
Adrenergic projection, 369
Adrenocorticotropic hormone, 362
Afferent fibers, 91
  in cranial nerves, 132
  groups, 87t
  gustatory, 268
  mechanoreceptive, 151
  primary vestibular, 307
  viscerosensory, 268
Afferent neurons, 40
AICA. See Anterior inferior cerebellar artery
Airway protective reflex, 263, 269
Akinesia, 331, 333
Allocortex, 50, 214–217
  lateral cortical surface of, 403f

Allodynia, 113
Alveus, 407, 465, 467, 471, 473, 495
Alzheimer disease, 3, 401
  cholinergic neurons and, 34
  key neurological signs, 5
Amacrine cells, 161
Amino acids, 7
Amnesia, 390
Amygdala, 13, 17f, 22, 120f, 220, 373, 386, 388f, 391f, 399f, 463, 469, 473, 477, 479, 495
  acute pain and, 121
  addiction and, 395f
  basolateral division of, 405

basolateral nuclei of, 393f
blood supply of, 60t
central division of, 405
central nuclei of, 393f
connections of, 393f
cortical division of, 404
cortical nuclei of, 393f
emotions and, 387
extended, 396
functional divisions of, 394
nuclear divisions in, 400f, 404–405
olfactory bulb projections and, 217
olfactory system and, 212
output pathways of, 405
parabrachial nucleus and, 109, 117, 146
salient stimuli and, 345
Amygdaloid complex, 494–495
Anastomosis, 65
Anastomotic channels, 66f
Anatomical planes, 26f
Aneurysm, 59, 79
Angiography, 68–69
Angular gyrus, 419, 421
Anorexia, 372
Anosmia, 212
Ansa lenticularis, 343, 346f, 473, 475
Anterior cerebral artery, 64–65, 64f–65f, 79, 243, 263, 481
  branches of, 67f
  cerebral cortex and, 68
  collateral circulation and, 66f
Anterior choroidal artery, 64, 243, 263, 348
  branches of, 67f
Anterior cingulate cortex
  acute pain and, 119–121
  pain pathways and, 121f
Anterior cingulate gyrus, 109, 402
  fMRI, 40f
  limbic loop and, 338f
  medial dorsal nucleus and, 119, 140
  noxious stimuli processing and, 123
Anterior circulation, 60, 61f, 79, 80
  cerebral angiography, 69f
  cerebral hemisphere blood supply and, 64–65
  diencephalon blood supply and, 64–65
  MRA of, 71f
  subcortical structures and, 66–68
Anterior commissure, 330, 341f, 343, 345f, 359f, 398f, 407, 425, 469, 473, 475, 477, 479, 484–485, 489, 491, 493, 495
Anterior communicating arteries, 65, 79
Anterior dimension, 20
Anterior dorsal thalamic nucleus, 396
Anterior inferior cerebellar artery (AICA), 62, 62f, 79, 187, 266
Anterior lobe, 301, 303f
Anterior nucleus, 46, 46f, 47t, 54, 388, 467, 471, 483
Anterior olfactory nucleus, 212, 217, 220, 481
Anterior perforated substance, 214, 220, 402
Anterior pituitary hormones, 361t

Anterior temporal lobe degeneration, 385–386, 386f
Anterior thalamic nuclei, 394, 407, 470–471, 482–483, 491
Anterograde amnesia, 390
Anterograde degeneration, 40
Anterolateral system, 109, 123, 435, 437, 439, 441, 443, 445, 447, 449, 451, 453, 455, 457, 459, 461, 465
  axons, 313f
  decussation of, 116f
  lesions, 269
  medial lemniscus and, 117
  pain pathways and, 121f
  projection neurons and, 113
  trigeminothalamic tract and, 139
Anteroventral cochlear nucleus, 196
Antidiuretic hormone (ADH), 362–364
Aortic arch, 142
Aphasia, 194–196
  global, 57
Apraxias, 239
Arachnoid granulations, 77f, 79, 80
Arachnoid mater, 19–20, 23, 25f, 73f
Arachnoid villi, 76, 79, 80
Arbor vitae, 301
Archicortex, 217
Arcuate nucleus, 361f, 362, 372–373, 397, 447, 451
Area postrema, 75f, 79, 431
Argyll Robertson pupils, 292
Arterial blood supply, 59
Ascending pathways, 32
Association areas, 102
Association complex, 15
Association cortex, 47–48
Associative loop, 337f, 338, 338f
Astrocytes, 8f, 9, 22, 134
Ataxia, 269, 309, 355, 357
  Friedreich's, 299–300, 300f, 304–307
Athetosis, 333
Auditory axons, 190–191
Auditory cortex
  defects, 194–196
  fMRI of, 193f
  higher-order areas, 184, 192–194, 193f, 196
    linguistics processing and, 194
  primary, 16, 184, 193f, 196
    Heschl's gyri and, 191–192
  secondary, 184, 192–194, 193f
    linguistics processing and, 194
Auditory system
  functional anatomy of, 183–184
  organization of, 185f
  organs, 184–187
  regional anatomy of, 184–196
  sensitivity, 189–190
Auricle, 186f
Autonomic control, 397f
Autonomic division, of peripheral nervous system, 9–10, 22, 373
Autonomic motor column, 257, 260–261
Autonomic motor fibers. See Visceral motor fibers